International Perspectives on Social Policy, Administration, and Practice

The Springer series International Perspectives on Social Policy, Administration and Practice puts the spotlight on international and comparative studies of social policy, administration, and practice with an up-to-date assessment of their character and development. In particular, the series seeks to examine the underlying assumptions of the practice of helping professions, nonprofit organization and management, and public policy and how processes of both nation-state and globalization are affecting them. The series also includes specific country case studies, with valuable comparative analysis across Asian, African, Latin American, and Western welfare states. The series International Perspectives on Social Policy, Administration and Practice commissions approximately six books per year, focusing on international perspectives on social policy, administration, and practice, especially an East-West connection. It assembles an impressive set of researchers from diverse countries illuminating a rich, deep, and broad understanding of the implications of comparative accounts on international social policy, administration, and practice.

More information about this series at http://www.springer.com/series/7

Steven L. Arxer • John W. Murphy
Editors

Community-Based Health Interventions in an Institutional Context

Springer

Editors
Steven L. Arxer
Department of Sociology and Psychology
University of North Texas at Dallas
Dallas, TX, USA

John W. Murphy
Department of Sociology
University of Miami
Coral Gables, FL, USA

ISSN 2625-6975 ISSN 2625-6983 (electronic)
International Perspectives on Social Policy, Administration, and Practice
ISBN 978-3-030-24653-2 ISBN 978-3-030-24654-9 (eBook)
https://doi.org/10.1007/978-3-030-24654-9

This Springer imprint is published by the registered company Springer Nature Switzerland AG
The registered company address is: Gewerbestrasse 11, 6330 Cham, Switzerland

Contents

Contributors

Steven L. Arxer is Associate Professor at the University of North Texas at Dallas in the Department of Sociology and Psychology. He has a PhD in sociology at the University of Florida. Arxer specializes in qualitative methods with a focus on minority populations, intersectionality, and gender. He is co-author of *Aging in a Second Language*.

Karen A. Callaghan earned a BA in sociology at La Salle University (Philadelphia) and MA and PhD in sociology at The Ohio State University. Callaghan's areas of interest include participatory community-based research, community organizing, and service-learning. Callaghan is currently Professor of Sociology and Dean, College of Arts & Sciences at Barry University, Miami Shores, Florida.

Jung Min Choi received his BA at UC Berkeley and finished his PhD at York University in Toronto, Canada. He is Associate Professor in the Department of Sociology at San Diego State University. He has published, all guided by anti-essentialist philosophies and community-based approaches, on critical pedagogy, race and racism, globalization and the bankruptcy of neoliberalism. He is currently President of The Dignified Learning Project, a nonprofit education-based organization in San Diego.

Kyaien O. Conner is Assistant Professor in the Department of Mental Health Law and Policy at the University of South Florida and a faculty affiliate of the Louis de la Parte Florida Mental Health Institute. She received her PhD, MSW, and MPH from the University of Pittsburgh and completed a postdoctoral fellowship in Geriatric Psychiatry at the Western Psychiatric Institute. Her research focuses on factors that influence disparities in mental health service utilization and treatment outcomes for African American older adults.

Ramsey Dahab holds various degrees in the Liberal Arts, including an MA in International Studies from Florida International University and a PhD in Sociology from the University of Miami. His areas of interest include nativism, global inequalities, and social theory—the incorporation/development of pedagogies that help to fulfill potential in the world.

Danielle Dukes is a third year medical student at Ohio University's Heritage College of Osteopathic Medicine. She has research interests in the social determinants of health, food insecurity, women's and infant health, and mental health issues. She obtained an MS in Biology and an MBA with a focus on Health Care Management, from Wright State University before matriculation into medical school.

Berkeley Franz is a medical sociologist whose research and teaching focus on health disparities, hospital–community relationships, and health policy. She is currently Assistant Professor of Community-based Health at Ohio University's Heritage College of Osteopathic Medicine, in Athens, Ohio. She received an MA in religious studies from the University of Chicago and a PhD in sociology from the University of Miami. Berkeley has worked both domestically and internationally on community-based research projects and has published extensively on the theory and development of community-based partnerships.

Dawn Graham serves as faculty in the Department of Social Medicine at Ohio University Heritage College of Osteopathic Medicine. She earned a Doctorate in Counseling Psychology from Purdue University in 2010 and Master of Arts in Applied Behavioral Science from Valparaiso University in 1999. Clinical experience includes work in the University of Chicago Hospitals, Michigan City Area Schools, Purdue University, Porter Starke Community Mental Health, and Logansport State Psychiatric Hospital. Previously, she served as the Principal Investigator on a multi-million dollar federal grant to promote maternal/child health in Southeastern Ohio with university and community partnerships in coordination with the Ohio Department of Health. She is a member of the American Psychological Association and previously acted as Chair of the Ohio Psychological Association Public Sector Issues committee. Graham has been involved in multiple studies involving the impact of compassion fatigue for health care professionals working with underserved patients. She conducts national and international talks on health, psychology, and research.

Charlene Holkenbrink-Monk received her MA in sociology from San Diego State University and is currently enrolled in a joint doctoral program (San Diego State University and Claremont). Her research interests include community-based education and critical pedagogy. Currently, she teaches at California State University, San Marcos, San Diego Mesa College, and San Diego City College.

Elaine Hsieh has been involved in research on bilingual health communication for over a decade. She has conducted ethnographic studies, in-depth interviews, focus groups, surveys, and multi-phase studies that examine the interactions between providers and patients who do not share the same language. The three aspects that she has investigated are: (a) the discrepancies between the beliefs and the practice of medical interpreters, (b) interpreters' influences on the quality of health care services, and (c) interpreters' mediation of conversational partners' identities and communicative goals. She also has received funding from the National Institutes of Health to further expand her Bilingual Health Communication model, exploring providers' expectations and needs for medical interpreters.

Lesli Johnson is Associate Professor. After a successful clinical career in mental health, Lesli joined Ohio University's Voinovich School of Leadership and Public Affairs in 1997 to lead the Planning, Evaluation, Education, and Research team, providing services to public and nonprofit organizations throughout the region and beyond. She has 20 years of experience working in community programs, including mental health, health, education, and child welfare. Dr. Johnson has been the lead evaluator on a number of state and federal efforts to improve health through community and integrated efforts. Areas of emphasis include promoting collaborative efforts, evaluating systems development, and engaging stakeholders in meaningful conversations and actions.

Eric Kramer has research interests that include mass media, international and intercultural communication. He is author of seven books including *Modern/Postmodern: Off the Beaten Path of Antimodernism*, *The Emerging Monoculture: Assimilation, and the "Model Minority"* and several journal articles and award winning papers. He has served on the review and editorial boards and has reviewed for several journals including *The Harvard International Journal of Press/Politics*, *The Journal of Communication*, *Communication Studies*, *The Journal of Applied Communication*, *The Journal of Intercultural Communication*, *Journal of International and Intercultural Communication*, *International Journal of Intercultural Relations*, *The Howard Journal of Communications*, and so forth.

Airín D. Martínez is Assistant Professor at the School of Public Health & Health Sciences at the University of Massachusetts—Amherst. Her research examines the sociopolitical and institutional arrangements that produce chronic disease disparities among Latinx immigrants and their US-born children. Her current research examines how the local implementation of immigration enforcement policies creates material deprivation and psychosocial stress among Latinx mixed-status families. She hopes her research can reverse policies excluding US immigrant populations and inform community-based prevention strategies.

Kathleen Moore is a research professor in the Department of Mental Health Law and Policy at the University of South Florida and Executive Director of the Louis de la Parte Florida Mental Health Institute. She received her MA and PhD in social/health psychology from Kent State University and completed a postdoctoral fellowship at Duke University Medical Center. For the past 20 years, she has worked on numerous community-based research projects with local addiction and mental health providers.

John W. Murphy has a PhD in sociology from Ohio State University. For the past 30 years he has been writing on and working in community-based projects in both the United States and several countries in Latin America. Most recently he worked on a health project on the Island of Grenada. Currently, he is Professor of Sociology at the University of Miami. Along with several of his colleagues, he is author of the book, *Narrative Medicine and Community-Based Health Care and Planning.*

Krista Mccarthy Noviski is a health coach and graduate student in the Department of Sociology and Anthropology at the University of Toledo in Toledo, Ohio. She received her BS in Pre-Medicine from Bowling Green State University in Bowling Green, Ohio and completed her health and wellness coach training through *Wellcoaches.* Her interests include social connection and health and the patient's experience of illness. Her current research is focused on empathy in medicine and the lived experience of teaching empathy to medical students.

Karie Jo Peralta is Assistant Professor in the Department of Sociology and Anthropology at the University of Toledo in Toledo, Ohio. She received her PhD from the University of Miami in Coral Gables, Florida. Her areas of interest are community-based research, third sector organizations, and applied sociology. Most recently, she worked in the Dominican Republic on a household survey of Haitian immigrant families and a growth assessment of their children.

Khary K. Rigg is Associate Professor in the Department of Mental Health Law and Policy at the University of South Florida and a faculty affiliate of the Louis de la Parte Florida Mental Health Institute. He received his PhD from the University of Miami and completed a postdoctoral fellowship in health services research from the University of Pennsylvania, Perelman School of Medicine. The overall goal of his research is to generate findings that improve the way drug prevention, treatment, and harm reduction interventions are developed and delivered.

Amanda Sharp is a PhD student in the College of Behavioral and Community Sciences at the University of South Florida. She received her BA from Humboldt State University and earned an MPH from Boston University. Her research focuses on how to make interventions more patient-centered through approaches such as motivational interviewing.

Kerri Shaw is the Social Work Field Director and the director of the Community Health Worker Training Program at Ohio University. She has been recognized as the 2014 Athens Foundation Woman of the Year for her work in the community, including the development of the Athens County Peanut Butter and Jelly Project. She earned both a bachelor's and master's degree in social work from Ohio University, is a Returned Peace Corps Volunteer, and is a fierce advocate and activist for women and children in Appalachia.

Daniel Skinner is Assistant Professor of Health Policy in the Department of Social Medicine at Ohio University, Heritage College of Osteopathic Medicine, on the Dublin, Ohio campus. He earned his PhD in political science from the City University of New York. The author of more than two dozen peer-reviewed academic articles in health policy, medical education, and political theory, Dr. Skinner is also co-editor of *Not Far from Me: Stories of Opioids and Ohio* (Ohio State University Press, 2019) and author of *Medical Necessity: Health Care Access and the Politics of Decision Making* (University of Minnesota Press, 2019).

Tashina J. Vavuris has a Master's in Sociology from San Diego State University where she explored educational inequities and community-based philosophy. Since then, she has been studying community-based practices and has collaborated in projects in Ecuador and Grenada centering on community health. Currently, she is a doctoral student at the University of California at Santa Cruz in the Environmental Studies Department, where she studies notions of sustainability, transformative pedagogical practices, and the process of community-based practices.

Chapter 1
Introduction

John W. Murphy

Community-based work is becoming quite popular nowadays. But since the passage of the Community Mental Health Act of 1963, health and other services were supposed to be attuned to the needs of communities (Lefkowitz, 2007). Local norms and definitions are important and should be consulted when planning interventions. This viewpoint was reinforced by the Alma-Alta conference in 1978 (Rifkin, 2009). As a result of this deliberation, local participation in service planning and delivery is deemed crucial for relevant and equitable health care.

Since Alma-Alta, two principles have come to characterize community-based projects (Murphy, 2014). The first is that local knowledge matters. The idea is that communities consist of reservoirs of knowledge that their members create and use as referents for judging health and illness, along with other elements of social life. Phenomenologists, for example, refer to these knowledge bases as "stocks of knowledge," while others refer to them as "worlds" (Schutz & Luckmann, 1973). In each case, the general theme is that persons define their situations, and that the accompanying values, beliefs, and commitments should guide the design, implementation, and evaluation of any program of action.

Community-based services should be built from the "ground-up" to enhance their relevance, due to the local nature of knowledge. To facilitate this strategy, the second principle of community-based work comes into play; that is, community members should control all projects. The goal of this change is to ensure that local customs and practices are not violated, and through their involvement communities are able to realize their skills and desires. Some critics refer to this outcome as empowerment (Geiger, 2016; Rappaport, 1984). But the practice is only logical: local persons understand the worlds that are operative and how they can be entered. Following this entrée, the assumption is that services or research will improve.

J. W. Murphy (✉)
Department of Sociology, University of Miami, Coral Gables, FL, USA
e-mail: j.murphy@miami.edu

S. L. Arxer, J. W. Murphy (eds.), *Community-Based Health Interventions in an Institutional Context*, International Perspectives on Social Policy, Administration, and Practice, https://doi.org/10.1007/978-3-030-24654-9_1

This shift in orientation represents a great advance. Not long ago local involvement was thought to be detrimental (Rifkin, 1996). After all, these persons are not professionals and thus lack essential skills. Recent research and practice, however, demonstrate that such claims are false. Local persons have exhibited skill levels thought to be beyond their station, and have been very helpful in dealing with health and related issues (Frank, 2010). Moreover, they have access to knowledge and social networks that are beyond the reach of outsiders, even those who are diligent and well-intentioned.

But a key element has been overlooked in those discussions of community-based work. Although community agency has been emphasized, the institutional framework of interventions has received scant attention. In other words, a key component has been ignored. That is, health and other interventions occur in institutional contexts that should receive attention. This conclusion is also consistent with the spirit of Alma-Alta. Despite this insight, the impact of community-based philosophy and practice on institutions is seldom mentioned. The purpose of this volume is to remedy this situation.

As might be suspected, emphasizing local participation changed the philosophy and configuration of service delivery. Practitioners, clients, and agencies, for example, are cast in a new light. Roles are changed and the usual organizational hierarchies are challenged. New sources of knowledge are exposed and consulted, while the nature of services and their delivery are rethought. For example, hospitals, research programs, training, and funding schemes are significantly altered. Nothing, in short, is unscathed by this shift to a community-based philosophy.

What Is an Institution?

Institutions have been conceived traditionally in realistic terms (Stark, 1963). Any organizations that have been institutionalized, therefore, have adhered to a particular formula designed to promote their legitimacy. Specifically, these organizations have been lifted above or removed from contingency. In other words, the illusion is created that they are divorced from partisan perspectives and thus provided with a unique, almost timeless status that reflects the common weal.

When portrayed in this way, institutions are bestowed with a "foundational" character (Fish, 1989). The point of this maneuver is to create a façade that can instill order and enlist loyalty. In fact, realists contend that order can be preserved only if institutions have a status superior to their inhabitants. As a result, these organizations appear to be normative and stable, beyond the political fray, and worthy of widespread recognition. Detached from any particular group or bias, institutions are presumed to have universal appeal.

To borrow from Herbert Marcuse, legitimate and lasting institutions have an "affirmative character" (Marcuse, 1969). Due to this status, they can impose durable customs and rules that stifle critique and thwart opposition. To make organizations seem substantial, and thus formidable, they are institutionalized through the use of structural imagery. Serious organizations, for example, have a chain of command, a system of roles and statuses, and communication channels that reflect a particular logic. Given these descriptives, threats to the prevailing order can be controlled relatively easily.

Organizations that are institutionalized in this way have so-called binding power (Funk, 1998). That is, they can restrict choices and establish a sense of cohesion. Behavioral parameters can thus be imposed with little resistance, because of the power and prestige attributed to these organizations. As described by Erich Fromm (2005), everyone is diminished by these institutions; their legitimacy is simply undeniable and overwhelming.

Basically, a state of asymmetry is established between these institutions and almost everyone else. Those with power, and cultural or economic supremacy, can claim some association with these organizations and related privileges. But the remainder of persons are expected to be intimidated and readily conform to institutional requirements. In this regard, institutionalized organizations are transformed effectively into idols (Sung, 1989). What this designation means, in this context, is that they are not necessarily worshiped but that their imperatives are uniformly followed and seldom questioned. Institutions speak with unrivaled authority.

Such organizations, according to Karl Marx, would be treated as alienating (Marx, 1973). In other words, they have assumed a timeless and adversarial character that is unwarranted. Nonetheless, most persons are enthralled and dominated by their creations. The obvious question, however, is how does this distortion occur? How are persons led to believe that the products of their labor should control their lives? At this juncture, the simple answer is that through a subtle philosophy, institutions are granted the illusion of autonomy.

Institutionalization and Dualism

At first glance, community-based work appears to be mostly a practical undertaking. Organizing an intervention, indeed, demands that attention be directed to solving various technical problems. Likewise, learning to navigate institutions requires pragmatic awareness, a tolerance of tedium, and a willingness to compromise. Philosophy seldom comes to mind when considering these issues.

Nonetheless, at the core of institutionalization is a philosophical theme that is problematic. How do institutions achieve the appearance of autonomy? The answer to this question rests on Cartesianism, or dualism (Bordo, 1987; Leder, 1992). As noted earlier, once an organization is institutionalized, a specific arrangement of roles, jobs, and norms is superior to other forms of human organization. Put differently, people and their associations that stand outside of institutions are contingent and lack the presumed stability and obligations intrinsic to institutions. Cartesian philosophy enters at this point, as institutions are understood to be severed from their creators, given their unique structural status.

Cartesianism encourages the separation of subjectivity from objectivity. The rationale behind this separation is that subjectivity, based on interpretation, represents an unreliable source of knowledge. Through scientific methodology, for example, subjectivity can be overcome, thereby bringing objectivity into view. In this Cartesian picture, not only is subjectivity problematic, this source of information must be overcome for truth to be encountered.

Dualism allows particular information, or processes, to be severed from basic human expressions, such as choices, values, or interpretations. An organization that is institutionalized, accordingly, can be treated as autonomous, as if human agency is ancillary to the rules or hierarchies that are enforced. Through dualism, however, these organizations can become impediments to the ambitions of individuals or communities. In the language of sociologist Emile Durkheim (1983), institutions come to be viewed as existing "sui generis" and capable of providing constraints.

As should be noted, this version of institutionalization is antagonistic to community-based work. When predicated on realism, institutions are regularly insensitive to local demands, while community initiative is treated as a threat. When institutions are viewed as autonomous, local history and participation pose challenges to the *status quo* and are dismissed as uninformed distractions (MacDonald, 2016). Sound policy reflects institutional standards that are objective and rational, thereby minimizing community input. Community control, of course, is not part of the agenda.

But because community-based projects emphasize participation, particularly local knowledge and control, Cartesianism is revealed to be untenable. Neither knowledge nor organizations are autonomous because the standard location of these abstractions no longer exists. In community-based philosophy, dualism is undermined by the insight that individuals and communities create worlds of knowledge and that these domains can never be objective or timeless in the Cartesian sense. In short, their significance is always situated.

Institutions, therefore, must be approached differently in community-based work than in the past. Rather than autonomous, they should be viewed as narratives that simply inscribe a perspective on valid knowledge, order, and how health or any other issues should be conceptualized and addressed (Polkinghorne, 1988). As narratives, the Cartesian influence on institutionalization is rendered passé. Nonetheless, institutionalization and the related organizations do not vanish, but instead must be approached in a manner compatible with the anti-dualism prescribed by local participation.

Institutions and Community-Based Work

Community-based work subverts dualism by placing participation, or human agency, at the center of knowledge production and institutional life. As a result, organizations and their supports are removed from the pedestal reserved traditionally for institutions. In the absence of their usual autonomous status, institutions are not prescriptions but possibilities linked to local practices. As some social philosophers might say, institutions are now local constructions (Gergen, 2009).

In the previous section, institutions were compared to narratives that serve to illustrate how social life might be ordered. Clearly, community-based work should thrive in this environment, since institutional control is transferred to local actors. But this recommendation depends on a particular thesis on language gaining recognition.

In terms of Cartesianism, language is envisioned to be a tool, particularly a pointer. The function of language, accordingly, is to highlight objects in the world, most notably their differences. Consistent with dualism, language does nothing but illustrate the traits of natural referents. The role of narratives, in this philosophy, is to describe the world in the most accurate way possible.

In a non-dualistic framework, on the other hand, language is not mimetic but creative. As Roland Barthes says, there is nothing outside of language that may emerge as objective (Barthes, 1977). There is no other option but to treat reality as a linguistic convention. Given the murkiness of language, narratives strive to bring clarity out of possible interpretations. Institutions, accordingly, stabilize a particular interpretation until further notice. Consequently, institutions are no longer ominous but subject to local control and (re)interpretation. The legacy of an organization, therefore, does not have to weigh heavily on an individual or community, but can be reinvented to meet local definitions and needs.

A hospital, neighborhood, clinic, or training center, for example, is expected to have a new identity and different relationship with clients. None of these institutions should be intrusive and obscure the worlds present in a community, but emerge from local interaction. Without support from dualism, organizations can return to being local constructions or stories, generated through discourse, that tell how a community defines health, the appropriate delivery of services, and acceptable outcomes (Charon, 2006). Such institutions are not obstacles but facilitate health care.

Organization of Book

This book examines as its central issue the impact that a community-based philosophy has on institutions and the institutionalization of community health delivery. Chapters in this volume explore how institutional arrangements can be rethought in ways conducive of a community-based approach. The volume considers how community partnerships, funding schemes, curriculum for health workers, the status of patients and clients, and community research programs, among other organizational features, are framed and designed from a community-based philosophy.

Chapter 2 addresses the broad question of what is a community-based organization. Here John W. Murphy explains how the focus of community-based work is local knowledge and community control of health projects. To deliver services in accordance with these principles, community-based organizations must be instituted. What these organizations require, separate from the past, is a different management style and unique division of labor. Most organizations that are employed to provide health services in a community-based manner, however, have a traditional structure, and thus have difficulty fulfilling their aims. A new organization must be created that is consistent with the philosophy that underpins community-based work. Such an organization, for example, would be less hierarchical and not focused on a specific division of labor as in the past.

In Chap. 3, Karen A. Callaghan discusses how community-based partnerships are established within a new institutional framework. Community-based health services are not provided by stand-alone organizations. Simply put, a network of providers must be available. Accordingly, a variety of organizations must enter into partnerships. This arrangement is not necessarily novel, but traditionally these associations have been fraught with conflicts and struggles for power, thus undermining their effectiveness. Community-based partnerships, on the other hand, must be predicated on dialogue and mutual respect. Instead of fighting for dominance in a community, these new organizations must be integrated around the plans established by communities. A new way of conceptualizing and carrying out this process must be established.

Jung Min Choi, John W. Murphy, Ramsey Dahab, and Charlene Holkenbrink-Monk, in Chap. 4, explore the issue of funding and budgeting. Often funds are directed to community organizations in ways that are either irrelevant or difficult to use. Additionally, budgets are formulated by agencies that are disconnected from the communities where services are needed. Community-based funding and budgeting, accordingly, are beginning to receive serious attention. Communities, accordingly, are given the latitude in some cases to establish budgets and spending strategies, along with identifying and pursuing sources of funds that are consistent ethically with these priorities and desires. Community-based funding and budgeting, in this way, are vital to supporting interventions in a community-sensitive manner.

Clearly, research plays a key role in community-based health work. Understanding the health needs of a community is vital to the success of any health-care project. From an organizational perspective, however, the focus of a research program is often methodological. That is, developing scientifically sound data collection instruments is often the focus. However, such an emphasis leaves little room for appreciating how knowledge is socially produced and legitimized. Moreover, an overemphasis on methodological concerns can diminish the ability of researchers to appreciate the underlying assumptions of a community's worldview and frustrate their entrance to that world. Chapter 5, by Steven L. Arxer, examines the philosophical and practical considerations of implementing a research program in health projects that preserves the knowledge production of community members.

Chapter 6 focuses on the training of community-based health workers from a participatory organizational perspective. Tashina Vavuris argues that health practitioners receive a significant amount of training before and after they enter the field. But often, this education is mostly pragmatic, that is, focused on how to conduct needs assessments, evaluate interventions, or implement accreditation standards. Of course, these tasks are important. But this education does not necessarily begin with the philosophy that sustains community-based work. When beginning with the principle that community knowledge matters, training must be initiated on how to enter the world constructed by a community's members. Every task, accordingly, must be thought of as a mode of engaging a community, instead of simply gathering data or making observations. Valid knowledge, communities, and norms, for example, must be rethought in the training process to produce persons who can work effectively in community-based interventions. This shift in orientation is not often the centerpiece of training.

Chapter 7 continues the discussion regarding health worker training, with Dawn Graham, Kerri A Shaw, and Leslie Johnson outlining key dimensions of developing a community-based curriculum for health worker training. The previous chapter explored the use of community-based health workers in interventions and the importance of integrating local experts into planning. In this chapter, they share the experience of developing a training curriculum for the State of Ohio. Given new rules regarding certification in different areas of the United States and internationally, developing a curriculum that can be approved and disseminated is of increasing importance. In these programs, significant institutional support is needed to develop curricula and train additional trainers, so that training can be shared with communities interested in integrating community health workers into their programming. The goal of this chapter is to present the challenges faced in creating a certified training curriculum and the potential for future curriculum development efforts.

Non-profit hospitals have the potential to be strong partners in community-based projects. Since the Affordable Care Act was passed in 2010, hospitals have new requirements to engage communities in identifying health needs and developing new community health programs. In Chap. 8, by Berkeley Franz, Daniel Skinner, and Danielle Dukes, a case study approach is used to explore how hospitals are developing new partnerships and the challenges they face in fostering relationships with the communities where they are located. Potential strategies will be suggested for improving communication between hospital employees and community members in the planning of community-based projects.

Karie Jo Peralta and Krista McCarthy Noviski investigate the political dimension of community-based organizations in Chap. 9. A central way institutions gain legitimacy and the ability to guide human behavior is through claims of value-neutrality and objectivity. Institutions are often thought to be bureaucratic and based on formal rules that facilitate decision-making in any sphere of life. In the case of health organizations, the language of science, technology, and standardization guide how community needs and the authority of health practitioners are understood. In this context, health professionals attain their unique status vis-à-vis patients and community members. But this dichotomy can contradict the aims of community-based health interventions. In particular, health organizations become the center of health assessments, while medical professionals attain greater power to direct health initiatives as opposed to patients. Nonetheless, community health workers, for example, require respect and legitimacy. In this chapter, the political dimension of community-based health organization is discussed, along with the challenges this model presents to conventional depictions of health institutions.

Chapter 10, by Khary K. Rigg, Amanda Sharp, Kyaien O. Conner, and Kathleen A. Moore, examines how the patient-provider relationship has evolved over the years. Patients are now thought to play a central role in the provision of treatment, especially within the context of community-based interventions. In both theory and practice, the role of the patient is supposed to differ from traditional biomedical approaches to treatment with patient input introducing a new level of transparency and relevance into service provision. Specifically, patients are to play an increasingly active role in health-care delivery and their backgrounds treated as central in any intervention. In short, a new form of participation between patient and provider is key to interventions that claim to be patient-centered and community-based. The current health-care system, however, does not promote such participation and obstacles to involving patients in their own care exist. The chapter traces the history of the patient-provider relationship and discusses the recent shift toward elevating the importance of persons receiving care. The authors also discuss obstacles to genuinely involving patients in their own treatment and make recommendations for how these barriers can be overcome. They conclude by discussing promising strategies for meaningfully involving patients in treatment, as well as how the role of patients in community-based care might be re-thought.

In Chap. 11, Elaine Hsieh and Eric Kramer focus on the health-care system, specifically highlighting the nature of debates about universal care. Of importance to the authors is not the arguments launched themselves but rather how polemics are being used to rationalize particular visions of health care. How communities are presented and imagined in relation to their work status, for example, is a central way in which arguments related to universal health care are forged and barriers erected. Hsieh and Kramer contend that a deeper examination of the philosophy behind current work-eligibility arguments to health care can promote dialogue on this hotly debated issue.

Airín D. Martínez continues the discussion regarding universal health care in Chap. 12. The focus is how a community-based health-care institution reimagines the basic operation of health care. Because a community-based model understands knowledge to be locally produced, the basic operations of identifying and exploring health needs changes, as well as the ways in which treatment is approached. Specifically, patients and communities do not internalize the directives of professionals, but rather collectively legitimize health initiatives and direct the process of community healing. Simply put, an entirely new model is proposed for identifying illness, formulating interventions, defining health, and evaluating outcomes.

The final chapter emphasizes the need for a re-evaluation of institutionalized health care. Drawing from the chapters described above, the benefits of institutionalizing community-based health projects is illustrated. To the extent that community-based efforts are described as substantially different from conventional health practices, health institutions must be conceptualized and operationalized anew to preserve the intentions of communities. Furthermore, an entirely new ethic of health care must be promoted. In short, a careful examination of how community-based projects can be institutionalized has the prospect for advancing effective strategies for community health planning.

Conclusion

The paradigm that has been operative in health care is changing (Foss, 2012). Persons and communities that were once marginal to this process are moving to the center. To paraphrase supporters of this move, local persons are becoming the experts (Kretzman & McKnight, 1993). But an overlooked facet of this process are the institutions where services are delivered. For this shift to be complete, these organizations must respond in a manner that is consistent with a community-based philosophy on research and treatment interventions.

Institutions can be resistant to change, however, when they are perceived to be autonomous. When conceived in this manner, these organizations are intimidating and may contravene local efforts to make health projects relevant and effective. But in the realist context, this obstinance is considered to be an asset for preserving tradition and order.

This autonomy, however, is sustained by a philosophy that is called into question by community-based work. Deprived of support from dualism, institutions are contingent, malleable, and adaptable to local worlds. In other words, these organizations can be treated as local inventions that serve persons and their communities. Researchers and health practitioners, accordingly, are no longer trapped by intractable institutional goals and practices. An open horizon of choices is thus presented to those who engage in community-based work. Therefore, in addition to dealing with human agency, community-based researchers and practitioners should focus on institutional factors that influence local participation.

With this new outlook on institutions, how will health projects be affected? How are typical organizational practices challenged? The aim of this volume is to provide some answers to these questions. In this way, another step can be taken to bringing community-based health care to fruition. The health-care system can thus be better grounded in the communities that are supposed to be served.

References

Barthes, R. (1977). *Image, music, text*. New York: Hill and Wang.

Bordo, S. (1987). *The flight of objectivity*. Albany, NY: SUNY Press.

Charon, R. (2006). *Narrative medicine: Honoring the stories of illness*. Oxford, UK: Oxford University Press.

Durkheim, E. (1983). *Pragmatism and sociology*. Cambridge, UK: Cambridge University Press.

Fish, S. (1989). *Doing what comes naturally*. Durham, UK: Duke University Press.

Foss, L. (2012). *The end of modern medicine: Biomedical science under the microscope*. Albany, NY: SUNY Press.

Frank, A. W. (2010). *Letting stories breathe*. Chicago: University of Chicago Press.

Fromm, E. (2005). *On being human*. New York: Continuum.

Funk, R. (1998). Erich Fromm's concept of social character. *Social Thought and Research, 21*(1–2), 215–229.

Geiger, H. J. (2016). The first community health center in Mississippi: Communities empowering themselves. *American Journal of Public Health, 106*(101), 1738–1740.

Gergen, K. J. (2009). *An introduction to social construction*. New York: Sage.
Kretzman, J., & McKnight, J. (1993). *Building communities from the inside out*. Chicago: Acta Publications.
Leder, D. (1992). *The body in medical thought and practice*. Dordrecht, Netherlands: Kluwer.
Lefkowitz, B. (2007). *Community health centers: A movement and the people who made it happen*. New Brunswick, NJ: Rutgers University Press.
MacDonald, J. J. (2016). *Primary health care*. Oxford, UK: Earthscan.
Marcuse, H. (1969). *Negations*. Boston: Beacon Press.
Marx, K. (1973). *The economic and philosophical manuscripts of 1844*. New York: International Publishers.
Murphy, J. W. (2014). *Community-based interventions: Philosophy and action*. New York: Springer.
Polkinghorne, D. E. (1988). *Narrative knowing and human sciences*. Albany, NY: SUNY Press.
Rappaport, J. (1984). Studies in empowerment: Introduction to the issue. *Prevention in Human Services, 3*(2), 1–7.
Rifkin, S. B. (2009). Lessons from community participation in health programmes: A review of the post- Alma-Ata experience. *International Health, 1*(1), 31–36.
Rifkin, S. B. (1996). Paradigms lost: Towards a new understanding of community participation in health programs. *Acta Tropica, 61*(2), 79–92.
Schutz, A., & Luckmann, T. (1973). *The structures of the life-world*. Evanston, IL: Northwestern University Press.
Stark, W. (1963). *The fundamental forms of social thought*. New York: Fordham University Press.
Sung, J. M. (1989). *La idolatría del capital y la muerte de los pobres [The idolatry of capital and the death of the poor]*. San José, Costa Rica: DEI.

Chapter 2
A Community-Based Organization

John W. Murphy

Introduction

Becoming community-based is not easy, although this idea has become quite de rigueur nowadays (Murphy, 2014). But most often, this maneuver is treated as logistical. Service agencies, for example, are placed in communities, while local persons are selected to sit on their governing boards. Although these steps are important, they deal mostly with technical matters. The aim of these and similar tactics is to bring services and any accompanying research closer to communities. Nonetheless, these changes overlook a significant factor in the process of becoming community-based.

There is no doubt that this shift in orientation requires that very pragmatic issues be addressed. Along with referral links, supervision, and treatment options, the location of a service center is important and should not be brushed aside. But with this focus on practical matters, the philosophy behind community-based work is regularly downplayed or missed. However, knowledge of this philosophy, and how to implement the related ideas, is crucial to successfully making this change.

The principle at the core of community-based interventions is participation (Fals Borda, 1988). The basic idea is that all persons create their respective realities in concert with others; no-one is an atom that acts alone. Broadly speaking, community-based philosophy is an off-shoot of constructionism (Gergen, 1999). Social facts and norms, accordingly, are not viewed to be objective but framed by communities in one way or another. The result is that communities consist of interpretive worlds that must be entered, if service or research is to have relevance (Gadamer, 1996). Local knowledge and control, therefore, are the cornerstones of community-based practice.

J. W. Murphy (✉)
Department of Sociology, University of Miami, Coral Gables, FL, USA
e-mail: j.murphy@miami.edu

S. L. Arxer, J. W. Murphy (eds.), *Community-Based Health Interventions in an Institutional Context*, International Perspectives on Social Policy, Administration, and Practice, https://doi.org/10.1007/978-3-030-24654-9_2

In philosophical terms, community-based work is anti-Cartesian, or non-dualistic (Bordo, 1987). Traditional planning, on the other hand, is dualistic, with a differentiation made regularly between subjectivity and objectivity. But within this typology, emphasis is placed on objectivity, since subjectivity is considered to be an unreliable source of information. The desire to enact "evidence-based" medicine is an example of this trend (Howick, 2011). The use of rigorous methodology, for example, is presumed to promote appropriate service delivery through the discovery of data divorced from the errors introduced by interpretation. Given this bias, communities participate minimally in planning activities, since they are situated and biased.

The elevation of local knowledge in importance reflects this anti-dualistic stance. Consistent with the outlook that persons are constructing knowledge, including so-called medical facts, the resulting body of information should guide all clinical interventions and research. In this sense, local knowledge matters, along with local control of any community project. With persons actively shaping their communities, and thereby specifying preferences and promoting select perspectives, these changes are entirely logical.

What is important is that community-based projects or interventions begin with an epistemological shift. Accordingly, the status of knowledge should be reviewed, along with the identity of evidence. Discussions should be initiated about local knowledge and how this information should be used, and why local guidance is imperative. For the most part, however, service planning and delivery does not begin in this manner. In short, philosophy does not play a foundational role.

This new philosophy, nonetheless, has not been applied to an important area, that is, the development of organizations that are expected to deliver health care and other services in a community-based manner (Lune, 2010). Most important to remember at this juncture, considering anti-dualism, is that communities should no longer be treated merely as places. Health-care facilities, additionally, should not be viewed as anchors that hold these locations together. This imagery obscures the existential or constructionist character of these organizations and their surroundings.

Contradicting a standard portrayal, a community-based organization is not a linchpin in communities that disseminates health services. What is omitted from this depiction is the participation that creates both organizations and communities, and in the end joins them together. A perspective on organizations must be unveiled that is compatible with this thesis, or health facilities will not become community-based. To use a pertinent term proposed by Philip Selznick (1948) some time ago, a community-based organization must have a proper "character." Specifically, a move must be made away from the realism that sustains the traditional rendition of organizations and toward a position that values human agency.

Realism Is Problematic

In the traditional description, organizations are expected to bring about stability and order. To accomplish this aim, they are provided with a unique status in the context of realism. Predicated on dualism, organizations are assumed to be autonomous;

they are touted to represent closed systems (Scott, 2002). With this stature, they are divorced from daily contingencies and can impose control. The survival of social order, in fact, depends on the lasting impact of this institutional effect.

A façade must be provided, in other words, that creates the illusion of organizational invulnerability. To have gravitas, organizations must appear to be substantial and transcend the uncertainties of everyday life. Rules, for example, must have universal legitimacy and should not favor a particular group or seem to be applied willy-nilly. Order will falter unless a sense of universality is cultivated and unbiased authority is maintained.

So, how is this image created? Usually, organizations are described by using structural metaphors (Perrow, 1979). In this way, their functioning and lines of authority are reinforced. A quick glance at an organizational chart in most healthcare facilities reveals the logic and chain of command that is operative. Most often, this imagery is hierarchical, with precise paths of interaction specified between departments. With such a depiction, the message is conveyed clearly that such an organization has a purpose and operates according to reliable principles.

Following such a realistic portrayal, persons are expected to adjust to organizational requirements (Fromm, 1959). Certain parameters are illustrated that should not be violated. For example, an organization is accorded fixed boundaries, an exact division of labor, and purposeful norms. Accordingly, all those who enter should know their place, the tasks they are supposed to perform, and the network of authority. These expectations are thus clear, without ambiguity, so that an organization operates smoothly.

Obviously, discipline can be enforced with this strategy, but other problems begin to arise. The desired autonomy, for example, begins to separate organizations from their communities. Specifically, organizational identity is sustained by focusing on their unique traits and capacities. In the case of health care, these organizations are thought to have specific functions that preserve a community. What they are expected to accomplish should not be confounded by the intrusion of demands associated with other organizations. Blurred boundaries can only cause problems—the meaning of health care cannot be institutionalized effectively if contested. The equilibrium of a community would be disrupted by such a mistake.

This realism also has impact on the internal operation of an organization (Burrell & Morgan, 1979). Due to the rigid division of labor, jobs are narrowly designed, while the range of persons who can perform specific roles is restricted. The result is the gradual professionalization of care delivery, with an accompanying hierarchy of knowledge (Freidson, 1970). As might be expected, emphasis is placed on professional medical education and the associated knowledge base.

As long as organizations are conceptualized in these ways, they will never become community-based. Indeed, their identities are secured by remaining autonomous. Becoming thoroughly integrated into a community would only cause confusion brought about by conflicting interpretations and demands. When couched in realism, a reliable organization must rise above this cacophony. For example, even choosing the name of a hospital may be problematic, with respect to identifying who is welcome and the tasks performed (Wu, 2011). A fuzzy identity is not helpful.

A proper sense of autonomy must be promoted to guarantee that a clear label or brand is presented.

The division of labor that is usually prescribed, however, militates against any significant change. The professionalization of most tasks means that local knowledge tends to be sidelined, along with the participation of everyday persons in meaningful ways in health-care organizations. So-called laypersons are thus consigned to the periphery of service delivery and, most likely, merely asked periodically for input that has little impact.

The standard realism must be abandoned before health-care organizations can become close to a community. New imagery is necessary that is less imposing and exclusionary. Organizational integrity must be preserved, but while incorporating local knowledge and control. In other words, a mode of organization must be proposed that is reliable, in the absence of the typical institutional effect brought about by realism.

Realism Is Not Needed

The general aim in community-based work is to make an organization concrete—accessible and reliable—without reification. Important to remember is that a community is not a place but comprised of various interpretive worlds (Dussel, 2008). Consistent with the principle of participation, a community should not be viewed as an object. What this discovery means is that a community must be engaged but not merely through contact with an organization. But rather, a form of entanglement must be achieved that is not possible with objects.

New imagery is needed that defies the bounded and structural character of traditional organizations. The purpose, however, is not to deconstruct organizations and transform them into an array of periodically interlocked activities. Although Karl Weick's (1976) position on sense-making, and loose-coupling, at first glance looks to be compatible with a community-based philosophy, such a conclusion would be premature. Simply calling for flexibility is not enough. Instead, and truly significant, persons must be able to construct and preserve an organization through their agency. Through their participation, they must be able to create an organization that has longevity and embodies the goals of a community.

As should be noted, dualism is overcome in a community-based model. There are no insiders or outsiders, but only those who unite, as an organization, to promote health care. Any job design that results, for example, is an outgrowth of the interaction that takes place during this process. The resulting organization is not merely loosely coupled but real and demanding, but only because of the agreements of the participants. In this regard, some critics argue that such organizations are held together by trust (Luhmann, 2017). But the glue that is present is not this vague. What unites these organizations is the solidarity that is engendered through the day-to-day activities of solving problems and achieving goals. In this portrayal, an organization is self-created.

Rosabeth Moss Kanter (1983), for example, was once on the verge of proposing this perspective on organizations. In the so-called matrix organization, persons are allegedly capable of writing their own jobs, while authority is dispersed. With this proposal, she wanted to unleash the entrepreneurial spirit of persons. Viewing the members of organizations as entrepreneurs was common during the 1980s, when she advanced this imagery.

But life in the matrix was never this creative. Those who proposed self-managed organizations, on the other hand, certainly had this outlook in mind (Rothschild & Whitt, 1986). In effect, a community-based model borrows from this orientation, whereby average persons are given the latitude to invent and control organizations. From this perspective, their exclusion in the past was not due to a lack of desire or talent but prejudices based on political and other reasons.

There are no organizational *a prioris* in a community-based strategy. The focus is on skill development and the dissemination of information, so that an organization never becomes autonomous and issues demands. Adaptation should thus be eclipsed by invention and self-direction, as an organization is dissolved into a community. True community-based organizations are not simply flexible but a product of their member's desires and actions. Rather than obtrusive, such organizations disappear into a community.

In reality, community-based organizations represent not only a change in the image of an organization but the nature of social relationships. Much more is advanced, in other words, than technical changes. In some ways, these new organizations embody a cultural revolution, a novel and shared vision of valid personal behavior, acting together, and creating knowledge and order.

A Few Practical Concerns

Traditional organizations are semi-permeable, with limited access granted to communities. Community-based organizations, on the other hand, are much more than permeable, although local access is greatly increased. And while access is important, a self-managed organization does more and encourages the exercise of a community's agency (Rothschild & Whitt, 1986). But going beyond access, the point is to promote total transparency through local control.

A community-based organization invites more than input; in fact, the term "invite" conveys the wrong impression. In this new framework, an organization is not autonomous, and thus does not generate opportunities for their members. There is no distance between persons and organizations that can lead to conflict with and, possibly, the oppression of their constituents. Rather, this form of organization spreads out laterally like a field (Bourdieu, 1990). There is no separation created by autonomy that is necessary for alienation to occur.

What happens, instead, is that a community-based organization is built from the ground-up, possibly beginning with a local health committee. This base establishes the framework, for example, to identify needs, the required services, and the general policies to be enacted. The delivery of services, simply put, is established from below. In many respects, the aim is to overcome the influence of the so-called "medical emperors" that have dominated service delivery and give more responsibility to those, in the past, who were merely the recipients of services (Cueto, 2004).

At this juncture, readers may begin to think of stakeholder participation (Stufflebeam, 2001). But community-based participants are different from stakeholders. Stakeholders, for example, are much more generic and, most likely, have little to do with the daily affairs of a community, or any organization that is established. Furthermore, their interests are often very personal, even idiosyncratic, and contravene the common good of a community. Community-based participants are neither strategic political appointments nor interested in receiving notice or praise. These persons work for the community and are attuned to the realities that are at play. In organizational parlance, they are mission driven.

Because of this involvement, a community-based organization is never finalized. The guidance provided by a community is ongoing and not restricted, as is often the case, to the beginning of a project or intermittent consultations with stakeholders. A constant flow of advice is underway, thereby preventing services from drifting away from a community.

Community-based organizations, accordingly, are a lot less professionally oriented than is usually the case. In short, these organizations are guided completely by local personnel. The awareness is promoted that local persons have valuable insights into their problems and the types of services that are appropriate. In other words, local knowledge is at the core of these organizations.

For some time, the attempt has been underway to employ in health agencies the members of the communities that are served (Lefkowitz, 2007). In this way, both patients and practitioners would share some history, thus making service delivery more palatable. But because the traditional conception of the organization was not seriously challenged, professionals often remained in control of interventions. Real effort had to be made to include laypersons (Ward Jr. & Geiger, 2017). But in most cases, a strategic plan was inaugurated to search for local professionals who had the requisite credentials, or to get local persons professionally trained. As a result, services may have been dispensed by local persons, but neighborhood control was seriously compromised.

At the outset of a project, however, professionals may be helpful. The point is not to disparage their skills, but to put them in the hands of local persons (Geiger, 2016). The plan, accordingly, should be to expand the knowledge base of a community, without overshowing local insights. And once locals are exposed to this new knowledge, they can decide how much of this information is relevant, the modifications that should be made, and how quickly implementation should proceed. A community-based strategy does not introduce information and cajole community members into accepting certain ideas and goals, but rather inaugurates a discussion that can advance in any number of directions.

Knowledge, in this sense, is not in the possession of any one group. A knowledge base is simply expanded, so that the most locally relevant decisions can be made. The problem is that such growth, often called capacity building, is undertaken regularly in a paternalistic manner (Kretzman & McKnight, 1993). That is, processionals descend on a project with a plan that they tout to be progressive and necessary for a problem to be successfully solved. Therefore, adoption is thought to be logical and thus almost foreordained, and any reluctance exhibited by a community is treated as irrational.

Evidence is mounting, in fact, that local persons can carry out many procedures that were formally restricted to the bailiwick of professionals (Behforouz, Farmer, & Mukherjee, 2004; Rifkin, 2009). Many of these activities are quite complex and require training that locals can master. In many ways, local persons are demonstrating abilities, and gaining expertise, that were thought to be beyond their range. But before this knowledge expansion can have significance in communities, a change in orientation must take place. Learning must be the focus of interventions, rather than looking to the usual, professional sources of knowledge. Many biases must be overcome pertaining to who has important knowledge and is capable of entertaining new or complex ideas and mastering new skills.

The resulting organization is non-hierarchical or, in managerial terms, flat (Lune, 2010). But a flat organization is not necessarily community-based; indeed, in managerial circles, flat organizations have been around for time. Typically, the designation flat simply signals that few status distinctions are made, although control of an organization may still remain in a few hands. Local control, accordingly, is not given serious consideration.

Community-based organizations are considered to be flat because jobs are invented, rotated, and leadership is situational (Murphy, 2014). Skills are learned as persons change jobs and encounter new situations. Hence, a loose division of labor is present. As a result of this practice, the knowledge base of everyone is enhanced.

At this juncture, "task shifting" may come to mind (Campbell & Kerry, 2011). This term is used regularly when discussing the dispersion of knowledge in community-based projects. Similar to job rotation, tasks that were monopolized by medical personnel are shifted to others. But in a community-based organization, tasks are shifted to unskilled persons. An entirely new theory of work is adopted, whereby locals are treated as experts, intensely trained, and encouraged to direct an intervention (Greenhalgh, 2009).

For many persons, however, the origin of their jobs remains a mystery. When they enter an organization, a structure already exists and their job assignments are prescribed. A weighty imagery and practice are present that stifles agency. Contrary to this condition, in a self-managed organization jobs are defined by the collectively negotiated goals and put into practice through the interaction that takes place. For this reason, these organizations are described as invented.

Additionally, in community-based organizations, different persons are expected to step in when leadership is needed. Rather than assume that leaders are born, or emerge from one social class of persons, the point is emphasized that leadership rests on expertise and interest. Therefore, one person may lead in a particular situation and another during a different task. In the end, however, skills are disseminated and support offered to the extent that leadership is no longer monopolized.

But especially noteworthy is that local persons write their jobs. In other words, they establish the division of labor. As mentioned earlier, Kanter (1983) broached this idea. This ability, however, is what makes an organization self-managed, a twist that Kanter never took seriously. In a self-managed scenario, a narrative is proposed that specifies the tasks, logic of production or performance, and the mode of evaluation, not to mention the style of authority. This entire process of organizing, therefore, is a collective invention.

As should be noted, the operation of a community-based organization is thoroughly dispersed. But tasks are not merely assigned to persons who were earlier on the periphery. When this is the case, dissemination likely has little to do with local invention and control. Authority may remain hierarchical and impose tasks. True dispersion, in line with a community-based philosophy, indicates that an organization reflects local agency. Governance is thus embedded in local interaction and represents the will of the community that constitutes an organization. As is required of community-based organizations, dualism is overcome and organizational autonomy is averted.

A Move Away from Philosophy

Organizations must change when they strive to become community-based. Particularly important is that they become completely transparent, with information flow unimpaired throughout the process of service delivery. Accordingly, as should be noted in the previous section, an organization and a community become thoroughly integrated when they are community-based.

At this juncture, a few concrete examples are introduced to illustrate this process. Questions are asked that attempt to illustrate how transparency and integration are achieved in community-based health organizations, such as hospitals or community clinics.

1. Is an organization hierarchical or flat? The goal of community-based organizations, of course, is to be as flat as possible. Can policy decisions and accompanying changes be led at any level of the organization? In this way, community sentiment can easily reach leaders, who are not ensconced in the world of administration. The organization, in other words, is not abstract and intimidating.
2. Are departments linked together, other than, perhaps, on the organizational chart? A real linkage should be in place that requires these groups to work together and share information. Rensis Likert (1967) called this a "linking-pin model." Do persons in specific departments collaborate with others, as a regular practice of conducting business? Do they coordinate their needs and efforts? In community-based organizations, departments should be interacting, for example, as they track clients when they receive services and move through an organization. In this way, a client's record is holistic, while the members of an organization gain a broad picture of service delivery.

3. Do local persons sit on departmental committees? Community members, for example, are often invited to be on hospital boards. But participating regularly in how these committees function represents something completely different. In their case, local knowledge is integrated into the everyday operation of an organization, rather than intermittently when a crisis may arise.
4. Is there active involvement with communities? Usually, most community contact is passive—locals may be consulted, for example, when a needs assessment is expected to be conducted. Community outreach is, likewise, passive, with attempts made to locate or contact persons. But the question remains: Do community members work regularly, for example, with clinicians or evaluators? Are they a normal part of these teams?
5. Is training available to local persons? The point is that local skill development is important, along with community participation. For example, learning how to navigate the administration of a hospital, become familiar with clinical nomenclature, and how to introduce significant input and make changes are important skills. Training should thus be extended to all those who are expected to shape an organization.
6. Are clinical practices—hospitals as well as neighborhood clinics—close to communities? Often these providers are spatially in or near to communities, but have the pathways been cleared to treatment? Is local knowledge used to define problems and accessibility, so that stigma is not attached to seeking care, for example, for mental health issues? Making sure that services are in a community must extend beyond logistical considerations. How a health organization interacts with a community should be a local determination.

Conclusion

The bottom line is that the delivery of health services is a group effort. But the nature of this group, or organization, is a key concern in the design of community-based interventions. By traditional standards, community-based organizations implode and dissolve into their respective communities. According to traditionalists, such organizations are insubstantial. But while these organizations may be unobtrusive, they are not flimsy.

An organizing principle certainly exists that is neither natural nor autonomous. A community-based organization is self-generating and represents collectively designed narratives about how health issues should be addressed. A community specifies what problems are important and how remedies should be applied. In fact, how these plans are executed constitutes a health-care organization. In terms of a community-based philosophy, this dispersed locus of organizing is vital.

In community-based work, a particular population becomes the organization. No facet of this process is treated as autonomous; nothing about service delivery is imposed. As a community becomes self-directed, and begins to focus on health care, an organization emerges that is dedicated to identifying and finding solutions to problems. In this regard, service delivery is thoroughly local.

At the root of this change is philosophy. Specifically important is that organizations must be imagined to exist without support from dualism. Within this new framework, at least initially, institutions may appear to be weak, even flighty. But without dualism, problems can be identified, plans made, and remedial strategies implemented in the absence of the usual formalized guidelines.

For this reason, community-based organizations are substantial but difficult to pin down. The community that invents these organizations knows the rules, has access, and recognizes transgressions, because local knowledge is operative. Outsiders, nonetheless, may declare in frustration that no organization exists, only a hodgepodge of persons and practices. Those who want to become community-based, however, should not fall prey to the stale imagery supplied by realism and settle for rigorous, clearly delineated but irrelevant health-care organizations, out of fear of not having a true organizational presence.

Community-based organizations hold a lot of promise. Health services can be provided in an effective way, thereby improving care. And somewhat related, communities can acquire skills and gain a sense of self-efficacy, so they can become agents of social change (Bandura, 1995). But these changes are not likely to occur unless service organizations are rethought. A new theory of organizing is needed, one that enhances local agency, knowledge, and, in the end, control. In this sense, philosophy is at the core of changing direction and becoming community-based.

References

Bandura, A. (1995). *Self-efficacy in changing societies*. Cambridge, UK: Cambridge University Press.

Behforouz, H. L., Farmer, P. E., & Mukherjee, J. S. (2004). From directly observed therapy to Accompagnateurs: Enhancing AIDS treatment outcomes in Haiti and in Boston. *Clinical Infectious Diseases, 38*, S429–S436.

Bordo, S. (1987). *The flight to objectivity*. Albany, NY: SUNY Press.

Bourdieu, P. (1990). *In other words*. Stanford, CA: Stanford University Press.

Burrell, G., & Morgan, G. (1979). *Sociological paradigms and organizational analysis*. London: Heinemann.

Campbell, C., & Kerry, S. (2011). Retreat from Alma-Ata? The who's report on task shifting to community health workers for AIDS care in poor countries. *Global Public health: An International Journal for Research, Policy, and Practice, 6*(2), 125–138.

Cueto, M. (2004). The origins of primary health care and SELECTIVE primary health care. *American Journal of Public Health, 94*(11), 1864–1874.

Dussel, E. (2008). *Ethics and community*. Eugene, OR: Wipf & Stock.

Fals Borda, O. (1988). *Knowledge and people's power*. New York: New Horizons Press.

Freidson, E. (1970). *The profession of medicine: A study of the sociology of applied knowledge*. Chicago: University of Chicago Press.

Fromm, E. (1959). *The sane society*. New York: Rinehart and Co.

Gadamer, H.-G. (1996). *The enigma of health*. Stanford, CA: Stanford University Press.

Geiger, H. J. (2016). The first Community Health Center in Mississippi: Communities empowering themselves. *American Journal of Public Health, 106*(10), 1738–1740.
Gergen, K. (1999). *An invitation to social construction*. Thousand Oakes, CA: Sage.
Greenhalgh, T. (2009). Chronic illness: Beyond the expert patient. *British Medical Journal, 338*, 629–631.
Howick, J. (2011). *The philosophy of evidence-based medicine*. West Sussex, UK: Wiley-Blackwell.
Kanter, R. M. (1983). *The change masters: Innovations in productivity in the American corporation*. New York: Simon & Schuster.
Kretzman, J. P., & McKnight, J. L. (1993). *Building communities from the inside out*. Chicago, IL: ACTA.
Lefkowitz, B. (2007). *Community health centers: A movement and the people who made it happen*. New Brunswick, NJ: Rutgers University Press.
Likert, R. (1967). *The human organization: Its management and value*. New York: McGraw-Hill.
Luhmann, N. (2017). *Trust and power*. Cambridge: Polity Press.
Lune, H. (2010). *Understanding organizations*. Cambridge, UK: Polity Press.
Murphy, J. W. (2014). *Community-based interventions: Philosophy and action*. New York: Springer.
Perrow, C. (1979). *Complex organizations*. Glenview, IL: Schott, Foresman, and Company.
Rifkin, S. B. (2009). Lessons from community participation in health programmes: A review of the post Alma-Ata experience. *International Health, 1*(1), 31–36.
Rothschild, J., & Whitt, J. A. (1986). *The cooperative workplace*. New York: Cambridge University Press.
Scott, R. W. (2002). *Organizations: Rational, natural, and open systems* (5th ed.). Englewood Cliffs, NJ: Prentice-Hall.
Selznick, P. (1948). Foundations of the theory of organizations. *American Sociological Review, 13*(1), 25–35.
Stufflebeam, D. L. (2001). The metaevaluation imperative. *American Journal of Evaluation, 22*(2), 183–209.
Ward Jr., T. J., & Geiger, H. J. (2017). *Out in the rural: A Mississippi health center and its war on poverty*. New York: Oxford University Press.
Weick, K. (1976). Educational organizations as loosely coupled systems. *Administrative Science Quarterly, 21*(1), 1–19.
Wu, C.-C. (2011). The impact of hospital brand image on service quality, patient satisfaction, and loyalty. *African Journal of Business Management, 5*(12), 4873–4882.

Chapter 3
Establishing Community-Based Primary Health Care

Karen A. Callaghan

Introduction

For many decades, global attention has focused on the need to deliver effective health care to all communities, including those that are impoverished and disenfranchised. Despite advancements in technology and medical science, disparities in health outcomes and access to care continue to persist (Weinstein, Geller, Negussie, & Baciu, 2017). In addition, the cost of providing health services continues to increase. These problems are particularly evident in the American health care system, where government resources are the only safety net for those who cannot acquire private insurance. This approach affects adversely lower income communities, since they are more likely to face financial, cultural, linguistic, and other barriers to accessing adequate health care. While this situation may seem dire, what is known as the primary health care movement may provide viable remedies.

According to the World Health Organization (WHO), primary health care requires reconceptualizing the very nature of health, illness, delivery modalities, and the status of medical professionals and patients. The WHO Alma-Ata Declaration (1978) stipulates that health refers to "complete mental, physical, and social well-being, and not merely the absence of disease or infirmity…" (section I). Focusing on "well-being" rather than the eradication of pathological conditions requires a thoroughly different approach to health services. Effective care must target a myriad of social, economic, and personal circumstances previously considered tangential to medical treatment and intervention. In addition, helping patients and communities achieve good health must involve an assessment of the quality of relationships, the environment, educational and employment opportunities, housing, finances, and

K. A. Callaghan (✉)
Barry University, Miami, FL, USA
e-mail: kcallaghan@barry.edu

S. L. Arxer, J. W. Murphy (eds.), *Community-Based Health Interventions in an Institutional Context*, International Perspectives on Social Policy, Administration, and Practice, https://doi.org/10.1007/978-3-030-24654-9_3

personal choices, as well as of the laws, policies, procedures, and social practices that affect access to relevant care and resources (Kickbusch, 2003).

The Alma-Ata Declaration went further, however, to ensure that health care would be tied closely to the concerns and circumstances of communities. One of the key tenets of the Declaration is "…maximum community and individual self-reliance and participation in the planning, organization, operation and control of primary health care…" (World Health Organization, 1978, section VII, 5). This statement reflects the endorsement by the Conference of authentic democratization of the health-care system. Such a maneuver requires that population health become a primary focus of government and nongovernment entities that control or influence related policies, planning, and the distribution of resources. The goal of this strategy is the coordination of health promotion and care across all sectors. When these efforts are accomplished with maximum community participation, relevant and effective services can be delivered more efficiently.

Subsequent WHO Conferences continued to emphasize this needed shift to health promotion, direct community participation, health focus in all policies, intersectoral coordination, and consideration of the social determinants of health. The Ottawa Charter for Health Promotion (1986), for example, states that:

> Health promotion works through concrete and effective community action in setting priorities, making decisions, planning strategies and implementing them to achieve better health. At the heart of this process is the empowerment of communities, their ownership and control of their own endeavours and destinies. (Strengthen community action section)

This Charter (1986) also emphasizes that the health-care system must "embrace an expanded mandate" to go beyond clinical interventions, emphasize health promotion, and "open channels" to address social, economic, and environmental barriers to well-being (Reorient health services section). Likewise, the Rio Political Declaration on the Social Determinants of Health (2011) calls specifically for more intersectoral cooperation and coordination and for support "to empower the role of communities and strengthen civil society" (section 12.2). An emphasis on local empowerment, collective responsibility, coordinated efforts, and "harnessing the potential of digital technology" to enhance participation can be found also in the Shanghai Declaration (2016, Health literacy empowers and drives equity section).

The fundamental assumptions of these Declarations are clear: if the purpose of health care is to maintain the well-being of all persons, then *all* of the circumstances jeopardizing that well-being must be addressed in ways that are meaningful and effective. Providing care in a one-dimensional, reductionist framework is a stopgap and ultimately a waste of resources, since health exists within a complex of social, economic, environmental, and personal situations that are unique to local communities.

The WHO Declarations should be understood as the formal culmination of various global movements dedicated to reducing disparities in health and in access to meaningful services and care. Inequities in health represent a threat to individuals who are suffering but also to the strength of democratic civil society (Brown, Harrison, Burns, & Ziglio, 2013). An inclusive society where persons participate fully in multiple levels of governance is predicated on facilitating their well-being and full development. Excluding entire segments of a population from meaningful participation due to a lack of resources, information, or support undermines democracy.

These very concerns gave rise to several movements in the American health care system that were intended to expand access, provide more effective care, become patient-centered, include community participation, and integrate social determinates of health. In other words, each of these reforms attempted to introduce an aspect of primary health care into the existing system. Examples of these projects include community health centers, community-oriented primary care, patient-centered medical homes, and the use of social determinants of health in formal diagnoses (Geiger, 2002). While each approach has helped to expand services within the context of a more holistic view of health, the question remains as to whether these practices are guided by a community-based philosophy. This type of conceptual framework is crucial for facilitating maximum community participation in the planning, implementation, and control of a primary health-care system.

Primary Health Care as Community-Focused Projects

Implementation of the Affordable Care Act (ACA) signaled renewed interest in primary health care in the United States (Klink, 2015). This legislation mandated providing access to health care for millions of new recipients, as efficiently and effectively as possible. While some critics have cast this legislation as unprecedented, the ACA should be understood as part of a history of reforms intended to provide accessible *community-focused* care (Chowkwanyun, 2018). For example, the ACA provision to expand Medicare and Medicaid eligibility clearly ties this approach to the development of community health centers, which was a strategy of the 1960s War on Poverty. While political struggles over the right to adequate health care are a necessary part of this process, the primary health-care movement depends also on efforts to reconceptualize the nature and practice of medical treatment and intervention.

Although instituted originally as part of the Public Health Services Act of 1965, community health centers (CHCs) continue to serve as an important care provider in many low income and poor communities (Wright, 2013b). According to the National Association of Community Health Centers (2019), more than 1350 federally qualified health centers annually serve approximately 28 million people. Approximately, 90% of these patients live in or near poverty, over 60% are Black or Hispanic, and more than 50% receive Medicaid or Medicare health benefits. In order to retain eligibility to receive federal funds, CHCs must provide care in designated high medical need areas, offer comprehensive "enabling" services, be affordable to everyone, and maintain a 51% patient member governing board (National Association of Community Health Centers, 2019, pp. 2–3). CHCs are expected to address population health issues, since many of their clients experience chronic conditions associated with racial-ethnic and income disparities (Stevens, 2016). As proponents note, "CHCs pride themselves equally on providing community-accountable and culturally competent care aimed at reducing health disparities associated with poverty, race, language, and culture" (Adashi, Geiger, & Fine, 2010, p. 2049).

Community accountability is obviously an important theme in the governance of CHCs. Serving on the governing or advisory boards is the primary mechanism for the community to exercise influence or control over operational and policy decisions. CHC governance is described as "community-based leadership" (Sharma, Huang, Knox, Willard-Grace, & Potter, 2018, p. 1070), a "grass roots governing structure" (Fiscella & Geiger, 2014, p. 2044), and as a means to "engage and empower patients" (Wright, 2013a, p. 430). While this approach appears to be moving toward full participation, several crucial issues should be addressed regarding the scope and nature of community input. The goals of CHCs are to effect positive clinical outcomes for individual patients and to bring about changes in the social determinants that are effecting the whole community. Those aims require different levels of community participation and even control over health projects. The CHC movement has struggled to understand how community involvement might require fundamental changes in the traditional biomedical approach to clinical care.

H. Jack Geiger (2002), one of the pioneers of the CHC movement, addressed the issue of how a "health program … could be deliberately fashioned as an instrument of community development and as a lever for social change" through the community-oriented primary care (COPC) model made famous by Sidney and Emily Kark's work in South Africa (pp. 1714–1715). The Karks' approach used community development techniques to address population health issues, which, as the WHO Declarations stipulate, are linked clearly to the social, environmental, and economic circumstances of any community. This project illustrated that community empowerment should be understood as an important first step to creating sustainable changes in overall well-being.

Since the 1950s and 60s, however, the implementation of COPC and the notion of community empowerment have undergone various changes. Proponents of COPC point to several key principles and practices that constitute the community-based nature of this approach. COPC begins with "a defined community" and delivers services based on "its assessed health needs" (Mullan & Epstein, 2002, p. 1750). Importantly, this care is delivered "through the planned integration" of public health and primary care practices (Mullan & Epstein, 2002, p. 1750). Since COPC assumes that health promotion practices are as important as clinical interventions, community engagement is a principle feature, since this involvement is needed to assist in assessing and prioritizing health problems and selecting feasible interventions. Community members' participation is usually accomplished via service on formal and informal advisory boards, on task forces or research groups, and as part of focus groups.

An additional influence of the ACA on primary health care models is the emphasis on delivering better quality services to patients through more efficient use of resources. In this context, the Patient-Centered Medical Home (PCMH) is considered a primary means to deliver high-value care to a wide range of clients. Through rigorous accreditation standards, PCMHs are required to provide services in a sensitive, responsive, relevant, and coordinated manner (Stange et al., 2010). Teams of professional and clinical staff provide care and treatment planning, which is supposed to ensure informed coordination of service. Patients and family members can expect to have direct continuous contact, via phone calls and electronic messages, with their care providers. In addition, group and home visits, drop-in services, same-day appointments, and referrals to non-clinical services are routine practices. Communication between service providers and patients is considered a key concern for services and relationships to be culturally informed, honest, and supportive.

PCMHs are expected also to be guided by Patient Advisory Councils that are composed of patients, family members, and caregivers. Typically, these Councils address issues related to "practice improvement," which can range from enhancing the physical comfort and look of the clinic waiting rooms to better quality communication about "bad news" regarding a patient's health status (Sharma et al., 2016, pp. 778–779). PCMHs are characterized also as employing a community-oriented approach. However, according to the US Agency for Healthcare Research and Quality, PCMH interventions are considered community-based when patients are referred to preventative services, located in their local neighborhoods, which typically involve screening and counseling (Dymek et al., 2013).

A final practice that should illustrate the community-based nature of these approaches to care and intervention is the recognition of the social determinants of health (SDH) in formal diagnoses and treatment planning. As illustrated in the WHO documents, addressing SDH is crucial for reducing health disparities and improving the well-being of communities. Many people are sick and suffering due to where they live, their social identities, whether they have a job, and their ability to pay for care. Effective interventions must include services to individual patients as well as comprehensive prevention and health promotion programs. New approaches to public health and social epidemiology have emerged in response to this shift (Awofeso, 2004). Public health models now call for the critical interrogation of the social and political changes that are needed to ensure better quality housing, food, water, sanitation, education, employment, and recreation, because these conditions are related directly to the health status of communities. Social epidemiologists have developed multidimensional eco-social frameworks to explain disease and health distribution. Krieger (2009), for example, recommends that epidemiological studies should routinely address salient factors such as stress related to living in lower income neighborhoods, structural and institutional privilege and oppression, and targeted marketing of unhealthy products and lifestyles.

The U.S. Centers for Disease Control (CDC) promotes a "place-based" framework for understanding and addressing SDH. Krieger's recommendations appear to be included as common issues that public health professionals should employ when designing health promotion activities. In addition, the CDC guidelines recommend that practitioners incorporate engagement strategies to "harness the skills and talents of a community" and "foster connectedness and trust" (Centers for Disease Control, 2013, p. 10). Examples of recommended community engagement methods include participation in interviews, focus groups, and forums; service on research teams and advisory boards; and employment in agencies or other community-based organizations.

Since community-oriented health projects are supposed to integrate public health and primary care practices, efforts are underway to use of SDH information in clinical care settings as well. The American College of Physicians recommends that medical professionals should become advocates for public policy and clinical interventions designed to ameliorate the negative effects of SDH (Daniel, Bornstein, & Kane, 2018). In addition, medical education should include training on the significance of SDH and on how to integrate this information into screening techniques and treatment planning.

As should be expected, CHCs have been at the forefront of the use of SDH in formal clinical intake and diagnoses. The widespread use of electronic health record (EHR) systems has presented new challenges for the focus on SDH. In order to ensure that patient-level SDH information is included in EHRs, the National Association of Community Health Centers and several other professional associations have launched national effort to adopt the Protocol for Responding to and Assessing Patient Assets, Risks, and Experiences (PRAPARE) (Gold et al., 2018). This assessment tool can be embedded in EHRs. After collecting information on 13 core SDH measures (for example, race-ethnicity, housing status, stress, employment status), clinical staff can use these data to determine if patients require referrals to additional services or need support to comply with treatment and care requirements (Gold et al., 2018, p. 403). According to the PRAPARE training manual, using this electronic assessment tool allows medical and other clinic staff to see the "increased complexity of patients," provide more targeted care, and "advocate for change at the community and national levels" (National Association of Community Health Centers, 2016).

These various attempts to develop a more responsive and holistic model of care seem to have embraced a community-based approach; however, significant barriers to full and authentic participation continue to exist. Even when the desire to offer effective primary care, prevention, and health promotion services is genuine, the task of connecting with and affording patients and communities maximum participation and control seems elusive. Giving patients direct access to medical professionals, providing care in pleasant surroundings, and taking into account the well-documented relationships between social indicators and health will result in providing services that are possibly more relevant and, therefore, effective. However, these practices do not support or reflect the exercise of sustained community participation, control, and self-reliance. Why then despite numerous attempts to allow more involvement and inclusion in the design, delivery, and control of health care services, do communities seem to remain on the periphery of important decision-making about their well-being?

Community-based approaches to research, planning, and intervention require not only the adoption of new practices, such as allowing patients to serve on an advisory board, but also, and more important, a dramatic re-thinking of certain philosophical assumptions. This conceptual shift requires a critical interrogation of the traditional biomedical, science-based approach to health and illness. The notion that everyday members of a community can play a significant role in the design and delivery of health projects makes little sense in this traditional framework. Nonetheless, from the biomedical standpoint, individuals and communities when supplied with the correct information can learn to make better choices about diet and exercise and they can help clinical staff understand how to make interactions less stressful. In addition, communities can create health-related support programs to help other residents. In this regard, communities can serve as important consultants for any medical practice. However, for communities to become the central driving force of primary health care systems, an important epistemological shift is imperative (Murphy, 2014).

The philosophical assumptions on which the biomedical model is based stress the importance of developing objective knowledge that is not tainted by subjective opinions or perspectives. In the medical context, this objectivity is expressed as "expert" knowledge that is developed through employing rigorous scientific methodology. Only persons with certain credentials can be authorized to interpret and use this knowledge, while they follow specific protocols for implementation. In this context, communities are incapable of producing or independently analyzing knowledge (Murphy, Franz, & Callaghan, 2015). In addition, intimate contact or engagement with those who may be the recipients of treatment or interventions is viewed as inappropriate or even harmful. Forming such relationships with communities is antithetical to the protocols that should be followed to produce the desired outcomes. Community input needs to be limited to those issues or aspects of care that are related to facilitating compliance with treatment regimens.

As with any paradigm based on dualism, only knowledge divorced from subjectivity should be used to make serious decisions. If any useful information exists within communities, certain methods must be used to extract what will become valid data. These empirical indicators can then be used by researchers and medical professionals to gain insights into individual and community needs, assets, and challenges. Community involvement with these data collection efforts is usually minimal. Persons may be asked to complete surveys or interviews, but in many cases, communities are often pre-defined by using zip codes and census tract data. The voices of actual persons are marginalized to preserve as much objectivity as possible.

Qualitative methodologies may appear to include more dynamic community participation; however, these approaches do not necessarily reject the dualistic scientific paradigm (Murphy et al., 2015). Common qualitative methods, such as key informant interviews and focus groups, do not preclude identifying the researchers and practitioners as the experts who must control the data collection, analysis, and interpretation. Focus groups, for example, are used typically to elicit feedback on specific questions or issues that have been identified as important by external parties. Often, the aim of this type of data collection is to determine how to generate community support or buy-in for projects. The personal viewpoints garnered through these techniques are often used as proxies for the community as a whole.

A more authentic democratic form of community participation requires a shift away from the biomedical-scientific paradigm and the underlying dualism of objectivity-subjectivity. When dualism is rejected, an alternative framework of how knowledge, community, and participation are constituted is possible. Within a community-based paradigm, full community participation not only makes sense but also is a necessary prerequisite for any primary health-care project (Murphy & Franz, 2017).

Participation, Dialogue, and Local Knowledge

An authentic community-based approach assumes that all knowledge is derived from particular interpretations and perspectives (Murphy, 2014). Professional experts may have knowledge and skills that are quite useful for many persons and communities. However, the true validity of that knowledge cannot be determined until close contact has been established with these persons. Developing such contact is not possible if a community is identified or understood through analysis of empirical referents or social indicators. For example, using zip code areas and census tracts to define communities creates a disembodied, abstract version of actual persons and the way they experience and interpret their lives. From a community-based perspective, a health project should begin with attempts to gain entrée to a new social world, rather than with plans for extracting data or objectively determining neighborhood boundaries.

When dualism is rejected, how communities are understood and approached is fundamentally changed. In order for community-based projects to be successful, what had been deemed previously as subjective, and therefore unreliable and unsubstantiated, viewpoints must be given full attention and consideration. As Berger and Luckman (1966) contend, a community is a life-world or a complex of meaning, which emerges as persons engage with others and try to make sense of their lives. Human agency or intentionality are evident in all aspect of community life (Berger & Luckman, 1966, pp. 20–21). How persons define or interpret health, well-being, and illness is revealed only through their narratives or stories, that is, through the meaning they have constructed about their lives.

Communities, then, have biographies, that is, complex narratives, that reveal persons' perspectives, values, and assumptions (Murphy, 2014, pp. 25–26). Any efforts to include community participation in research, planning, and interventions must allow these stories to be told. This assumption underscores the importance of gaining entrée and using dialogue as a primary means to developing sustained relationships with communities. Soliciting community feedback on an occasional basis to ensure that new projects have support will create relationships that are fragmented, unreliable, and not worthy of much attention or trust. Furthermore, community members need time to reflect on how the services of a clinic or the effects of an intervention might serve a meaningful purpose in their lives. Authentic dialogue requires, therefore, that the biographies of communities be taken seriously, that is, as legitimate knowledge that can not only inform but also direct the planning and delivery of primary health care and interventions (Fals Borda, 2013, p. 160; Fals Borda, 1988).

The ultimate aim of community-based approaches is to allow researchers, medical professionals, and local residents to co-constitute services, interventions, planning, and further investigations (Freire, 1992, p. 97). What has been considered "expert" knowledge must play a role in this process but only as one type of narrative, developed by professional communities as they construct interpretations of specific problems and remedies. This knowledge can be introduced to communities once trust and intimacy have been established. However, medical practitioners must enter communities with humility and respect and with a genuine interest in learning. Regardless of their credentials or experience, these professionals are novices in each unique community. They must be open to grasping and affirming the multiple layers of social reality that are revealed by the narratives of a community's history, conflicts, victories, defeats, alliances, and challenges. These stories can be dynamic, confusing, and contradictory but they must be understood to form sustained, productive relationships. Medical practitioners must learn to understand the world from the standpoint of the community. In other words, once dialogical relationships have been established, practitioners and residents can begin to explore democratically the feasibility of various interventions and services (Solomon, 1976).

Community-Based Primary Health Care

The global efforts to institute primary health care systems that allow maximum participation reflect the commitment to empower individuals and communities to become directly responsible for sustaining their own well-being. Empowerment, in this context, does not mean that communities are disorganized and helpless and must rely on more powerful outsiders to secure the information and resources needed to address their problems (Rappaport, 1987). An authentic community-based approach begins by forming dialogical relationships in order to reveal local knowledge, rather than merely asking residents to react to or "consume" the ideas and strategies of others (Freire, 1992, p. 100). Communities can be empowered when their histories, values, perspectives, and interpretations are taken seriously and not dismissed as trivial information that gets in the way of sound medical practice. This epistemological shift requires significant changes in the common strategies that have been used in the past to provide more community-accountability, grassroots leadership, and community development as key components in primary health care.

Primary care projects must begin with identifying a target community. In fact, one of the key processes for creating COPC involves "defining (geographically, members registered in a practice or as a sociological construct) and characterizing the community to determine health needs…" (Gofin, Gofin, & Stimpson, 2015, p. 128). Interestingly, COPC practitioners admit that the "idea of community" can be an "elusive concept" and that "simple geography" is not a sufficient means to identify a target community (Mullan & Epstein, 2002, p. 1750). However, the remedy proposed to resolve this dilemma is to make better use of electronic tools for mapping rates of chronic health problems, mortality and natality rates, and socio-demographic data to understand community boundaries and health concerns (Hayashi, Bazemore, & McIntyre, 2011, p. 62; Mullan & Epstein, 2002, p. 1752).

While the use of Geographic Information Systems and electronic databases can readily identify the spatial clustering of resources, services, and various social, economic, and health problems (Sampson, Morenoff, & Gannon-Rowley, 2002), a community cannot be defined through these methods. Reliance on empirical indicators creates a disembodied schematic of community life that may have little relevance for the persons actually living in these areas. While the data garnered through electronic means may have some utility for planning processes, the communities in question must first be identified through direct contact.

Participatory community-based mapping processes can be used to begin a dialogical process that allows residents to define the space, relationships, and commitments of their community life (Murphy et al., 2015). Gaining entrée to initiate this process may begin with local clubs, churches, and community-based agencies. However, the purpose of mapping is to become continuously more inclusive to avoid relying on the perspectives of select groups or leaders. Communities consist of multiple realities, and the particular connections, issues, and possibly contested interpretations of certain groups and associations cannot be considered the sole arbiter of local knowledge (Blumenthal, Hopkins III, & Yancy, 2013; Elwood, 2006). Participatory mapping allows the residents to take the lead, literally, on a project or discussion. In this context, residents are cast not as patients or research subjects but as co-investigators who provide direction and original thinking for the project.

COPC practitioners may feel that defining a community is a slippery task if they are expecting to discover a fixed, stable entity that readily conforms to objective referents. Communities' identities are dynamic and reflect diverse viewpoints, conflicts, and disputes as well as solidarity and consensus. Participatory mapping processes can provide opportunities for residents to reflect critically on an identity and begin to consider the perspectives and aims of practitioners and researchers. Further, multiple maps can be created to represent the diversity and various dimensions of residents' lived experiences. These different maps can be discussed and critiqued to reach a strategic consensus on how to define and prioritize health problems (International Fund for Agricultural Development, 2009). As part of this process, residents can consider how the resources and services available from a health center or medical interventions might be of use to the community.

Having patients and residents serve on advisory and governing boards is also a way that local knowledge can have a direct impact on decision-making about health services. However, in practice, the role of local representatives on these boards is usually marginalized in favor of those who can contribute more professional expertise, particularly in the areas of law and finance. Wright and Martin (2014) refer to this situation as the "expertise gap" that governing boards may face when trying to foster direct community involvement. As a result, local representatives are viewed as "non-professionals" and their input is construed often as a type of consumer feedback (p. 932). These dynamics reflect clearly the dire need for a community-based framework for health-care governance. Without this framework, local knowledge is understood as nothing more than feedback on personal experiences. However, CHC boards, for example, need information about the community they serve. As a result, local representatives are often criticized as "… being too particular in their perspectives and interests, and therefore unable to provide the breadth of insights about the needs and views of the wider community" (Wright & Martin, 2014, p. 943). This contradiction is tied directly to status of what is considered subjectivity in the traditional biomedical model. As a result, the role of patients in governance is undermined, since from an epistemological standpoint they have nothing to offer as board members.

If COPC projects and CHCs, in particular, are serious about fostering grassroots leadership, then community-based models of co-governance must be implemented. The nature of and need for "expertise" should be critically explored. The fact that community representatives may not already possess certain information should not diminish their status. Must all board members have the same depth of knowledge about finances, legal statutes, and accreditation issues? Community participants can be trained in these issues as they can learn to guide research projects and medical interventions. Participatory budgeting practices can be used to facilitate all board members' commitment to ensuring that community priorities are reflected in their work (Hagelskamp, Schleifer, Rinehart, & Silliman, 2018). In this regard, all board members should be trained on the use of authentic community-based techniques to develop sustained relationships with the community being served. Indeed, local representatives can serve as the facilitators for this process (Minkler, Garcia, Williams, LoPresti, & Lilly, 2010).

Obviously, building sustained and close relationships is key to ensuring that communities increasingly become more involved and eventually assume full responsibility for health-care planning and implementation. However, facilitating sustained community participation requires fundamentally rethinking and reorganizing the roles, processes, and even facilities associated with medical care. Creating and maintaining vibrant health committees and employing community health workers are practices that can facilitate the development and organizing that are important for expanded community control (Pérez & Martinez, 2008).

Local health committees can be organized as part of the mapping processes that should accompany the initial entrée to a community. As local residents discuss and debate their identity, aspirations, and challenges, these committees can begin to coordinate and communicate salient information to medical practitioners, planning and advisory boards, and government agencies. But communities should decide how health committees are composed and members are appointed or elected. Local activists and leaders play important roles in this process and local health practitioners should participate as well.

In addition, health committees can function most effectively when supported by community health workers (CHWs) (Murphy, Franz, & Callaghan, 2016).

Community members can be trained as CHWs and conduct health surveys and assessments, serve on health committees, and accompany local patients through the health system as advocates. The ACA includes provisions for expanding the role of CHWs, but with primary focus on their capacity to provide support and referral services to individual patients and their families (Malcarney, Pittman, Quigley, Horton, & Seiler, 2017; Shah, Heisler, & Davis, 2014). Although CHWs are viewed as important liaisons between the clinic staff and patients, their communication is often limited to addressing SDH issues as the "social barriers" that might limit the effectiveness of services (Thomas-Henkel & Shulman, 2017).

However, CHWs can also assume leadership roles in conducting community-based research and community development projects and ensuring that an ever-expanding number of residents are included as co-investigators in these endeavors (Murphy et al., 2016). Researchers and practitioners can assist with these processes by sharing their related knowledge and skills about how to collect and organize information and to interact effectively with decision-making authorities. Medical professionals and other clinic staff can ensure that CHWs are taken seriously, as recognized advocates for the community who can share information that is vital to providing effective care. Whenever possible, clinics and other facilities should be made available to health committees, CHWs, and other groups for meetings, training sessions, and similar gatherings. The clinic or heath center can become a hub for a wide range of community activities and as such become an embodied space for care, support, and meaningful action (Krieger, 2005).

As community residents become involved in co-designing and conducting research projects, collaborating on developing proposals for policy changes, and coordinating service delivery, what Kiefer (1984) calls their "participatory competence" is enhanced (p. 9). This development represents more than the acquisition of better technical skills. As communities engage in mapping processes, open debates and dialogues, and research projects, they reflect critically on their identity, self-efficacy, assets, aspirations, and challenges. Consequently, as Freire (1992, pp. 95–96) notes, persons can then "see and act differently toward the world," as they assess how certain personal and social changes and interventions may improve their well-being. Likewise, as medical professionals, researchers, and clinic staff appreciate the nature and importance of local knowledge, they should see and act differently toward communities. From a community-based perspective, practitioners do not enter a community simply to deliver ready-made health services. On the contrary, a community-based approach requires that health projects be initiated by finding opportunities for practitioners to share their knowledge and skills through close collaboration with communities.

Furthermore, practitioners should see their potential collaborators as not only as those (patients) who visit a medical facility but as all local residents who are in need of advocacy to promote their well-being. From a population health standpoint, for example, all residents who are effected by SDH should be viewed as the community served by a clinic or practice. SDH issues are typically addressed only on an individual patient level through referrals to support services. While those remedies are still needed, organizing and advocating for specific social and political changes might provide more sustainable solutions to chronic health problems. Prominent groups such as the National Association of Community Health Centers and the College of Physicians call for significant legal and policy changes at the local and national level. CHCs and medical practitioners should be at the forefront in supporting community activism to address SDH (Daniel et al., 2018; National Center for Community Health Centers, 2016). Practitioners and governing boards should be willing to work with health committees and CHWs to develop action plans to address these needs of communities. Working collaboratively with communities, they can help define the policy changes that would create more access, openness, and democracy in the planning and delivery of health care.

Conclusion

The primary health care movement, globally and in the United States, calls for reducing health disparities, including inequities in access to services. In addition, as advocated by the WHO, primary health care is effective only when the design and delivery of services has included the maximum participation of individuals and communities. The point is that the well-being of neglected and marginalized communities can be assured only when they are able to exercise direct control of their health care. In essence, primary health care should be derived from a community-based model.

In the American health care system, CHCs and other models of COPC have been implemented to ensure that services are culturally appropriate, accessible, affordable, and representative of the patient population. However, the strategies for achieving these goals have been well entrenched in the traditional biomedical model. The focus is still on individual patients and their immediate health needs. When patients serve on decision-making councils, they are treated more like consumers with limited knowledge of the real workings of the clinic or health center.

An authentic community-based model for health care requires practitioners to be ready to form close bonds with communities based on solidarity and respect. The community cannot be understood simply as a location from which to deploy services. Entering into a relationship with a community must begin with dialogue and openness. Practitioners must divest themselves of the notion that their medical knowledge and skills provide automatically insights into the life-world of a community. Only by listening carefully to the stories of local residents will the various perspective, values, interpretations, and commitments be revealed. Medical professionals must be willing to take local knowledge seriously, if interventions are to have any appeal or impact.

In addition, from a community-based approach, community empowerment and development are as important as any clinical interventions for creating well-being (Moore, 2018). Practitioners should be able and willing to facilitate enhancing community capacity for research, advocacy, and organizing by supporting health committees, CHWs, and sustained collaborations with activists and community-based organizations. In other words, practitioners must assume that communities, regardless of their challenges or lack of resources, are capable of sophisticated analysis of their circumstances, effective self-advocacy, and creative problem solving.

References

Adashi, E. Y., Geiger, H. J., & Fine, M. D. (2010). Health care reform and primary care - the growing importance of the community health center. *New England Journal of Medicine, 362*, 2047–2050. https://doi.org/10.1056/NEJMp1003729

Awofeso, N. (2004). What's new about the "new public health"? *American Journal of Public Health, 94*(5), 705–709.

Berger, P. L., & Luckman, T. (1966). *The social construction of reality: A treatise in the sociology of knowledge*. New York: Doubleday & Co.

Blumenthal, D. S., Hopkins III, Y., & Yancy, E. (2013). Community-based participatory research: An introduction. In D. S. Blumenthal, R. J. DiClemente, R. L. Brauthwaite, & S. S. Smith (Eds.), *Community-based participatory health research: Issues, methods, and translation to practice* (2nd ed., pp. 1–34). New York: Springer Publishing.

Brown, C., Harrison, D., Burns, H., & Ziglio, E. (2013). *Governance for health equity*. Copenhagen, Denmark: Regional Office of the World Health Organization.

Centers for Disease Control and Prevention – Division of Community Health. (2013). *A practitioner's guide for advancing health equity: Community strategies for preventing chronic disease*. Atlanta, GA: US Department of Health and Human Services.

Chowkwanyun, M. (2018). The war on poverty's health legacy: What it was and why it matters. *Health Affairs, 37*(1), 47–53. https://doi.org/10.1377/hlthaff.2017.1328

Daniel, H., Bornstein, S. S., & Kane, G. C. (2018). Addressing social determinants to improve patient care and promote health equity an American College of Physicians position paper. *Annals of Internal Medicine, 168*, 577–578. https://doi.org/10.7326/M17-2441

Dymek, C., Johnson Jr., M., Mardon, R., Hassell, S., Carpenter, D., McGinnis, P., et al. (2013). *Clinical-community relationships measures atlas*. Rockville, MD: Agency for Healthcare Research and Quality. Retrieved from https://pcmh.ahrq.gov

Elwood, S. (2006). Negotiating knowledge production: The everyday inclusions, exclusions, and contradictions of participatory GIS research. *The Professional Geographer, 58*(2), 197–208.

Fals Borda, O. (1988). *Knowledge and people's power*. New York: New Horizons Press.

Fals Borda, O. (2013). Action research in the convergence of disciplines. *International Journal of Action Research., 9*(2), 155–167.

Fiscella, K., & Geiger, H. J. (2014). Caring for the poor in the 21st century: Enabling community health centers for a new era. *Journal of Health Care for the Poor and Underserved, 25*(4), 2044–2052.

Freire, P. (1992). *Pedagogy of the oppressed*. New York: Continuum.

Geiger, H. J. (2002). Community-oriented primary care: A path to community development. *American Journal of Public Health, 92*(11), 1713–1716.

Gofin, J., Gofin, R., & Stimpson, J. P. (2015). Community-oriented primary care (COPC) and the affordable care act: An opportunity to meet the demands of an evolving health care system. *Journal of Primary Care & Community Health, 6*(2), 128–133.

Gold, R., Bunce, A., Cowburn, S., Dambrun, K., Dearing, M., Middendorf, M., et al. (2018). Adoption of social determinants of health EHR tools by community health centers. *Annals of Family Medicine, 16*, 399–407. Retrieved from https://doi.org/10.1370/afm

Hagelskamp, C., Schleifer, D., Rinehart, C., & Silliman, R. (2018). Participatory budgeting: Could it diminish health disparities in the United States? *Journal of Urban Health, 95*, 766–771. Retrieved from https://doi.org/10.1007/s11524-018-0249-3

Hayashi, A. S., Bazemore, A., & McIntyre, J. (2011). Transforming community health and primary care education using clinical and administrative data and geographic information systems. *Journal of Map and Geography Libraries, 7*, 61–70.

International Fund for Agricultural Development. (2009). *Good practices in participatory mapping, a review prepared for IFAD*. Rome: IFAD.

Kickbusch, I. (2003). The contribution of the World Health Organization to the new public health and health promotion. *American Journal of Public Health, 93*(3), 383–388.

Kieffer, C. (1984). Citizen empowerment: A developmental perspective. In J. Rappaport & R. Hess (Eds.), *Studies in empowerment: Steps toward understanding and action* (pp. 9–36). New York: Haworth Press.

Klink, K. (2015). Incentives for physicians to pursue primary care in the ACA era. *American Medical Association Journal of Ethics, 17*(7), 637–646.

Krieger, N. (2005). Embodiment: A conceptual glossary for epidemiology. *Journal of Epidemiology and Community Health, 59*, 350–355.

Krieger, N. (2009). Putting health inequities on the map: Social epidemiology meets medical/health geography—An ecosocial perspective. *GeoJournal, 74*(2), 87–97.

Malcarney, M.-B., Pittman, P., Quigley, L., Horton, K., & Seiler, N. (2017). The changing roles of community health workers. *Health Services Research, 52*(1), 360–382.

Minkler, M., Garcia, A. P., Williams, J., LoPresti, T., & Lilly, J. (2010). Sí se puede: Using participatory research to promote environmental justice in a latino community in San Diego, California. *Journal of Urban Health, 87*(5), 796–812. https://doi.org/10.1007/s11524-010-9490-0

Moore, A. (2018). *Partnerships for health equity and opportunity: A healthcare playbook for community developers*. Build Healthy Places Network. Retrieved from https://www.buildhealthyplaces.org/resources/partnerships-for-health-equity-and-opportunity-a-healthcare-playbook-for-community-developers//

Mullan, F., & Epstein, L. (2002). Community-oriented primary care: New relevance in a changing world. *American Journal of Public Health, 92*(11), 1748–1755.

Murphy, J. W. (2014). *Community-based interventions: Philosophy and action*. New York: Springer.

Murphy, J. W., & Franz, B. (2017). The patient-centered medical home as a community-based strategy. *The Permanente Journal, 21*, 17–002. Retrieved from https://doi.org/10.7812/TPP/17-002

Murphy, J. W., Franz, B. A., & Callaghan, K. A. (2015). Is community-based work compatible with data collection? *Journal of Sociology and Social Welfare, XLII*(4), 9–21.

Murphy, J. W., Franz, B. A., & Callaghan, K. A. (2016). Group maturity in a community-based project. *Social Work in Public Health, 31*(5), 341–347. https://doi.org/10.1080/19371918.2015.1125320

National Association of Community Health Centers. (2016). *Understand the PRAPARE project*. Retrieved from http://www.nacha.org/PRAPARE

National Association of Community Health Centers. (2019). *Community health center chartbook*. Retrieved from http://www.nachc.org/wp-content/uploads/2019/01/Community-Health-Center-Chartbook-FINAL-1.28.19.pdf

Pérez, L. M., & Martinez, J. (2008). Community health workers: Social justice and policy advocates for community health and well-being. *American Journal of Health, 98*(1), 11–14.

Rappaport, J. (1987). Terms of empowerment/exemplars of prevention: Toward a theory of community psychology. *American Journal of Community Psychology, 15*(2), 121.

Sampson, R. J., Morenoff, J. D., & Gannon-Rowley, T. (2002). Assessing "neighborhood effects": Social processes and new directions in research. *Annual Review of Sociology, 28*, 443–478.

Shah, M., Heisler, M., & Davis, M. (2014). Community health workers and the Patient Protection and Affordable Care Act: An opportunity for a research, advocacy, and policy agenda. *Journal of Health Care for the Poor and Underserved, 25*(1), 17–24. https://doi.org/10.1353/hpu.2014.0019

Sharma, A. E., Huang, B., Knox, M., Willard-Grace, R., & Potter, M. B. (2018). Patient engagement in community health center leadership: How does it happen? *Journal of Community Health, 43*, 1069–1074.

Sharma, A. E., Willard-Grace, R., Willis, A., Zieve, O., Dubé, K., Parker, C., et al. (2016). How can we talk about patient-centered care without patients at the table? Lessons learned from patient advisory councils. *Journal of the American Board of Family Medicine, 29*(6), 775–784. https://doi.org/10.3122/jabfm.2016.06.150380

Solomon, B. B. (1976). *Black empowerment: Social work in oppressed communities*. New York: Columbia University Press.

Stange, K. C., Nutting, P. A., Miller, W. I., Jaén, C. R., Crabtree, B. F., Flocke, S. A., et al. (2010). Defining and measuring the patient-centered medical home. *Journal of General Internal Medicine, 25*(6), 601–612.

Stevens, D. (2016). Health centers after 50 years: Lessons from the health disparities collaboratives. *Journal of Health Care for the Poor and Underserved, 27*, 1621–1631.

Thomas-Henkel, C., & Shulman, M. (2017). *Screening for social determinants of health in populations with complex needs: Implementation considerations*. Center for Health Care Strategies, Inc. Retrieved from https://communityactionpartnership.com/external_resources/screening-for-social-determinants-of-health-in-populations-with-complex-needs-implementation-considerations/

Weinstein, J. N., Geller, A., Negussie, Y., & Baciu, A. (2017). *Communities in action: Pathways to health equity*. The National Academies of Science, Engineering, and Medicine: The National Academies Press.

World Health Organization. (1978). *Declaration of Alma-Ata*. International Conference on Primary Health Care, Alma-Ata, USSR. Geneva, Switzerland: World Health Organization.

World Health Organization. (1986). *Ottawa charter for health promotion*. Geneva, Switzerland: World Health Organization.

World Health Organization. (2011). *Rio declaration on social determinants of health*. Geneva, Switzerland: World Health Organization.

World Health Organization. (2016). *Shanghai declaration on promoting health in the 2030 agenda for sustainable development*. Geneva, Switzerland: World Health Organization.

Wright, B. (2013a). Do patients have a voice? The social stratification of health centers governing boards. *Health Expectations, 18*, 430–437.

Wright, B. (2013b). Who governs federally qualified health centers? *Journal of Health Politics, Policy, and Law, 38*(1), 27–55. https://doi.org/10.1215/03616878-1898794

Wright, B., & Martin, G. P. (2014). Mission, margin, and the role of consumer governance in decision-making at community health centers. *Journal of Health Care for the Poor and Underserved, 25*, 930–947.

Chapter 4
Community-Based Funding and Budgeting: Participatory Budgeting as a Transformative Act

Jung Min Choi, John W. Murphy, Ramsey Dahab, and Charlene Holkenbrink-Monk

Why Community-Based Budgeting?

Since the 1980s, when Ronald Reagan aggressively rolled back the gains made by the various civil rights groups in the 1950s and 1960s, many people have been disillusioned about the state of our democracy (Katznelson, 2005). Citizens are often dissatisfied and frustrated at the dysfunction of the government shrouded in an oversized bureaucratic machine. And for years, everyday citizens have felt disconnected from the neoliberal government that caters mostly to millionaires and multinational corporations who lobby solely for personal profit (Chomsky, 1999).

Partly in response to an unresponsive government, people in different cities across the country have engaged in, and supported, participatory policy reforms. Borrowing from the general framework found in community-based work (CBW), people are experimenting with direct democracy to improve their communities through policy (Lerner, 2014). An aspect of CBW that is drawing the bulk of attention recently is called Participatory Budgeting (PB). While PB has its roots in Porto Alegre, Brazil, it is a growing trend throughout the world, including the United States. In some cities, like New York and Chicago, citizens engaging in participatory budgeting where community members have a direct say and control over the budget for community improvement is becoming commonplace. In fact, the

J. M. Choi (✉)
Department Sociology, San Diego State University, San Diego, CA, USA
e-mail: jchoi@sdsu.edu

J. W. Murphy · R. Dahab
Department of Sociology, University of Miami, Coral Gables, FL, USA

C. Holkenbrink-Monk
Department of Sociology, California State University, San Marcos, CA, USA

S. L. Arxer, J. W. Murphy (eds.), *Community-Based Health Interventions in an Institutional Context*, International Perspectives on Social Policy, Administration, and Practice, https://doi.org/10.1007/978-3-030-24654-9_4

New York Times has recently called participatory budgeting "revolutionary civics in action," noting that Participatory Budgeting in New York City (PBNYC) is the fastest growing participatory budgeting process in the United States. According to the Ash Center for Democratic Governance and Innovation at the Harvard Kennedy School, over 51,000 local residents voted on implementing and overseeing projects to improve their neighborhoods to the tune of 32 million dollars in 2014–2015 through the Participatory Budgeting in New York City.

A Community-Based Philosophy

Quite often, community projects encourage participation and involvement of people in producing an outcome. Along the way, strangers may become acquaintances and acquaintances may become friends. The point is that intimacy among community members is nurtured and cultivated. A variety of persons and groups can participate in a community project as stakeholders or partners. While this sentiment seems to portray a positive trajectory toward democratic planning, on closer examination, traditional community projects continue to operate under atomistic philosophy with altruism as the default mechanism that supposedly ties its members as a collective.

Unlike traditional community projects, the philosophy of community-based work rests on two major principles that are very important. The first is that local knowledge should guide any project (Fals-Borda, 1988). Second, *full* participation by community members is a prerequisite to any community-based work. Accordingly, a crucial epistemological shift is made by true community-based initiatives.

Traditionally, community projects have been based on dualism (Bordo, 1987). Specifically, the assumption is made that subjectivity can be divorced from objectivity. In fact, this separation is necessary to acquire reliable data. After all, objective information is the accepted standard. Within this dualistic framework, methods are designed to overcome subjectivity. With this source of error transcended, sound data can be gathered and reliable decisions made. In effect, subjectivity is a distraction that must be left behind if a project is to be based on real evidence. In the absence of subjectivity, facts are available for scrutiny.

Community-based projects, on the other hand, eschew this dualism; this separation is thought to be impossible to justify. What actually occurs, instead, is that persons are intimately connected with everything that is known. Specifically, they interact and give meaning to their lives and act on the basis of these interpretations. In this sense, interpretation and other modes of human agency are impossible to sidestep.

Communities are thus comprised of what Kleinman (2010) calls "moral worlds," that is, norms and expectations that are constructed and modified as those persons see fit. The implication is that rather than objective, facts are invented and tied intimately to language use and the narratives communities create to make sense of their history and prospects. Hence, as some critics say, facts are "biographical" (Berger & Luckmann, 1967).

What this rejection of dualism suggests is that local knowledge is essential to the success of any project. The values, beliefs, and commitments of a community's members are not illusory but provide insight into how they define themselves, important issues, and a successful intervention. Local knowledge, in short, reveals how a project should be designed to fit neatly and effectively into a community.

The second big principle is participation (Murphy, 2014). Clearly, community projects rely on local volunteers. But most often, these persons are mainly consulted or invited periodically to meetings. In reality, they are manipulated to gain their approval or access to resources, such as funds or land. A community-based project moves far beyond this minimal level of involvement.

Advocates of community-based projects, accordingly, argue that local persons should participate intimately in every phase of the project. Some go so far as to argue that they should control these endeavors. Given the importance accorded to local knowledge, this degree of participation only makes sense. Every opportunity, in short, should be available for this reliable information to be utilized.

But equally important is that this participation enhances the sustainability of a project. The research in social psychology demonstrates that real inclusion increases a community's commitment to an activity (Lune, 2010). For example, such "buy-in" helps to guarantee the longevity and quality of a project (Kaplan, 1973). Because of their continuous input, neighbors will take pride in their work, demand to make suggestions, and assume key responsibilities.

Most community projects do not address the issue of dualism. This epistemology often labors silently, however, to marginalize local input and lessen participation. Most community projects, after all, are very practical rather than philosophical affairs. Nonetheless, despite this initial conception, a significant theoretical shift is at the core of community-based work.

What Is a Community?

Almost none of the discussions of traditional community projects begin with the question: what is a community? This omission seems to indicate that the answer is obvious. In fact, they adopt the two usual options. But both of these versions, due to the influence of dualism, treat communities in a very superficial manner. Most projects are thus integrated into a community haphazardly.

A community is envisioned typically to be either a group or a collection of individuals (Murphy, 2014). And because of dualism, both identities are specified by objective traits that link these persons to a particular location. For example, racial, ethnic, and other markers are understood to identify persons from a particular locale. In most cases, a community is associated with demographic features and a location.

Recent research, on the other hand, reveals that this perspective is shortsighted. What is missed by the traditional objective indicators is the process whereby persons become connected and form a community (Land, 1983). Persons, stated simply, are united through their commitments. They define themselves as existing together, as sharing key elements or experiences, and gradually establish bonds that reflect these beliefs. At times, conventional identity markers may refer to a community that mimics these traits, but at others, these characteristics may have little or nothing in common.

A community is thus fairly elusive but not impossible to discover. From a community-based perspective, however, this finding is very important. No longer can a project be predicated on merely making contact with a community and trying to establish workable and cordial relationships. Something more profound is necessary, since a community is not an object but a domain of commitment (Chavis & Newbrough, 1986). A community-based viewpoint takes into account that persons constructed and continue to construct this association.

The point now is not simply to find or enter but engage a community. This process can begin with the standard "walk about," in order to become visible, interact with residents, and understand the environment. But the goal of these efforts goes beyond familiarity or friendship.

Eventually, discussions, meetings, maps, and any other means must lead to a dialogue that reveals why certain persons formed a community. From the inception of a community-based project, the world created by persons is the focus of attention (Minkler & Wallerstein, 2011). Access to this domain, or a true meeting, is necessary to understand why a community exists and how to engage these persons in meaningful relationships. Clearly without local knowledge, this style of engagement will not likely occur. Indeed, the basic premise of participatory budgeting is to best capture the elusive local knowledge of different communities (often forgotten or underserved) so that the needs of that community are met according to the priorities set by its community members.

Participatory Budgeting (PB): Beyond Traditional Budgeting

Traditionally budgets have been out of the hands of the public and made behind closed doors. The standard practice of budget making usually involves publicly elected officials consulting experts or bureaucrats in the allocation of tax dollars. The dualistic nature of traditional budgeting is quite clear: the demarcation of managers of money (politicians) and recipients (the public) of money. This benefactor/beneficiary relationship is sustained and legitimized through what Durkheim calls "rituals" where things are categorized distinctly between the sacred (experts) and the profane (lay community members) (Durkheim, 2001).

Nevertheless, due to many years of dysfunction and misuse of the tax money, the public is now clamoring for increased transparency. Due to economic fluctuations, and poor budget decisions, local needs have been overlooked. Select segments of cities, for example, have been ignored, while money is readily available in other parts for neighborhood improvements (Lerner, 2014). Such inequities have begun to erode confidence in governmental planning. Many surveys report government dysfunction as one of the most serious problems faced by the American public.

The outcry for a new budget process is not merely a technical issue. The point is not merely the elimination of corruption or bias, or to streamline matters, but to democratize the budget process. Only a "thin democracy" is in place if communities cannot play a role in determining how tax money is allocated (Barber, 1984). Given that the economy is central to social life, anything less than full participation of the citizenry poses serious questions about whether democracy exists at all. And a democratic polity seems to have widespread appeal.

Participatory budgeting burst on the scene in Porto Alegre, Brazil (Abers, 1998, 2000). As part of the worldwide movement to create a more equitable and sustainable world, a revolutionary way of creating, implementing, and evaluating city budgets was initiated. Through their local councils, persons who were formerly excluded from this process—including the poor and marginalized—were suddenly thrust into the forefront of formulating budgets. A strategy for allocating funds, accordingly, began to percolate up from neighborhoods, including specific projects that were identified as having priority. And because of this change, services were greatly improved in underserved areas (Pape & Lerner, 2016).

Once this process began, local persons felt empowered and demanded more inclusion (Rappaport, 1981; Wampler, 2007b). Simply put, they began to understand the connection between the economy and their freedom. If they could control city spending, many of the barriers to personal and collective growth could be eliminated.

The benefits of participatory budgeting began to be recognized beyond Brazil (Abers, 1998, 2000). Although a radical idea, many cities examined the process. One of the more famous examples in the United States is Chicago. Although tried seriously in only one ward, the concept began gradually to spread. Many citizens throughout the city, accordingly, began to raise questions about how government spending could be made more pertinent and equitable.

But many fears plagued this process. Specifically noteworthy is that persons will be selfish and only look out for themselves. Those who are most powerful, furthermore, will likely dominate this activity (Lerner, 2011). Hence, the budget process will no longer be rational but a free-for-all, whereby persons and communities battle one another to secure advantages.

While such dire scenes were never witnessed, why budget participants should collaborate was never made clear. At times, appeals were made to altruism and community spirit (Sousa, 1998). But another rationale is available that has not received much attention, although this idea is central to community work. This principle is solidarity, and can offer an appropriate moral framework for participatory budgeting.

While altruism and community spirit are sometimes effective in supporting participatory budget formation, these notions are notoriously vague. Solidarity, likewise, can be misunderstood, unless the philosophical maneuver presupposed by this notion is explained, along with the practical implications. In other words, simple appeals for solidarity will not likely advance the cause of participatory budgeting.

The aim of this chapter, accordingly, is to address solidarity to supply participatory budgeting with a necessary moral framework (Pateman, 1970; Jordan, 2016). Of course, there is never a guarantee that persons or communities will adhere to moral guidelines, but having a framework is certainly better than not. Additionally, one that is attuned to the participatory nature of budget formation would be especially important.

Participatory Budgeting Must Do More than Simply Reform

Clearly, there are many benefits to participatory budgeting. In addition to improved transparency, proponents claim that relations are improved within and between communities, not to mention with governmental representatives (Lerner, 2014). Democracy seems to spread, in other words, as persons learn about the needs and ambitions of their neighbors and engage them in dialogue about budget priorities. In this regard, even the World Bank has identified participatory budgeting as a valuable best practice (Lerner, 2017).

In democratic societies, local participation in institutions is encouraged. Town meetings and involvement on school boards, for example, are part of the mythology, along with grassroots activism. Nonetheless, budgets have been almost sacrosanct and developed mostly by professionals. The assumption is that when carried out in this way, the process will be reasonable, follow set guidelines, and be value-free. In short, rationality will prevail.

For the most part, the formation of budgets remained out of sight. But even when reviewed publicly, the process seems vague, mysterious, and mostly incomprehensible. After all, for the most part, the public has had little or no experience in these affairs. Only a select group has had access to these deliberations and grasps the technicalities of assembling a budget.

Critics, accordingly, began to call for increased accountability, and local participation seemed to be a logical solution. In different places, the theories and motivations varied, but in the end, grassroots guidance was considered to be necessary and viable. The required budget information is thus disseminated throughout a community, along with the requisite skills, so that local persons can act as experts and direct the budgeting process (Wampler, 2007a). Over time, these persons acquire the confidence and skills necessary to be in complete charge of this activity.

Most often, a community group is formed that guides this activity. Following this step, meetings are called where budget information is discussed, projects are proposed and evaluated, and votes are taken. Like most community discussions, this process is not necessarily neat and can be tedious. Constructing a local budget, accordingly, can take up to 6 months. But communities seem to enjoy the process and like the outcomes (Cabannes, 2004).

The anticipated result is that due to this participation, money will be spent wisely and that communities will be satisfied with the results. Local projects, in other words, will be supported in the long term, due to the commitment of community members. Simply put, participation confers a sense of ownership that culminates regularly in increased sustainability (Souze, 2001). In the literature on this topic, this support is referred to as "buy-in," and is recognized as vital to the success of a project.

While communities do not have access to the entire budgets of cities, even in Brazil, a lot of money is available—usually up to 15% of a city's budget. Most important, however, is that this amount has been sufficient to foster significant change (Kasdan & Markman, 2017). Indeed, the cumulative effect has been impressive. But can these non-professionals perform such a task, even with the necessary training? The general fear is that they are undisciplined, untested, and likely to make either stupid or self-serving decisions. What must guide this process, therefore, to avert disaster?

Cultural Challenges of Participatory Budgeting

In many respects, participatory budgeting resembles a utopian project. That is, given how persons usually behave, how can this process ever succeed? Local participation may be a nice, and even a captivating idea, but the likelihood of average persons dedicating themselves to a long-term, voluntary endeavor and cooperating is slim. In fact, this idea contradicts the cultural norms that are currently in place (Harvey, 2005).

The standard expectation is that most persons or communities will focus on their personal interests. For the most part, they are encouraged to follow this path and believe that such behavior is entirely warranted. After all, in the United States, they are taught to look out for themselves first, and if inclined to engage later in charity. Concern for the collective good, however, is optional. Any other policy is simply irresponsible.

For participatory budgeting to succeed, therefore, neighbors must be forced or enticed to cooperate. Pressure must be applied so that they see the wisdom of working together. This socialization may take the form, for example, of moral appeals or something more stringent, such as legal mandates. The problem is that these and similar enticements result often in resentment, and even spawn additional conflict.

Why does this situation appear to be so entrenched? The simple answer is that America is a capitalist society. Even though democracy is touted, and the common good applauded, persons are consumers first and then citizens. What this distinction means in everyday affairs is that they succeed or fail through their own efforts and owe little to others. Persons are expected to make sound decisions that advance their own aims, and perhaps those of their families, while according others the freedom to pursue their goals.

Although capitalism certainly contributes to minimizing the communal character of daily life, there is another, more profound philosophy that contributes to this condition. Specifically, the Western tradition is replete with atomism (Mathews, 1991). The basic idea is that reality, including society, is comprised of isolated units, or atoms, that may combine under certain conditions. Their traditional behavior, however, is that they adhere to individual trajectories and, at times, crash into one another. Any association, and resulting configuration, is tenuous.

Clearly, capitalism is consistent with this outlook, since relationships are mostly strategic to secure advantages at the market place. But what about participatory budgeting? In this case, persons can be expected to behave like self-interested egos, who calculate and strategize to protect their individual interests.

A neighborhood, accordingly, will likely act like a composite of interest groups, who focus on their immediate concerns (Herrnson, Deering, & Wilcox, 2013). Any suggestion that they should cooperate is not appealing, due to the sacrifice that may be involved. As interest groups, almost by definition, they have unique agendas that must be given priority. In fact, within this framework, cooperation may even be treated as unnatural, or at least an unwarranted intrusion or burden.

With this atomistic imagery in place, participatory budgeting will be difficult to implement. Persons can be presumed to bicker constantly and become easily frustrated with the dedicated interaction required by the process. When people believe that they must be brought together, and view these appeals as coercive, any collective action is going to be resisted and breed resentment. Participatory budgeting, accordingly, will likely be approached as an idealistic scheme, with little chance of success.

The Philosophical Thrust of Participatory Budgeting

The problem is that atomism conveys an illusion. In effect, persons are not, and never have been, atoms. They are not fundamentally cut off from one another, and only by chance come into contact. Social existence, in other words, does not consist of mostly accidental encounters, interspersed with chance alliances (Taylor, 1985). At the basis of social existence is a bond.

Basically, atomism is sustained by faulty imagery, and, most recently, a particular economic ideology. In reality, persons are open to others and share a common space. In many ways, accordingly, their fates are joined, even when the communal nature of social life is denied. Even when persons or communities strive to assert their individuality, and stress their unique virtues and successes, they cannot escape the influence of others.

But given this connection, how is the illusion of atomism maintained? Stated simply, this imagery persists because of dualism. Although fundamental to Western philosophy, dualism came to the forefront with Rene Descartes (Bordo, 1987). To supply a sound, unequivocal foundation for truth, he claimed that the mind and objects occupy categorically distinct realms. In more contemporary terms, subjectivity is separated from objectivity, along with facts from values. As a result, reliable knowledge is available that is uncontaminated by personal flaws or opinions.

Although dualism is treated by various contemporary philosophers as defunct, this viewpoint prevails in many areas, including descriptions of social life. In this specific case, persons are subjects while others are objects and vice versa. The result is solipsism, whereby each person is presumed to occupy a unique bubble (Strauss, 2008). A lot of ink has been spilt by philosophers, accordingly, trying to explain whether the minds of others can be known. Any authentic solidarity is thus difficult to imagine.

Bringing persons together is fraught with difficulty. Various schemes have been proposed, such as the state or contract, which assume a gap exists between persons. But also presumed, for example, is that persons are bound together sufficiently to form a state or establish a contract. That is, even before persons are saved from chaos by these schemes, they are open to others and able to cooperate.

What these newer writers are saying is that social philosophy traditionally has begun in the wrong place (Levinas, 1998). In other words, persons were never separate and unable to establish relationships, without the aid of governmental or legal frameworks. For this reason, the term intersubjective is used regularly nowadays to describe the basic human condition. Persons are not subjects severed from others, or objects, but instead are always intertwined with others and able to interact.

A more holistic image is thus appropriate for describing a community (Bauman, 2008). A new way of thinking about moral order is also implied, one that supports participatory budgeting. An entirely different message about motivation and goals is possible than is associated with atomism. Most important is that the ideology of the "individual first" loses credibility, with the ascendance of communitarian viewpoint. Starting from intersubjectivity, instead of the individual, inaugurates a new approach to understanding social responsibility (Mijuskovic, 1992). Instead of rare, simply put, cooperation is the norm. Solidarity, accordingly, is not beyond the pale.

Communal Budgetary Discourse: A New Moral Framework

Simply because persons or communities are open to others, and have impact on one another, does not mean that they have similar priorities. In contrast, the assumption is that they have different perspectives and ambitions. Conflict is thus likely. Nonetheless, even in view of these differences, a discussion about budgets diverges significantly from past discourse. The key realization is that persons are in this budget process together.

As a result, the first important change in their initial response is not self-enhancement. The traditional view that persons are on the prowl constantly to seek advantages and hoard opportunities no longer makes sense, given the communitarian character of social life (Cohen & Arato, 1992). Such avariciousness would be a scandal and hardly normative. Those who exhibit such behavior would no longer be cheered but criticized.

On the most basic level, the morals of society would change. The usual rip-off ethic would be viewed as leading to chaos. How could everyone looking out mostly for themselves, and taking advantage of others, have a positive outcome? Society would consist of barking dogs who exhibit only the most superficial concern for others, such as avoiding direct confrontations. All the time, however, they scheme against their adversaries (Lewis & Weigert, 1985).

But contrary to this unfortunate situation, the second change is that compromise is not treated as defeat. When in their adversarial mode, interactions are tactical and disingenuous. Persons or communities listen to others simply to circumvent their positions and gain the upper hand. Taking the views of others into consideration in a more genuine way is treated as naïve and, in general, unproductive (Harvey, 2005).

In a more communal situation, a different outlook and outcomes are expected. Rather than a loss of freedom or autonomy, compromise is logical. Because behavior has impact far beyond the individual in the absence of atomism, divergent views should be equitably reconciled. After all, who has the unlimited freedom required to usurp the positions of others? Persons are now expected to act in concert, because of their fundamental connection.

As a result, and third, a moral budget emerges from honest negotiation that recognizes possibly different aims. The basic view of this process is that everyone's view counts and should never be violated (Sen, 1999). A realistic budget, therefore, resembles a mosaic rather than a consensus. The aim, in other words, is not to distill positions until a bottom line is achieved, but to incorporate as many proposals as possible. Basically, a different logic of negotiation is operative than is usually the case. Instead of imposing a framework a priori that restricts, and thus eliminates proposals, persons strive to adjust their respective positions until the largest range of possible projects is included. Multiple interests are thus encouraged, rather than mergers that may reflect power or a mythical imperative and require the marginalization of many proposals.

During this process, for example, some persons may realize that, at this time, the proposals of others are more important for the commonweal. Such deferment is not a personal loss, but a gain that everyone will realize. Remember that the basic point, from the beginning, is not personal enhancement but a more expansive project, that is, the promotion of all participants. The representation of diverse positions in the final budget product entails a new logic, as opposed to a zero-sum game (Thurow, 1981). Such a restrictive game, in fact, represents the old imagery of separate competitors who strive to control the budget process.

In the end, the participants make a budget. And indeed, this process is only nominally economic but social, since budget restrictions depend on how persons or communities want to treat one another and use their collectively generated resources. With persons negotiating within the confines of the common good, and the accompanying diversity, they can make any adjustments they see fit to fulfill their goals (Dussel, 1988). Budgetary *a prioris*, in other words, are passé in a truly participatory or communal environment (Baiocchi & Ganuza, 2013).

Conclusion

Clearly, budgeting is a very practical activity to determine how money will be spent. Nonetheless, the participants should not be lulled to sleep by the apparent mundane nature of this process. A change of philosophy is advanced that is crucial to the success of participatory budgeting. If this shift is not appreciated, this approach to forming a budget is in jeopardy.

Particularly noteworthy is that past imagery has been antagonistic to this mode of budgeting, not to mention misrepresenting social life. Persons are not atoms, thereby invalidating the "me-first" reaction to opportunities for gain. As atoms, the collective response necessary for participatory budgeting to succeed is difficult to envision. The personal gains of persons or communities take precedence over everything else.

But a different imagery, and accompanying philosophy, is available that is more supportive of this novel economic process and solidarity. In the absence of atomism, persons and communities must now negotiate in a framework that encourages collective action, and even sees such a response as perfectly rational. A new moral outlook is thus possible, in contrast to adversarial relationships.

Rather than focusing on personal gain that may translate into the common good, a more direct approach is suggested to dispensing funds (Baiocchi, 2005). That is, through dialogue, a fair and representative budget can be developed. Through a fully participatory process, each proposal can be treated with dignity. The result is a budget mosaic that includes a range of proposals, without pre-conceived mandates (Lerner, 2014). The end product can thus be representative, rather than a distillation of input.

But as mentioned earlier, this new imagery requires a serious discussion of philosophy. At first, such an assessment maybe resisted. After all, in the traditional context of framing budgets, such an analysis is a distraction. In participatory budgeting, on the other hand, a reassessment of philosophy is essential. Participants must understand, for example, why atomism is unworkable, inaccurate, and generally silly. An opposing position, based on intersubjectivity, must make sense and be applied appropriately. Participatory budgeting, in fact, depends on the moral position that accompanies this change in philosophy. Participatory budgeting without this philosophy will not likely come to full realization.

References

Abers, R. (2000). *Inventing local democracy: Grassroots politics in Brazil*. Boulder, CO: Lynne Rienner.

Abers, R. (1998). From clientelism to cooperation: Local government, participatory policy, and civic organizing in Porto Alegre, Brazil. *Politics and Society, 26*(4), 511–523.

Baiocchi, G. (2005). *Militants and citizens*. Palo Alto, CA: Stanford University Press.

Baiocchi, G., & Ganuza, E. (2013). Participatory budgeting as if emancipation mattered. *Politics and Society, 42*(1), 29–50.
Barber, B. R. (1984). *Strong democracy: Participatory politics in a new age*. Berkeley, CA: University of California Press.
Berger, P., & Luckmann, T. (1967). *The social construction of reality*. Garden City, NY: Doubleday.
Bordo, S. (1987). *The flight to objectivity*. Albany, NY: SUNY Press.
Bauman, Z. (2008). *Does ethics have a chance in a world of consumers?* Cambridge, MA: Harvard University Press.
Cabannes, Y. (2004). Participatory budgeting: A significant contribution to participatory democracy. *Environment and Urbanization, 16*(1), 27–46.
Chavis, D. M., & Newbrough, J. R. (1986). The meaning of community in social psychology. *Journal of Community Psychology, 14*(4), 335–340.
Chomsky, N. (1999). *Profit over people: Neoliberalism and global order*. New York, NY: Seven Stories Press.
Cohen, J. L., & Arato, A. (1992). *Civil society and political theory*. Cambridge, MA: MIT Press.
Durkheim, E. (2001). *The elementary forms of religious life*. Oxford, UK: Oxford University Press.
Dussel, E. (1988). *Ethics and community*. Eugene, OR: Wipf and Stark.
Fals-Borda, O. (1988). *Knowledge and people's power*. New York, NY: New Horizons.
Harvey, D. (2005). *A brief history of neo-liberalism*. Oxford, UK: Oxford University Press.
Herrnson, P. S., Deering, C. J., & Wilcox, C. (2013). *Interest groups unleashed*. Thousand Oaks, CA: Sage.
Jordan, B. (2016). Building student power through participatory budgeting. https://www.thenation.com/article/building-student-power-through-participatory-budgeting/
Kaplan, R. (1973). Some psychological benefits of gardening. *Environment and Behavior, 5*, 145–161.
Kasdan, A., & Markman, E. (2017). Participatory budgeting and community-based research: principles, practices, and implications for impact validity. *New Political Science, 39*(1), 143–155.
Katznelson, I. (2005). *When affirmative action was white*. New York, NY: W.W. Norton and Company.
Kleinman, A. (2010). Four social theories for global health. *The Lancet, 375*(9725), 1518–1519.
Land, K. C. (1983). Social indicators. *Annual Review of Sociology, 9*, 1–26.
Lerner, J. (2017). Conclusion: Time for participatory budgeting to grow up. *New Political Science, 39*(1), 156–160.
Lerner, J. (2014). *Everyone counts: Could participatory budgeting change democracy?* Ithaca, NY: Cornell University Press.
Lerner, J. (2011). Participatory budgeting: Building community agreement around tough budget Decisions. *National Civic Review, 100*(2), 30–35.
Levinas, E. (1998). *Entre nous: On thinking-of-the-other*. New York, NY: Columbia University Press.
Lewis, J. D., & Weigert, A. J. (1985). Social atomism, holism, and trust. *The Sociological Quarterly, 26*(4), 455–471.
Lune, H. (2010). *Understanding organizations*. Cambridge, UK: Polity Press.
Mathews, F. (1991). *The ecological self*. London, UK: Routledge.
Mijuskovic, B. (1992). Organic communities, atomistic societies, and loneliness. *The Journal of Sociology and Social Welfare, 19*(2), 147–164.
Minkler, M., & Wallerstein, N. (2011). *Community-based participatory research: From processes to outcome*. San Francisco, CA: Jossey-Bass.
Murphy, J. W. (2014). *Community-based interventions: Philosophy and action*. New York, NY: Springer.
Pape, M., & Lerner, J. (2016). Budgeting for equity: How can participatory budgeting advance equity in the United States? *Journal of Public Deliberation, 12*(2), 9. https://www.publicdeliberation.net/jpd/vol12/iss2/art9

Pateman, C. (1970). *Participation and democratic theory*. Cambridge, MA: Cambridge University Press.

Rappaport, J. (1981). In praise of paradox: A social policy of empowerment over prevention. *American Journal of Community Psychology, 9*(1), 1–15.

Sen, A. (1999). Democracy as a universal value. *Journal of Democracy, 10*(3), 3–17.

Sousa, B. (1998). Participatory budgeting in Porto Alegre: Toward a redistributive democracy. *Politics and Society, 26*(4), 461–509.

Souze, C. (2001). Participatory budgeting in Brazilian cities: Limits and possibilities in building democratic institutions. *Environment and Urbanization, 13*(1), 159–184.

Strauss, D. F. M. (2008). Atomism and holism in the understanding of society and social systems. *Koers, 23*(2), 187–205.

Taylor, C. (1985). Atomism. In *Philosophical papers* (pp. 187–210). Cambridge, UK: Cambridge University Press.

Thurow, L. C. (1981). *Zero-sum Society*. New York, NY: Penguin Books.

Wampler, B. (2007a). A guide to participatory budgeting. In A. Shah (Ed.), *Participatory budgeting* (pp. 21–54). Washington, DC: The World Bank.

Wampler, B. (2007b). *Participatory budgeting in Brazil: Contestation, cooperation and accountability*. University Park, PA: Penn State University Press.

Chapter 5
Aims of a Community-Based Research Program

Steven L. Arxer

Introduction

The theoretical considerations related to community-based planning and organization discussed so far in this volume extend to community research. A new community-based philosophy suggests a different methodology and approach to conducting research. In some ways, community-based research is defined by the shift away from positivism. Rather than adopting the assumptions and tactics of the natural sciences, community-based researchers often prefer the tactics advanced by the cultural sciences. And while a movement away from positivist science is notable, community-based research presents new aims that are broader than conventional methodological debates.

The debate between positivism and cultural sciences has been a prominent issue in the Western intellectual tradition. At the center of this controversy is a question about the nature of reliable knowledge. To the extent that human perception is filled with values, assumptions, and commitments, then particular methodologies should be used to acquire the facts leading to truth. Reminiscent of early Greek thinkers such as Plato, *doxa* must be overcome if information is not to remain muddled by opinion. A more certain basis of knowledge is needed, at least with respect to a scientific world-view.

In this way, Western philosophy has been identified with a realistic view of nature that leads to positive science. This realism means that an ahistorical ground, separate from bias and quotidian issues, should be the source of knowledge. Hughes and Sharrock (1997, pp. 97–100) describe this discussion in Western philosophy as the *Natur- Geisteswissenschaften* debate. While experience is the root of knowledge,

S. L. Arxer (✉)
Department of Sociology and Psychology, University of North Texas at Dallas, Dallas, TX, USA
e-mail: steven.arxer@untdallas.edu

S. L. Arxer, J. W. Murphy (eds.), *Community-Based Health Interventions in an Institutional Context*, International Perspectives on Social Policy, Administration, and Practice, https://doi.org/10.1007/978-3-030-24654-9_5

the focus of research is on nature and not cognition, interpretation, or other human sources (de Man, 1983, pp. 2–35). To borrow from Stanley Fish (1989, p. 30), the aim of science is to "anchor the universe and thought from a point above history and culture." Positivism asserts that valid knowledge must be severed from everyday subjectivity so that the true nature of things can be illuminated. Moreover, researchers should adopt specific methodologies to guarantee valid judgments about facts. In practice, this strategy entails using data collection techniques that are primarily empirical and capture the quantifiable characteristics of objects. With respect to the social sciences, an empirical methodology fosters certitude about the structure of society, institutions, and communities.

To be sure, the central tenants of positivism have not gone unscrutinized. Social scientists have grown skeptical of positivism, particularly following the "linguistic turn" in philosophy (Tucker, 1994, p. 13). Simply put, access to a primordial foundation, such as nature, is precluded given the symbolic texture of reality. Humans cannot be disinterested observers, since all information is derived from assumptions that guide the perception of reality. Michel Foucault (1989, p. 42) refers to this symbolic domain as "epistēmē" while drawing attention to the cultural presuppositions that are endemic in any outlook. Through language and communication, persons cultivate meaning for themselves and their environment. Basically, persons intervene in their world and are active participants in the creation of knowledge.

Some see this methodological debate as culminating in quantitative and qualitative researchers occupying different camps. As Fred Kerlinger once noted, "There is no such thing as qualitative data. Everything is either 1 or 0" (quoted in Miles & Huberman, 2002, p. 40). On the other side, for instance, D. T. Campbell has stated that "All research ultimately has a qualitative grounding" (Miles & Huberman, 2002, p. 40). Community-based philosophy has generally been characterized as more compatible with a "qualitative version," which focuses on community participation and community biographies (Murphy, 2014 p. 77). Describing communities as places where persons enact their values and behavioral modalities seems to be an appropriate lens to understand communities, as opposed to as empirical locations. In this vein, community-based participatory research (CBPR) has emerged as the methodology of community-based researchers (Minkler, 2005). As McTaggert (1991) notes, CBPR attempts to center the voices and actions of community members, thereby avoiding a reductionist empirical view of social life.

This chapter explores the ways in which CBPR moves community-based research beyond the quantitative and qualitative debate. In particular, quantitative and qualitative approaches still share a preoccupation with successful strategies for collecting data. As Dabbs Jr. (1982, 31–63) writes, "Qualitative and quantitative are not distinct." Dabbs Jr. (1982, p. 31–63) differentiates between qualitative and quantitative investigations noting that qualitative research refers to the collection of "meanings, concepts, definitions, characteristics, metaphors, symbols and descriptions of things…" while arguing that quantitative research generates "counts and measures of things." In both cases, the focus is on a data collection strategy and in refining the tools of this process. Although the issue of accurate data acquisition is important to CBPR, a community-based research agenda pays attention to research activism among community members to gather information and effect social change. Accordingly, Minkler (2005, p. ii3) defines CBPR as "participation, research, and action."

So as to better appreciate the unique methodological orientation proposed by CBPR, some historical roots to this practice are presented and compared to positivist and qualitative methods. Given that the aim of CBPR is to involve community members in research projects, as a way to better plan and deploy healthcare projects, the way that participation is conceptualized by quantitative and qualitative methods must be explored. The goal is to address how a preoccupation with data collection techniques and rigor marginalizes persons not identified as experts in methods. In this way, both approaches miss the important step of promoting community-directed plans because they adhere to traditional views on knowledge production that center professional experts in the research process.

Against Positivism and Realism: Roots of Community-Based Participatory Research in Health

The difficulties associated with health problems in marginalized communities, such as the urban poor, helped to give rise to a community-based approach to solving healthcare issues. The complexity of these problems and the need for more "authentic" community partnerships meant that traditional approaches, driven by "outside experts," were viewed as insufficient to address healthcare needs in locally relevant ways (Minkler & Wallerstein, 2003). The historical roots of CBPR can be found in the action research of social psychologist Kurt Lewin in the 1940s (Lewin, 1946). He emphasized the cyclical process of data collection, participant action, and investigative reflection. Perhaps to a greater extent, CBPR is tied to the revolutionary intellectual approaches put forth in countries in South America, Asia, and Africa in the 1970s (Hall, 1992). For example, the ideas of Brazilian adult educator Paulo Freire (1970) and of Fals-Borda (1987) focused on co-learning and action-based inquiry. These scholars developed their approaches to inquiry in light of, and as a way to counter, the colonial experience of oppressed communities. Within this broad intellectual and geo-political context, new research approaches grew to address community development problems in areas of health and inequality, among others (Minkler & Wallerstein, 2003).

At the core of participatory action methods is a rejection of positivistic logic and method. While participatory action research is identified as a "political process," driven by the commitments and social practices of community participants (McTaggert, 1997), positivism seeks to distinguish facts from values. Knowledge for positivists exists "outside the mind" and is related most closely to physical events (Durkheim, 1965, p. xiii). Unhampered direct experience, accordingly, is of paramount importance in discovering truth.

Because nature is the source of facts, knowledge is only available to those who can perceive nature accurately. The degree to which physical properties contain knowledge suggests that careful observation and perception are necessary. For this reason, positivists view knowledge and the acquisition of information to be a rigorous affair. As Reid (1994) notes, positivists view legitimate knowledge to be derived from serious experimentation. Most commonly, this viewpoint means that research should adopt the scientific method as a way to temper the mind and minimize perceptual errors. Only after rigorous training is perception trusted, since the human element is always a liability. Consequently, the mind is given a passive role in this methodology, in that knowledge is both objective and only obtainable through the use of specific techniques and steps.

Once in the hands of expert practitioners, data collection can be considered sound and result in information treated as objective. Information that is empirical in nature and highlights objective properties is thought to be valid. Methodology that narrows the mind through instrumentation and natural observation helps persons discard their biases (Lake, 1993). A key assumption of positivism is that methodological techniques are value-free. Lyotard (1984) claims that these tools are treated as "prosthetic aids" that enable researchers to better contact the world. Simply put, interpretation is presumed to be overcome through strict pursuit of standardized techniques. Research proceeds in a rigorous stepwise manner, because judgments are replaced by methodological rubrics, operations, and calculation. Data are transformed into autonomous, objective *things*. All that is needed to obtain facts are skilled researchers who can follow methodological guidelines that are neutral. (Hughes & Sharrock, 1997, p. 28).

Positivism's focus on standardized protocols is significant in community work. When this approach is applied to studying communities, a hierarchy can easily develop between researcher practitioners and community members. An emphasis on specialized skills—such as identifying research questions, methodological design, and statistical analysis—raises the stature of trained professionals who gain control of local projects. The implied training deemed necessary for research inquiry defines professionals as the "experts" and indispensable to social planning (Gilgun, 2005). A type of surrogate vision on behalf of communities is encouraged, for otherwise data may be sullied by the beliefs and values of the everyday observer.

The end product of this situation is twofold. First, in order to avoid being guided by unsubstantiated ideas, expert researchers must be at the center of the research process. After all, what training does the layperson possess that is sufficient to encounter the real world in a dispassionate manner? Often enough, interpretive judgments and personal experiences are presumed to be the starting point of community members' understanding. However, a key tenant of CBPR is that community inquiry should be a "'co-learning process' to which community members and outside researchers contribute equally" (Minkler, 2005, p. ii4).

Second, an abstract or realistic view of the social world is created. Specifically, the social world is associated with empirical properties, such as demographic factors, social networks, and capacity levels, that characterize a community. However, researchers become disconnected from the social world they study. Their role as practitioners is merely to gather and analyze data, because methodology has been overly formalized. A community is thus imagined to be a complex of variables that can be collected in a mechanistic way.

In contrast, community-based research assumes that expert knowledge is not a priori superior to that of community members and their worldviews. Rather than dispassionate, researchers must be deeply involved, as opposed to taking a passive stance, when encountering communities and tap into local knowledge. Researchers should, as Minkler (2005, p. ii4) states, show "a lifelong commitment to self-evaluation and self-critique" in relation to assumptions about community life. After all, communities are not obtrusive things to be observed but rather a political terrain shaped by local and external discourses. In a way, expert knowledge may be a hindrance to local projects to the extent that their presumed superiority marginalizes community viewpoints.

Qualitative Approaches and the Rejection of Grand Designs

A number of different intellectual traditions, such as phenomenology, ethnography, symbolic interactionism, and postmodernism, claim that the philosophical basis of positivism is simply untenable. Specifically, the Western philosophy of dualism that has separated truth from opinion and has sought to identify select methodological approaches as superior is passé. As Derrida (1978, p. 282) argued, the positivist grand design of knowledge and method is "forced to stop considering itself as the culture of reverence." This incredulity toward the scientific enterprise is due to what some call the "linguistic turn," which reimagines the way the human presence relates to facts, truth, method, and reality.

Central to this new epistemology is that reality is symbolic, that is, represents a constellation of "language games" that mediate perception (Lyotard, 1984, pp. 9–11). The upshot of this argument is that reality is linguistically constituted by the way persons interpret themselves and their surroundings. It is worth mentioning that this thesis on language replaces the "indexical view" used by positivists. Indexicality refers to the idea that language basically "points to" or "indicates" what is real in the world. A natural reference still exists, distinct from speech acts; the role of language is simply to express the way an empirical world is already organized. This portrayal of language is still dualistic, because reality retains a distinct status outside of symbolic interpretation (Rorty, 1991). Put differently, language merely puts reality on display for researchers.

Qualitative approaches contend that discourse does not stand for reality, but rather shapes the nature of human perception. As Derrida (1976, p. 156) once stated, "nothing exists outside of the text." Reality and discourse are intertwined in a fundamental way that requires what is meant by reality and truth to be rethought. The schism between facts and values is extremely difficult to retain, because linguistic interpretation precludes a neutral standpoint. As Roland Barthes (1977, p. 30) writes, there is "no other side" to language, no autonomous reference point to anchor truth.

Because reality is a discursive practice, the traditional methods used by positivists to acquire knowledge are jettisoned by qualitative researchers. In this respect, the use of structural metaphors to describe the arrangement of the social world and the instrumentation used to access facts are abandoned. Indeed, the mechanistic imagery that suggests standardized techniques neatly separate judgments from facts is not suitable in a linguistically constituted world. As Lyotard (1984, p. 36) notes, "knowledge has no final legitimacy outside of serving the goals envisioned by the practical subject." Because reality is mediated by language and no longer exists a priori, all knowledge emerges from the locally conceived rules of language. Scientific and other models of reality are thus the result of different language games that draw the boundaries of reality. To borrow from Kuhn, science is a "paradigm" that represents one model of reality. Truth, therefore, is tied to the rules of speech that sustain a particular community.

In this context, technical competence is not sufficient to procure knowledge. Positivists understand technical rigor to be the antidote to the biases imposed by subjectivity and assume that with methodical tools in hand, facts can be revealed as a detached reality. However, qualitative researchers view this methodology as counterproductive to the discovery of truth, because of the abstract portrayal of knowledge (Lacan, 1977, p. 282). Language subtends reality; thus, the assumptions that frame discourse become the focus point of inquiry. Rather than obscuring values through instrumentation, the goal of research is to apprehend the symbolic dimensions of reality. Derrida (1980, p. 48) makes this point when he claims that researchers need to consult the epistemological interests that accompany data. The concern is that researchers who prioritize scientific refinement in the name of objectivity may distort data. At worst, researchers marginalize the persons they study when the assumptions that accompany a particular linguistic community are overshadowed by a structural rendition of community identity.

The New Language of Qualitative Research: Cultural Competence

Rather than technical competence, qualitative researchers often strive to develop their communicative competence instead. This "new language of qualitative method" becomes the focal point of analysis (Gubrium & Holstein, 1997). At the center of a qualitative research is an appreciation that facts are not things, but rather "accomplishments" reached through social interpretation (Pollner, 1991). Values and beliefs, therefore, imbue facts. Qualitative methods thus introduce a new element in knowledge acquisition. Gubrium (2009), for example, notes that communication is the focus of data collection. Through various methods, such as interviewing and participant observations, qualitative researchers try to gain access to how communities build their social worlds through collaborative speech.

This shift is important for community-based research. The empirical character of a community (e.g., demographics, geography, levels of capital, etc.) should not be taken as the sole cause of behavior and experience. Put differently, variables have primarily a social significance for a community. Reminiscent of the symbolic interactionist Herbert Blumer (1969), behavior is viewed by qualitative researchers to be the result of how persons give meaning to their worlds. Community assessments, for instance, are evaluated in terms of the intentions, beliefs, and commitments of community members. Claims related to community needs are validated from within the constellation of priorities established by these persons. This is to say that the knowledge production of a community should not be ignored in favor of expert insights. The patina of scientific objectivity does not carry the status required to obscure other sources of knowledge, given that a "disinterested logic of inquiry" is impossible (Foucault, 1975, p. 8).

The problem with positivism, according to qualitative researchers, is that simply having numerical data collection does not guarantee that the meaning of a phenomenon will be obtained. Instead, a qualitative approach asks researchers to exhibit sensitivity to the "domain assumptions" (Gouldner, 1970, p. 46) that contextualize a community. In some circles, this practice has come to be known as "intercultural competence" or cultural sensitivity (Deardorff, 2009). Either way, this practice implies that the researchers understand a person's or community's actions by exploring the presuppositions they make about reality. Murphy (1986) describes this activity as "epistemological participation" and distinguishes this activity from the procedural issues that are the hallmark of positive science.

In the field of health care, the idea of cultural competence has gained widespread attention as a possible way to improve the quality of care, as well as reduce social inequalities (Betancourt, Green, Carrillo, & Park, 2005). But to the extent that professionals still control research and services, local knowledge may be marginalized, even though emphasis is placed on communication (Betancourt et al., 2005). Nonetheless, exhibiting some awareness of the value of local input may improve planning, although a community may not play a large role in this process.

Beyond Cultural Sensitivity and Toward Praxis

While qualitative methodologies are most closely tied to community-based research, there are reasons why this strategy is not necessarily suggestive of a community-based approach. As Minkler (2005, p. ii5) cautions, there are "dangers of co-optation" related to certain research and intervention proposals. Of concern here is the reintroduction of traditional top-down research approaches that obscure the real intent of community-based planning and CBPR in particular.

McTaggert (1997, p. 79) identifies several core principles of CBPR. One is the notion of "self-critical communities." In practice, community-based research requires that community participants be engaged in inquiry and reflection, and not just professional researchers. In short, everyday persons should be deeply involved in the research process, or in what some call "theory-making" (Minkler, 2005, p, ii5). The issue for CBPR is the status of laypersons in the research process and not just the nature of knowledge.

While qualitative research emphasize the symbolic side of reality and encourages exploration of how communities frame issues, this aim does not guarantee that a community-based model will be adopted in the research process. After all, community members may be solicited to share their stories through interviews and focus groups, but a qualitative project may still be driven primarily by professionals. A community project may still be designed and managed by the researcher who develops the study question, conducts interviews and observation, codes and analyzes data, and produces findings (Heron & Reason, 1997).

The issue is that promoting cultural sensitivity does not address the assimilation of laypersons into the scientific enterprise. As opposed to such assimilation, CBPR seeks to develop a "partnership synergy" between community and researcher (McTaggert, 1997). Moreover, this relationship is not superficial and based merely on the transference of information from subject to researcher. As explained by Lasker et al. (2001, pp. 1799–205),

> [T]he synergy that partners seek to achieve through collaboration is more than a mere exchange of resources. By combining the individual perspectives, resources, and skills of the partners, the group creates something new and valuable together—something that is greater than the sum of its parts.

The challenge with both quantitative and qualitative methods is that they do not directly address the issue of inequality in the dialogue between researchers and community members. Qualitative investigations may remain led by professional researchers and thus communication is limited. Since the researcher directs what is asked, who is asked, and how to interpret community stories, certain viewpoints may be missed. In the end, the community is asked to adjust to the structure of the research process, because professionals are assumed to be best trained to collect the narratives of communities and distill pertinent information through elaborate coding schemes.

Although in-depth observations and narrative data can provide some context to a community, the values and perspectives of these persons may remain hidden without their thorough participation in a project. Cornwall and Jewkes (1995, pp. 1667–1676) highlight this concern by noting that community-based research should be alert to the "the attitudes of researchers, which in turn determine how, by and for whom research is conceptualized and conducted and the corresponding location of power at every stage of the research process." For this reason, CBPR argues for a participatory methodology that more fully centers community members' praxis, as authentic and full participants in the research process.

Conclusion

This chapter examines the epistemological and methodological backdrop to developing community-based research. The philosophical shift away from positivism toward more qualitative approaches highlights the trends within healthcare research to adopt methods that are attuned to local communities and their needs. In particular, methods that sensitize researchers to the communities they study and serve have become de rigueur in some circles, as professionals begin to see the value of local input. In many ways, health planners have begun to recognize that communication with communities is vital to successful health plans.

At the same time, these efforts to sensitize health professionals have a long way to go. To borrow from Stanley Fish (1989), cultural sensitivity does not "go all the way down," in that this strategy may not necessarily promote local control of health research. In particular, rejecting the epistemological hierarchy between local and expert knowledge is only part of the solution. Also needed is a shift that places local persons at the center of how and why knowledge is produced, managed, and used. CBPR suggests that professional researchers should no longer be presumed centerpieces of research projects; instead, community members should be given fuller participation in this knowledge economy.

References

Barthes, R. (1977). *Image, music, text*. New York, NY: Hill and Wang.

Betancourt, J. R., Green, A. R., Carrillo, J. E., & Park, E. R. (2005). Cultural competence and health care disparities: Key perspectives and trends. *Health Affairs, 24*(2), 499–505.

Blumer, H. (1969). *Symbolic interactionism: Perspective and method*. Englewood Cliffs, NJ: Prentice-Hall.

Cornwall, A., & Jewkes, R. (1995). What is participatory research? *Social Science & Medicine, 41*, 1667–1676.

Dabbs Jr., J. M. (1982). Making things visible. In J. Van Maanen (Ed.), *Varieties of qualitative Research* (pp. 31–66). Beverly Hills, CA: Sage.

de Man, P. (1983). *Blindness and insight*. Minneapolis, MN: University of Minnesota Press.

Deardorff, D. K. (2009). *The SAGE handbook of intercultural competence*. California, USA: Sage Publications.

Derrida, J. (1976). *Of grammatology*. Baltimore, MD: Johns Hopkins University Press.

Derrida, J. (1978). *Writing and difference*. Chicago, IL: University of Chicago Press.

Derrida, J. (1980). *The archeology of the frivolous: Reading Condillac*. Pittsburgh, PA: Duquesne University Press.

Durkheim, E. (1965). *The rules of sociological method*. New York, NY: The Free Press.

Fals-Borda, O. (1987). The application of participatory action-research in Latin America. *International Sociology, 2*, 329–347.

Fish, S. (1989). *Doing what comes naturally*. Durham, NC: Duke University Press.

Foucault, M. (1975). *The birth of the clinic*. New York, NY: Vintage Books.

Foucault, M. (1989). *The archaeology of knowledge*. London, UK: Routledge.

Freire, P. (1970). *Pedagogy of the oppressed*. New York, NY: Seabury Press.

Gilgun, J. F. (2005). The four cornerstones of evidence-based practice in social work. *Research on Social Work Practice, 15*(1), 52–61.
Gouldner, A. W. (1970). The coming crisis of Western sociology. New York: Basic Books.
Gubrium, J. F., & Holstein, J. A. (1997). *The new language of qualitative method.* New York, NY: Oxford University Press.
Gubrium, J. F. (2009). *Analyzing narrative reality.* Thousand Oaks, CA: Sage.
Hall, B. L. (1992). From margins to center: The development and purpose of participatory action research. *The American Sociologist, 22*, 15–28.
Heron, J., & Reason, P. (1997). A participatory inquiry paradigm. *Qualitative Inquiry, 3*(3), 274–294.
Hughes, J., & Sharrock, W. (1997). *The philosophy of social research.* New York, NY: Longman.
Lacan, J. (1977). *Ecrits.* New York, NY: Norton.
Lake, R. W. (1993). Planning and applied geography: Positivism, ethics, and geographic information systems. *Profess in Human Geography, 17*(3), 404–413.
Lasker, R. D., Weis, E. S., & Miller, R. (2001). Partnership synergy: A practical framework for studying and strengthening the collaborative advantage. *Milbank Quarterly, 79*, 179–205, III–IV.
Lewin, K. (1946). Action research and minority problems. *Journal of Social Issues, 2*, 34–46.
Lyotard, J. F. (1984). *The postmodern condition: A report on knowledge.* Minneapolis, MN: University of Minnesota Press.
McTaggert, R. (1991). Principles for participatory action research. *Adult Education Quarterly, 41*(3), 168–187.
McTaggert, R. (1997). Sixteen tenants of participatory action-research. In Y. Wadsworth (Ed.), *Everyday evaluation on the run.* Sydney, Australia: Allen & Unwin.
Miles, M. B., & Huberman, M. A. (2002). *The qualitative researcher's companion.* Thousand Oaks, CA: Sage.
Minkler, M. (2005). Community-based research partnerships: Challenges and opportunities. *Journal of Urban Health, 82*(2), ii3–ii12.
Minkler, M., & Wallerstein, N. (2003). *Community based participatory research for health.* San Francisco, CA: Jossey-Bass.
Murphy, J. W. (1986). Phenomenological social science: Researcher in the public interest. *Social Science Journal, 23*(3), 327–343.
Murphy, J. W. (2014). *Community-based interventions.* New York, NY: Springer.
Pollner, M. (1991). Left of ethnomethodology: The rise and decline of radical reflexivity. *American Sociological Review, 56*(3), 370–380.
Reid, W. J. (1994). The empirical practice movement. *Social Service Review, 68*(2), 165–184.
Rorty, R. (1991). *Objectivism, relativism, and truth.* Cambridge, MA: Cambridge University Press.
Tucker, W. (1994). *The science and politics of racial research.* Urbana, IL: University of Illinois Press.

Chapter 6
Training Community-Based Health Workers

Tashina J. Vavuris

Introduction

Community-based work (CBW) has the potential to transform the scope of research, which is an aspect of CBW that needs to be addressed and reflected to include non-traditional perspectives and different forms of knowledge (Smith, 2012, p. 1). But this potential transformation takes time and energy to deconstruct ways of knowing that stem from histories where research has been hierarchical and one-dimensional—where the experts contact and unleash their own knowledge to transfuse what they presume to be problematic. Moving beyond this type of engagement, community-based practitioners (researchers, students, professors, and those alike) must undergo a philosophical shift, one that redirects their understanding of knowing. Further, allowing practitioners to disengage from traditional knowledge to embrace the ways of understanding operative in a given community is central to any community-based initiative.

The training and educational shift that is needed to foster community engagement in a genuine manner incorporates dialogue, respect, empathy, collaboration, commitment, and solidarity and allows *critical praxis* to form (Ferreira, 2017; Freire, 1970, 2000; Murphy, 2014). Placing the community at the center of a project allows for community members to self-identify their needs and engage every facet from start to finish. This specific aspect of training cannot be overlooked, since community members are not just participants, but are intertwined in all aspects of a project. This type of practice is essential for community engagement to be self-sustaining and the goals of a project to be continuously re-worked. Accordingly, training for genuine community engagement to take place is crucial from the beginning of a project and cannot be a mere afterthought.

T. J. Vavuris (✉)
Department of Environmental Studies, University of California, Santa Cruz,
Santa Cruz, CA, USA

S. L. Arxer, J. W. Murphy (eds.), *Community-Based Health Interventions in an Institutional Context*, International Perspectives on Social Policy, Administration, and Practice, https://doi.org/10.1007/978-3-030-24654-9_6

Additionally, there is an important ethical commitment to embrace communities, one where practitioners move beyond the dominant status quo and embrace ethics where "passionate solidarity and informed empathy" can take precedence (Lykes, 2013). Thus, practitioners must adopt a *new vantage point* through vital epistemological shifts (Tuck, 2009, p. 55). A new paradigm thus enables and incorporates personal histories to understand individual biases and reimagine a future that encompasses a *deeper awareness* and understanding of the everyday lived experiences of people in their communities (Torre & Ayala, 2009). This *deeper* awareness must encourage the critique necessary for local knowledge to support a project.

Given the assumption that current social programs do not meet the needs of most people, they can feel alienated and, at first, be reluctant to participate in local community affairs (Murphy, 2014). Alienation is not an abstract term, but sheds light on the modes of disconnect between persons and their daily experiences. In this regard, María Elena Torre and Jennifer Ayala examine the importance in acknowledging the role of the researcher by stating:

> Participation, action, and research are not neutral, value-free terms…with the recognition that knowledge production is a political activity and that researchers come from particular communities with their own historically rooted relationships to research and power. (Torre & Ayala, 2009, p. 388)

Indeed, Torre and Ayala (2009) state that there is a "liberatory potential" in community engagement practices. In addition, the ethical role of the practitioner/researcher is essential in community work, with the aim of reinventing the current situation and promoting social change (Cahill, 2007). Hence, when community engagement is carried out with the ideals described above, personal and collective agency can be nurtured to bring about transformative and collective praxis (Murphy, 2014, p. 3).

In this chapter, several concepts will be explored. First, the idea of traditional community-based practices, where pragmatic training methodologies are endorsed, will be introduced. Second, a brief overview of community-based philosophy will be examined to illustrate the need to move beyond the traditional ways of training CBW practitioners. Third, community knowledge will be examined and explored to reveal how this information can reinforce the shift to prioritizing local knowledge. And finally, the chapter will end with a summary of how the essential components of CBW can be interwoven in the training of health workers.

Overall, there are many fields that speaks to varying degrees of community engagement (CBW, Y-PAR, PAR, Community-initiated PAR, Student-led community-engaged research, Community-initiated student research, Community-based design research, and so on). Nonetheless, there are similarities between community engagement practices, but there are also distinct ways in which community work is conceptualized and practiced. This discussion in no way is an end to community engagement pedagogy, but rather a continuation of conversation that has already taken place within various fields and by many authors (Murphy, 2014; Tuck, 2009; Tuck & Guishard, 2013; Torre & Ayala, 2009; Munck,2014; Medin & Bang, 2014; Kretzman & McKnight, 1993). Community engagement draws from various disciplines such as sociology, psychology, and community well-being, in addition to various histories of activism that embrace topics such as liberatory pedagogy, decolonial methods, feminism, black liberation, and so on. All that said, this chapter is limited due to space and will not be able to address all the necessary dimensions for community-based involvement, but will summarize basic aspects of engaging in ethical and liberating community work.

Traditional Community-Based Pedagogy

Traditional training education is mostly pragmatic, that is, focused on how to conduct needs assessments, evaluate interventions, or implement accreditation standards. Of course, these tasks are important, but must be expanded to include a critical epistemological dimension. This shift in orientation is not often the centerpiece of training; hence, the goal of this chapter is to expand on how training can support community-engaged practices.

Specifically important is that the traditional style of training and education is not in line with community-based philosophy. While pragmatism is important when engaging in community-based practices, especially when the overarching topic is community health, there is a shift that needs to be at the forefront for CBW to undergo a philosophical alignment. Practitioners should not only learn about a range of research and organizational tasks but also acknowledge the new outlook that accompanies community-based projects. In fact, training must go beyond technical and practical preparation to address some key philosophical themes.

The education regularly received often lacks concern for community members and their needs, more so, their dreams and desires. The ideal community education breaks down the traditional hierarchy and focuses on the members that are being served with a given project. This task does not follow a straight line, but rather is fluid and adheres to a community's views and aspirations. As a result, training is not about teaching the community, but more about recognizing how understanding the perspective operative in a community is a resource to more fully engaging the community. Once this change is understood, the goals of a community can come into focus. Accordingly, the community must be treated in a manner that allows each member to have the potential to contribute to a project. The point is to inaugurate a reflexive process where community members become the new experts who solve problems. But the traditional approach adopts a methodology that attempts to make a given community more like a researcher or practitioner, and thus projects are disconnected from these persons and fail inevitably to be community-based.

Pedagogical approaches in community-based interventions must understand the theoretical implications behind the work. To bring about change that community members see fit, the pedagogical practices need to be rethought. One of the facets of training that needs to be stressed is how learning is situated and includes various levels of knowledge. Most often, the researchers' questions and ways of knowing dominated an inquiry, as well as the classroom (Gutiérrez & Vossoughi, 2010,

p. 101). In this regard, education can be a "tool to produce and dispossess the other," which for obvious reasons has the potential to further alienate communities (Tuck, Smith, Guess, Benjamin, & Jones, 2014, p. 53). To avoid this problem, Gutiérrez and Vossoughi (2010) state how the process they employ in community work is one

> in which *experiment* is reclaimed and reframed as open and creative, in ways that creates spaces to experiment pedagogically, to design collective Third Spaces that heighten the potential for deep learning to occur and for the development of powerful literacies that facilitate social change (p. 102).

Liberating pedagogy (among other names) and ways of critical thinking, as outlined by many, but mostly credited to Paulo Freire, are interwoven into critical frameworks and pedagogical practices that embrace the idea of recreating worlds based on the needs and perspectives of communities (Freire, 1970). While there are limitations to Freire's critical pedagogical thought, his strategy has influenced pedagogical practices and social research methods, including participatory community engagement approaches. Freire's aim is to question the production of knowledge and who benefits from this activity (Fals Borda, 1979, 1987). Interweaving liberating pedagogy with the training of community workers has benefits, especially for researchers who want to engage local knowledge. Specifically, this engagement can act as a form of resistance by revealing any hierarchies of knowledge. For example, Caitlin Cahill (2007) states, "As an ethic of inclusion, participatory research potentially represents a challenge to white privilege's [white supremacist] investment in maintaining and producing racial hierarchies in the normative production of knowledge" (p. 363). As many activists have claimed, community engagement, when genuinely embraced, can begin to celebrate diverse knowledge bases and widespread inclusion.

In this fashion, there has been an extensive history that tends to favor elites' knowledge within education, with a range of others marginalized in both research and planning (Darder, 1994). As a remedy, CBW can be used to reveal some of these historical patterns and unearth how the world and society do not function on their own, but rather are socially created. The upshot of this reorientation is that there is potential to bolster the needs and imaginaries of communities. Consequently, as outlined by Antonia Darder (1994):

> Educational conditions promoting inequality have been made possible by the underlying philosophical assumptions that inform traditional research methodology, namely, the acceptance of a dualistic, objective, value-free, hierarchical, and instrumental perspective regarding knowledge. It is a view that sees human beings as separate from nature, and thus, as objectifiable, observable, quantifiable, predictable, and controllable. Through objectifying human beings into "things," human behavior can be treated as if it existed according to a predetermined set of universal rules, independent of the contexts in which the behavior takes place. (p. 23)

Moving beyond this trap needs to be at the forefront of community-engaged training and practice. Training should pursue the demystification of knowledge hierarchies and question the origins and implications of knowledge histories to bring communities into planning routines. CBW should embrace pedagogy practices that facilitate community members actively participating in their own production of their knowledge, by elevating in importance the meaning of their lived experiences and how they construct their situations (Darder, 1994; Murphy, 2014).

The Need for Community-Based Philosophy

A nondualistic framework is needed in order to shift into a new paradigm (Krieger, 2011). Understanding the separation of objectivity and subjectivity is a necessary part of training to act appropriately. When communities are viewed within this binary, the idea that community members use subjective information identifies a community's perspectives as false information. In academia, especially in regards to research-focused institutions, the emphasis falls on "value neutrality and a positivist objectivity as prerequisites for 'serious science'" (Fals Borda, 1987, p. 330). Thus, a reorientation is required to alter the traditional scope of research. Specifically important, community members should not be dismissed because their perspectives of the world are needed to promote change. True community practitioners peruse local narratives in order to understand how a given issue is locally constructed. Nonetheless, for this shift to take place, practitioners must learn to treat knowledge as biographical, that is, as a product of local discourse and related commitments (Berger & Luckmann, 1967; Schutz, 1967). This adventure of understanding how a community constructs their lived experiences and reality is part of a community-engaged philosophy.

Understanding the philosophical importance of community-based work is imperative when engaging in communities that have been historically marginalized for various reasons. Especially important is the idea of dismantling the normative ethos about the nature of a community. In CBW, the concept of *community* should be a key starting point. Further, being able to redefine the meaning of *community*, which should be defined by the community, lays the groundwork for developing an *authentic commitment* to a project (Fals Borda, 1987; Murphy, 2014). And, the community has the opportunity to interact through meaningful dialogue and genuine collaboration.

In this case, dialogue is not merely reduced to communication or an intimate relationship, although, these notions are also important. As Hans-Georg Gadamer (1996) states, dialogue requires taking a risk and entering the worlds of other persons, and thus presumes that people enter into a truly living relationship. This activity is realized by persons reflecting on their own stories, that is, placing them at risk, and thereby recognizing their boundaries. As a result, they can begin to entertain others' narratives and read them as their authors intend. In other words, practitioners can overcome their own stories and enter the world created by the narratives enacted by communities. Dialogue, however, is not value-neutral, but represents the ability to shift from one world to another through reflection.

The identity of a community moves beyond geographical location or a common trait, but reflects a commitment to a particular new order. This idea is revolutionary in the sense of how communities have been constructed over the years and within the realm of community work (Murphy, 2014). In the traditional understanding of communities, people are grouped together by geographical location, skin color, cultural identity, language, economic status, and so on. While these identifiers are potential unifiers, community members should not be limited to these "qualifying" markers without consulting how a sense of solidarity is created through dialogue and agreement. With this new way to understand communities, entrée occurs when certain signs or indicators are read in the manner intended by the participants. In a manner or speaking, communities are authors.

The idea is to reimagine a space where local knowledge aligns with research goals and that critique becomes a regular part of community training practices. Radical and liberating strategies have been utilized throughout time, but have not been given priority in community engagement practices (Fals Borda, 1988). Indeed, the goal is not to reinforce an existing system, but to open the opportunity for communities to establish their own agendas. Thus, CBW requires training that incorporates local experts into planning, and thus rethinking the concept of "expert status." But this task is done not by leading, but rather learning and assisting when needed (Murphy & Casanova, 2018, p. 18). When thinking of community interventions, there are many ways that this expectation can be implemented to provide a project with an appropriate framework (Gutiérrez & Vossoughi, 2010; Murphy, 2014). Especially important, the necessity is that these practices are continuous throughout a project and guided by community members (Gutiérrez & Vossoughi, 2010; Murphy, 2014).

To understand this change further, there are basic principles that sustain CBW to nourish a community's transformation. Throughout the philosophical shift, there are two distinct components that are vital for a community project to be genuine and sustainable. The first is that community or local knowledge is valid and already exists prior to a project taking form (Murphy, 2014). Frequently, community engagement uses terms such as *empowerment* to explain that the project will allow community members to have a voice. The assumption, however, is that community members did not have power prior to the project, and were merely granted this power based on the researchers' largess. The term empowerment, according to Wallerstein and Bernstein (1994), is defined as: "a social action process in which individuals and groups act to gain mastery over their lives in the context of changing their social and political environment" (p. 142). Furthermore, this concept is extended not only to individuals but communities to uproot oppressive situations (Wallerstein & Bernstein, 1994). But the issue remains: with their ability to define themselves, communities do not need outsiders to acknowledge their skills or power to (re)create their futures.

Hence, communities need to be viewed as assets rather than deficits that need to be fixed, overcome, or empowered (Chambers, 1997; Kretzman & McKnight, 1993). Through community engagement practices, these assets can be activated as expanded. The basic idea is that community-based philosophy illustrates a community's agency and encourages further involvement in the planning process. Furthermore, through collaboration and critical praxis, community-based projects can bolster community members to be active agents of change within their own communities. Here praxis is not just theory and action as discussed by Freire (1970), but political action and community organizing (Fals Borda, 1979).

The second principle is the importance of community members being engaged in every aspect of the project (Murphy, 2014). The key to authentic participation is an intimate connection to a project, rather than token, periodic consultation. Taking this a step further is insuring that a project is truly dictated by community members, rather than seeing persons as simply the focus of a project. Community members, for example, should establish a project design, how this undertaking is evaluated, and formulate any policies that may be deemed important. The more the community is connected to and leading a project, sustainability is increased and the prospects for positive outcomes improved.

Engaging a Community

As mentioned in the previous section, local knowledge needs to be infused into a project from the start to hold true to community-based practice (Murphy, 2014). Learning from the community and the *already present knowledge* is essential for a project to be properly situated (Medin & Bang, 2014; Murphy, 2014). As Gutiérrez and Vossoughi state, "it is important to highlight the principles that orient and help organize the work, always mindful of the need to situate the project in ways that privilege the standpoint of nondominant communities to whom the learning project is oriented" (2010, p. 102). Thus, and as mentioned in previous sections, standard notions of expertise need to be confronted with the recognition that "everyday people carry deep knowledge and analysis about conditions of their lives and should lead in determining meaningful research questions, designs, methods, analyses and products" (Torre & Ayala, 2009, p. 388).

In this context, the concept of participation needs to be explored further, given the power dynamics present and who should dictate the flow of a project (Munck, 2014). Many projects claim to be participatory, but challenges remain (Murphy, 2014). What is distinct here is that participation means more than increasing numbers of participants. True collaboration and co-generation of a project should incorporate the values, beliefs, and commitments of a community into a project (Murphy, 2014).

For example, a community-based project should embrace personal narratives as teaching tools, helping to produce a model of "meaningful, complex, and sometimes disrupted" lived experiences, rather than focusing on deficits that encourage the "painful stories" to be re-lived for the sake of research (Tuck et al., 2014, p. 60). Therefore, to engage a community in an authentic way self-reflection must be ongoing. Once personal and communal biases are acknowledged, interaction can proceed in an honest and genuine way. As Murphy (2014) reminds us:

> Prejudices must be addressed, for example, that portray certain persons as unintelligent or unmotivated, so that participation is widespread and ideas that were formerly unknown may receive serious attention. Planning can thus begin to reflect a community. (p. 10)

Without an honest reflection, the harm that can be done by social projects, and well-intentioned practitioners, will go unnoticed. Accordingly, reflection on existing injustices is an aspect of CBW that needs to be prioritized, along with communities and their ambitions (Long, Ballard, Fisher, & Belsky, 2016). But respect should not be reduced to superficial treatment, such as decorum, but rather suggest a deeper commitment to others (Buber, 1958). Moving in a similar direction is the idea of social reflexivity, which allows for community collaborators to reflect through and with one another. By engaging one another in this way, participants can come together despite biases and personal narratives that are potentially fixed in history and rooted in many forms of discrimination (Cahill, Sultana, & Pain, 2007).

Community knowledge is a way to move beyond social relationships that continue to oppress communities, especially poor and minority communities. As mentioned by Eileen R. Carlton Parsons (2017) and Richard Delgado (1989), *counterstories* are a way for people who have been marginalized to reflect on obstacles to self-development, regain their integrity, and move in a new direction. Therefore, the goal of a project should not be to measure the community, but rather embrace dialogue and communicate effectively (Murphy, 2014). The difference here is the epistemological framing of how communities are defined and how the community knowledge is used in a project. The important question at this juncture is: whose reality is important? A community-based project, simply put, celebrates local participants and the agenda that emerges.

Conclusion

Valid knowledge, communities, and norms are some of the key items that will need to be rethought in the training process to engender effectiveness in community-based interventions. Community practitioners need to be sensitive and self-reflective to have success in these projects. In addition, being able to understand and incorporate a philosophical shift that allows community knowledge to be imbedded into every facet of a project is as crucial, but is often an overlooked aspect of training. Education of practitioners should include reflection on the struggle of communities to maintain their integrity in the face of attempts at marginalization and insults.

In terms of CBW, a reflective question is *who is benefiting from the research*? (Whitman, Pain, & Milledge, 2015). Bringing together narratives that have undergone meaningful connections to bring about change in a community is a vial facet of CBW. Thus, through "sovereignty, contention, balance, and relationship" a move can be made to a new vantage point to engage in new ways of understanding (Tuck, 2009, p. 47).

In sum, there needs to be a shift in understanding of community-based work and interventions. To truly connect with a community in a non-oppressive manner, a philosophical change in the training of practitioners is critical. By engaging in dialogue and continual praxis, communities can be approached in a more honest way, thereby celebrating community knowledge and projects. Training should reflect these aims and become transformative.

References

Berger, P., & Luckmann, T. (1967). *The social construction of reality*. New York, NY: Anchor Books.

Buber, M. (1958). *I and thou*. New York, NY: Scribner.

Cahill, C. (2007). Repositioning ethical commitments: Participatory action research as a relational praxis of social change. *ACME: An International E-Journal for Critical Geographies, 6*(3), 360–373.

Cahill, C., Sultana, F., & Pain, R. (2007). Participatory ethics: Politics, practices, institutions. *ACME: An International E-Journal for Critical Geographies, 6*(3), 304–318.

Chambers, R. (1997). *Whose reality counts? Putting the first last*. London,UK: Intermediate Technology Publications.

Darder, A. (1994). Institutional research as a tool for cultural democracy. *New Directions for Institutional Research, 1994*(81), 21–34.

Delgado, R. (1989). Storytelling for oppositionists and others: A plea for narrative. *Michigan Law Review, 87*(8), 2411–2441.

Fals Borda, O. (1979). Investigation reality in order to transform it: The Colombian experience. *Dialectical Anthropology, 4*(1), 33–55.

Fals Borda, O. (1987). The application of participatory action research in Latin America. *International Sociology, 2*(4), 329–347.

Fals Borda, O. (1988). *Knowledge and people's power*. New York, NY: New Horizons.

Ferreira, F. (2017). Critical sustainability studies: A holistic and visionary conception of socioecological conscientization. *Journal of Sustainability Education*, 13.

Freire, P. (1970). *Pedagogy of the oppressed*. New York, NY: Continuum.

Freire, P. (2000). *Pedagogy of freedom: Ethics, democracy, and civic courage*. Lanham, MD: Rowman & Littlefield Publishers.

Gadamer, H.-G. (1996). *The enigma of health: The art of healing in a scientific age*. Stanford, CA: Stanford University Press.

Gutiérrez, K., & Vossoughi, S. (2010). Lifting off the ground to return anew: Mediated praxis, transformative learning, and social design experiments. *Journal of Teacher Education, 61*(1–2), 100–117.

Kretzman, J., & McKnight, J. (1993). *Building communities from the inside out*. Chicago, IL: Acta Publications.

Krieger, N. (2011). *Epidemiology and the people's health*. New York, NY: Oxford University Press.

Long, J., Ballard, H., Fisher, L., & Belsky, J. (2016). Questions that won't go away in participatory research. *Society and Natural Resources, 29*(2), 250–263.

Lykes, M. B. (2013). Participatory and action research as a transformative praxis: Responding to humanitarian crises from the margins. *American Psychologist, 68*(8), 774–783.

Medin, D. L., & Bang, M. (2014). The cultural side of science communication. *Proceedings of the National Academy of Sciences of the United States of America, 111*(Supplement 4), 13621–13626.

Munck, R. (2014). Community-based research: Genealogy and prospects. In R. Munck, L. McIlrath, B. Hall, & R. Tandon (Eds.), *Higher education and community-based research* (pp. 11–26). New York, NY: Palgrave Macmillan.

Murphy, J. W., & Casanova, F. (2018). *Community-based work and the accompanying changes in sociology*. Unpublished Manuscript, Department of Sociology, Miami University.

Murphy, J. W. (2014). *Community based interventions: Philosophy and action*. New York, NY: Springer.

Parsons, E. R. C. (2017). Interfaces between critical race theory and sociocultural perspectives. In I. Esmonde & A. Booker (Eds.), *Power and privilege in the learning sciences: Critical and sociocultural theories of learning sciences* (pp. 24–46). New York, NY: Routledge.

Schutz, A. (1967). *The phenomenology of the social world*. Evanston, IL: Northwestern University Press.

Smith, L. T. (2012). *Decolonizing methodologies: Research and indigenous peoples*. New York, NY: Zed Books.

Torre, M. E., & Ayala, J. (2009). Envisioning participatory action research entremundos. *Feminism and Psychology, 19*(3), 387–393.

Tuck, E. (2009). Re-visioning action: Participatory action research and indigenous theories of change. *The Urban Review, 41*(1), 47–65.

Tuck, E., & Guishard, M. (2013). Uncollapsing ethics: Racialized sciencism, settler coloniality, and an ethical framework of decolonial participatory action research. In T. M. Kress, C. S. Malott, & B. J. Portfilio (Eds.), *Challenging status quo retrenchment: New directions in critical qualitative research* (pp. 3–27). Charlotte, NC: Information Age Publishing.

Tuck, E., Smith, M., Guess, A. M., Benjamin, T., & Jones, B. K. (2014). Geo-theorizing Black/Land: Contestations and contingent collaborations. *Departures in Critical Qualitative Research, 3*(1), 52–74.

Wallerstein, N., & Bernstein, E. (1994). Introduction to community empowerment, participatory education, and health. *Health Education Quarterly, 21*(3), 141–148.

Whitman, G. P., Pain, R., & Milledge, D. G. (2015). Going with the flow? Using participatory action research in physical geography. *Progress in Physical Geography, 39*(5), 622–639.

Chapter 7
Creating a Community Health Worker Training Program

Dawn Graham, Kerri Shaw, and Lesli Johnson

CHW Importance in the Region

The role of Community Health Workers (CHWs) cannot be understated. Their roles include outreach, programming, prevention, and linkages to healthcare access for the wider population. This emerging occupation is critical as noncommunicable, chronic, and preventable disease rates continue to rise. For a successful implementation, community organizations and university partnerships must work efficiently and in tandem in order to enhance service delivery. CHWs serve a key role in facilitating access to services in rural areas. By developing a certified CHW training program, healthcare providers are creating a strong workforce that aims to improve overall health outcomes in the region. Promotion of health and wellness combined with preventing the adverse effects of noncommunicable disease states prove an important advancement in the health and well-being of the Southeastern Ohio region. In partnership with the Athens City-County Health Department and colleges from across Ohio University, we promote and extend the CHW efforts within the region. In this chapter, we discuss the implementation, challenges, and resilience that contribute to a successful CHW program.

D. Graham (✉)
Social Medicine, Heritage College of Osteopathic Mediicne, Athens, OH, USA
e-mail: grahamd@ohio.edu

K. Shaw
Social Work, Ohio University, Athens, OH, USA

L. Johnson
Voinovich, Ohio University, Athens, OH, USA

S. L. Arxer, J. W. Murphy (eds.), *Community-Based Health Interventions in an Institutional Context*, International Perspectives on Social Policy, Administration, and Practice, https://doi.org/10.1007/978-3-030-24654-9_7

Community Health Worker (CHW) trainings are offered throughout the Appalachian region of Ohio, which suffers from at-risk and distressed economies, high poverty rates, declining population demographic trends, and a workforce that often lacks the skills needed in emerging business sectors. Additionally, these counties have low levels of educational attainment, relative lack of access to health-care services, and sparse health-promoting community infrastructure. A key social determinant that influences health outcomes is the level of economic distress. Athens County is the poorest county in Ohio according to data from the 2010 US Census, and neighboring counties experience similar levels of economic distress. Adjacent to Athens County, Vinton County is the second poorest in the State of Ohio. In Vinton County, approximately 1 out of 5 (20.6%) residents is living in poverty and in nearby Meigs County, 22.4% of residents are living in poverty (quickfacts.census.gov). Perry County ranks 78th out of Ohio's 88 counties; Washington County ranks 34th out of the 88 counties. The healthcare needs of this population are greatly impacted by its poverty (Kliegman, 1992). Lack of access to care combined with high rates of uninsured contribute to overall acute and chronic health concerns.

The Appalachian Region

The distinct needs of Appalachian Ohio and the unique cultural elements of our service area provide a key context for the training design. This uniqueness of culture is highlighted at a state level, as the Ohio Development Services Agency partners with the Governor's Office of Appalachia to enhance strategic initiatives to promote health, wellness, and strengthen both the health and economic development of this underserved region of Ohio (Ohio Development Services Agency, 2019). Specifically, the focus areas include increasing job opportunities, reducing isolation, and most important, strengthening the capacity of regional infrastructure and the ability of people to be competitive in the global economy. The proposed community health worker program enhances these strategic principals by augmenting social support networks (decreasing social isolation) and connecting our population with access to healthcare.

Access to healthcare services is a critical need throughout Perry, Meigs, and Vinton Counties and specifically in the rural areas of Athens and Washington Counties. Vinton, Washington, and Perry are designated as federally underserved areas for primary care, dental care, and mental healthcare, while Athens County is underserved for dental and mental health. Perry and Vinton Counties also lack adequate hospitals, urgent care facilities, and emergency departments. The targeted counties also rank poorly in the Robert Wood Johnson 2016 County Health Rankings. Among the 88 Ohio counties, Athens (68th), Perry (54th), Meigs (79th), Muskingum (71st), and Vinton (85th) all rate in the lower half in terms of measured health outcomes.

Developing a New Curriculum

One of the major challenges in developing a new curriculum was to first explore what other training programs were doing successfully, and then develop a plan to integrate these ideas into our existing organization in an efficient way. The CHW program was an interprofessional, university-community collaboration joining the Athens City-County Health Department, the Ohio University College of Health Professions, and the Heritage College of Osteopathic Medicine. The community health work is at an intersection of social work and health professions, and we recognized the need to work across disciplines to meet the training needs of our community. Additionally, the Athens City-County Health Department was already involved in community health work and was a willing partner thanks, in part, to successful past collaborations Logistically, the three organizations held regular face-to-face meetings to develop a curriculum that aligned with the Ohio Board of Nursing's competencies and our own community needs. We created a shared electronic depository for the creation of e-materials.

The Northeast Ohio Medical University (NEOMED) granted us access to the materials they had developed. In addition, as the planning team collected and amended materials found throughout the curriculum "road trip," we took to assess other community health worker programs and inform our own. Working within the university system, the curriculum is technically university property. Our colleagues at NEOMED were gracious in granting access to the documents and materials they used in order to implement their own training program. In fact, throughout the State of Ohio, there is a formalized library cloud into which various organizations can download and disseminate research and materials to one another for increased efficiency in programming.

Currently, there are 15 certified community health worker training programs throughout the State of Ohio (Ohio Board of Nursing, 2019). Certification is a challenge, since the Ohio Board of Nursing has the duty to accommodate the needs of healthcare organizations throughout the state, while still adhering to strict standards of competency. Since the educational level of CHW trainees ranges from GED-level students to individuals with college degrees, the curriculum must be set up to make CHW training didactics understandable and portable across various agencies and regions within the state. As we talked to colleagues around the state, the most basic lesson learned was that there was no standardized curriculum that existed due to CHW as an emerging profession.

The OU CHW Training Program received certification by the Ohio Board of Nursing in January 2017. The curriculum content focuses on culturally competent care within a patient-centered, rural Appalachian Ohio community. Participants learn how to provide relational-based care to patients as generalists, while learning about chronic care issues prevalent in the rural community such as Type 2 Diabetes, and COPD. Participants also develop a knowledge base of the resources available to community members to help them meet basic needs and tackle social determinants of health. Due to the high poverty rate, ingrained behavioral health patterns, and isolated population, the program's development leadership specifically recruits participants with a deep commitment to serve and understand the distinct population.

The Appalachian Region and Stakeholders

There are three key stakeholder groups and two related groups within the Appalachian region related to CHW programming. Primary stakeholders include the programs and organizations that utilize or seek to utilize CHWs to increase access and improve health outcomes, including health departments and Federally Qualified Health Centers. Others include individuals who could potentially become certified and employed as CHWs and those who are part of a vulnerable population who could benefit from the effective use of CHW services. Secondary stakeholders include the OU CHW certification, providers, and Medicaid/managed care organizations. In order to address these critical health outcomes, we offered a training and master training program throughout the region. The master training program was delivered to us by Northeastern Ohio Medical University. As master trainers are developed in each region, they are able to sustain programming efforts by working collectively and offering low or no cost training to other healthcare sites interested in the curriculum.

History of the Program

In the fall of 2015, faculty across Ohio University were invited to discuss a potential grant that would allow greater access to healthcare agencies and services to local community members. The authors have years of experience in the healthcare system and have experience in this Appalachian region. The main charge was to begin setting up the infrastructure that would later become Ohio University's more standardized and formal curriculum. Eventually, we were able to develop, train, and disseminate both a standardized community health worker curriculum and a master training program for long-term sustainability of CHWs across the area. The purpose of this critical grant funding opportunity (Ohio Medicaid and Technical Assistance and Policy Program) is to help train healthcare professionals to work with the large population of Medicaid-assisted patients in order to improve the overall health metrics in the State of Ohio.

The Ohio University Community Health Worker Program is well-received throughout the region to date and, has developed a strong working partnership with the Athens City-County Health Department and its Director of Community Health Worker Development, who serves as a primary trainer for the OU CHW Program. In 2016, the Athens City-County Health Department conducted a Communities

Preventing Chronic Disease Assessment (CPCDA), which identified if and how local healthcare providers utilize CHWs in their practices to link patients to community resources that promote the self-management of blood pressure. As a result of this assessment, participants in Year 2 identified evidence-based lifestyle change programs (42.9% Yes) and prevention of type 2 diabetes (28.6% Yes). Holzer Clinic, Ohio University Community Health Program Free Clinic, OhioHealth O'Bleness Athens Medical Associates OB/Gyn, University Medical Associates, Inc., O'Bleness Ohio Health Residency Clinic, and Hopewell Health Center (FQHC) were included in the CPCD Assessment. This information was used toward setting the goals of creating CHW field placements and workforce development opportunities moving forward.

In August 2016, nine professionals completed Community Health Worker and Master Trainer programs. These trainers are community members serving their home communities in public health and are committed to offering CHW training programs in their counties, as well as supporting efforts in other identified counties. These nine professionals represented:

- Ohio University College of Health Sciences and Professions
- Ohio University Heritage College of Osteopathic Medicine Department of Social Medicine
- Athens City-County Health Department
- Muskingum County Health Department
- Washington County Health Department
- Unique Services Logistics Career Academy, LLC (Columbus)

In addition to the professional organizations listed above, additional agencies are coordinating efforts. The Athens City-County Health Department and Washington and Meigs County Health Departments were recipients of a POWER (Partnerships for Opportunity and Workforce and Economic Revitalization) grant through Marshall University. Through this opportunity, the CHW trainers focused on creating healthcare professionals who specifically target clients with chronic health concerns including decreasing A1C levels in patients with diabetes. Although training will continue to expand, we currently have CHWs working in a regional Mennonite community, a local FQHC, and a WIC office.

CHW Regional Training and Utilization

In March 2016, *State Reform*, an online resource sponsored by the Robert Wood Johnson Foundation, provides up-to-date information about how different states are addressing the use of community health workers (State Community Health Worker Models 2016). Ohio has a certification process in place through the Board of Nursing, as well as a number of certified training programs. However, compared to other states, Ohio has not yet identified a funding mechanism or appropriate CHW roles. Currently, there are a number of efforts throughout Ohio University and

Southeast Ohio to utilize CHWs. Several local health departments, some physician practices, and The Diabetes Institute among others have requested or received funding to support CHWs within their organizations. Since the CHW Program was initiated in 2015, opportunities for research collaboration, workforce development, and community partnerships have arisen. For example, the Diabetes Institute submitted a HRSA expansion grant, *A New Approach to Diabetes Navigation in Rural Appalachia*, to train and employ community health workers in tandem with Diabetes Navigators to expand the reach of services in the region to include children with diabetes while also providing a sustainable source of employment for community members.

Additionally, Marietta Senior High School is offering a year-long course to graduating seniors, taught by a CHW Master Trainer. The training program serves as a pipeline for workforce development in this poverty-stricken region. This course allows graduating students to be eligible for the Ohio Board of Nursing certificate, thereby making them more competitive in the job market. The training offers them experience and practice in the healthcare field while serving as a pathway to higher education in healthcare professions. The course falls under the administrative auspice of Ohio University.

Stakeholder Needs

The primary stakeholder groups benefit from shared information, role clarification, education, and potential collaboration. As the CHW pipeline progresses, the stakeholders could use a common marketing platform to spread word to the public. The OU CHW certification provider could use information for continuous program improvement and to support the clinical training requirement, while managed care organizations benefit from more cost-effective services. Further, some exploration of opportunities to network and potentially collaborate could be beneficial to the various stakeholder groups. Finally, exploring strategies for sustainability is key to the continued development of this effort. Otherwise, current efforts will be fragmented and time-limited. We utilize a multipronged approach, beginning with contacts with organizations, currently or potentially employing CHWs, to identify the following: what current programming efforts are in place, challenges, successes, evaluation activities, and current needs, otherwise known as an environmental scan. After this initial step, we propose a facilitated stakeholder meeting to explore opportunities, needs, and barriers to collaboration.

We explored the feasibility of creating a regional network that would include organizations that are using or plan to utilize CHWs and identify potential opportunities for collaboration and the creation of community health improvement strategies. Another objective is to standardize the curriculum already approved by the Ohio Board of Nursing to create user-friendly, replicable lesson plans and training manual for the CHW training program. To date, we have completed a comprehensive training manual, and e-based trainings continue around the region. Experimental courses were offered to Ohio University students beginning in fall 2018.

Diversity of Programs

We discovered that CHW training programs were as diverse as the communities in which they were implemented. In an urban, northern Ohio, CHW trainings were offered to high school students as a way to help promote community advocacy, as well as give these students a skill set upon graduation. With graduation rates in Ohio currently at 84% (nces.ed.gov), the implementation of new certification upon graduation would serve to set up high school seniors for success.

From an organizational perspective, this program is also a strong workforce development pipeline. As the national rhetoric focuses on affordability and accessibility, the timing of our local implementation could not be more perfect. In a sense, we are training people to implement access to healthcare services at a lower cost at the same time insurance companies and managed care organizations are ramping up ways to cover the cost of preventative services. One of our first steps in information gathering was to visit existing programs around the state to see how they were training and implementing their CHW curriculums. Two sites within Ohio included Cleveland State University and the University of Cincinnati Nursing programs. Of note, the Cincinnati program focuses on decreasing infant mortality rates. Our purpose is to create a generalist program that allows each student to specialize on a target population (maternal/child health, developmental disabilities, diabetes management, etc.) These two institutions were gracious in helping us to develop ideas that could work in our rural, Appalachian region.

Logistical Challenges

One of the main challenges of managing the ongoing training program is to find a graduate assistant who is passionate and available to provide support with the certification process, literature review, and curriculum development. Throughout the life of the program, we have been fortunate to hire graduate assistants who have been instrumental in helping with day-to-day duties and moving the project forward. The College of Health Sciences houses a series of graduate students from health professions to help us organize and document the developing curriculum. They have also conducted and transcribed interviews as part of the regional assessment process.

Another challenge of implementing our community health work has been learning how to market the service. In the early days, we received feedback from other health professionals worried about "turf" issues. More specifically, public health professionals were worried that community health workers would target the same communities that receive services from the local health departments (i.e., immunizations). But, through cultivating relationships and building trust, we were able to understand how to best market the value of community health workers. In fact, that marketing is still in process. We had to learn to explain to our colleagues that the role of CHWs is to serve as a liaison to connect community members to services. Oftentimes, the role of the CHW can be seen as overlapping with public health and nursing professionals. Time was needed to help CHW trainees understand how to market themselves as a help to other service providers while making the case that the CHW serves as a pipeline for patient populations that would otherwise have not accessed these health services. This understanding was critical to developing a meaningful relationship that emphasized the outcome of services while strengthening the healthcare workforce. In addition, we had to recruit community partners who would help us train with minimal recompense due to limited resources.

The concept of community health workers as culturally competent conduits of health information and access to care, is especially useful in rural areas where people may be reluctant to trust outsiders and tend to rely on family and friends for health information. Oftentimes, especially in rural areas, people are reluctant to trust outsiders. In addition, if someone has what is perceived to be a bad experience in a healthcare setting, that person is likely to avoid the organization and spread this information to their friends and family members.

Scope of Work/Timeline

The chart below outlines the timeline and scope of work as the program continues to evolve throughout Ohio University and the larger Southeastern Appalachian region of Ohio.

Year 1 Fall July–Dec 2017	Year 1 Spring Jan–Jun 2018	Year 2 Fall July–Dec 2018	Year 2 Spring Jan–June 2019
Training #1 (2 simultaneous cohorts)	Curriculum Implementation (cohorts 1 and 2)	Training #2 (2 simultaneous cohorts)	Curriculum implementation (cohorts 3 and 4)
Student recruitment for year 1 spring	Student recruitment for year 2 fall	Student recruitment for year 2 spring	Focus group interviews for student experience
Community site recruitment	Community/student match (cohorts 1 and 2)	Community/student match (cohort 2)	Community/student match (cohorts 3 and 4)
Evaluation data setup and planning	Pre-evaluation for cohorts 1 and 2	Post-evaluation for cohorts 1 and 2	Pre-evaluation for cohorts 3 and 4 (post upon completion)

Year 1 Fall July–Dec 2017	Year 1 Spring Jan–Jun 2018	Year 2 Fall July–Dec 2018	Year 2 Spring Jan–June 2019
Identifying content experts to provide specialized training across years (cultural competency, etc.)	Motivational interviewing training and cultural competence training for cohorts 1 and 2	Motivational interviewing training and cultural competence training for cohorts 3 and 4	Post-evaluation for cohort 2
CHW site travel and discussions	Active recruitment of cohorts 3 and 4 for year 2	Preliminary data gathering and assessment	Dissemination and write up of data research to academic journals/conferences

CHWs Addressing Health Disparities

The community health worker can fulfill multiple roles in helping clients to access services. According to Snyder (2016), the roles of a CHW include the following: addressing social determinants of health affecting care, increasing care access, providing educational services, assisting in care coordination, and sharing cultural and economic characteristics with community members. The CHWs can provide and share access to screenings, focus on chronic disease management such as Diabetes, and promote maternal and child health.

An important component of the responsibilities of a community health worker include helping clients educate themselves on the importance of preventative health. Most insurance companies, including Medicaid, cover basic health screenings such as colon cancer screens and pap smears. Many community members do not realize that these prevention services are fully covered by Medicaid and private insurance. A large number of local community health workers promote screenings as critical prevention tools to help diagnose and treat problems before they result in a serious and chronic health condition or illness.

Program Metrics

Program outcome measures allow us to continue to monitor quality improvement processes and make sure that the program is having an impact on patients. Outcome measures are also key to sustainability for financial purposes. By talking with colleagues around the state and contracting with the Ohio University Voinovich School for Leadership and Public Affairs, we were able to come up with key program metrics. They include the following below:

Patient demographics	Process measures	Patient behaviors	Intervention outcome measures
Age	# receiving education	Program education process	Specific health outcomes (i.e., blood pressure, A1C levels)
Gender	# outside referrals to local agencies	Changes in daily activities	Consumer satisfaction
Specific health problems (i.e., type 2 diabetes, asthma)	# patients screened	Presence of compliance and self-management	Increase in health issue awareness as evidenced by survey data
Physical activity	# educational programs facilitated by CHWs	Office visits to primary care/ preventative medicine	Cost savings metrics (i.e., lower ED visit utilization)

In addition to program metrics, conducting continuous quality improvement processes is crucial to increasing sustainability efforts and efficiency in program delivery. In coordination with local agencies, we determined the key strengths, weaknesses, opportunities, and threats to program sustainability. The strengths identified included:

- Ohio University's CHW Program is now certified by the Ohio Board of Nursing and remains a platform for sustainable workforce development within the Southeastern Ohio region.
- An already existing master trainer program allows for expansion of services wherever demand is greatest.
- Local media and word of mouth has expanded the knowledge of our programming efforts in surrounding counties outside of Athens.
- Community partnerships and support for the CHW program have expanded in the form of providing participants, sites, and resources for training.
- The relationship with Athens City/County Health Department continues to grow and strengthen, thus extending financial resources and in-kind capacity to expand the CHW work throughout the region.

Weaknesses identified are as follows:

- This is an intensive training program with a significant time commitment; scheduling is challenging for trainers and trainees.
- Uncertainty in local and federal funding makes it difficult to plan for sustainability of programming efforts.
- The inability to have a full-time worker devoted to CHW training and development causes logistical difficulties in coordinating training efforts.
- The application turnaround was very quick for the first cohort, which might explain small cohort number.

New partnerships with health departments in neighboring counties are emerging:

- New Washington County partnerships extend programming across the region.

- Ongoing relationships with CHWs in Franklin County provide greater opportunity for training in urban areas.

  Threats:

- Ambiguity of sustainable funding sources causes greater uncertainty in planning future training opportunities.
- Political climate around Medicaid funding and other organizations and impact on rural service providers makes it difficult to plan future programming.

The Curriculum

As the curriculum continues to refine individual modules and flexibility in course delivery, the original program goals stay consistent. Namely, the objectives are fivefold:

1. Increase enrollment and completion of community health worker programming for community members who may not otherwise have access to professional development opportunities that are offered in population dense areas.
2. Expand enrollment and completion of community health worker programming for community members who may not otherwise have access to professional development opportunities that are offered in population dense areas.
3. Increase, sustain, and maintain a community population in line with the community strategic initiative for economic development, patient recruitment, and overall public health prevention services.
4. Promote educational activities across multiple healthcare serving agencies.
5. Enhance community members' opportunities for professional development along the adult developmental spectrum.

Community-Based and Experiential Learning Curriculum

The existing CHW program emphasizes adult learning strategies that engage learners with community organizations in a systematic and engaging way. The Ohio University CHW Training Program emphasizes cultural competence throughout its curriculum, including a training session facilitated by FQHC Hopewell Health Center, *Appalachian Culture and Poverty,* which utilizes author Ruby Payne's materials from *Bridges Out of Poverty* (2001) to frame socioeconomic issues, social determinants of health, and communication styles in Appalachia to develop empathy and understanding in care providers. Twenty of the 100 hours of in-class didactic content focus on cultural competence implementing a curriculum developed by a faculty member of the Ohio University Social Work Program with an additional 130 hours completed while immersed in community-based field placements.

Students also complete a module of motivational interviewing training. The theory of motivational interviewing is a unique addition to the community health worker program in Appalachian Ohio. Motivational interviewing is an evidence-based practice that promotes behavior change with a patient-driven perspective that originated in the treatment of patients with substance abuse issues (Carroll et al., 2006). The practice employs an "OARS" approach to promote healthy behaviors and will be actively learned and implemented by all community health workers. The "OARS" approach allows for Open-ended questions; utilizes Affirming statements to promote patient empowerment; utilizes Reflective listening to confirm beliefs and challenges that prevent clients from making healthy choices; and Summarize concerns and feeling about healthcare in general (Berthold, Avila, & Miller, 2009). Motivational Interviewing is a systematic, learner-friendly approach to empowering patients for long-term, positive impact.

The Ohio University CHW Training Program is a model of interprofessional participation that utilizes trainers from diverse backgrounds, including public health, social work, psychology, and nursing with a focus on experiential learning practices. Ohio University has a unique approach of interprofessional learning, since it holds a yearly interprofessional education (IPE) forum for students and healthcare workers alike. Community health workers will have ready access to programming efforts and educational opportunities offered by Ohio University. Examples of IPE learning opportunities for community health workers include access to Global Health programming, interdisciplinary research symposiums, and practicum placement in integrated community health settings. In addition, the certified CHW curriculum has IPE examples and readings embedded into the training.

Identification of Students and Community Partners

Over the past 2 years, relationships have been cultivated with over 20 organizations in the region, and the CHW Program has been received with success and enthusiasm. Members of the recruitment team include a Social Work Field Liaison and the Director of Campus and Community Relations, both of whom have strong ties and histories with agencies and organizations in the region. These relationships have facilitated conversations and commitments from potential field placements and employers.

For example, students will be recruited through Ohio University, Hocking College, local social service agencies, healthcare institutions, and the AmeriCorps/COMCorps program. COMCorps is housed in the Ohio University Heritage College of Medicine Community Health Program and has a mission to increase access to:

- Evidence-based nutrition education
- Healthy fresh food

- Physical activity
- Preventative and primary healthcare services

The first training cohort began in February 2017 in Athens with six participants. These persons were recruited from local partner agencies that are supportive of the Community Health Worker training program. Participants represent the following organizations that serve Athens, Vinton, and Hocking counties:

- AmeriCorps/COMCorps – Athens City/County Health Department & Live Healthy Appalachia
- Vinton County Help Me Grow
- Ohio University College of Family Medicine
- Hopewell Health Center (FQHC)
- HAVAR, an agency that provides in-home daily living support to individuals with disabilities

Evaluation Plan

Students complete knowledge-based assessment surveys pre- and post- the training period. Demographic data are also collected, including employment history and the significance of obtaining the CHW certificate. Data are regularly compiled and analyzed into a longitudinal dataset via statistical analysis and through qualitative data coding. Participant feedback is collected after the completion of each training module and during field visits to enhance programming and continuous quality improvement practices. The Voinovich School of Leadership and Public Affairs is managing the evaluation plan and providing annual reports. Employment status and benefits of obtaining the CHW certificate will be tracked across time by the Voinovich School.

In addition, change in social empathy is assessed using a Social Empathy scale. The purpose of this study is to understand the level and dimensions of social empathy in community health worker trainees. Using the Social Empathy Index (Segal, 2011), information will be gathered when participants enter and complete the program. Participants will complete the SEI in the first class of the program and then again in the final class. The pre and post-assessments will be examined for changes generally in social empathy and specifically in areas of strength and weakness for the student group at entrance and completion. This analysis will contribute to understanding of community health worker education, social empathy in participants, and the concept of social empathy generally.

Social empathy adds dimensions of understanding system-level barriers and broader self-other knowledge to interpersonal empathy: "interpersonal and social empathy [are] tools for us to improve our own lives and other people's lives, as well as to promote social well-being" (Segal, 2011). The community health worker program is focused on improving access to care and increasing education related to all aspects of health—physical, mental, and social. Cultural competence is required to provide quality, effective service and is a key element of the program.

Proposed Partnerships

The community health worker program that has been established through MEDTAPP currently has over 21 linkages within the Southeastern region of Ohio. These referral networks will be enhanced by each cohort trained throughout the next 2 years (approximately 8 additional training sites). By utilizing existing trained community health workers, we will continue to utilize and expand our reach for engaging providers. In addition, former MEDTAPP partnerships established in the local trauma informed care initiative have allowed us to expand outreach opportunities for local providers. For example, current training at Hopewell Health Centers, a local Federally Qualified Healthcare Center that also serves as a Community Mental Health Center, has been working with our local team and has access to providers in over 19 Ohio counties throughout the region. Our plan to expand partnerships includes the following steps:

1. Ask known established entities (i.e., Hopewell) about potential providers who are apt to utilize and/or communicate the usefulness and effectiveness of community health worker services.
2. Reach out to existing providers and providing brief education about the CHW program.
3. Utilize the marketing/communication toolkit to inform existing patients about the benefits and services existing within the community.
4. Track referral sources by existing community health workers through an already existing shared documentation platform through Ohio University's MEDTAPP programs.

Placement Sites

To date, over eight local rural agencies have agreed to be a secure placement site for regional trained community health workers, including a drug/alcohol addiction center, a geriatric nursing facility, two health departments, a local WIC agency, and a local Primary Care and dental clinic. As current community health workers continue to be certified in the region, part of their charge will be to identify additional site placements (including current employment sites). In addition, the current community health worker program through the Athens Health Department will utilize additional existing funding streams to help place CHWs in the surrounding rural areas.

In tandem, we will continue to enhance and develop community partnerships with managed care plans. Current leadership maintains existing partnerships with several of the local managed care plans through the work of former maternal and child health grants throughout the region. These existing linkages include Molina, Paramount, Caresource, and United. As CHWs are placed within the region, existing linkages with these managed care outreach workers will be called on for ongoing communication and potential employment opportunities to serve in the rural regional healthcare sites. In addition, managed care plans are invited to regional collaboration meetings for updates and information sharing between university and community partnerships.

Addressing Social Determinants of Health

Helping students understand the nuances of a community and community needs plays an integral role in the success of this program. The students need to understand the social determinants that affect the community members' decisions to seek or not to seek medical attention. The core instructors, given their extensive experience working in these communities, along with exposure through supervised practicums, will help develop these skills. Understanding the social determinants surrounding the healthcare of a community is paramount in the success of the CHW and the overall outcomes of the curriculum.

The social determinants of health that the CHW training program will utilize are taken from the evidence-based practice contributed by the Office of Disease Prevention and Health Promotion (HealthyPeople.gov). Leading health indicators such as poverty, local graduation rates, statistics on violence, and unemployment are emphasized and highlighted throughout the already approved curriculum through the Ohio Board of Nursing. Multiple pre-/post-outcome measures that include social empathy, concrete health knowledge, and developmental warning signs are measured on a quarterly basis to help track knowledge, attitudes, and outcomes. Culturally sensitive education involving the complexities of health disparities in this rural, Appalachian region is of the highest priority when training local CHWs. One CHW training participant shared that she is asked at every home visit where she is from and who her relatives are. Because of her cultural training, she understands that this is a way her patients build rapport and identify her as an "insider."

CHWs are embedded automatically into interprofessional experiences at each placement site. A unique aspect of the rural healthcare systems within Appalachian Ohio includes the ongoing coordination and programming between health professionals from several disciplines. Utilizing the existing infrastructure within Ohio University's College of Health Sciences and Professions, CHW cohorts are exposed to ongoing efforts across the region to make interprofessional experiences available. A specific example will be the inclusion of speakers from Hopewell

Health Centers, Inc. Hopewell Health Centers is a regional Federally Qualified Healthcare Center that also serves as a certified Community Mental Health Agency with 15 separate locations within the Southeastern Ohio. Hopewell is an established partner and has been providing integration and cultural competence training for our agencies throughout the past decade.

Implementation Timeline

Year 1 fall July–Dec 2017	Year 1 spring Jan–Jun 2018	Year 2 fall July–Dec 2018	Year 2 spring Jan–June 2019
Training #1 (2 simultaneous cohorts)	Curriculum implementation (cohorts 1 and 2)	Training #2 (2 simultaneous cohorts)	Curriculum implementation (cohorts 3 and 4)
Student recruitment for year 1 spring	Student recruitment for year 2 fall	Student recruitment for year 2 spring	Focus group interviews for student experience
Community site recruitment	Community/student match (cohorts 1 and 2)	Community/student match (cohort 2)	Community/student match (cohorts 3 and 4)
Evaluation data setup and planning	Pre-evaluation for cohorts 1 and 2	Post-evaluation for cohorts 1 and 2	Pre-evaluation for cohorts 3 and 4 (post upon completion)
Identifying content experts to provide specialized training across years (cultural competency, etc.)	Motivational interviewing training and cultural competence training for cohorts 1 and 2	Motivational interviewing training and cultural competence training for cohorts 3 and 4	Post-evaluation for cohort 2
CHW site travel and discussions	Active recruitment of cohorts 3 and 4 for year 2	Preliminary data gathering and assessment	Dissemination and write up of data research to academic journals/conferences

Future of the Training Program in Southeast Ohio

In 2017, funding priorities for MEDTAPP shifted and the Ohio University Community Health Worker Training Program went from being grant-funded to support a university endowment fund through the College of Health Sciences and Professions. This change has allowed the program director to focus on information gathering and visioning during 2018–2019. In collaboration with the Voinovich

School, an environmental scan of the work being done by community health workers in the region has been completed and analyzed in preparation for a Stakeholders Convening to be held in June 2019. The CHW Program is supported strongly by the University leadership and is included in several community-university grant proposals. As more data are collected and shared about the benefits and efficacy of community health workers in our region, we are hopeful that a consistent funding stream for employment will be identified; that the workforce will continue to grow and flourish; and that our communities will become more engaged in healthier lifestyle choices through access to resources and information as a result of their relationships with community health workers.

Acknowledgments Athens City-County Health Department: Ruth Dudding, Josh Scakacs, Jack Pepper

Cari Hollenbeck

Gemini Wright

Ohio Medicaid and Technical Assistance and Policy Program (MEDTAPP)

Marietta High School: Kim Depue and Mary Ella Bauer

Dr. Sarah Garlington

Dr. Jeff DiGiovani

Dr. John McCarthy

Dr. Randy Leite

References

Berthold, T., Avila, A., & Miller, J. (Eds.). (2009). *Core competencies in community health.* Oakland, CA: Jossey Bass.

Carroll, K., Ball, A., Nich, S., Martino, C., Frankforter, S., Farentinos, T., et al. (2006). Motivational interviewing to improve treatment engagement and outcome in individuals seeking treatment for substance abuse: A multisite effectiveness study. *Drug and Alcohol Dependence, 81*, 301–312.

Kliegman, R. (1992). Perpetual poverty: Child health and the underclass. *Pediatrics, 89*(4), 585–588.

Ohio Board of Nursing. (2019, March). *Community health workers.* Retrieved from URL http://www.nursing.ohio.gov/CommunityHealthWorkers.htm

Ohio Development Services Agency: Governor's Office of Appalachia. (2019, March). *Appalachian Regional Commission.* Retrieved from URL https://development.ohio.gov/cs/cs_goa_rc.htm

Payne, R., DeVol, P., & Smith, D. (2001). *Bridges out of poverty: Strategies for professionals and communities.* Highland, TX: Aha! Process.

Segal, E. (2011). Social empathy: A model built on empathy, contextual understanding, and social responsibility that promotes social justice. *Journal of Social Service Research, 37*(3), 266–277.

Chapter 8
Is the Affordable Care Act Encouraging Hospitals to Engage their Communities? Experiences from Appalachian Ohio

Berkeley Franz, Daniel Skinner, and Danielle Dukes

Scholars often describe hospitals as contained and unified social institutions. In fact, some of the most prominent social theorists of medical institutions, from Erving Goffman to Michel Foucault to Paul Starr, have chronicled the Western hospital as though it is a mostly homogenous institution governed by an internal logic (Foucault, 1973; Goffman, 1961; Starr, 1982). Although there is much that unites traditional inpatient hospitals in terms of their mission of providing acute patient care and organizational structure, they exhibit diversity as well. Variation owes to differences in hospitals' financial arrangements, organizational environments, regional locations, and unique histories.

The need to bring analytic nuance to the study of hospitals has gained renewed importance in an era of American health care defined in large part by passage of the Affordable Care Act (ACA) in 2010 (Jacobs & Skocpol, 2012; Starr, 2013). Yet, while the political landscape has been shaped by attempts to repeal the bill since early 2017 – with each repeal followed closely in media coverage – the bill's provisions concerning hospitals are rarely discussed. The extent to which they are understood among the general public is unknown. Among the more important and promising of these provisions are those requiring that nonprofit hospitals, roughly 56% of all hospitals in the United States (AHA, 2019), increase and more rigorously structure their "community benefit" activities as a condition of maintaining their 501(c)(3) nonprofit tax exempt status.

Although all nonprofit hospitals have been required by the IRS since the 1960s to document the ways in which they benefit their communities, over 85% of this benefit has traditionally been provided in various forms of charity patient care,

B. Franz (✉)
Heritage College of Osteopathic Medicine, Ohio University, Athens, OH, USA
e-mail: franzb@ohio.edu

D. Skinner · D. Dukes
Heritage College of Osteopathic Medicine, Ohio University, Dublin, OH, USA

S. L. Arxer, J. W. Murphy (eds.), *Community-Based Health Interventions in an Institutional Context*, International Perspectives on Social Policy, Administration, and Practice, https://doi.org/10.1007/978-3-030-24654-9_8

including the subsidization of costs associated with the care for patients covered by Medicaid and over government insurance programs (Folkemer et al., 2011; Young, Chou, Alexander, Lee, & Raver, 2013). The ACA nudges – even pushes – hospitals outward in stating that they must reach beyond their typical patient population and engage the communities beyond hospital walls. This move uses community benefit requirements to expand the hospital's role into traditional public health activities and beyond direct patient care.

Specifically, the ACA requires that nonprofit hospitals, in consultation with the communities they serve, undertake Community Health Needs Assessments (CHNAs) every 3 years to understand their communities' most pressing health needs and then publicly disseminate their findings (Evashwick, 2013). In response to these identified health needs, hospitals must develop an implementation strategy (Internal Revenue Service, 2013). The results of new programs and initiatives formed from the strategy are to be reported annually to produce accountability in community benefit programming. In mandating this process, the ACA is part of a broader trend that is encouraging hospitals to take on local population health needs in addition to providing patient-level care. For those that lack a commitment to the process, the ACA, through Section 4959 of the Internal Revenue Code, authorizes an excise tax of up to $50,000 per year (Rosenbaum, 2015) in addition to the possible revocation of their federal tax exemption status. In 2018, the IRS demonstrated that it actively audits nonprofit hospitals for CHNA compliance in the private letter ruling that revoked a hospital organization's section 501(c)(3) status for failing to comply with requirements (Internal Revenue Service, 2018).

Beginning in 2012, the first 3-year cycle of CHNAs and subsequent community investments created new opportunities for expanding the reach of hospitals' community benefit activities. Although preliminary reports suggest that hospitals are using a variety of different approaches to meet these new requirements such as collecting primary data and utilizing secondary data sources (Burke et al., 2014), less is known about the experiences of hospitals as they take on new community benefit activities, especially when addressing underserved and rural populations. As a result, our study aims to provide a thorough analysis of the community benefit and CHNA efforts of hospitals across the Appalachian region of Ohio. This sample includes a diverse subset of hospitals including small county hospitals, large urban hospitals, and hospitals within health systems of varying sizes.

Although preliminary reports indicate that US hospitals are responding to the new ACA requirements by developing various community partnerships and programs in response to CHNA findings and using multiple methodologies (e.g., collaborations between hospital facilities and public health agencies or consultant-led CHNA processes) to complete reports (Beatty, Wilson, Ciecior, & Stringer, 2015; Pennel, McLeroy, Burdine, & Mataritta-Cascante, 2015; Wilson, Mohr, Beatty, & Ciecior, 2014), few studies have documented the experiences of rural hospitals or, more specifically, hospitals within the Appalachian region of the USA. This region is particularly notable for distressed socioeconomic conditions, but more recently significant health disparities have been documented as a result of widespread unemployment and low income households, a prevalence of risky health behaviors, environmental factors, and lack of access to medical care (Borak, Salipante-Zaidel, Slade, & Fields, 2012; Halverson & Bischak, 2008; Hendryx, 2009; Hendryx & Ahern, 2009; Ludke & Obermiller, 2012; Morrone, Kruse, & Chadwick, 2014; Smith & Hollorman, 2011; Wewers, Katz, Fickle, & Paskett, 2006). As such, this region particularly stands to gain from increased population health activity if hospitals are able to implement new programs in underserved communities.

To understand hospital experiences with CHNAs in this underserved region, the first two authors conducted interviews with hospital staff, administrators, and consultants, and evaluated formal documents associated with the CHNA and implementation process. Specifically, we sought to understand how these new activities are informing community health engagement in surrounding communities. These findings make clear that the ACA has formalized community-benefit requirements; accordingly, we outlined how those tasked with taking on CHNAs have experienced the subsequent changes. As we explain, our interviews revealed a complex set of challenges, as well as muted optimism, regarding the possibility that ACA-mandated CHNAs will positively impact population health in a region that lacks material resources and faces a myriad of other challenges. Our results provide insight into the process of community-benefit activities and how such requirements might be improved in future health policy debates in order to successfully engage local communities in improving population health outcomes.

Methods

Overview of Study

The purpose of our study was to understand how hospitals in Appalachian Ohio have adjusted to new ACA requirements to conduct CHNAs and develop programming to respond to local needs. Using grounded theory methodology, we conducted in-depth interviews with hospital personnel and outside consultants who worked on CHNAs in either 2013 or 2016 in this region. In accordance with grounded theory principles, we did not begin with specific hypotheses, but rather guiding research questions that informed our interview guide (Charmaz, 2006). Specifically our questions were:

1. What steps have been taken and methods employed to carry out CHNAs in the years since the ACA was implemented?
2. How do hospitals evaluate the effectiveness of these new community benefit activities?
3. What are the significant challenges to improving health outcomes in rural, Appalachian communities?

The goal of this methodology is to begin with general questions that allow findings to emerge from participants' perspectives. After submitting a protocol outlining this study, we were cleared by the Ohio University Institutional Review Board on May 9, 2015.

Recruitment and Sampling

Appalachian Ohio's 32 counties include 26 nonprofit hospitals. We made initial contact with hospitals either by email or phone. Although hospitals are required to make their CHNA results public, often the persons responsible for these activities are not identified. Therefore, at times we had to initiate contact by calling the hospital's general number or by filling out comment forms on hospital web pages. Determining who was responsible for CHNAs was thus challenging given the fact that few of the hospitals in this region had dedicated full-time staff to these activities. Despite the challenges associated with making initial connections, consent was ultimately received from 17 research participants who had either worked or were currently working on post-ACA CHNAs. Fifteen participants were hospital employees while working on CHNAs, and two were external consultants. Participants represented 21 different hospitals, some of which were independent and others which were part of large, often multistate health systems. Of the 21 hospitals included in our sample, 12 were affiliated with nine health systems.

Data Collection and Analysis

Interviews occurred by phone and lasted between 30 and 60 minutes. After each interview was completed, the audio files were transcribed by a professional transcriptionist. In line with grounded theory methodology, preliminary coding began after each interview was transcribed and the results were used to inform future recruiting. Because there was a fixed sample size due to the region chosen for the study, preliminary coding was used to identify hospitals in the region who may be different or offer divergent perspectives than the existing hospitals who had not yet agreed to participate. Five additional hospitals were added to the sample through follow-up contact after theoretical sampling occurred (Charmaz, 2006). We continued to interview and analyze data until no new categories emerged. This stage, dubbed "theoretical saturation" by grounded theory experts, was reached after 17 interviews, spanning 21 hospitals. This sample size is within the normal range for grounded theory research (Charmaz, 2006).

Interviews were coded by the authors using the web-based data analysis software Dedoose. Following grounded theory procedures, coding was undertaken in three phases (Walker & Myrick, 2006). The first stage, open coding, requires line by line descriptors be applied throughout the transcript. The next step is for the researchers to complete "axial coding" where initial line by line descriptors are grouped into similar clusters. Finally, theoretical coding occurs and involves identifying overall emerging themes and describing a causal structure of relationships between these themes. Certain procedures are often employed at each stage of coding to ensure that data analysis is rigorous and consistent between researchers. In this project, the researchers engaged in cross-coding to improve reliability, in addition to the collaborative questioning of categories, memo-writing, and word-analysis (Strauss & Corbin, 1998). This method of coding was used to foster creativity and reduce bias while generating themes in a systematic approach.

Findings

Our findings concern the specific challenges of undertaking CHNAs for hospitals serving rural, underserved, and vulnerable populations, as well as the degree of optimism that interviewees displayed regarding the capacity of post-ACA CHNAs to positively effectuate change in their communities. Our interviews revealed significant challenges in studying and working with rural populations, notably demographic and geographic diversity, resources in both hospitals and communities, and other barriers to implementing the kind of programming required to address problems impacting these populations. In our analysis of the attitudinal dispositions held by interviewees regarding the CHNA process and future of community benefit, we consider participant perspectives on whether local health outcomes can be improved by hospital community benefit work, which range from the somewhat negative to muted, qualified optimism. The barriers described were relevant both in producing the official CHNA reports which are due every 3 years and also in developing the required implementation programs from the needs identified through the CHNA process. In order to ensure the anonymity of participants, we deploy pseudonyms for all data presented.

Challenges

Low-Resource Communities

In many ways, the successful undertaking of a CHNA requires cooperation not only with community organizations and health institutions, but community members themselves who are able to engage despite structural disadvantages they may face. Donna explained that the large county in which her hospital is located "is almost an entirely different world" than areas just on the other side of a major highway, adding:

we have pockets of the county that don't have cell service. We have pockets of the county that don't really have access to broadband to have access to the internet. Seems unreal in 2016, but it's true. There were households that didn't have great running water, those are things that you've got people who, again, our unemployment rated always higher than the state/national average, which means people don't have the disposable income to really take control of their own health. Running advocates for themselves, because they're deciding whether or not I can eat today, or whether I can go to the doctor.

As Sharon noted:

reaching…some of the population that we need to in this market is tough. You know, you really have to be out into the communities and where the people are that you need to reach… Reaching that population with the messages that we need to and helping them through, we do a lot of nutrition education and we have cooking classes at the library, things like that. But really getting the message to the people that we need to is a challenge for us.

In many cases, difficulty in reaching and working with local populations was cast as a communication issue. As Stacy noted, "access is always a challenge because our patients have access issues and communication sometimes can be an issue."

Jackie added:

I would say that…the health needs are different. I mean, there's a huge problem with smoking…and of course, where there's a large proportion of smoking, you've got great incidence of lung cancer. In fact, lung cancer is the number one cause of death in those counties. So then what we have to do is we have to look at, you know, how can we motivate people to be tested, to do smoking cessation, how do we deal with some of the social determinants? You know, they don't have transportation, they don't have this, they don't have that. So there's a lot more extenuating resources that have to be provided if we really want to be successful.

Here Jackie is pointing out that while finding a relevant population health problem to address might be simple, finding the range of resources needed to provide effective intervention is not.

Rural Geography

Geography, for several reasons, creates additional barriers to working with local populations. Most of these ways, moreover, tend to be drawn in comparison with the contexts posed by urban populations. As Amy noted:

I think it's much easier if you've got a concentrated population, to know how to do a few things and be able to get to people. When people are spread out all over the place, it's much more difficult to go into areas and to be able to provide services. It's more costly, it's less efficient to serve a rural community as opposed to urban.

In some cases, geographic challenges manifested in problems accessing data. Jennifer, for example, who oversaw a CHNA that spanned multiple states, notes:

…when you would talk to people at the state level…Kentucky had decent data, but it wasn't as current as Ohio. But Indiana, we often just had trouble even figuring out what data had rolled up…So I think in a small town, there's a few places, not too many, but there are a few places that they were so small that the numbers were suppressed because you'd be able to figure out who was the person who had Hep-C.

The expansiveness of rural populations also presented challenges when developing implementation plans to respond to identified health needs. As Nancy noted:

> delivering the programming is always a challenge when you're serving a rural community because you don't have condensed areas of population, they have to be able to travel to get to it. There's also a lot more difficulty getting into the schools to do health programming, we have that. We try to get creative, like, we do a lot of summer programming at the public library...Those programs have like feeding programs during the summer, they serve lunches and that type of thing, so we can get upwards of 40 or 50 kids in a spot to do stuff. So that's an example of just trying to reach the population when it's spread out and not able to travel to what you're trying to do. So delivering the programming, that part of it, that's always a challenge. Budgeting for it to make sure that you're able to provide the services, particularly for us when you're talking about a health system that serves [multiple] counties. In those counties, for example, we have 31 school districts, over 100 schools. How do we provide equitable programming to all those places? We're not doing it. And it's not because we won't, it's because we can't. Trying to get the resources, the human resources and the monetary resources to do all of that is, it's not easy.

CHNAs directed at areas with large numbers of traditionally underserved populations, framed the experience for many of our interviewees. While most hospital personnel we interviewed reported difficulties in data collection, often because of what they saw as challenges with reaching distant populations. Lauren, however, reported the opposite, noting:

> we had great response, like I said, other than us not being probably as aware of some of our populations like we talked about with the Guatemalans and the Amish. I think we had great response, sometimes I think maybe being a smaller county may have worked to our advantage.

A minority of respondents, therefore, emphasized the unique advantage that Appalachian hospitals may have in that they often are an important institution in their county with existing community relationships in place which may facilitate successful CHNAs – something that urban hospitals might have to put more effort into.

Hospital Resources

These geographic and demographic factors result in clear challenges in carrying out CHNAs. Because most of the hospitals whose employees we interviewed tended to be undercapitalized when compared to their urban counterparts, many employees tasked with doing CHNAs must balance multiple duties, making focus on the CHNAs difficult. For example, Nancy estimated that working on CHNAs accounts for only a third of her time: "I am also the grant writer and grants manager for the health system, I am the government relations officer, I am also their community outreach person." Nancy added that this is probably unique to the Appalachian setting of her hospital. In other hospitals, "Those are all full-time jobs. These are all full-time jobs, even here. But we don't have the resources…." Patricia added:

> You know, going into this, that's something that we didn't necessarily anticipate. Having these new requirements, while they could be positive, they also are a new requirement that is a lot of work. So that's been quite striking. And you're right, it really does vary among the hospitals; some hospitals can afford to pay consultants to produce big reports.

Donna identified staffing as a problem, noting that while "obviously we staff to extremely safe levels and that sort of thing," she also lacked:

> a staff that is just then dedicated to doing community outreach, community benefits, community health. So it was difficult for us to implement some of the programs that we took a look at. For example, we have a problem with women who smoke in their first trimester. Part of it is…getting people to take advantage of the programs that we offered was a struggle….

Sharon added to this theme of problems associated with staffing, noting "you know, it's a mandate that we're required to provide that, we really just don't have the staffing."

Melanie agreed and explained how her institution had been creative to meet these new requirements with limited resources. Her solution was to leverage community partnerships to complete the CHNA and develop an implementation strategy:

> You know, we agreed for example, last community needs assessment, we agreed that obesity prevention was gonna be our one common strategy that we all tried to address over a 3-year period of time. It was based on how each organization would tackle the issues, but we did agree that it would be a common, top-of-mind strategy to improve population health. Again, there's a common purpose, a common theme for all of the activities if that makes sense.

Implementing Programs

For many interviewees, the social context of their hospitals also posed challenges for implementing strategies for addressing those needs. For example, Stacy noted, "that where we need the support is after the assessment is done, what are we gonna do about it? That's where the support needs to come in." Nancy added:

> They want us to be effective in impacting the health, but if there's not a lot of good models for us to follow to do it…I don't know. At the end of the day, I don't know how effective many of us are going to be. I spent a lot of time researching programming that we think will work and trying to develop community programs around clinical stuff we do that we know works, but how can we make it so it reaches the broader community?

For Sarah,

> Carrying out the assessment is not an issue, it's coming up with programs and getting people to participate and be interested in making lifestyle changes. And that may be, I would say some of that is maybe a personal bias in that I've lived and worked in a large metropolitan area as well as living and working here and, you know, the difference is dramatic. As far

> as, you know, the barriers that you're working with here in the Appalachian counties as opposed to some of the others are significant.

Sarah sees problems, as well, in the fact:

> ...that there's requirements to do the assessment and then requirements involved in that with determining actions to help improve the health of the community that you serve. And then, as were defined later as many things as can be objectively measured in regards to the types of things that you're doing to help improve the health of the community, but there's no real funding in essence for that.

Cautious Optimism About CHNA Process and Effects

Doubting that CHNA Process Will Positively Affect Communities

Because of the significant challenges many participants faced in carrying out CHNAs and implementation programs to address needs, our interviews revealed a fairly wide spectrum concerning the degree to which those carrying out CHNAs were optimistic about the impact the new CHNA process was likely to have on local health outcomes. Nancy, when asked whether the CHNA process might improve health outcomes, let out an audible sigh before speaking. She responded:

> if I had to rate it on a scale, I probably would be right in the middle but just slightly to the left on the 'I don't think so'. And again, it has to do with the fact that, you know, what community programs, what types of outreach can you do that is going to be effective to the community that you serve? I find great examples, but many of them are in urban areas. The rural culture and Appalachian culture is something that you have to take into consideration here. You know, health literacy.... I'm not optimistic, not because I don't think people care and don't want to do the work; I'm not optimistic because I don't know that there's evidence-based models out there that are gonna be effective for us and our population.

Her mixed assessment was in large part a reaction to the particular challenges in programming that rural hospitals face, as well as a perceived lack of an evidence base to help them overcome those challenges.

Patricia was also not optimistic, and viewed the process largely as a burden that was likely to have few positive effects. Her view is:

> it's just a lot of paperwork for us to do. I really don't know that the people that really need it, you know, the low-educated people, the people that are in the system on welfare, I don't think they're getting anything out of it.... Yeah, the issues are out there and whether they're getting rectified or not I think we're all trying to take steps towards them, but they're tough. Especially with no funding available for them.

Hillary also exhibited mixed feelings about the process, explaining "I'm not saying that we wouldn't get information back from this that we couldn't use, but I don't know that it's really gonna shape how we are delivering our services." In Hillary's view, converting CHNA findings into tangible change in hospital services is perhaps more challenging than the CHNA process itself.

Describing Change as Slow in Community Health

Though not necessarily a pessimistic view, Amy emphasized the difficult, and at times imperceptibly slow, process of changing health outcomes and behaviors. Addressing smoking and tobacco use, for example, she asked:

> how many years has it taken us to really start seeing a decline? You know, it's like 20, 25, 30 years ago they started that process and you're seeing the benefits today. And I think it's the same thing with doing these community health needs assessments and working to impact communities. I think it's gonna be a slow process but, you know, I think it'll get there in time…Long-term, yes. With anything, you have so much ingrained and embedded issues, so many issues help determine the lifestyle. And it really takes a long time, long-term work in order to make impact. I think that, you know, re-doing this every three years, you're really not gonna see dramatic changes in what those community needs are or what direction you're going. But I think, you know, when you start going and looking 20 years back, when we reach that point I think yes, you will see that.

Chantelle similarly expressed optimism attenuated by what she perceived as socioeconomic realities. At the same time, there were worse consequences to not attempting to take on these challenges now, however difficult change would be. She explained:

> I think when you deal with the magnitude of the problems that have been identified, like substance abuse, for us to even move the needle even if everybody is fully resourced, is going to be really hard. But I think it gives us direction and I think if we can collaborate on an ongoing basis with our community partners, maybe we can be more strategic in the way we address some of these massive needs. And these are just such huge problems that honestly, if we don't get worse, that would be progress in some ways.

Believing CHNAs will Improve Local Health Outcomes

Sarah, whose institution had a more complicated view of the CHNA process, was more optimistic, but, like others in our sample, that optimism was muted by her perceptions of socioeconomic conditions. She noted, for example:

> I would like to think that it, you know, I think that we believe that it will have some impact. Again, I'm not sure if we're 100% convinced that we have enough resources and enough funding, particularly in Appalachia given the fact that if you look at most of the counties in Ohio that fall into that category, we tend to have lower income, more uninsured and then higher rates of poor lifestyle choices and higher rates of chronic disease. Again, cultures that are, you know, have maybe been rooted for a while that are more rooted in unhealthier lifestyle. Um, so I think that we hope that it'll do that, I don't know if we have enough resources to be able to counteract some of the things we have working against us. That's certainly our hope and our intention, but I can't, I don't think any of us could say with certainty…you know, that we could ultimately, compared to again other areas of the state that may not be, there's non-Appalachian areas of the state that may not have quite the same level of issues.

Stacy, however, is optimistic that the work invested in health education in the community will pay off over time. She explains:

> I think certainly the efforts that we've put out there have been beneficial. You know, we also know that our region is, you know, less healthy. And regions around us, movement on

patient behavior is slow. So us having to do these guidelines are not gonna change people's desire to change their health, but you know, our hope is that having resources and education...you know, we've been doing it for years and we keep plugging away and over time that's gonna have an impact.

Susan's optimism is rooted in her institution's comparatively high level of capitalization and commitment to the CHNA process. Though she finds some aspects of the process to be "burdensome," her institution responded by hiring additional staff to support this work. She explained: "it's burdensome for only a short time and then when you see the impact that it makes, you realize that it was the right thing to do and that it was worth it."

Lauren recast the question of the effects that the CHNA she led was poised to make on her community as, "do we think this has been worth it?" which she posed to her colleagues. She reports, "And really the consensus from that group was yes."

Discussion

Given that socioeconomic and geographic challenges are very much part of the Appalachian context, the fact that barriers to improving health emerged as some of the most significant findings is unsurprising. However, an unexpected finding was that optimism about the impact of CHNAs varied across hospitals despite recognized and oftentimes similar challenges. To the extent that the ACA promises to bring about change in some of the USA's high need areas, Appalachia represents one of the greatest challenges, as well as a site in which improvements may be most impactful. In other words, in Appalachia we may be able to more acutely observe whether or not the ACA's various mechanisms – of which CHNAs and new community benefit rules are merely one piece – can drive positive changes in health outcomes.

Although several major findings emerged related to the experience of conducting CHNAs in the Appalachian context, several distinctions are worth exploring. For example, concerns about financial resources underlie most hospital employees' perspectives on the CHNA process, and undercut many efforts at addressing health needs identified in the reports. Furthermore, hospitals within our sample were situated differently with regard to the number of employees dedicated to the CHNA process and financial resources available for both producing the official CHNA report and for supporting follow-up implementation activities. One particularly interesting finding was that employees from hospitals that are part of larger systems felt that there were adequate resources at their disposal, but faced challenges engaging the local community, whom they at times felt distanced and disconnected from.

Some hospital systems, for example, conducted CHNAs from one primary location, resulting in difficulties developing the relationships necessary to partner with local social service organizations, health departments, and residents to implement programs. As a result, financial resources should be seen as only one challenge underlying community health improvement in this region. Equally important is for hospitals who do not currently have ties to the communities they serve to focus their efforts on establishing pathways for communicating with local organizations who are already enmeshed in a community. Our interviews further suggest that an awareness of this challenge is a critical step toward ensuring that hospitals that are part of larger systems adequately represent community perspectives in their report. Because CHNAs produced by large systems must make sense of needs across large geographic areas, it is difficult to appreciate the diversity of local contexts and to facilitate the relationships necessary to develop site-specific interventions that will benefit all locales equally.

At the same time, however, many of the smaller hospitals that either were not part of a system, or whose CHNAs were not being done in coordination with their system, reported benefits stemming from their smaller status, especially as regards their knowledge of the community. In some cases, these hospitals felt that their closeness to community members and organizations yielded higher response rates in data collection and an advantage in developing the partnerships necessary to carry out CHNAs and subsequently develop collaborative implementation projects. In other words, although larger systems are better capitalized financially for large-scale CHNAs and general community benefit funding, smaller hospitals may subsidize their community benefit work through the social and cultural capital developed by virtue of their status within a rural community. This positioning may allow independent rural hospitals to expand existing relationships in the promotion of new community health initiatives. Likewise, larger health systems that possess the capital and lack the community relationships needed to implement their plan could use their capital to form relationships with stakeholders across their service area to foster social capital – instead of focusing on using the financial advantage they do have on a few site-specific interventions.

In addition to distinguishing between the different types of challenges that various hospitals face in this region, our findings also suggest important differences in the optimism that exists regarding the ability to improve health outcomes through hospital–community engagement. For many hospital employees, the opportunity to undertake CHNAs with the formal rigor required by ACA and IRS guidelines, serves as an opportunity to make good on their passion for public health. For these individuals, post-ACA CHNAs are seen as an opportunity to realize hospitals' ultimate goals of preventing illness and actively seeking out opportunities to tackle large, even seemingly intractable problems. Although most interviewees made clear that low resources and other challenges were significant impediments to progress, the process itself made sense to them and provided them with clear questions about what it would take to use the CHNA and post-CHNA programming to positively impact health outcomes and address social problems.

In contrast, some hospital employees and consultants were not confident that either CHNAs or the programs their results encourage would be enough to move the needle on local health outcomes. Our interviews suggest four main reasons for this pessimism. In each case, these attitudes reflected not only the CHNA process itself, but specific conditions owing to the challenges of doing CHNAs in underserved, rural areas such as Appalachian Ohio.

First, some participants believe that rural and Appalachian culture produces something of a culture of complacency that will result in hospital outreach falling on deaf ears. More specifically, many participants suggested that providing support for good health will not be effective if individuals do not take personal responsibility for their own health. In this way, some interviewees' perspectives reflected a common ideological thread in American health policy and politics, namely, an emphasis on individual behaviors and choices over systemic, socioeconomic, and structural conditions. These views draw upon ongoing debates about the cause of disparities, wherein those involved in devising solutions attempt to ascribe weight to quite different factors in an attempt to steer solutions toward one area over another (Resnik, 2007). For example, when attempting to address a disparity that is widely discussed as a function of individual behaviors – like physical activity or diet – the solutions to the problem will likely be focused on changing the behavior, not the conditions that caused the behavior. Thornton and colleagues explain that "if one's neighborhood is unsafe even during daylight hours and an individual lacks the resources to move to a safer neighborhood, interventions targeting outdoor physical activity are unlikely to be effective" (Thornton et al., 2016).

The reliance on personal factors as an explanation for inequality has been described as a "dominant ideology" among Americans (Kluegel & Smith, 1986). More specifically related to health, neoliberal ideology has been cited as an important framework for downplaying structural support for addressing health inequalities in favor of individual actions (Peacock, Bissell, & Owen, 2014). The language of personal responsibility has long been central to American identity (Franklin & Seavey, 2008; Lavin, 2008) and has persisted during ACA legislative debates and implementation (Gollust & Lynch, 2011). Instead of focusing only on this lens, however, some participants working on CHNAs emphasized individual-level factors such as motivation as major drivers of health outcomes *in addition to* structural barriers such as unemployment, access to care, or proximity of healthful, quality food outlets. Unsurprisingly, given these seemingly intractable barriers, many hospital employees believe that their efforts with CHNA and community benefit will only take hold if significant changes in individual behavior take place as well.

Second, some interviewees appeared to be weighing the potential population health benefits to the bureaucratic and resource intensiveness of the CHNA process. In these comments there is a palpable sense of being overwhelmed by the CHNA process itself, but also the conditions under which they, at their mostly under-resourced hospitals, were expected to carry out the process. Although not all of our participants described financial strain, there is evidence that taking on CHNAs might produce more challenges for small, rural hospitals which have fewer beds, staff, and more narrow profit margins than their urban counterparts (Kaufman et al., 2016; Younis, 2013). As a result, allocating personnel to carry out CHNAs or finding resources for developing new programs may be difficult for some hospitals. In addition, rural hospitals tend to be located within populations that have a disproportionate amount of aging residents, poverty, and morbidity (National Rural Health Association, 2016). The cumulative result of these factors may mean that if significant health issues arise in CHNA reports, hospitals may not have the resources to address problems if they are outside of existing expertise, require significant investment of resources, or rely on dedicated staff to engage geographically dispersed communities.

Third, while many interviewees expressed positivity regarding the CHNA process and what was required of hospitals, some were less than optimistic about the prospects of converting that process into tangible programs due to a lack of institutional buy-in. Here, it appears, our research illuminates a major crossroads for medicine, in general, and for nonprofit hospitals more specifically, as the latter adjust to quite different institutional contexts and even a revision of the traditional hospitals' mission. By expanding hospitals' responsibilities to the surrounding community in addition to specific patient populations, the CHNA process requires a willingness to reorganize existing community benefit practices and adjust both staffing and strategic planning. In addition, the potential inclusion of nonmedical social determinants of health as areas of focus for hospitals stands to radically change the role of hospitals – a change that cannot be done without buy-in. The extent to which hospitals are willing to change existing and ingrained practice models will likely mediate the effectiveness of new CHNA requirements in changing health outcomes and reducing health care costs (Rosenbaum, 2016).

Fourth, the most optimistic interviewees in our sample, we found, held this view for clear reasons. In particular, hospital employees whose professional backgrounds were based in community health, community benefit, or nursing departments, were consistently more optimistic than those located in business, marketing, or development. In this way, a sense of hope in our sample was seemingly related to whether a hospital connected community benefit activities with public health or with business practices tied to retaining nonprofit status. Institutional culture, in other words, may play a role in determining whether community benefit inspires a shift toward community health programming or retains a traditional focus on direct patient care with community benefit as a pesky side-requirement. In making progress toward community-level investments, we argue that optimism may play an important role. The motivational aspect of progress may be especially critical when those carrying out day-to-day efforts are residents of the communities they serve or facing barriers to improving significant health disparities.

Conclusion

The ACA's community benefit requirements stand to effectuate change in local communities by requiring nonprofit hospitals to assume new roles in the promotion of population health through community engagement. Yet, although the regulations themselves apply to nonprofit hospitals in general, our qualitative study finds that their impact varies – in some cases widely – depending on context. It is therefore difficult to make large claims about community benefit and CHNAs without engaging the contexts and particulars of hospitals as they are located in specific communities, with varying resources and histories. In the case of the present study, focused on Ohio's Appalachian region, we have underscored the specific challenges of undertaking CHNAs in rural and vulnerable communities, where expansive geographic space, low socioeconomic status, and access to health care present significant challenges. Despite these barriers, however, our study suggests that many hospital employees tasked with overseeing the CHNA process see promise, even if their optimism about the prospect of improving health conditions is muted in light of regional challenges. In each case, the degree of optimism can be read as thoughtfulness not only about the CHNA process, but the socioeconomic realities facing these hospitals. Given the contemporary embrace of population health interventions, and innovative strategies for investing in programs that promise to reduce health disparities, the possibility exists for well-capitalized funding sources – including and perhaps especially those emanating from the federal government – to see value in providing increased support for hospital-initiated programs that promise to promote wellness and reduce disparity in rural and vulnerable populations.

References

American Hospital Association. (2019). *Fast Facts on U.S. Hospitals, 2019*. https://www.aha.org/statistics/fast-facts-us-hospitals

Beatty, K. E., Wilson, K. D., Ciecior, A., & Stringer, L. (2015). Collaboration among Missouri nonprofit hospitals and local health departments: Content analysis of community health needs assessments. *American Journal of Public Health, 105*(S2), S337–S344.

Borak, J., Salipante-Zaidel, C., Slade, M. D., & Fields, C. A. (2012). Mortality disparities in Appalachia: Reassessment of major risk factors. *Journal of Occupational and Environmental Medicine, 54*(2), 146–156.

Burke, J. G., Truong, S., Albert, S., Steenrod, J., Gibert, C., Folb, B., et al. (2014). What can be learned from the types of community benefit programs that hospitals already have in place? *Journal of Healthcare for the Poor and Underserved, 25*(1 Suppl), 165–193.

Charmaz, K. (2006). *Constructing grounded theory: A practical guide through qualitative data analysis*. London, UK: Sage.

Evashwick, C. J. (2013). *Hospitals & community benefit: New demands, new approaches*. Chicago, IL: Health Administration Press.

Folkemer, D. C., Spicer, L. A., Mueller, C. H., Somerville, M. H., Brow, A. L. R., Milligan, C. J., & Boddie-Willis, C. L. (2011). *Hospital community benefits after the ACA: The emerging federal framework*. The Hilltop Institute Issue Brief, January.

Foucault, M. (1973). *The birth of the clinic* (A. M. Sheridan, Trans.). New York, NY: Vintage.

Franklin, B., & Seavey, O. (2008). *Autobiography and other writings*. Oxford: Oxford University Press.

Gollust, S., & Lynch, J. (2011). Who deserves health care? The effects of causal attributions and group cues on public attitudes about responsibility for health care costs. *Journal of Health Politics, Policy and Law, 36*(6), 1061–1095.

Goffman, E. (1961). *Asylums: Essays on the social situation of mental patients and other inmates*. New York, NY: Anchor Books.

Halverson, J. A., & Bischak, G. (2008). *Underlying socioeconomic factors influencing health disparities in the Appalachian region*. Washington, DC: Appalachian Regional Commission. Available at: http://www.arc.gov/assets/research_reports/socioeconomicfactorsinfluencinghealthdisparitiesinappalachianregion5.pdf

Hendryx, M. (2009). Mortality from heart, respiratory, and kidney disease in coal mining areas of Appalachia. *International Archives of Occupational and Environmental Health, 82*(2), 243–249.

Hendryx, M., & Ahern, M. M. (2009). Mortality in Appalachian coal mining regions: The value of statistical life lost. *Public Health Reports, 124*(4), 541–550.

Internal Revenue Service. (2018). *Private letter ruling: Certified mail -return receipt*. Dallas, TX: Tax Exempt and Government Entities Division. Available at: https://www.irs.gov/pub/irs-wd/201829017.pdf

Internal Revenue Service. (2013). *Community health needs assessments for charitable hospitals*. Federal Register, available at: https://www.federalregister.gov/articles/2013/04/05/2013-07959/community-health-needs-assessments-for-charitable-hospitals

Jacobs, L. R., & Skocpol, T. (2012). *Health care reform and American politics: What everyone needs to know*. Oxford, UK: Oxford University Press.

Kaufman, B. G., Thomas, S. R., Randolph, R. K., Perry, J. R., Thompson, K. W., Holmes, G. M., et al. (2016). The rising rate of rural hospital closures. *Journal of Rural Health, 32*(1), 35–43.

Kluegel, J., & Smith, E. R. (1986). *Beliefs about inequality*. New York, NY: Aldine de Gruyter.

Lavin, C. (2008). *The politics of responsibility*. Urbana, IL: University of Illinois Press.

Ludke, R. L., & Obermiller, P. J. (Eds.). (2012). *Appalachian health and well-being*. Lexington, KY: University of Kentucky Press.

Morrone, M., Kruse, N. A., & Chadwick, A. E. (2014). Environmental and health disparities in Appalachian Ohio: Perceptions and realities. *Journal of Health Disparities Research and Practice, 7*(5), 67–81.

National Rural Health Association. (2016). *What's different about rural health care?* http://www.ruralhealthweb.org/go/left/about-rural-health

Peacock, M., Bissell, P., & Owen, J. (2014). Dependency denied: Health inequalities in the neoliberal era. *Social Science and Medicine, 118*, 173–180.

Pennel, C. L., McLeroy, K. R., Burdine, J. N., & Mataritta-Cascante, D. (2015). Nonprofit hospitals' approach to community health needs assessment. *American Journal of Public Health., 105*(3), e103–e113.

Resnik, D. B. (2007). Responsibility for health: Personal, social, and environmental. *Journal of Medical Ethics, 33*(8), 444–445.

Rosenbaum, S. (2015). Additional requirements for charitable hospitals: Final rules on community health needs assessments and financial assistance. *Health Affairs Blog, 23*.

Rosenbaum, S. (2016). Hospital community benefit spending: Leaning in on the social determinants of health, 94(2), 251–254.

Smith, L., & Hollorman, C. H. (2011). Health status and access to health care services: A comparison between Ohio's rural non-Appalachian and Appalachian families. *Family and Community Health, 34*(2), 102–110.

Starr, P. (1982). *The social transformation of American medicine: The rise of a sovereign profession and the making of a vast industry*. New York: Basic Books.

Starr, P. (2013). *Remedy and reaction: The peculiar American struggle over health care reform*. New Haven, CT: Yale University Press.

Strauss, A., & Corbin, J. (1998). *Basics of qualitative research: Techniques and procedures for developing grounded theory* (2nd ed.). Thousand Oaks, CA: Sage Publications.

Thornton, R. L. J., Glover, C. M., Cené, C. W., Glik, D. C., Henderson, J. A., & Williams, D. R. (2016). Evaluating strategies for reducing health disparities by addressing the social determinants of health. *Health Affairs*. (Project Hope),, *35*(8), 1416–1423.

Walker, D., & Myrick, F. (2006). Grounded theory: An exploration of process and procedure. *Qualitative Health Research, 16*(4), 547–559.

Wewers, M. E., Katz, M., Fickle, D., & Paskett, E. D. (2006). Risky behaviors among Ohio Appalachian adults. *Preventing Chronic Disease, 3*, 1–8.

Wilson, K. D., Mohr, L. B., Beatty, K. E., & Ciecior, A. (2014). Describing the continuum of collaboration among local health departments with hospitals around the community health assessments. *Journal of Public Health Management and Practice, 20*(6), 617–625.

Young, G. J., Chou, C., Alexander, J., Lee, S. D., & Raver, E. (2013). Provision of community benefits by tax-exempt U.S. hospitals. *The New England Journal of Medicine, 368*, 1519–1527.

Younis, M. Z. (2013). A comparison study of urban and small rural hospitals financial and economic performance. *Online Journal of Rural Nursing and Health Care, 3*(1), 38–48.

Chapter 9
Community-Based Political Interventions

Karie Jo Peralta and Krista McCarthy Noviski

Introduction

Community control is key for interventions to address local health concerns (World Health Organization, 1986). For this authority to be established, community participation is necessary. Underlying this element is an appreciation of a community's ability to contribute knowledge and skills to the planning and implementation of health initiatives (Israel, Checkoway, Schulz, & Zimmerman, 1994). Community-based projects thus take into consideration the capacities of individuals to communicate their intimate understandings of their well-being, grasp medical information, learn preventative measures, and implement primary care techniques (e.g., Rahman et al., 2019; Smallwood et al., 2015).

There are many examples of community-based training and capacity building efforts in community-based health initiatives. Typically, they aim to increase popular knowledge of medical issues, improve health-care delivery, and strengthen the research skills of individuals, organizations, and communities (Cueva, Cueva, Revels, & Dignan, 2018; Ruiz et al., 2012; Saad-Harfouche et al., 2011). What is often lacking in these endeavors is a focus on their institutional contexts and how they may prevent self-determination and local control.

This chapter addresses this gap by applying a community-based framework to examine structures that shape community health projects and their links with local participation. Special attention is given to the political dimension of traditional and community-based health organizations. The purpose is to illustrate how institutional facets may either undermine or support communities in taking charge of their health.

K. J. Peralta (✉) · K. McCarthy Noviski
Department of Sociology and Anthropology, The University of Toledo, Toledo, OH, USA
e-mail: Karie.Peralta@utoledo.edu; Krista.Mccarthy@rockets.utoledo.edu

S. L. Arxer, J. W. Murphy (eds.), *Community-Based Health Interventions in an Institutional Context*, International Perspectives on Social Policy, Administration, and Practice, https://doi.org/10.1007/978-3-030-24654-9_9

This analysis is important for identifying and demystifying oppressive structures in community health initiatives, as well as crucial for recognizing how institutions may be designed to reinforce a community's authority over its health.

At the outset of this chapter, the theoretical framework that guides the present analysis is described. Next, institutional barriers to community participation are explained, followed by a discussion of structures that support a community's control over its well-being. The last section concludes by stressing the importance of community-based theory for creating conditions that encourage communities to direct their own health progress.

Analytical Framework

A community-based lens reveals transformative possibilities for organizations and projects to become aligned with the aspirations of communities. In health contexts, using a community-based framework can bring into view aspects that obstruct a community's ability to make decisions about its well-being. Furthermore, applying this perspective can expose prospects for local participation, which is at the heart of community-based health initiatives (World Health Organization, 1986).

Central to community-based philosophy (Murphy, 2014) is its rejection of realism and dualism (Delanty, 1997). What is particularly problematic with realism is its assumption that there is a domain independent from individuals where principles and values reside, and these elements regulate human behavior and promote social order (Durkheim, 1974). Along these lines, the realities of a community are considered in structural terms (Parsons, 1951) and understood to be separate from its members (Delanty, 1997).

In this view, structures are believed to be objective and, given their universal and absolute basis for action, have a powerful influence over individuals (Durkheim, 1974). Realism may be at play in medical situations when, for example, nurses follow their rounding schedules and protocols for providing care, even when they see that they have a negative effect on the patient experience. These job-related conditions may appear to be solidified and not within the nurses' power to change (Berger & Luckmann, 1966), and so they continue their service as if they were unable to make adjustments in their schedules and tasks.

With regard to dualism, community-based philosophy takes issue with the assumption that value-free information exists in a realm outside persons (Murphy, 2014). The notion that the mind is separate from the body informs the belief that personal perspectives are invalid, due to their subjective nature (Bordo, 1987). Accordingly, objectivity is promoted as the gold standard. Dualism therefore grounds the positivist approach that suggests that only individuals with scientific training have the ability to grasp unbiased knowledge. The reason is that science entails following systematic procedures that remove prejudices and partialities (Delanty, 1997).

When health-care organizations operate according to dualism, efforts to humanize interventions are undermined from the start. Take empathy training in medical schools, for example. Teaching medical students to show empathy toward their patients is challenged by the dualistic biomedical model that physicians are expected to follow. This issue causes tension when diagnosing a medical condition and developing an understanding of a patient's life experience with illness (Pedersen, 2010).

Adherence to dualism results in two general issues that prevent institutions from truly supporting communities in the realization of their health goals. The first is the weakening of the belief in community agency through affirmations of the realist illusion that the social world is detached from individuals (Bourdieu, 1990). For example, organizational problems are seen as natural and, therefore, beyond human control. Communities may thus consider themselves to be incapable of creating change. The second issue is the marginalization of local knowledge through assertions that cling to ways of knowing that disregard individual and interpersonal understandings grounded in daily life experiences (Fals Borda, 1988).

Unlike dualism, a community-based view emphasizes social constructionism and participation (Murphy, 2014). The core idea is that communities co-create their social worlds and critical consciousness of their worlds through dialogue (Freire, 1970). Therefore, community members are not subjected simply to impinging social forces, such as norms, that shape their experiences. Nor are they ever severed from what is known. Rather, they construct their realities and knowledge and linguistically give meaning to them in an interpersonal and cooperative manner (Merleau-Ponty, 1968; Wittgenstein, 1958).

A participatory vision of health care positions the community at the center of interventions (World Health Organization, 1986). All guiding ideas, forms of organizing, and decisions emanate from the group and stem from the negotiated interpretations of its members (Minkler & Wallerstein, 2012). Despite the technical knowledge that medical experts may be able to offer, these persons do not dominate the scene. While their insights may be eventually deemed to be important by the community for an initiative, the indigenous knowledge (Fals Borda, 1988) co-generated by community members through intersubjective communication (Gadamer, 1975) is what establishes communal plans and actions.

Power in community-based projects is thus shared between all community members (Minkler & Wallerstein, 2012), including medical professionals committed to the group's health. Because all individuals are inextricably linked to knowledge, identifying and making sense of symptoms, as well as interpreting lived experiences of illnesses, are accomplished through face-to-face dialogue (Buber, 1970). In this way, community members are empowered and viewed as having the capacity to contribute significantly to processes intended to improve their health outcomes in forms other than merely checking boxes in a health history form or following a doctor's order. In a community-based sense, such actions are always up for discussion between all groups potentially affected by the decisions being made.

The next section applies this analytical framework to assess institutional facets of traditional organizations and projects. Determinations are made with respect to how they may inhibit community participation. Particular attention is given to elements that are typically taken-for-granted, but are, nevertheless, critical for recognizing necessary structural changes, if a project is to become community-based.

Institutional Barriers to Community Participation

Norms that Constrain Community Participation

Institutions are imbued with social norms that consist of expectations that guide the actions of group members. In the Western philosophical tradition that supports traditional health organizations, norms fall under the category of "social facts" (Durkheim, 1982/2013, p. 29). Durkheim (1982/2013) explains that social facts should be regarded as "things" (p. 29) that are disconnected from individuals. Accordingly, norms are believed to hold an objective status with an imposing influence that motivates people to behave in uniform ways and, thus, stabilizes an organization by producing social order.

When formally institutionalized in medical settings, norms become written rules and policies for practitioner conduct (Borkowski, 2015). Most health-care organizations, for example, have established procedures that range from proper practices for attending to patients to processes for executing successfully a community health needs assessment. When these official norms are broken, the result is often reprimand, if not punishment.

Informal norms, on the other hand, are the implicitly, shared understood standards for behaving and interacting (Durkheim, 1982/2013). For instance, Barnato, Tate, Rodriguez, Zickmund, and Arnold (2012) observed critical care physicians accept passively the instructions of specialists. They considered this submissiveness to be attributed to the general understanding of informal norms that allude to appropriate ways to respond to individuals with greater decision-making power.

From a community-based perspective, norms in and of themselves are not problematic. After all, they are significant cultural elements that can facilitate interactions and the co-generation of popular knowledge (Geertz, 1973). In endeavors intended to be community-based, however, norms that constrain community participation are the concern. Such norms likely originate from the dualistic view that assumes a division between communities and their knowledge bases and, therefore, do not give credence to the principles and ethics that are determined by community members. This issue typically plays out in a health context where there is a preoccupation with information that is value-neutral and when outlooks on treatments and healing are expected to be unbiased and free from emotion.

These objective data and views are believed typically to be acquired through the use of the scientific method that involves the implementation of standardized procedures and rules (Delanty, 1997). The emphasis is on applying the language of science to verify truths and confirm logical beliefs about empirical data (Sankey, 2000). In the ordinary medical environment, solely physicians and other health experts are thought to be capable of obtaining factual and, therefore, useful information because of their high-level technical education and scientific literacy. Consequently, the participation of regular community members would be judged to be a distraction to making and evaluating observations, based on the notion that these rules-based approaches for rationalization require specialized knowledge and sound methodological techniques of which average citizens are not aware.

In conventional health-care organizations, actions guided by norms that elevate professional perspectives over local insight restrict community contributions and participation on a regular basis in simple, yet important, ways. For example, patients are often made to feel more like a number than an individual. Their stories about their experiences of sickness are seldom given adequate time and attention by physicians, because of scheduling policies and the subjective nature of patient experiences (Rhodes, McFarland, Finch, & Johnson, 2001).

In sum, there is a need to recognize the issue with the traditional understanding of norms. When they are considered to be an external force, beyond the power of individuals, and seemingly natural (Durkheim, 1982/2013), there leaves little hope for realigning health organizations with a humanistic orientation. Planners informed by a community-based viewpoint do no buy into the function of norms as controlling a community. Rather, they presume that interpretation mediates understandings of norms (Barthes, 1987) and appreciate the ability of individuals to engage one another in the creation and maintenance of local arrangements (Berger & Luckmann, 1966) that encourage behaviors consistent with a community's ideals.

Schemes that Sideline Community Members

Traditional health-care organizations typically strive to be effective by operating in accordance with Fayol's (1949) management principles. They include the establishment of order and a hierarchy of positions. Individuals are expected to employ their technical skills and carry out specialized tasks, while following administrative rules and codes of conduct. These bureaucratic elements support a top-down chain of command. Power is thus centralized at the top ranks (Weber, 1978).

This imagery is consistent with the realist framework that presumes reality is controlled by an elevated base where social norms and power exist (Durkheim, 1982/2013). Organizations constructed according to this assumption are likely led by persons with high qualifications, extensive training, and substantial proficiency, who are believed to be capable of offering unbiased and fair assessments geared toward increasing productivity. Accordingly, the expectation of low-status organizational members is that they obey directives and complete their duties without thinking critically about them.

At this point, the concept of roles is in need of consideration. Realists view roles as being interdependent parts of a social system. The functioning of the system is reliant on the execution of the responsibilities assigned to each role. When roles are not fulfilled, the connections between them weaken and, as a result, the system becomes unbalanced and may even fail. The purpose of social norms is then to guide role behaviors with the aim of ensuring order, and the system is set up in a way to discourage anyone from doing more or less than what their role requires (Parsons, 1951).

To illustrate, the organization of health departments is depicted commonly in the shape of a pyramid. The commissioner is often at the peak. This supervisory role is supported by a board committee that is full of medical professionals who advise on policy matters, provide guidance on programs and services, and handle the budget. Below this group is the administrative staff with managerial responsibilities, followed by the providers, who implement the services. What is evident in this case is not only the hierarchy but also the interdependence of roles. For example, the service providers count on the board to oversee responsibly the department's finances, otherwise there would be a reduction of services. At the same time, their position restricts them from implementing consequences if the higher-ups mismanage the organization. In the event that any role goes unfilled, there is bound to be instability, at least temporarily, because there is a low likelihood of anyone stepping seamlessly into another role.

These schemes are not consistent with a community-based orientation, because they impede community members from holding meaningful organizational positions and taking on leadership roles. Moreover, they exclude local persons from taking part in decision-making processes that concern their lives. A case in point is when a panel of researchers meet to discuss a virus that is spreading through a region and consider options to combat the epidemic without any community members present. In this example, the opinions of various professionals are taken into account and the pros and cons of different approaches to fight the outbreak are debated without the perspectives of the community.

The essence of community-based endeavors is community members and, without their direction, projects run the risk of being insensitive to a group's needs (Minkler & Wallerstein, 2012). Writing on his community-based efforts in Colombia, Fals Borda (1979) noted that "when the actual level of consciousness of the situation encountered (that of the members of the basic communities) was taken into account as a starting point for action…, political errors caused by excessive activism or ignorance were avoided" (p. 50). His work exemplifies how community-based projects are rooted in communal ideas and understandings, rather than in colonizing and imperialist assertions that dehumanize community members and relegate them to the periphery of their own realities.

Even seemingly minor symbols in traditional health-care intuitions should be reconsidered such as the sliding window in waiting rooms and online patient portals used for disseminating test results. These features may be interpreted as barriers between individuals and their care. Technology, in fact, is often assumed to be a tool to enhance neutrality, which is part of the positivist tradition (Delanty, 1997) and may impede local participation.

Routines that Restrain Community Action

Greenwood, Oliver, Sahlin, and Suddaby (2008) define a routine as a "more-or-less taken-for-granted repetitive social behavior that is underpinned by normative systems and cognitive understandings that give meaning to social exchange and thus enable self-reproducing social order" (pp. 4–5). In organizations, these context-specific behavioral patterns facilitate the coordination of individuals and transfer of information with minimal mental effort (Becker, 2004). Furthermore, institutionalized recurrent actions are believed to create organizational stability (Howard-Grenville, Rerup, Langley, & Tsoukas, 2016).

Essentially, this common view of routines relies on realism. Bourdieu (1990) explains that what allows behaviors to become repetitive over time and, eventually, institutions, is the dependence on seemingly autonomous structures for guidance. Individuals therefore perform routines as if they were merely mindless, passive actors. Because human agency is distinct from structure, the maintenance of the status quo is almost guaranteed.

Routines are commonplace in health-care settings (O'leary & Mhaolrúnaigh, 2012). To a large extent, patients can predict accurately how their appointments in a health clinic will come to pass. From check in to check out, routines are enacted continuously. Any deviation from expected patterns of behaviors is likely to be viewed as problematic, suspicious, or awkward. For example, a patient would probably feel uneasy if prescribed medicine before being examined thoroughly.

From a community-based standpoint, routines in health-care projects are not inherently troubling. Rather, they become concerning when they are reinforced by dualism and, thus, believed to be unalterable. Additionally, this understanding overlooks the abilities of individuals to innovate and create new practices (Howard-Grenville et al., 2016). In health-care institutions, dehumanizing routines are bound to undermine the self-determination of persons. This issue becomes evident when health professionals are so worried about upholding rules that they continue to follow them even while their actions undermine their ability to reach organizational goals (Merton, 1939).

In a public health survey, for instance, interviewers are expected to administer the questionnaire in the same way with each respondent. Because the principle of objectivity underpins this process, entertaining the perspectives of participants will only sidetrack researchers and taint the results. Therefore, what is not usually built into this standardized information gathering routine are opportunities for respondents to explain their health experiences in detail.

A community-based approach, however, would not view such a break from the routine as a distraction. In fact, this action would be common practice. Because knowledge is mediated by language (Lyotard, 1984), dialogue with survey participants is considered necessary for obtaining insight into local realities. Such engagement allows the interviewer access to the community's biography (Berger & Luckmann, 1966), which is composed of the interlinked meanings that individuals attach to their group's culture, history, and prospects for their collective future. Given the emphasis on anti-dualism in community-based philosophy (Murphy, 2014), accessing and correctly interpreting a community's biography should be standard in community-based projects.

Institutions that Support Community Authority

The rest of this chapter explores how community-based institutions foster local participation. Of primary focus are values, formations, and communication that center communities in health interventions. In contrast to a dualistic view that considers these institutional elements as autonomous and controlling (Durkheim, 1982/2013), a community-based perspective facilitates an understanding of these features as always interpretive and socially constructed (Berger & Luckmann, 1966). This theoretical shift is necessary to create institutional contexts that support social action and sustain community momentum.

Values that Promote a Community's Vision

Interventions that are community-based adhere to local values (Fals Borda, 1988). Therefore, community-based planners should learn the residents' ideals and ethics, as well as the meanings that they give to them. Only then may a planner begin to grasp a community's logic and contribute meaningfully to the design of project goals. Nonetheless, in a truly community-based initiative, a group's health aims are always determined by its members and are founded on their understandings of what objectives may be possible to meet. This process integrates the unique standpoints of community members by respecting their personal perspectives, interpretations of their collective experiences, and the lessons that they have learned from their everyday lives (Hancock & Minkler, 2012).

Traditional medical professionals and health practitioners, who rely on positivist procedures for project development, tend not to operate with this appreciation. These persons typically enter a community with the belief that their objective knowledge is what may serve the group best. For example, public health consultants may propose drafts of policies for medical clinics without engaging their communities of practitioners and patients together in dialogue about their health-care service experiences. In these cases, there is little reason to engage a community in the creation of health plans, because neutral information derived from the generalizable results of scientific research is what is considered important. Accordingly, conventional approaches involve the imposition of values that hold in high regard technology and strategies for obtaining unbiased data.

What a community-based lens brings into view is how social norms, including morals and customs, are established through "joint action" (Blumer, 1969, p. 17).

Moreover, behavioral patterns are believed to spring from arrangements of social action (Blumer, 1969). The implication for the development of community-based organizations is that institutional rules and expectations that are commonly thought to be outside the control of individuals, in actuality, may be created from local interpretations. Structures, therefore, may be grounded in the agreed upon meanings that group members give to their realities and, in turn, may be designed to be consistent with a community's vision.

From a community-based perspective, what is important to note is that traditional understandings of institutions are problematic, particularly with respect to who and what guides a project. When a medical organization is the result of local, interpersonal creations (Berger & Luckmann, 1966), the aspirations of a community to be free of environmental health hazards and disease may be articulated in ways that promote group "buy-in" (Woods, 2013) and, thus, allows for community participation to be the centerpiece of a project (Fals Borda, 1988).

In short, values that are generated by communities provide the appropriate guidance for their activities (Berger & Luckmann, 1966). Significantly, a community-based approach encourages communities to use their power to socially construct institutions that support local involvement. At the same time, this orientation takes into account the meanings that individuals give to these institutions, so that they may be (re)shaped in ways that promote local leadership.

Formations that Foster Community Leadership

Community members are the main leaders of community-based projects (Sandmann & Vandenberg, 1995). Without their guidance, interventions are not likely to be effective. Institutions with a community-based focus thus need a type of organization that espouses local control. Traditional organizations, with their top-down hierarchy, do not usually support this objective. Decision-making power is centralized and enacted by upper-level administrators and executives (Weber, 1978), who are often far removed from direct patient care, settings with barriers to health care, and the challenging realities of residents. This condition tends to marginalize communities in health initiatives and undermines their capabilities to lead.

A horizontal structure, however, intends to eradicate dominating relationships, encourage local participation, and allow for potentially any community member to step up, albeit temporarily, to contribute their skills to a project (Ramnarayan, 2011a). Local residents, for example, provide guidance on the activities of neighborhood health centers and ensure grassroots planning and supervision (Cooper et al., 2016). When power is decentralized (Ramnarayan, 2011a), communities have the opportunity to oversee their health development and take ownership of initiatives that are supposed to benefit them. Moreover, there is a collective commitment to the belief that shared decision-making is in the group's best interest (Locke, 2003) and an appreciation of the stock of local resources that can be drawn from for community improvement purposes (Ramnarayan, 2011b).

Because the ability to lead is not considered to be an inherent quality, persons are seen as capable of learning new skills and training others (Van Wart, 2003). Along these lines, all community members, not only individuals with a high-level proficiency and advanced education, are thought to have the capacity to take on responsibilities in planning and implementation processes (Raelin, 2003). In community-based organizations, even timid individuals who are not considered usually to make good leaders may feel encouraged to offer their voices and talents, rather than go ignored or wait to be asked by an authority figure for their opinion or to assist in an initiative.

Community health workers are a prime example of everyday people engaged in leadership positions (Cooper et al., 2016). These individuals may have low literacy skills and little experience in the health field, but what makes them ideal community leaders is that they have considerable familiarity with a locale, earned respect from their neighbors, and a strong desire to serve others. Their local knowledge may help to create an interpretive frame for identifying community issues and conceptualizing possible interventions (Fals Borda, 1988), while their solid social relationships and dedication to their community may be important unifying factors in a project. Indeed, community health workers have been found to be successful in implementing health services around the world and are valued by many health associations (Cooper et al., 2016; Kim, Farmer, & Porter, 2013; Rahman et al., 2019).

To be clear, health researchers, clinical practitioners, and other medical specialists may hold, at some point, important leadership positions during an initiative. However, they are not conferred high status in projects based on their academic background and medical expertise (Raelin, 2003). In fact, the egalitarian foundation of community-based projects provides an orientation that aims to empower everyone involved and facilitate democratic organization for constructing community knowledge and programs.

Communication that Creates Community Knowledge and Cohesion

Communication is a crucial aspect of participatory processes and community building initiatives (Walter & Hyde, 2012). Writings on practices for open and strategic communication abound in the body of literature on community health interventions. The emphasis is usually on developing technical skills, such as active listening, for effective communication (Li et al., 2018; Tran et al., 2004) and, therefore, considers communication in merely instrumental terms (Mumby, 1997). Clearly, these practical competencies are important, but community-based health promotion recognizes the need to consider health concerns using a discursive understanding of communication in conjunction with social constructionist views of community and culture (Ford & Yep, 2011).

Regarding communication as constitutive calls for engagement with how communities linguistically interpret health and illness and their experiences of these issues (Mokros & Deetz, 1996; Mumby, 1997). This anti-dualist orientation calls for dialogue that is rooted in reflexivity and focused on achieving shared understanding (Cunliffe & Easterby-Smith, 2004). Reflexivity involves the suspension of judgment (Buber, 1970) and the examination of personal assumptions and parameters of perspective. By becoming aware of one's stance and its limits with reference to a particular cultural frame, the foundation is formed for engaging the viewpoints of others (Gadamer, 1975). The challenge, then, becomes arriving at mutual comprehension, which requires grasping the realities of community members. This aim may be achieved through entering into open, reciprocal relationships and recognizing others as fully human (Buber, 1970).

When community members are committed to dialogue, they may discursively build prejudice-free, democratic spaces that allow all community members to express their ideas and challenge one another's views in what Habermas (1984) calls, "the ideal speech situation" (p. 25). In health contexts, a community-based approach involves linguistically contesting and undermining privileged perspectives on disease and medical concerns, so that ideas that are typically marginalized have a chance to be considered fully (Mokros & Deetz, 1996; Mumby, 1997). Accordingly, diversity of thought and the existence of different knowledge bases are not feared, because community members have the ability to understand divergent logics and can agree to disagree (Habermas, 1996). Any differences in statuses among the group are not given any meanings that could influence the marginalization of voices, advance authoritarian views, or result in manipulated consensus. What does rise are the ideas and arguments that stem from authentic communal agreement (Habermas, 1984), which provides the basis for a cohesive effort.

For illustrative purposes, a medical researcher who merely indicates that children need a healthier diet, based on where their measurements fall on a growth chart, may be viewed as futile information when their households lack food for days at a time. In such cases, the children's experiences of hunger would likely be more telling of the kinds of interventions needed than height and weight statistics. That is not to say that empirical and seemingly unbiased data should be disregarded completely. Rather, they should be generated and interpreted using a community's knowledge and logic.

No matter how critical and straightforward information may appear to be to a community's well-being, such as the contamination of a local water source or simple hand washing methods for preventing sickness, health professionals should understand that their knowledge needs to be conveyed in a way that is consistent with a community's worldview. In order to do so, they will need to engage in culturally sensitive ways and comprehend the community's modes of thinking (Airhihenbuwa, 1995).

Conclusion

This chapter explored the political side of health interventions by applying a community-based perspective. Using this lens revealed problems with placing confidence in the ability of traditional health organizations to address the well-being of communities. These institutions tend to be sustained through taken-for-granted assumptions about the organizational power of structures to encourage conformity and bring about order. Their abstractness conveys the image that they are beyond human influence, which leaves individuals and communities subject to domination (Berger & Luckmann, 1966). The "natural attitude" (Husserl, 1913/2014, p. 48) is to accept institutions as they exist. As a result, ineffective, and even irrelevant, organizations and interventions may persist (Berger & Luckmann, 1966).

A shift from dualism, however, reveals that organizations are a social product. Institutional transformation is thus predicated on justifications that are grounded in human action (Berger & Luckmann, 1966). This understanding should evoke a sense of optimism about community-based health initiatives. Community members can (re)construct norms to facilitate their participation in health projects and promote dialogue about their well-being. They can also make organizational arrangements that allow them to take on leadership responsibilities and make locally informed decisions about their group's future health. Of course, all of these activities are political. Yet, when a community-based approach is employed, the possibility is opened for the "people's power" (Fals Borda, 1988) to prevail.

References

Airhihenbuwa, C. O. (1995). *Health and culture: Beyond the western paradigm*. Thousand Oaks, CA: Sage.

Barnato, A. E., Tate, J. A., Rodriguez, K. L., Zickmund, S. L., & Arnold, R. M. (2012). Norms of decision making in the ICU: A case study of two academic medical centers at the extremes of end-of-life treatment intensity. *Intensive Care Medicine, 38*(11), 1886–1896.

Barthes, R. (1987). *Criticism and truth*. Minneapolis, MN: University of Minnesota Press.

Becker, M. (2004). Organizational routines: A review of the literature. *Industrial and Corporate Change, 13*(4), 643–677.

Berger, P. L., & Luckmann, T. (1966). *The social construction of reality*. New York: Doubleday.

Blumer, H. (1969). *Symbolic interaction: Perspective and method*. Englewood Cliffs, NJ: Prentice-Hall, Inc..

Bordo, S. (1987). *The flight to objectivity: Essays on Cartesianism and culture*. Albany, NY: State University of New York Press.

Borkowski, N. (2015). *Organizational behavior, theory, and design in health care*. Burlington, MA: Jones & Bartlett Publishers.

Bourdieu, P. (1990). *In other words: Essays towards a reflexive sociology*. Stanford, CA: Stanford University Press.

Buber, M. (1970). *I and thou* (2nd ed.). New York: Charles Scribner's Sons.

Cooper, L. A., Purnell, T. S., Ibe, C. A., Halbert, J. P., Bone, L. R., Carson, K. A., et al. (2016). Reaching for health equity and social justice in Baltimore: The evolution of an academic-

community partnership and conceptual framework to address hypertension disparities. *Ethnicity & Disease, 26*(3), 369–378.
Cueva, K., Cueva, M., Revels, L., & Dignan, M. (2018). Culturally-relevant online education improves health workers' capacity and intent to address cancer. *Journal of Community Health, 43*(4), 1–7.
Cunliffe, A. L., & Easterby-Smith, M. (2004). From reflection to practical reflexivity: Experiential learning as lived experience. In M. Reynolds & R. Vince (Eds.), *Organizing reflection* (pp. 30–46). Burlington, VT: Ashgate Publishing Company.
Delanty, G. (1997). *Social science: Beyond constructivism and realism.* Minneapolis, MN: University of Minnesota Press.
Durkheim, E. (1974). *Sociology and philosophy* (D. F. Pocock, Trans.). New York: Free Press.
Durkheim, E. (1982/2013). *The rules of sociological method* (W. D. Halls, Trans.). New York: The Free Press.
Fals Borda, O. (1979). Investigating reality in order to transform it: The Colombian experience. *Dialectical Anthropology, 4*(1), 33–55.
Fals Borda, O. (1988). *Knowledge and people's power: Lessons with peasants in Nicaragua, Mexico and Colombia.* New York: New Horizons Press.
Fayol, H. (1949). *General and industrial management* (C. Storrs, Trans.). London: Pitman.
Ford, L. A., & Yep, G. A. (2011). Working along the margins: Developing community-based strategies for communicating about health with marginalized groups. In T. L. Thompson, A. Dorsey, K. I. Miller, & R. Parrott (Eds.), *The Routledge handbook of health communication* (pp. 241–261). Mahwah, NJ: Lawrence Erlbaum Associates.
Freire, P. (1970). *Pedagogy of the oppressed* (M. B. Ramos, Trans.). New York: The Continuum International Publishing Group Inc.
Gadamer, H. G. (1975). *Truth and method* (2nd ed., J. Weinsheimer & D. Marshall, Trans.). New York: The Continuum Publishing Company.
Geertz, C. (1973). *The interpretation of cultures: Selected essays*. New York: Basic Books.
Greenwood, R., Oliver, C., Sahlin, K., & Suddaby, R. (2008). Introduction. In R. Greenwood, C. Oliver, K. Sahlin, & R. Suddaby (Eds.), *The SAGE handbook of organizational institutionalism* (pp. 1–46). London: Sage.
Habermas, J. (1984). *Theory of commnicative action: Reason and the rationalization of society* (Vol. 1) (T. McCarthy, Trans.). Boston, MA: Beacon Press.
Habermas, J. (1996). *Between facts and norms: Contributions to a discourse theory of law and democracy* (W. Rehg, Trans.). Cambridge, MA: MIT Press.
Hancock, T., & Minkler, M. (2012). Community health assessment or healthy community assessment: Whose community? Whose health? Whose assessment? In M. Minkler (Ed.), *Community organizing and community building for health and welfare* (pp. 153–170). New Brunswick, NJ: Rutgers University Press.
Howard-Grenville, J., Rerup, C., Langley, A., & Tsoukas, H. (2016). Introduction: Advancing a process perspective on routines by zooming out and zooming. In J. Howard-Grenville, C. Rerup, A. Langley, & H. Tsoukas (Eds.), *Organizational routines: How they are created, maintained, and changed* (pp. 1–22). Oxford, UK: Oxford University Press.
Husserl, E. (1913/2014). *Ideas I* (D. O. Dahlstrom, Trans.). Indianapolis, IN: Hackett Publishing Company, Inc.
Israel, B. A., Checkoway, B., Schulz, A., & Zimmerman, M. (1994). Health education and community empowerment: Conceptualizing and measuring perceptions of individual, organizational, and community control. *Health Education Quarterly, 21*(2), 149–170.
Kim, J. Y., Farmer, P., & Porter, M. E. (2013). Redefining global health-care delivery. *The Lancet, 382*(9897), 1060–1069.
Li, L., Hien, N. T., Liang, L. J., Lin, C., Lan, C. W., Lee, S. J., et al. (2018). Efficacy of communication training of community health workers on service delivery to people who inject drugs in Vietnam: A clustered randomized trial. *American Journal of Public Health, 108*(6), 791–798.
Locke, E. A. (2003). Leadership: Starting at the top. In C. L. Pearce & J. A. Conger (Eds.), *Shared leadership: Reframing the hows and whys of leadership* (pp. 271–284). Thousand Oaks, CA: Sage.

Lyotard, J. F. (1984). *The postmodern condition*. Minneapolis, MN: University of Minnesota Press.
Merleau-Ponty, M. (1968). *The visible and the invisible*. Evanston, IL: Northwestern University Press.
Merton, R. K. (1939). Bureaucratic structure and personality. *Social Forces, 18*(4), 560–568.
Minkler, M., & Wallerstein, N. (2012). Improving health through community organization and community building: Perspectives from health education and social work. In M. Minkler (Ed.), *Community organizing and community building for health and welfare* (3rd ed., pp. 26–51). New Brunswick, NJ: Rutgers University Press.
Mokros, H. B., & Deetz, S. (1996). What counts as real?: A constitutive view of communication and the disenfranchised in the context of health. In E. B. Ray (Ed.), *Communication and disenfranchisement: Social health issues and implications* (pp. 29–44). Mahwah, NJ: Lawrence Erlbaum Associates.
Mumby, D. (1997). Modernism, postmodernism, and communication studies. *Communication Theory, 7*(1), 1–28.
Murphy, J. W. (2014). *Community-based interventions: Philosophy and action*. New York: Springer.
O'leary, D. F., & Mhaolrúnaigh, S. N. (2012). Information-seeking behaviour of nurses: Where is information sought and what processes are followed? *Journal of Advanced Nursing, 68*(2), 379–390.
Parsons, T. (1951). *The social system*. New York: Free Press.
Pedersen, R. (2010). Empathy development in medical education – a critical review. *Medical Teacher, 32*(7), 593–600.
Raelin, J. A. (2003). *Creating leaderful organizations: How to bring out leadership in everyone*. San Francisco: Berrett-Koehler Publishers, Inc..
Rahman, A. E., Perkins, J., Mazumder, T., Rifat Haider, M., Bakkar Siddiquel, A., Capello, C., et al. (2019). Capacities of women and men to improve maternal and newborn health: Effect of a community-based intervention package in rural Bangladesh. *Journal of Global Health, 9*(1), 1–16.
Ramnarayan, S. (2011a). Is your organization ready for change? In S. Ramnarayan & T. V. Rao (Eds.), *Organization development: Accelerating learning and transformation* (2nd ed., pp. 320–329). Thousand Oaks, CA: Sage.
Ramnarayan, S. (2011b). Participation: Considerations for designing process. In S. Ramnarayan & T. V. Rao (Eds.), *Organization development: Accelerating learning and transformation* (2nd ed., pp. 267–276). Thousand Oaks, CA: Sage.
Rhodes, D. R., McFarland, K. F., Finch, W. H., & Johnson, A. O. (2001). Speaking and interruptions during primary care office visits. *Family Medicine, 33*(7), 528–532.
Ruiz, Y., Matos, S., Kapadia, S., Islam, N., Cusack, A., Kwong, S., et al. (2012). Lessons learned from a community–academic initiative: The development of a core competency–based training for community–academic initiative community health workers. *American Journal of Public Health, 102*(12), 2372–2379.
Saad-Harfouche, F. G., Jandorf, L., Gage, E., Thélémaque, L. D., Colón, J., Castillo, A. G., et al. (2011). Esperanza y Vida: Training lay health advisors and cancer survivors to promote breast and cervical cancer screening in Latinas. *Journal of Community Health, 36*(2), 219–227.
Sandmann, L. R., & Vandenberg, L. (1995). A framework for 21st century leadership. *Journal of Extension, 33*(6), 1–9.
Sankey, H. (2000). The language of science: Meaning variance and theory comparison. *Language Sciences, 22*(2), 117–136.
Smallwood, S. W., Freedman, D. A., Pitner, R. O., Sharpe, P. A., Cole, J. A., Hastie, S., et al. (2015). Implementing a community empowerment center to build capacity for developing, implementing, and sustaining interventions to promote community health. *Journal of Community Health, 40*(6), 1122–1129.
Tran, A. N., Haidet, P., Street Jr., R. L., O'Malley, K. J., Martin, F., & Ashton, C. M. (2004). Empowering communication: A community-based intervention for patients. *Patient Education and Counseling, 52*(1), 113–121.

Van Wart, M. (2003). Public-sector leadership theory: An assessment. *Public Administration Review, 63*(2), 214–228.

Walter, C. L., & Hyde, C. A. (2012). Community building practice: An expanded conceptual framework. In M. Minkler (Ed.), *Community organizing and community building for health and welfare* (3rd ed., pp. 78–90). New Brunswick, NJ: Rutgers University Press.

Weber, M. (1978). *Economy and society: An outline of interpretive sociology*. New York: Bedminster Press.

Wittgenstein, L. (1958). *The blue and brown books*. New York: Harper and Row.

Woods, K. (2013). *Handbook on volunteer management*. Retrieved from http://www.ctcconnect.org/images/files/file/Volunteer%20Handbook%20For%20Lumity%20CTC%20Partners%20May-2013%20B.pdf

World Health Organization. (1986). Ottawa charter for health promotion. *Canadian Journal of Public Health, 77*(6), 425–430.

Chapter 10
Re-examining the Role of Patients in Community-Based Interventions

Khary K. Rigg, Amanda Sharp, Kyaien O. Conner, and Kathleen A. Moore

Introduction

The relationship between a healthcare provider and a patient has evolved over time. Until recently, this relationship consisted of a patient seeking treatment from a provider and the patient tacitly adhering to the provider's directives. In this traditional model of the patient-provider relationship (PPR), the provider uses his/her clinical expertise to select the intervention most likely to restore the patient's health. Patients play a passive role in this process and simply wait to be told by the provider what their pathology is and how to mitigate their issue.

This provider-dominated model of the PPR can probably be traced back as far as 1000 B.C. (Cushing, 2016). In fact, Edelstein (1937) proposed that the origins of this type of PPR model can be found in the priest-supplicant relationship, thus retaining the ideology of a parent-figure who manipulates events on behalf of the patient. Others point to medieval Europe as the beginning when physicians were thought to be healers imbued with "magical" powers (Kaba & Sooriakumaran, 2007). Again, providers are situated in a very high-ranking position that relegates patients to passive participants.

Another time period that laid the groundwork for the provider-dominated model of the PPR was the late eighteenth century when hospitals emerged as places to treat underprivileged patients (Jewson, 1976). Individuals of low socioeconomic status were widely regarded as inherently listless, which helped perpetuate a picture of the helpless patient (Kaba & Sooriakumaran, 2007). The emergence of the hospital coincided with the rapid growth of microbiological knowledge, which gave way to a new type of orientation to healthcare, one that focused on the accurate diagnosis

K. K. Rigg (✉) · A. Sharp · K. O. Conner · K. A. Moore
Department of Mental Health Law & Policy, University of South Florida, Tampa, FL, USA
e-mail: rigg@usf.edu

S. L. Arxer, J. W. Murphy (eds.), *Community-Based Health Interventions in an Institutional Context*, International Perspectives on Social Policy, Administration, and Practice, https://doi.org/10.1007/978-3-030-24654-9_10

of pathological abnormalities inside the body – the biomedical model of illness (Cushing, 2016). The biomedical model required an examination of the patient's body and the expert clinical knowledge possessed by the provider to produce a diagnosis. This arrangement made the patient highly dependent on the provider's expertise, while keeping the patient, once again, in a position of passivity.

Indeed, the provider-centric model of the PPR has remained the norm for some time, but starting in the 1950s, this relationship was increasingly criticized for being paternalistic. Hellin (2002) described this paternalism as analogous to the parent-infant relationship in which the patient is entirely dependent on the parent for decision-making. Thus, the provider's role involved acting in the patient's best interests, with providers regarding a "good patient" as one who submissively accepted the role of the infant (Hellin, 2002). As these criticisms became stronger throughout the 1950s, the deficiencies of such a paternalistic PPR became more apparent. This change also occurred when several psychoanalytic and psychosocial theories began to emerge that further conceptualized the patient as an active participant in the clinical relationship. With the popularization of writers like Parsons, Freud, Szasz, and Balint, coupled with the emergence of psychology and sociology, a shift was proposed to a more "therapeutic" model of the PPR that emphasized the importance of listening to the patient (Balint, 1969a, 1969b; Breuer & Freud, 1955; Parsons, 1951; Szasz & Hollender, 1956). This newfound interest in patients elevated the importance of engaging them in the therapeutic process and re-introduced them into the clinical conversation as active participants.

Towards Involving Patients in Their Own Care

In the mid-twentieth century, psychology and sociology joined the discourse about the PPR, mostly targeting the physician-patient relationship (Kaba & Sooriakumaran, 2007). With these new ideas inserted into the conversation, the proper nature of the PPR was now up for debate. Michael Balint, who was trained in both medicine and psychoanalysis, attempted to combine ideas from these new disciplines. Balint's work was hugely important in redefining the PPR because he was one of the first to argue that patients needed to be "understood as a unique human being" rather than entities that simply needed fixing. He argued that illness was as much a psychosocial phenomenon as a biological one (Balint, 1969a, 1969b). He encouraged doctors to look past the physical symptoms reported and focus on the patient's unique psychological and social context, thereby allowing them to understand the "real" reason for the consultation (Cushing, 2016). He also proposed that the unique emotional relationship that develops between provider and patient over many clinical encounters is a critical component of both the therapeutic and diagnostic process.

Important to note is that Balint was influenced by Thomas Szasz's model of mutual participation (Szasz, Knoff, & Hollender, 1958). In Szasz's model, the provider does not profess to know exactly what is best for the patient. Additionally, for mutual participation to exist, the interaction between patient and provider is based on both having equal power, mutual independence, and equal satisfaction. This ultimately creates a situation where the patients can take care of themselves. This model, therefore, provides the patient with a great degree of agency, is characterized by a high degree of empathy, and has elements often associated with friendship and partnership, in addition to imparting expert clinical advice.

George Engel and Carl Rogers expanded on the work of Balint and Szasz by viewing the PPR through the lens of "dynamic psychology" (Heidbreder, 1945). Engel advocated the need for a new medical model that linked science and humanism and used the term "bio-psychosocial-cultural" (Engel, 1977). This integrated information concerning *what was the matter with the patient* and *what mattered to the patient* (Cushing, 2016). Rogers, a humanistic psychologist, maintained that for patients to heal, they need an environment that provided genuineness, acceptance, and empathy (Rogers, Stevens, Gendlin, Shlien, & Van Dusen, 1967). Hence, any provider in a PPR needs to demonstrate unconditional positive regard, openness, warmth, and a willingness to listen and understand the patient (Rogers, 1961).

At their core, all of these writers advocate for a new way of looking at the PPR. One that calls for providers to communicate genuinely and involve their patients in their own care. The idea is that by incorporating patient perspectives into the diagnostic and treatment process, clinical outcomes will improve (Rigg & Murphy, 2013). This notion, first raised by Szasz and Balint, then further conceptualized by Engel, Rogers, and others, is now referred to in the literature as "patient-centered care." In fact, patient-centered care (PCC) appears with regularity in the medical, psychological, counseling, and social work literature (Kovacs, Bellin, & Fauri, 2006; McDaniel & Fogarty, 2009). The term is invoked to describe a type of healthcare where treatment is driven by the agenda of the patient. Other concepts such as "person-centered," "patient-led," and "personalized" care also exist for describing this type of PPR (Carey & Mullan, 2007; Fajt & Wenzel, 2015).

Although some of these concepts have slightly different emphases and definitions, they all generally refer to an idea that the "whole person" needs to be taken into account for proper treatment to occur. Most of the variations of PCC share the following components: (a) exploring both the illness and the patient's experience of that illness, (b) understanding the whole person within his/her social context, (c) finding common ground, (d) sharing power and responsibility, and (e) therapeutic alliance. PCC and its variants are clearly a departure from traditional models of PPR and call for greater involvement of patients in their own treatment. Fortunately, there is growing appreciation that such involvement will lead to improved health outcomes for patients, but questions still remain regarding the best ways to involve patients.

Obstacles to Genuine Patient Involvement

One barrier to involving clients meaningfully in their own care is the way that PPR quality is measured. Quality measures have been traditionally narrow, focusing mostly on accuracy in diagnosis and treatment outcomes (Chapman et al., 2011).

Indeed, quality measures are intended to standardize a high level of care across services, but some have argued that current measures do not accurately assess true PPR quality or address clinical meaningfulness (Blumenthal & McGinnis, 2015; Lindenauer et al., 2014). Research shows that provider and client characteristics may most accurately predict positive outcomes and satisfaction with care (Chaitoff et al., 2017; Johnson & Russell, 2015; Manary, Boulding, Staelin, & Glickman, 2013; Rigg & Wilson, 2013). As such, the question is whether current measures for quality of care actually enrich person-to-person interactions, or merely simplify them to an inflexible and externally dictated process. Therefore, the next incarnation of PPR quality metrics should probably represent a patient-centered skill set and be aligned with values like collaboration, empathy, and support for autonomy (Chaitoff et al., 2017; Manary et al., 2013; Zolnierek & Dimatteo, 2009).

Currently, the most popular indicator of PPR quality is patient satisfaction. For example, the Hospital Consumer Assessment of Healthcare Providers and Systems (HCAHPS) is a widely used patient satisfaction assessment that contains 32 questions that measure nine key topics: communication with doctors; communication with nurses; responsiveness of hospital staff; pain management; communication about medicines; discharge information; cleanliness of the hospital environment; quietness of the hospital environment; and transition of care (Centers for Medicare & Medicaid Services, 2019). Research supports a link between HCAHPS scores and profitability (Herrin, Mockaitis, & Hines, 2018), but their connection to genuine quality of care remains dubious. In fact, studies have shown that several of the HCAHPS measures have no relationship to patient satisfaction, thereby raising serious questions about whether these measures are meaningful to patients.

Existing payment models are another barrier to authentic patient involvement. For example, the traditional fee-for-service model, which charges for each step in the process from diagnostics to treatment, means that not only is a sick patient worth more than a healthy patient, but care is often fragmented, uncoordinated, and redundant (Saver et al., 2015). The fee-for-service model incentivizes quantity over quality by motivating providers to see as many patients as possible to increase reimbursements and profits. Within this model, providers are not rewarded for ensuring strong PPRs and positive patient experiences.

A value-based payment model has emerged as an alternative and potential replacement for fee-for-service reimbursement. Within value-based payment models, providers receive financial incentives for higher quality care and are penalized when their quality of care is low. Ostensibly, quality is accounted for by both measures of patient outcomes and patient satisfaction, so the focus on the PPR becomes a top priority (Srinivasan & Desai, 2017; Timbie et al., 2017; Unützer et al., 2009). Value-based payment models are still not widespread, however, and the fee-for-service structure continues to dominate the delivery of care in the United States (Kaufman, Spivack, Stearns, Song, & O'Brien, 2019; Miller et al., 2017).

Patient-Centered Communication for Improved Experience

Increasing calls for a patient-centered approach continues to drive the shift from an outcome-driven focus to one that is experience-driven. The point is not to advocate that healthcare providers should focus only on patient experience to the detriment of clinical outcomes, but that the execution of the former becomes much more compelling when the issue becomes clear about the control clinicians have over quality improvement. Evidence has shown that effective communication and engagement yield improved patient satisfaction, and that patient outcomes and patient satisfaction are correlated (Hibbard, Greene, & Tusler, 2009; Linden, Butterworth, & Prochaska, 2010; Manary et al., 2013; Tsai, Orav, & Jha, 2015). Research has also demonstrated success in establishing meaningful patient-centered communication skillsets among providers in relatively short periods of time (Carpenter et al., 2012; Chéret et al., 2018; DiRosa, Gupta, & DeBonis, 2017; Noordman, van der Weijden, & van Dulmen, 2012). An improved patient-centered communication style that enhances patient satisfaction is one in which the patient not only becomes more informed, but also feels supported and engaged (Zolnierek & Dimatteo, 2009). Clinician characteristics such as empathy, compassion, support for autonomy, and collaboration are congruent with evidence-based approaches for patient-centered care and are shown to yield improved patient satisfaction (Butterworth, Linden, & McClay, 2007; Chaitoff et al., 2017).

Effective communication that has been shown to support PPRs includes technical characteristics such as information sharing and clear questioning, as well as psychosocial and interpersonal characteristics such as rapport building (Butterworth et al., 2007; Chaitoff et al., 2017; Noordman et al., 2012; Zolnierek & Dimatteo, 2009). These traits align with a patient-centered communication approach and a strong therapeutic alliance that can determine positive outcomes when associated with effective client engagement (Barber et al., 2001; Campbell, Guydish, Le, Wells, & McCarty, 2015; Epstein et al., 2005; Matalon, 2008; Moyers, 2014; Smith, Dwamena, Grover, Coffey, & Frankel, 2011). In multivariate models, the goal factor of a therapeutic alliance emerged as a significant and independent predictor of greater change in patient activation scores (Allen et al., 2017).

Empathy is one specific characteristic that has been repeatedly linked to improved patient outcomes (Del Canale et al., 2012; Elliott, Bohart, Watson, & Greenberg, 2011; Hojat et al., 2011). Empathic listening is not only a core component of cultural competence and therapeutic alliance, but a marker of overall clinical effectiveness. In one study (Del Canale et al., 2012), a physician's empathy scores were compared with the occurrence of disease complications. The researchers concluded that clinicians who were more empathetic generally had patients with better clinical results and less medical complications. Unfortunately, the current medical system does not place a premium on cultivating this clinical skill. In a systematic review of studies that looked at the empathy of medical students and residents, the authors concluded that empathy declines during medical school and residency and gradually threatens healthcare quality (Neumann et al., 2011). Also, clinicians do not seem to be able to accurately self-assess their own empathy during patient interactions (Miller, Yahne, Moyers, Martinez, & Pirritano, 2004); therefore, there is a need for additional interventions and training in this area.

Re-thinking Cultural Competence for Providers

Provider training today continues to focus heavily on the technical aspects of healthcare, thus resulting in many graduates who are deficient in skills important to clinical practice, including cultural competence. Cultural competence has become a staple of contemporary clinical education, but this concept is often deployed simplistically. Many training programs seemingly take the position that exposing trainees to static, prepackaged ideas of "culture" will assist them in estimating patient behaviors or preferences. But the idea that providers can diagnose patients by spending only a few minutes with them, and then quietly infer their cultural belief system, is unrealistic.

Therefore, rather than cultural competence that narrowly views patient preferences as a series of generalized stereotypes, training programs should embrace frameworks that do not attempt to "fit" patients into preconceived cultural rubrics (Chang, Simon, & Dong, 2012). Cultural humility is one such framework (Miller, 2009). This approach shifts the focus from providers to patients and community members. In other words, cultural humility recognizes the complexity of cultural identity and belief, inaugurates a lifelong commitment to self-evaluation and critique to redress the power imbalances in the patient-provider dynamic, and develops mutually beneficial and non-paternalistic partnerships (Tervalon & Murray-Garcia, 1998).

Similarly, structural competency addresses cultural competency's failure to look beyond the patient-provider dyad. Specifically, structural competency contends that many health-related factors previously attributed to culture also represent the downstream consequences of decisions about larger structural contexts, including healthcare and food delivery systems, zoning laws, local politics, urban and rural infrastructures, structural racism, or even the very definitions of illness and health (Metzl & Hansen, 2014). Both cultural humility and structural competency are important frameworks for preparing student clinicians to become competent providers. In view of the need for community-based interventions, these approaches should be adopted by more training programs as a component of a more overarching reorganization of clinician training.

Promising Strategies for Involving Patients in Treatment

Evidence has shown that a more engaged patient is a healthier patient, and because of this awareness the role of the patient continues to evolve. Whereas patients were once expected to be passive recipients of their care, with little to no personal agency, patients are now identified as active, equal partners in managing their health.

This new engaged patient feels more empowered to take charge, more activated to follow-through, and has a high sense of self-efficacy. While procedural components of health delivery systems like payment models, quality measurements, and provider education, may still be transitioning to embody these emerging patient roles, there are some current community-based interventions being implemented that do align with these objectives.

Partners in Health Model

Partners in Health (PIH) is an international health services organization that has successfully integrated the role of the patients, their cultural worldviews, and community-based needs into a healthcare delivery model (Katigbak, Van Devanter, Islam, & Trinh-Shevrin, 2015). Founded by Paul Farmer and a team of world-renowned global health researchers and providers, PIH has introduced modern medical interventions to parts of the world where people would otherwise go without these services (Furin et al., 2006). What is most person-centered about PIH is their commitment to the integration of culturally competent approaches for sustainable interventions (Drobac et al., 2013). PIH is grounded in the belief that charity alone cannot solve health disparities, but that partnerships and solidarity with the communities they serve can strengthen the capacity for local health systems to move beyond simply introducing temporary, clinician-led interventions.

This focus on long-term collaboration rather than the provision of immediate but short-term solutions is the organizational equivalent to the Chinese proverb, "give a man a fish and he will eat for a day; teach a man to fish and he will eat for a lifetime" (DePasse & Lee, 2013). They have intentionally shifted away from other imperialistic service models that adopt a hierarchical approach (wherein a foreign entity provides for a less equipped, impoverished community) and have instead focused their resources on establishing partnerships that promote self-sufficiency (Carlson et al., 2010). This model is not only a microcosm of the more empowered patient role witnessed in contemporary variants of patient-centered care, but also operationalizes key principles seen in the patient activation model. The patient activation model (PAM), developed by Judith Hibbard and colleagues, asserts that activation is developed with the presence of three key patient characteristics: (1) confidence, (2) knowledge/skills, and (3) empowerment (Hibbard, Stockard, Mahoney, & Tusler, 2004). Being equipped with these strengths, whether on an individual or community level, is likely to improve activation.

Community Health Workers/Promotores de Salud

In their pursuit for culturally competent collaboration, PIH, like many other national and international health entities, promotes the use of community health workers (CHWs). CHWs, also called lay health workers, or in Spanish, *promotores de salud*, typically serve as local advocates that link the voices and needs of their community members to relevant healthcare information and services (Andrews, Felton, Wewers, & Heath, 2004). At PIH, they hire and train CHWs who are themselves members of the communities they are serving. This practice is consistent with a systematic review of the definitions of CHWs that describes them as paraprofessionals (or lay individuals) with comprehensive knowledge and understanding of a community's culture and language (Tilahun et al., 2017). They receive standardized job training that is shorter than health professionals, and their principal purpose is to provide culturally appropriate health services to their community (Olaniran, Smith, Unkels, Bar-Zeev, & van den Broek, 2017).

Research has shown that not only do CHWs supplement an otherwise strained health services workforce, but they actually improve access to healthcare for underserved areas and marginalized populations (Lewin et al., 2005). In 2006, the World Health Organization (WHO) declared a global health crisis due to severe shortages in the health workforce and inappropriate skill-sets for the needs of mostly rural and low/middle-income communities around the world (World Health Organization, 2006). The WHO has since identified the use of CHWs as a method to help address the shortage of clinicians and to bridge the gap in health inequity on a global scale (Lehmann & Sanders, 2007). Additionally, in October 2018, The Patient-Centered Outcomes Research Institute (PCORI) invested nearly $300 million in support of 79 clinical effectiveness studies of CHW intervention projects (PCORI, 2018). One such project found that the use of CHWs improved patient satisfaction and reduced hospital stays (Kangovi, Mitra, Norton, et al., 2018). This project used CHWs to bridge communication between patients and their clinical providers, thus allowing more individualized attention and time for collaborative goal-setting. With CHWs acting as an intermediary between health professionals and their patients, there can be more opportunities to operationalize those person-centered communication strategies that leverage patient motivation and engagement. Ultimately, CHWs, while not new, are a promising evidence-based strategy for improving not only patient outcomes, but patient empowerment and community involvement in healthcare.

OurNotes

Taking shared goal-setting and self-care management a step further is a newly piloted program called OurNotes (OpenNotes, 2017). OurNotes is a documentation platform that changes traditional doctor visit notes by taking what has been traditionally a one-sided process and turning it into a partnership. The technology involved in OurNotes gives patients access to the notes their doctors write about them after a visit and allows them to modify their records, thus offering patients a more active role in their clinical care. The intention of this service is two-fold, to reduce the burden of documentation for providers and to increase patient engagement. The intention is that patient contributions will help the clinician to focus on what is most important to the patient by allowing them to provide a written interval history between visits and establish a shared agenda for upcoming visits (OpenNotes, 2017). A pilot study of the program used expert interviews to assess the feasibility and perception of usefulness for OurNotes among practitioners. The results, overall, were positive, with most participants valuing OurNotes as an option for improving patient engagement (Mafi et al., 2018).

Narrative Medicine

Narrative medicine also bears mention. Charon (2001a), often called the mother of narrative medicine, defines this activity as the ability to recognize, absorb, interpret, critically understand, and be moved by a patient's story of illness. More than simply an expanded medical history, the point is to discover the meaning or the existential character of illness (Murphy, 2015). This strategy places a premium on the patient's voice, and ensures not only that they are heard, but that their worldviews are valued in a way that informs the care they receive. Narrative medicine, now offered as a master's degree at schools like Columbia University, is medicine practiced with the competence to identify and operationalize the story of the patient's experience (Charon, 2001a).

With roots in public health and social justice, narrative medicine may exemplify the professional evolution needed to more fully embody a patient-driven healthcare system. Research has suggested that narrative considerations increase the capacity for practitioners to understand their patients and reflectively engage with them (Charon, 2001b). Charon describes narrative medicine not as a new specialty but as a new clinical framework that can give physicians the theory, methods, skills, and texts to permeate their practice with the individual needs of their patients (Charon, 2001b). Through training in narrative medicine, practitioners may improve the skills necessary to engage in authentic discourse with patients like empathy, support for autonomy, and cultural competency. These are skills that, as previously mentioned, are essential to involving patients authentically in their own treatment.

Conclusion

Patient-centered care and community-based interventions have become quite popular over the last several decades. The core idea is to embed interventions as much as possible in a community so that treatment is accessible and appropriately designed. Also important is to involve patients in the development and implementation of interventions, so that a new level of relevance is introduced into service provision. Their input is supposed to provide the insights necessary to increase treatment effectiveness and ensure interventions are not harmful. Although there is widespread appreciation that collaboration between patient and provider is key to interventions that claim to be patient-centered and community-based, the current healthcare system does not promote such collaboration, and obstacles to genuinely involving patients in their own care exist (e.g., fee-payment structures).

In an effort to help achieve these goals, several recommendations were made in this chapter. We call for more clinicians to be trained on communication styles known to foster collaboration and patient involvement (e.g., empathetic listening). Additionally, we argue that the healthcare system would benefit from a rethinking of cultural competence. Even though cultural competence has become a staple of contemporary clinical education, the concept is often deployed too simplistically. Instead, training programs should embrace frameworks, such as structural competency and cultural humility, as part of a broad reorganization of provider training. We also identified several promising strategies for involving patients in their own treatment (e.g., CHWs, OurNotes, narrative medicine). And while most of these approaches are not new, they have failed to become mainstream in healthcare and are still viewed as ancillary. These approaches have unique potential to bring the experiences of patients into conversations about clinical practice and help transform the PPR to become truly collaborative.

In sum, patient-centered services are the product of genuine partnership between patient and provider. From the earliest phases, an intervention should be defined and controlled by the patient. Therefore, their participation establishes the reality that informs the identification of needs, the development of interventions, and the criteria for determining a successful program of services. The role of the patient, in other words, is to have an active voice in every stage of an intervention, and not merely to be consulted periodically throughout their care. After all, their input provides the blueprint for diagnosing illness and successfully formulating appropriate treatments.

References

Allen, M. L., Lê Cook, B., Carson, N., Interian, A., La Roche, M., & Alegría, M. (2017). Patient-provider therapeutic alliance contributes to patient activation in community mental health clinics. *Administration and Policy in Mental Health and Mental Health Services Research, 44*(4), 431–440.

Andrews, J. O., Felton, G., Wewers, M. E., & Heath, J. (2004). Use of community health workers in research with ethnic minority women. *Journal of Nursing Scholarship, 36*(4), 358–365.

Balint, E. (1969a). The possibilities of patient-centred medicine. *The Journal of the Royal College of General Practitioners, 17*, 269e76.

Balint, E. (1969b). The possibilities of patient-centered medicine. *The Journal of the Royal College of General Practitioners, 17*(82), 269.

Barber, J. P., Luborsky, L., Gallop, R., Crits-Christoph, P., Frank, A., Weiss, R. D., et al. (2001). Therapeutic alliance as a predictor of outcome and retention in the National Institute on Drug Abuse Collaborative Cocaine Treatment Study. *Journal of Consulting and Clinical Psychology, 69*(1), 119.

Blumenthal, D., & McGinnis, J. M. (2015). Measuring vital signs: An IOM report on core metrics for health and health care progress. *JAMA, 313*(19), 1901–1902. https://doi.org/10.1001/jama.2015.4862

Breuer, J., & Freud, S. (1955). Studies in hysteria. In *The standard edition of the complete psychological works of Sigmund Freud* (Vol. II). London, UK: Hogarth Press, Ltd..

Butterworth, S. W., Linden, A., & McClay, W. (2007). Health coaching as an intervention in health management programs. *Disease Management & Health Outcomes, 15*(5), 299–307. https://doi.org/10.2165/00115677-200,715,050-00004

Campbell, B. K., Guydish, J., Le, T., Wells, E. A., & McCarty, D. (2015). The relationship of therapeutic alliance and treatment delivery fidelity with treatment retention in a multisite trial of twelve-step facilitation. *Psychology of Addictive Behaviors, 29*(1), 106.

Carey, T. A., & Mullan, R. J. (2007). Patients taking the lead. A naturalistic investigation of a patient led approach to treatment in primary care. *Counselling Psychology Quarterly, 20*(1), 27–40.

Carlson, J. W., Lyon, E., Walton, D., Foo, W. C., Sievers, A. C., Shulman, L. N., et al. (2010). Partners in pathology: A collaborative model to bring pathology to resource poor settings. *The American Journal of Surgical Pathology, 34*(1), 118–123.

Carpenter, K. M., Cheng, W. Y., Smith, J. L., Brooks, A. C., Amrhein, P. C., Wain, R. M., et al. (2012). "Old dogs" and new skills: How clinician characteristics relate to motivational interviewing skills before, during, and after training. *Journal of Consulting and Clinical Psychology, 80*(4), 560–573. https://doi.org/10.1037/a0028362

Centers for Medicare & Medicaid Services. (2019). *Hospital consumer assessment for healthcare providers and systems*. Retrieved from http://www.hcahpsonline.org

Chaitoff, A., Sun, B., Windover, A., Bokar, D., Featherall, J., Rothberg, M. B., et al. (2017). Associations between physician empathy, physician characteristics, and standardized measures of patient experience. *Academic Medicine, 92*(10), 1464–1471. https://doi.org/10.1097/ACM.0000000000001671

Chang, E. S., Simon, M., & Dong, X. (2012). Integrating cultural humility into health care professional education and training. *Advances in Health Sciences Education, 17*(2), 269–278.

Chapman, J. R., Norvell, D. C., Hermsmeyer, J. T., Bransford, R. J., DeVine, J., McGirt, M. J., et al. (2011). Evaluating common outcomes for measuring treatment success for chronic low back pain. *Spine, 36*, S54–S68.

Charon, R. (2001a). Narrative medicine: Form, function, and ethics. *Annals of Internal Medicine, 134*(1), 83–87.

Charon, R. (2001b). Narrative medicine; a model for empathy, reflection, profession, and trust. *Journal of the American Medical Association, 286*(15), 1897–1902.

Chéret, A., Durier, C., Noël, N., Bourdic, K., Legrand, C., D'Andréa, C., et al. (2018). Motivational interviewing training for medical students: A pilot pre-post feasibility study. *Patient Education and Counseling, 101*(11), 1934–1941. https://doi.org/10.1016/j.pec.2018.06.011

Cushing, A. (2016). History of the doctor–patient relationship. In *Clinical communication in medicine* (pp. 6–20). Chichester, UK: Wiley.

Del Canale, S., Louis, D. Z., Maio, V., Wang, X., Rossi, G., Hojat, M., et al. (2012). The relationship between physician empathy and disease complications: An empirical study of primary care physicians and their diabetic patients in Parma, Italy. *Academic Medicine, 87*(9), 1243–1249. https://doi.org/10.1097/ACM.0b013e3182628fbf

DePasse, J. W., & Lee, P. T. (2013). A model for 'reverse innovation' in health care. *Globalization and Health, 9*(1), 40–47.

DiRosa, L., Gupta, A. K., & DeBonis, S. (2017). Effectiveness of a clinically oriented motivational interviewing training program in increasing skills & changing perceptions. *Osteopathic Family Physician, 9*(3).

Drobac, P. C., Basinga, P., Condo, J., Farmer, P. E., Finnegan, K. E., Hamon, J. K., et al. (2013). Comprehensive and integrated district health systems strengthening: The Rwanda Population Health Implementation and Training (PHIT) Partnership. *BMC Health Services Research, 13*(2), S5.

Edelstein, L. (1937). Greek medicine in its relation to religion and magic. *Bulletin of the Institute of the History of Medicine, 5*(3), 201–246.

Elliott, R., Bohart, A. C., Watson, J. C., & Greenberg, L. S. (2011). Empathy. *Psychotherapy (Chicago, Ill.), 48*(1), 43–49. https://doi.org/10.1037/a0022187

Engel, G. L. (1977). The need for a new medical model: A challenge for biomedicine. *Science, 196*(4286), 129–136.

Epstein, R. M., Franks, P., Fiscella, K., Shields, C. G., Meldrum, S. C., Kravitz, R. L., et al. (2005). Measuring patient-centered communication in patient-physician consultations: Theoretical and practical issues. *Social Science and Medicine, 61*(7), 1516–1528. https://doi.org/10.1016/j.socscimed.2005.02.001

Fajt, M. L., & Wenzel, S. E. (2015). Asthma phenotypes and the use of biologic medications in asthma and allergic disease: The next steps toward personalized care. *Journal of Allergy and Clinical Immunology, 135*(2), 299–310.

Furin, J. J., Farmer, P., Wolf, M., Levy, B., Judd, A., Paternek, M., et al. (2006). A novel training model to address health problems in poor and underserved populations. *Journal of Health Care for the Poor and Underserved, 17*(1), 17–24.

Heidbreder, E. (1945). Toward a dynamic psychology of cognition. *Psychological Review, 52*(1), 1.

Hellin, T. (2002). The physician–patient relationship: Recent developments and changes. *Haemophilia, 8*(3), 450–454.

Herrin, J., Mockaitis, K. G., & Hines, S. (2018). HCAHPS scores and community factors. *American Journal of Medical Quality, 33*(5), 461–471. https://doi.org/10.1177/1062860618765977

Hibbard, J. H., Greene, J., & Tusler, M. (2009). Improving the outcomes of disease management by tailoring care to the patient's level of activation. *American Journal of Managed Care, 15*(6), 353–360.

Hibbard, J. H., Stockard, J., Mahoney, E. R., & Tusler, M. (2004). Development of the Patient Activation Measure (PAM): Conceptualizing and measuring activation in patients and consumers. *Health Services Research, 39*(4 Pt 1), 1005–1026.

Hojat, M., Louis, D. Z., Markham, F. W., Wender, R., Rabinowitz, C., & Gonnella, J. S. (2011). Physicians' empathy and clinical outcomes for diabetic patients. *Academic Medicine, 86*(3), 359–364. https://doi.org/10.1097/ACM.0b013e3182086fe1

Jewson, N. K. (1976). Disappearance of the sickman from medical cosmologies 1770–1870. *Sociology, 10*, 225e44.

Johnson, D. M., & Russell, R. S. (2015). SEM of service quality to predict overall patient satisfaction in medical clinics: A case study. *Quality Management Journal, 22*(4), 18–36. https://doi.org/10.1080/10686967.2015.11918448

Kaba, R., & Sooriakumaran, P. (2007). The evolution of the doctor-patient relationship. *International Journal of Surgery, 5*(1), 57–65.

Kangovi, S., Mitra, N., Norton, L., et al. (2018). Effect of community health worker support on clinical outcomes of low-income patients across primary care facilities: A randomized clinical trial. *JAMA Internal Medicine, 178*(12), 1635–1643. https://doi.org/10.1001/jamainternmed.2018.4630

Katigbak, C., Van Devanter, N., Islam, N., & Trinh-Shevrin, C. (2015). Partners in health: A conceptual framework for the role of community health workers in facilitating patients' adoption of healthy behaviors. *American Journal of Public Health, 105*(5), 872–880.

Kaufman, B. G., Spivack, B. S., Stearns, S. C., Song, P. H., & O'Brien, E. C. (2019). Impact of accountable care organizations on utilization, care, and outcomes: A systematic review. *Medical Care Research and Review, 76*(3), 255–290.

Kovacs, P. J., Bellin, M. H., & Fauri, D. P. (2006). Family-centered care: A resource for social work in end-of-life and palliative care. *Journal of Social Work in End-of-Life & Palliative Care, 2*(1), 13–27.

Lehmann, U., & Sanders, D. (2007). Community health workers: What do we know about them? The state of the evidence on programmes, activities, costs and impact on health outcomes of using community health workers. University of the Western Cape. *Evidence and Information for Policy, Department of Human Resources for Health Geneva.*

Lewin, S. A., Dick, J., Pond, P., Zwarenstein, M., Aja, G., van Wyk, B., et al. (2005). Lay health workers in primary and community health care. *The Cochrane Database of Systematic Reviews, 25*(1), CD004015. ISSN 1469-493X.. https://doi.org/10.1002/14651858.CD004015.pub2

Linden, A., Butterworth, S. W., & Prochaska, J. O. (2010). Motivational interviewing-based health coaching as a chronic care intervention. *Journal of Evaluation in Clinical Practice, 16*(1), 166–174. https://doi.org/10.1111/j.1365-2753.2009.01300.x

Lindenauer, P. K., Lagu, T., Ross, J. S., Pekow, P. S., Shatz, A., Hannon, N., et al. (2014). Attitudes of hospital leaders toward publicly reported measures of health care quality. *JAMA Internal Medicine, 174*(12), 1904–1911. https://doi.org/10.1001/jamainternmed.2014.5161

Mafi, J. N., Gerard, M., Chimowitz, H., Anselmo, M., Delbanco, T., & Walker, J. (2018). Patients contributing to their doctors' notes: Insights from expert interviews. *Annals of Internal Medicine, 168*, 302–305. https://doi.org/10.7326/M17-0583

Manary, M. P., Boulding, W., Staelin, R., & Glickman, S. W. (2013). The patient experience and health outcomes. *New England Journal of Medicine, 368*(3), 201–203. https://doi.org/10.1056/NEJMp1211775

Matalon, A. (2008). Person centered care or public health improvement. *BMJ, 337*, 1355.

McDaniel, S. H., & Fogarty, C. T. (2009). What primary care psychology has to offer the patient-centered medical home. *Professional Psychology: Research and Practice, 40*(5), 483.

Metzl, J. M., & Hansen, H. (2014). Structural competency: Theorizing a new medical engagement with stigma and inequality. *Social Science & Medicine, 103*, 126–133.

Miller, B. F., Ross, K. M., Davis, M. M., Melek, S. P., Kathol, R., & Gordon, P. (2017). Payment reform in the patient-centered medical home: Enabling and sustaining integrated behavioral health care. *American Psychologist, 72*(1), 55–68. https://doi.org/10.1037/a0040448

Miller, S. (2009). Cultural humility is the first step to becoming global care providers. *Journal of Obstetric, Gynecologic, & Neonatal Nursing, 38*(1), 92–93.

Miller, W. R., Yahne, C. E., Moyers, T. B., Martinez, J., & Pirritano, M. (2004). A randomized trial of methods to help clinicians learn motivational interviewing. *Journal of Consulting and Clinical Psychology, 72*(6), 1050.

Moyers, T. B. (2014). The relationship in motivational interviewing. *Psychotherapy (Chicago, Ill.), 51*(3), 358–363. https://doi.org/10.1037/a0036910

Murphy, J. W. (2015). Primary health care and narrative medicine. *The Permanente Journal, 19*(4), 90.

Neumann, M., Edelhäuser, F., Tauschel, D., Fischer, M. R., Wirtz, M., Woopen, C., et al. (2011). Empathy decline and its reasons: A systematic review of studies with medical students and residents. *Academic Medicine, 86*(8), 996–1009.

Noordman, J., van der Weijden, T., & van Dulmen, S. (2012). Communication-related behavior change techniques used in face-to-face lifestyle interventions in primary care: A systematic review of the literature. *Patient Education and Counseling, 89*(2), 227–244. https://doi.org/10.1016/j.pec.2012.07.006

Olaniran, A., Smith, H., Unkels, R., Bar-Zeev, S., & van den Broek, N. (2017). Who is a community health worker? - a systematic review of definitions. *Global Health Action, 10*(1), 1272223.

OpenNotes. (2017). *The next step for OpenNotes is OurNotes*. Retrieved from https://www.opennotes.org/news/the-next-step-for-opennotes-is-ournotes/

Parsons, T. (1951). *The social system*. New York, NY: Free Press.

Patient-Centered Outcomes Research Institute. (2018). Retrieved from https://www.pcori.org/research-results/2012/does-program-focuses-lifestyle-changes-reduce-heart-disease-risk-factors-rural#/

Rigg, K. K., & Murphy, J. W. (2013). Storylines as a neglected tool for mental health service providers and researchers. *International Journal of Mental Health and Addiction, 11*(4), 431–440.

Rigg, K. K., & Wilson, G. (2013). Can patient-physician race concordance improve health outcomes for African-American HIV patients? Evidence, insights, and implications. In M. S. Harris (Ed.), *African-American perspectives: Family dynamics, healthcare issues, and the role of ethnic identity* (pp. 155–168). New York, NY: Nova Science Publishers.

Rogers, C. R. (1961). *On becoming a person: A therapist's view of psychotherapy*. Boston, MA: Houghton Mifflin.

Rogers, C. R., Stevens, B., Gendlin, E. T., Shlien, J. M., & Van Dusen, W. (1967). *Person to person: The problem of being human: A new trend in psychology* (p. 56). Lafayette, CA: Real People Press.

Saver, B. G., Martin, S. A., Adler, R. N., Candib, L. M., Deligiannidis, K. E., Golding, J., et al. (2015). Care that matters: Quality measurement and health care. *PLoS Medicine, 12*(11), e1001902. https://doi.org/10.1371/journal.pmed.1001902

Smith, R. C., Dwamena, F. C., Grover, M., Coffey, J., & Frankel, R. M. (2011). Behaviorally defined patient-centered communication--a narrative review of the literature. *Journal of General Internal Medicine, 26*(2), 185–191. https://doi.org/10.1007/s11606-010-1496-5

Srinivasan, D., & Desai, N. R. (2017). The impact of the transition from volume to value on heart failure care: Implications of novel payment models and quality improvement initiatives. *Journal of Cardiac Failure, 23*(8), 615–620. https://doi.org/10.1016/j.cardfail.2017.06.005

Szasz, T., & Hollender, M. (1956). A contribution to the philosophy of medicine: The basic model of the doctor-patient relationship. *Archives of Internal Medicine, 97*, 585e92.

Szasz, T. S., Knoff, W. F., & Hollender, M. H. (1958). The doctor-patient relationship and its historical context. *American Journal of Psychiatry, 115*(6), 522–528.

Tervalon, M., & Murray-Garcia, J. (1998). Cultural humility versus cultural competence: A critical distinction in defining physician training outcomes in multicultural education. *Journal of Health Care for the Poor and Underserved, 9*(2), 117–125.

Tilahun, D., Hanlon, C., Araya, M., Davey, B., Hoekstra, R. A., & Fekadu, A. (2017). Training needs and perspectives of community health workers in relation to integrating child mental health care into primary health care in a rural setting in sub-Saharan Africa: A mixed methods study. *International Journal of Mental Health Systems, 11*(1), 15.

Timbie, J. W., Bogart, A., Damberg, C. L., Elliott, M. N., Haas, A., Gaillot, S. J., et al. (2017). Medicare advantage and fee-for-service performance on clinical quality and patient experience measures: Comparisons from three large states. *Health Services Research, 52*(6), 2038–2060. https://doi.org/10.1111/1475-6773.12787

Tsai, T. C., Orav, E. J., & Jha, A. K. (2015). Patient satisfaction and quality of surgical care in US hospitals. *Annals of Surgery, 261*(1), 2–8. https://doi.org/10.1097/sla.0000000000000765

Unützer, J., Schoenbaum, M., Katon, W. J., Fan, M.-Y., Pincus, H. A., Hogan, D., et al. (2009). Healthcare costs associated with depression in medically ill fee-for-service medicare participants. *Journal of the American Geriatrics Society, 57*(3), 506–510. https://doi.org/10.1111/j.1532-5415.2008.02134.x

World Health Organization. (2006). *Working together for health: The World Health Report.* Retrieved at https://www.who.int/whr/2006/whr06_en.pdf?ua=1

Zolnierek, K. B., & Dimatteo, M. R. (2009). Physician communication and patient adherence. *Medical Care, 47*(8), 826–834.

Chapter 11
Work as Health: Tensions of Imposing Work Requirements to Medicaid Patients in the United States

Elaine Hsieh and Eric Kramer

Economic and political systems are reflections of dominant culture: its values, beliefs, expectations, motivations, and practices. Culture is expressed as an operant worldview. In the modern world, healthcare has shifted from being an expression of *religiō* to increasingly an economic-technological complex with political overtones. It may seem that issues of ethics and values have been reduced to the quantification of actuaries and accounting systems. But such calculations are means to other ends. Judgment is as pronounced as ever even as it has a veneer of objectivity. As individualism increases, the utilitarian ethics of hedonic calculus (I want to feel "good") and of mass averaging (economies of scale) constitute a rhetoric to justify decision-making and judgments. We wish to look behind the justifications to expose the values and motives at work.

This paper seeks to expose the true motives behind healthcare policy rhetoric and policy. We want to call attention not to argumentation per se but how arguments are being used (Toulmin, 1958). A pragmatism is in effect that cynically exploits and directs logic and argumentation turning philosophical analytics itself into a mere tool of mytho-ideological purpose that itself remains largely implied. The making of philosophical analytics into a mere means in the service of pursuing ulterior goals also functions to whitewash motives and obscure genuine purposes and goals. Effective arguing can make motives and goals appear "innocent" and even inevitable, objective, and natural. By implication contrary arguments are made to appear unnatural, subjective, contingent ("political"), and uselessly deluded. This process of this paper is to turn the logic of values upside down and recognize the value of logic as use-value employed for irrational means (Kramer & Kim, 2009). Argumentation, specific to this paper, arguments against universal access to

E. Hsieh (✉) · E. Kramer
University of Oklahoma, Norman, OK, USA
e-mail: ehishe@ou.edu

S. L. Arxer, J. W. Murphy (eds.), *Community-Based Health Interventions in an Institutional Context*, International Perspectives on Social Policy, Administration, and Practice, https://doi.org/10.1007/978-3-030-24654-9_11

healthcare, involves exploitation of analytical techniques and moral traditions to promote interests that have nothing to do with reason, logic, natural law (instinct), or classical morality. If effective, this critique should offer a path for a rhetoric of exposure, a process that would uncover the motives behind the arguments and the tropes they deploy and also expose the hypocrisy of those tropes. If effective, this will also suggest a means of defeating arguments by turning their axiomatic antecedents against them. Hence, arguments against universal access to healthcare are self-contradicting. But to show this, the gambit must be launched using the same traditions and language exploited by those seeking to justify denial of coverage individually and categorically.

Healthcare Cost Trends

Medicaid represents a public health insurance program that involves collaborations between the federal and state governments to provide "health coverage to millions of Americans, including eligible low-income adults, children, pregnant women, elderly adults and people with disability" (Centers for Medicare & Medicaid Services, n.d.-a). As of November 2018, 66 million Americans were enrolled in Medicaid and nearly 6.6 million children are enrolled in Children's Health Insurance Program (CHIP; Centers for Medicare & Medicaid Services, n.d.-b). In total, more than 35.4 million children are enrolled in CHIP or Medicaid, representing 50.6% of total Medicaid and CHIP enrollment (Rudowitz & Garfield, 2018). Medicaid covers one in five Americans and plays a critical role for certain populations, covering "nearly half of all births in the typical state; 76% of poor children; 48% of children with special health care needs and 45% of nonelderly adults with disabilities (such as physical disabilities, developmental disabilities such as autism, traumatic brain injury, serious mental illness, and Alzheimer's disease); and more than six in ten nursing home residents" (Rudowitz & Garfield, 2018).

One of the primary objectives of Medicaid is to enable each State to furnish "medical assistance on behalf of families with dependent children and of aged, blind, or disabled individuals, whose income and costs are insufficient to meet the costs of medically necessary services" ("Social Security Act," 2019). Medicaid represents the ideals of American federalism through which state and federal governments collaborate to provide health services to states' poorest, elderly, and disabled citizens. Simply put, Medicaid is an essential social safety net for many marginalized and vulnerable populations to access services that are critical to maintaining their health (Hahn, 2018).

Medicaid represents a significant portion of federal and state budgets. In 2017, the total Medicaid spending reached $582 billion, accounting for 17% of the total national health expenditure (Centers for Medicare & Medicaid Services, 2018b). In 2010, the Affordable Care Act enabled states to opt-in Medicaid expansion, providing states significant incentives to expand Medicaid coverage to more people with low incomes. In particular, the federal government would pay 100% of the cost of Medical expansion during 2014–2016, and the state portion will gradually phase in, capping at 10% of the total Medicaid expansion budget by 2020. Despite the strong federal incentives, only 32 states in the United States have adopted Medicaid expansion as of February 2019 (Centers for Medicare & Medicaid Services, n.d.-b). This is because Medicaid already represents a significant portion of state budgets. While the percentage of Medicaid in state budget can vary significantly (from 26% in Missouri to 7% in Oregon), 21 states reported that Medicaid accounts for at least 15% of their total state budget (Kaiser Family Foundation, 2019a). In addition, Medicaid is projected to grow 5.8% per year in spending in 2017–2026 due to the increasing number of aged and disabled enrollees. As a result, many worried that any increase in Medicaid expenditure can pose substantial pressure to states' already strained financial status. "Ten percent of $5 billion is a lot of money," said one state representative (Leonard, 2015). Despite the immediate benefits of providing health access to individuals who otherwise would not have health access due to low income, states' reluctance highlights their concerns of limited resources and other priorities (e.g., education and infrastructures). The commitment to provide health access to "as many people as possible" may not be a sustainable goal to states who already face budgetary concerns.

Reducing Access Through Work Requirements

Because health spending is projected to grow 1 percentage point faster than gross domestic product and that state Medicaid budget increases due to Medicaid expansion, both the federal and state governments have proposed creative strategies to limit health expenditures. One of the strategies proposed is Medicaid work requirement. In January 2018, the Centers for Medicare and Medicaid Services (CMS) issued new guidance for state Medicaid waiver proposals that incorporates requirements in Medicaid as a condition of eligibility. When eligible individuals fail to meet the Medicaid work requirements set by the state, they are disenrolled from the Medicaid and barred from reenrolling for a certain period (e.g., usually a few months) even when they are otherwise eligible for Medicaid. As of February 2019, Arizona becomes the seventh state to receive approval from CMS to impose a work requirement: state citizens have to have a job and get employment training or community service to be eligible for Medicaid (The Commonwealth Fund, 2019). Another eight states have work requirement proposals currently under review by CMS (Kaiser Family Foundation, 2019b; The Commonwealth Fund, 2019).

Requiring welfare recipients to work as an eligibility requirement to participate in welfare programs is not new. Imposing a work requirement is consistent with the celebrated virtues of self-reliance and self-sufficiency (e.g., "God help those who help themselves") in western, capitalistic, individualistic societies (Greene, 2008). The famed "Protestant work ethic," a myth spread by social science as well as civic and religious leaders throughout the twentieth century, undergirds the ideology justifying work requirements. Harboring racist and ethnocentric biases, this myth expresses the notion of the White Man's burden to teach Others the value of work as a pseudo-religious virtue. Salvation comes from labor. This construct implies that Others (the poor) are lazy, stupid, and deceitful. This trope also expresses social Darwinian notions that poverty and the poor are a burden to the larger community. Labor is thus seen as little more than the largest cost to doing business, a necessary evil that can be minimized with consolidation, automation, and export of work. Otherwise, labor is nothing but a liability to the overall economic system. Of course most labor is accomplished by poor and working-class individuals who must sell their labor to those who can profit from it so that everything labor produces costs more than they are paid to produce it making the economic cycle of production/consumption a process by which labor loses value with each transaction.

As a result of the 1996 welfare reform law and debates in the 2000s, federal cash assistance (i.e., Temporary Assistance for Needy Families [TANF]), nutrition assistance (i.e., Supplemental Nutrition Assistance Program [SNAP], also known as food stamps), and some housing assistance agencies currently incorporate work-related requirements of some kind (such as that the recipient be engaged in a job search, job training, or employment and community engagement activities) as a condition of program eligibility (Falk, McCarty, & Aussenberg, 2016). The rationale for imposing work requirements involves four primary goals: "offsetting work disincentives inherent in social assistance programs; promoting a culture of work rather than one of dependency; rationing scarce taxpayer dollars to the truly needy; and combating poverty" (Falk et al., 2016, p. 2). Work requirements in these welfare programs have been carefully investigated with irrefutable findings (see also Hahn et al., 2017): (1) work requirements carry high administrative costs (Hahn, Kenny, Allen, Burton, & Waxman, 2018), and (2) the complex administration yields high error rates that deny otherwise eligible individuals benefits, including individuals living with disabilities and chronic illnesses (USDA Office of Inspector General, 2016). Previous studies also have demonstrated that some states would attempt to maximize the work participation rate by closing cases rather than helping welfare recipients find and maintain steady work (Kauff & Derr, 2008).

Work requirements for Medicaid recipients, however, are much more complicated than other welfare programs. For one, Medicaid is designed to ensure healthcare access for the most vulnerable and marginalized citizens of a state, whose health (and access to healthcare) is often faced with significant barriers (e.g., health status, old age, and poverty). In other words, modifications to existing Medicaid programs must not create barriers to achieve its legislative mandates and objectives. CMS argued that the work requirements, including community engagement such as job training and public service, can "strengthen" Medicaid programs by helping "non-disabled, working-age Medicaid beneficiaries" to "improve health and wellbeing and achieve economic self-sufficiency" (Centers for Medicare & Medicaid Services, 2018a). By reframing the meanings and functions of work, CMS further argued that "[t]his policy is anchored in historic CMS principles that emphasize work to promote health and well-being." Many of the state proposals have highlighted similar emphasis, noting how requiring individuals to engage with the society through work, job training, or public services can enhance their psychological well-being and social awareness.

Work requirements for Medicaid recipients are an intriguing proposal for another reason: the policy targets an extremely small number of participants. A large percentage of the nonelderly, non-dual, non-SSI Medicaid recipients are already working (i.e., 60%; 42% working full time and 18% working part time), at school (6%), or unable to work due to illness or disability (14%) (Musumeci, Garfield, & Rudowitz, 2018). Another 11% are not working due to caregiving responsibilities (e.g., single mothers with young children), which is often included as an exempted category in state proposals (Garfield, Rudowitz, & Musumeci, 2018). This leaves roughly 6% of the population to be subjected to the Medicaid work requirements. It is intriguing that stage governments are willing to design and implement complex reporting systems to implement Medicaid work requirements despite the anticipated high administration costs and the small percentage of targeted population. So much ado about 6% of the population indicates that this is a political, more than serious substantive, gambit.

Those within the effected population are being used by conservatives to demonstrate their bona fides as responsible budget hawks. A dichotomy is suggested between irrational, emotional sentimentality, the bleeding heart liberal who is increasingly presented as a weak individual, and the rational, mature, and responsible manager of scarce resources, presented as the strong "adult-in-the-room" who is capable of making "hard choices" for the greater good of all. Two issues are presumed by this trope: first that resources are scarce and second that, therefore, choices must be made that ration access to healthcare. The rationing process demands criteria of those who deserve healthcare and those who do not. And according to the work ethic, to deserve something means to have earned it through work.

As a wedge issue, it purports to pit the hardworking good citizen against the lazy welfare cheat. Two wedges are at work: one that separates hardworking good people from lazy thieves and one that separates the vulnerable from the robust. The conservative rallying against such "theft" is thus presented as not merely a responsible steward of public funds but as a heroic leader of virtuous principle in accordance with the Protestant work ethic. In public pronouncements they, being good Christians, concede that vulnerable people, so long as they are citizens, must be helped. As during the 2016 presidential campaign, Trump stated that we cannot let people "die in the streets." A moral imperative to help the weak while punishing the wicked is promoted. But this is a double façade.

The puzzle gets more complicated when one realizes that for some states, their proposed Medicaid work requirements not only seek to punish the sins of sloth, envy, and greed but to also sacrifice to save the deserving too weak to fend for themselves, to be "my brother's keeper." While punishing the sinful who would take what they do not deserve is presented as noble, a lie is also revealed. For in fact some states do not promote these vulnerable populations' health or health access at all.

An analysis from Kaiser Family Foundation found that in Kansas and Mississippi, due to their Medicaid income-eligibility requirement, "meeting Medicaid work requirements through 20 hours of work per week at minimum wage could lead to loss of Medicaid eligibility. In addition, these jobs are unlikely to have health benefits" (Musumeci et al., 2018). In these states, individuals who are subject to work requirements are put in an impossible situation: "Damned if you do, damned if you don't" – If they do not meet the work requirements, they lose their Medicaid eligibility and access to health care; if they meet the minimum standard of work requirements, they will lose Medicaid eligibility, have no health insurance, and stuck with an income that barely supports basic cost of living, let alone health access. It would seem that such policy designs were not about "emphasiz[ing] work to promote health and well-being," as suggested by CMS, but about driving people out of Medicaid programs.

Insights into this puzzle are illuminated when one considers that as a health policy, Medicaid work requirements may simply be the pretext to minimize the financial burdens of Medicaid programs. Kentucky, the first state to receive CMS's approval to incorporate work requirement, projects that the policy will save the state and the federal government $2.2 billion over a 5-year period with an initial 3% decline in adult Medicaid enrollment in year 1 growing to 15% by year 5. By year 5, it's anticipated that nearly 100,000 will lose coverage (Meier, 2017; Solomon, 2018). In anticipation of the increasing costs of healthcare expenditure in Medicaid and the high administration costs for enforcing work requirements, large coverage losses allow the states' Medicaid programs limit state's expenses while maintaining budget neutrality (i.e., the cost to the federal government is not greater than the costs before incorporating work requirement; Hill, 2018), a necessary condition for CMS to approve states' Medicaid work requirement proposals. In other words, reducing the number of enrollees is essential to the cost-control elements *and the success* of the proposed Medicaid work requirement programs.

The experiences from Arkansas' Medicaid program, Arkansas Works, can provide some insight into the individuals who lose their Medicaid eligibility. Arkansas implemented its Medicaid work requirement in June 2018. By the end of October 2018, a total number of 15,081 individuals lose their Medicaid coverage, among whom only 3815 were due to noncompliance with work requirements (Arkansas Department of Human Services, 2018). However, work requirements are likely to be the reasons for many others to lose their Medicaid eligibility. For example, 28% of the participants lose their eligibility because they "failed to return requested information," another 25% were caused by "unable to locate client or moved out-of-state," 5% of enrollees requested to leave Medicaid, and 5% were listed as noncompliance. In contrast, only 13% listed their household increased income as the reason for becoming ineligible for Medicaid. While "churn" in Medicaid (i.e., individuals entering and leaving a welfare program) is normal, Arkansas experienced a larger percentage decrease of enrollees than any other state that expanded Medicaid (Hardy, 2018). To satisfy Medicaid work requirements, eligible Arkansans not only need to work at least 80 hours a month but also have to report their work activities monthly online, detailing hours spent in different eligible activities (e.g., working, education, volunteering, job training, or job search hours) (Arkansas Department of Human Services, n.d.). Given that Medicaid recipients who are subject to work requirements are individuals with low income, their lack of Internet access and technological literacy are likely to impose additional barriers to their ability and willingness to participate in *reporting* their work activities in order to remain in Medicaid. From this perspective, Medicaid work requirements is an over-inclusive policy, resulting in loss of eligible participants beyond the targeted population. This is not new, however. "[TANF] cash assistance program and from SNAP (food stamps) shows that considerable numbers of people who were working or should have qualified for exemptions from work requirements lost benefits because they didn't complete required paperwork or couldn't document their eligibility for exemptions" (Solomon, 2018).

By imposing work requirements, the state Medicaid programs can expect that more participants will leave the program than the actual number of people are targeted by the work requirements policy. For example, Kentucky anticipates "individuals with little to no claims activity choose to leave [Medicaid] rather than pay premiums" when they were not able to meet the work requirements. In a recent analysis, Kaiser Family Foundation explained, "Work requirements in Medicaid will *primarily affect people already working or exempt non-workers* by imposing new reporting requirements to document either their compliance or exemption with the rules regarding work [italics added]" (Garfield et al., 2018). Because the majority of Medicaid adults are already working or exempted, they will constitute the majority of people who are disenrolled under the Medicaid work requirements "even if they may lose coverage at a lower rate than those who are not already working but subject to work requirements" (Garfield et al., 2018). Depending on the different projected scenarios, Kaiser Family Foundation expected that between 1.4 and 4 million people may be disenrolled from Medicaid due to work requirements, among whom 77–91% are expected to be people who remain eligible but lose coverage due to new administrative burdens (e.g., not reporting work activities or exemption) (Garfield et al., 2018). By reducing the number of people covered by Medicaid and adopting a facially neutral yet over-inclusive-as applied policy, state governments can successfully control health expenditures while allowing the most vulnerable, marginalized citizens to "voluntarily disenroll" from Medicaid.

Unlike other welfare program that offers direct support (e.g., cash or food) to everyday life, Medicaid is ultimately a health insurance that provides access to healthcare – a recipient does not benefit from the welfare program until he or she utilizes healthcare services (i.e., Medicaid has no value to a person until one is ill or requires preventive care).

A New Rhetoric of Exposure

Our goal is to expose the motives behind the arguments. This paper presents a set of arguments based on common belief (culture), not moral principle or scientific fact, that must be acknowledged if policy change is to be successful. Deploying economic arguments against moral arguments, for instance, is mixing apples with oranges or, more accurately, competing in an apple-juice contest by using orange juice and expecting to win. We propose using apple-juice but in a different way. Headway in progressive healthcare reform must come from the grassroots.

We argue that one should make no mistake. Work requirements for medical aid are based on the Protestant work ethic and a common belief system that lies deeper than this contingent cultural-historical ideology. In this paper, we are not interested in arcane academic discussions of ethics and morality but rather the rhetorical sphere common to public communication and understanding. Thus, to understand the public sentiment about such policies, we must directly confront the cultural antecedents that motivate efforts to justify and demand rationing of healthcare. To do this we must directly access the mythological/cultural presumptions underlying such justifications. Hence, we recall the ideological complex variously canonized as the seven deadly sins and seven virtues presumed but rarely overtly stated that are the justifications for the policies discussed herein. But this ideological complex may emerge from and intertwine with an even deeper set of motives.

Ultimately, behind the value judgments and policy positions that limit access to healthcare is the belief that those who take what they do not deserve are selfish and being selfish encompasses all the capital vices (or cardinal sins). A concept of self is presumed and with it a construct of merit. Those with merit should be given aid. Merit involves the perceived worth of a person. The overall debate also presumes a zero-sum game. What I take is gone forever and is not available to you for sharing. It assumes a winner-takes-all hedonic calculus rooted in a particular cultural version of the self as a consumer.

Curiously, the United States and its people feel it necessary for the State to provide legal expertise to those who cannot afford it and who are charged with a crime, but this generosity does not extend to healthcare. Access to medical expertise for those who suffer an accident or disease is not similarly guaranteed. Why? Why do we choose to assure expert aid in one case but not the other?

Because, from the early US State's position, illness was beyond human interference. But a court could render great harm to a citizen through corruption. The Sixth Amendment thus provides for a jury of one's peers. This and other assumptions are obsolete and challenged herein.

It is true that the accused criminal is facing the power of the State for purported malicious actions against private or public goods, while the ill person faces the fates, often, in fact typically, without malign intent. Their illness may even be a just punishment by supernatural forces. Consequently, the State, *logically and justly*, has presumed that it has no role in health, illness, and healthcare. One would do better to throw oneself on the mercy of the fates or gods than the State. But this basic presumption no longer holds. In both cases the government has a hand in managing responses, and healthcare has become a very powerful economic and technological complex that demands regulation.

This divergence between care for the accused criminal and care for the patient is rooted in a fragmentation and divergence of the world splitting into what is morally good and what is legal, what is sacred and what is secular power, and what is right and what is economical. The shaman was both a healer and lawgiver. But these poles have diverged to the point of becoming competing spheres of interests. The modern secular State sees its dominion over human affairs and law, not nature or supernatural domains. This allows State actors to claim innocence with regard to moral and ethical issues. They deal only with legalities. Certainly, justice is inherent in law, but many legal experts will argue that unjust laws exist and that it is not the role of courts, judges, and juries to define law but to follow it. If you have a problem with a law, take it up with the legislative branch of government which has the power to make law. So, it is here, among the elected, that morality and ethics are exposed in the formulation of law. Too often underlying issues of what is right are brought up in courts where they are dismissed.

Therefore, the State (that saw itself as separate from the interests and purview of religion) seeks to limit its own power in the case of legal prosecution. The citizen must be protected from State power, and the State should have no influence over natural and supernatural domains. However, this dichotomy is increasingly erased as illness increasingly becomes an issue of science and economics: human pursuits where regulation is called for. Furthermore, what is natural is increasingly recognized as a matter of conceptualization; in other words "nature" has become recognized as a cultural artifact conceived as a resource base for technological manipulation, ownership, and management. Genetics is a prime example.

The argument is that the natural laws of market forces should determine access. State failure to recognize the need for regulation of healthcare access, or more to our point herein, State failure to be responsible stewards of public needs, belies a failure to recognize that illness is not an issue of religion or the fates but rather highly correlated with social and economic processes within the purview of secular power and administration. Being ill is less and less regarded as a function of god's will or luck. And yet this dichotomy persists. Consequently citizens facing State power in the courts are deemed to be deserving of attention and worthy of expert counsel, while citizens facing the random fates of accident or illness are not. Furthermore, when citizens are in the control of the State, such as incarceration, they are then afforded access to healthcare as a function of administrative responsibility.

Essentially, one ideology has dominated the regulatory process which insists that government is not responsible for the health and well-being of its citizens unless they are "wards of the State." We suggest a set of arguments based on the comparison between legal aid and healthcare aid. As noted, we argue that this incongruity is rooted in common beliefs and perhaps deeper motives. There are a few possible explanations. The distinction between the two, that one is the domain of State power while the other is the rightful domain of market forces and divine intervention, must be collapsed because this distinction is the structure that justifies denial of State power to "interfere" in healthcare. The call to "keep nanny government out of our lives" surrenders healthcare administration to the predatory practices of market forces and/or God's preordained plan (fatalism). Government, essentially, is the instrument of free humans to exercise agency over their own lives rather than passively submit to the cliché "that's just business," as if no other possibilities exist.

Instinct as Justification for Limiting Access to Healthcare

We propose that one explanation for the divergent appeal for aid between the criminal and the patient is social Darwinian. The US policy states that a person, citizen, or noncitizen should not be compelled to engage in forensic defense without the aid of legal counsel. But the US policy does not extend medical aid to those who cannot afford it and who are in need of it. This is rooted in a cultural proclivity to see weakness in others as not worthy of support. It may even be an instinctual response and part of evolutionary psychology. Weakness is not seen as having any merit. The daring criminal is more esteemed than the sick worker. Going to prison generates "street cred." But going to the hospital may, at most, generate empathy or pity. In the former case status is elevated. Some prisoners become celebrities. No one becomes a celebrity for being a patient. In the latter, the ill person is regarded as weak and passive. They may even be vilified if it is believed that they seek attention by faking illness. On the other hand, the criminal is perhaps misguided but bold and enterprising. I may secretly understand that what separates me from the thug is my own lack of courage and strength. I appeal to the police to fight my battles for me. Being a member of the sheep herd, I need the guard dog to fight the wolf for me. The wolf may be many things, but he is not weak or cowardly. The wolf's story is entertaining. The sheep's story is not interesting. The savior is willing to stand up to the bully. The greatest sin of all is of being weak, passive, and inert – uninteresting as Nietzsche (1987 Ger./1974 Eng.) put it. Criminal activity "makes the news." Unless you are already a celebrity, illness does not.

Maligning and attacking such perceived weakness may even be part of evolutionary biology. We fear the illness that may be contagious and hence the contagious person. A sick army is a weak army. One must respect the power of the corrupt king but not of the sick king. I may respect the tenacity, daring, and intellect of my enemies but I fear, pity, or disregard the sick. History books are filled with the nefarious activities of powerful people, but their illnesses are barely mentioned unless they impact the overall story or take on a scale, such as a plague, as to pique the interest of the writer. Becoming ill is never a strategy for "success." Illness and frailty are not paths to fame and fortune.

Hence, it may be that support for the sick is not nearly as sexy as tacit support if not adulation for the courageous and "genius" criminal. The deeds of the organized crime boss make "good copy." The more heinous, the more popular. But his illnesses do not make the cut. Illness, to the contrary, is mundane. The criminal mastermind pits herself against the wits of the law. The antiauthoritarian in us secretly, or even openly, cheers for the criminal, especially if her rebellious actions are seen as just. We enjoy the drama of a "worthy opponent." The sick are not worthy. The sick resist no one. The sick compete with no one. Illness does not project agency or bravado. Who will "outlive" who is part of the larger evolutionary game of success? People take pride in the longevity of their "good genes." We want to live longer and longer but only if in robust health. Aging as the frailty of mind and limb is regarded as an illness too, and so there is a constant tension between committing resources to the young, to the future, or to the old, to past glories (Kramer & Hsieh, 2012).

The rhetoric of instinct is a naturalizing language that implies inherent permanence. It is debunked already by modern biology that recognizes the interaction between environment and genetic *predispositions* or tendencies (not predetermination). In lay rhetoric, instinct is used as a pseudoscientific synonym for fatalism. It is hopeless to suggest we can change our nature. Throwing money at certain defective persons is simply a waste of resources. In short, it is hopeless. This rhetoric can be intercepted by basic arguments from the very humanism that modern industrialists and capitalists claim as their procreant cradle. While religion may not offer strong cross-examination, humanism itself does. Here the rhetoric can be challenged by the trope of free will that capitalists espouse. Their rhetoric can be used against them. And it is not difficult to see a tropic landscape where such a battle can be waged. Furthermore, rewards and punishments are meted out in a belief that behavior can be modified. So the threat of withholding healthcare is expected to motivate people to work. Clearly, then, according to capitalists themselves, things are not preordained, genetically or spiritually.

Medical science is focused on extending human longevity. From the earliest magic to the most modern and complex technical treatments, healthcare has always been a process of confronting and attempting to defeat natural and supernatural forces. Healthcare is the application of human agency and ingenuity to defeat those forces that would threaten our desired quality and quantity of life. So to punt, to surrender to an argument from "instinct," is a direct contradiction of the rhetoric of free will and enterprise so central to capitalist mytho-ideology.

Mytho-ideology

As myth takes the form of written canon, it becomes disputative and ideological. Another aspect of the dichotomy between the worthy criminal and the unworthy patient has to do with Protestant (Calvanist) *ethics* as an evolution of older Catholic morality (themselves in part borrowed from Plato and Aristotle's *Nicomachean Ethics* via Thomism). Aristotle's modernistic take on ethics involved the introduction of an analytical mindset presenting "the good" as a strategic necessity for social stability. Rather than stating a virtue or vice without context as an absolute, Aristotle and later Kant, following in his mode, asked a more social question. What if everyone else acted in the same way? Thus, pragmatics via social stability enters into an ethical and moral judgment. Ethics becomes an issue of reliable consistency.

"The good" is not "in itself" sui generis, but a matter edging toward quantification: moral calculus. The hedonic characterization of this calculus would be added later with the utilitarianism of the Benthamites who shifted focus from collectivistic to individualistic reckoning. It violates its own attempts at generalized truth by elevating personal desires to the status of ultimate criteria. Thus, the calculus changes fundamentally and what is good, what is rational pivots on personal wants and needs rather than group wants and needs. What is rational becomes synonymous with what is the most efficient means to achieve personal wants and needs. This then is linked to the "greater good for the greater number" by means of production and identification of the self with the group via economic common ground, a sort of inescapable membership. Membership suggests personal choice like selecting one's church or religion, a process basically impossible in earlier times. As individualism and free will emerge with modernization, identities proliferate. Religious affiliations multiply. Sectarianism and fragmentation increase. But what all have in common is the growing market economics and labor.

As production became the dominant organizing structure of society (industrial society), the needs of the self become identified with the needs of one's firm or corporation – even nation. Fortunes rise and fall together. The unfortunate are those who have no affiliation and are typically careerless/homeless (literally and figuratively). They wander among us as people with no country (Kramer & Hsieh, 2019). While presented as an objective Darwinian process, the outcomes are utterly personal and strike at the core of character assessment and identity. Those "outside the system" are labeled "aimless." As burdens on the system, moral judgment follows with repercussions such as denial of access to systemic healthcare. Debtor's prisons have been replaced by even more inescapable economic profiles, credit ratings, job histories, criminal records, educational attainments, and so forth. The virtual person is more permanent and believable (consequential) than the actual one. And its identity is more economic, spiritual, social, or psychological.

Being unemployed is the most common crack through which individuals fall. Without a "safety net," they languish in a purgatory, present yet denied entrance into the shelter of civil society. This includes access, or the lack thereof, to basic healthcare. This is not seen as immoral but quite the contrary. Such denial of the unproductive is expressly justified by moral criteria. The only way to combat this situation is to recognize the rhetoric and implied morality and confront it at that level of judgment and in those terms. Only then can inconsistency, hypocrisy, and contradiction be clearly drawn. This is what we call the rhetoric of exposure. It is more than a rhetoric of values or motives (Burke, 1969). And it is more than mere storytelling as ontogenesis (Fisher, 1984; Kramer, 2013). It is the use of analytical skills to demonstrate the hypocrisy of an argument over time. Within the dialectic one finds the contradicting logic that decenters such claims to ultimate validity such as instinct, exposing a field for free will and innovation. It disrupts the orderly "coordination" of meaning. Healthcare for all is hardly a hopeless pipedream as some claim based on various warrants and claims.

The Presumed Criteria: The Linguistic Ground Staked Out and Where Disputation Must Engage

The seven deadly sins are *Luxuria* (Lust), *Gula* (Gluttony), *Avaritia* (Greed), *Acedia* (Sloth), *Ira* (Wrath), *Indvidia* (Envy), and *Superbia* (Pride). The seven corresponding virtues are *Castitas* (Chastity), *Moderatio* (Temperance), *Caritas Liberalitas* (Charity – Generosity), *Industria* (Diligence), *Patientia* (Patience), *Gratia* (Gratitude), and *Humilitas* (Humility). As this paper unfolds, you will see how these fundamental cultural presumptions are operant in justifying rationing access to healthcare. Because they are fundamental and only tangentially exposed in public pronouncements, they are very powerful antecedents to policy debates. They are powerful because they are uncritically presumed. Three such "sins" strongly influence policy justifications: greed, envy, and sloth. These are attacked in policies that ration access to healthcare. Concurrently and implicitly, those who attack such sins also present themselves as champions of the corresponding virtues of charity, diligence, and gratitude. Those who are not deserving of healthcare are portrayed as lazy greedy cheats. Those who warrant such help are presented as "vulnerable" and therefore deserving of charity given from the industrious, charity that should be received with humility and gratitude. This is the basic structure of the values-discussion underpinning policy debates and ultimately justifying selective access to healthcare.

In previous times health included cosmic balance involving ritualized respect for the sacred, what Cicero called *Cultum deorum*, "the proper performance of rites in veneration of the gods" (Cicero, 1933, p. 28.). Health had much to do with notions of balance and harmony between the temporal and the timeless, and in collectivistic societies, it was a community-wide condition. With secularization and increasing individualism, *religiō* became, as Max Weber put it, disenchanted and a new system for meaning- and value-creation emerged, namely, science. But as the larger rationalization and mathematical reduction of all things deconstructed all previous sources of meaning and value-creation, they themselves offered no unifying principles but rather an endless fragmentation of incompatible value spheres. All truths are destined to become obsolete as antithesis counters thesis in an endless process, an absurd process of progress with no final goal.

Science was not the answer. Rather, what came to be the answer to the traditional human questions of existence increasingly were answered by labor. The human as philosopher died along with the great existential questions, and the human as producer/consumer was born. Order no longer came from transcending criteria but from increased calls for self-discipline. The modern sees herself as an instrument of production. Use-value came to dominate industrial culture so that people could come to be seen as "useless" and "useful." A simple positivism emerged. You were either measurably profitable to the firm or you were not. The body came to be seen less as the receptacle of an eternal soul and more as an instrument of contingent production. "What have you accomplished for me lately" is the new measure of value. The grand durée has been supplanted by "time famine" and a chronic sense of urgency (Kramer, 1992, 2013; Levine, 1997). Even capitalism is suffering as day-trading has accelerated to algorithmic automatic nanosecond trading, making entrepreneurial planning increasingly difficult. The system is characterized by a "time famine" (Levine, 1997) and "temporal anxiety" (Gebser, 1985), distressing all involved.

The Body as Material Production

Maintenance of the body is now driven so that athletes can keep "producing stats" and workers can keep laboring through illness and injury. Measurable performance is the ultimate truth. Pain management is a relatively new idea. It emerges with the modern individual and industrial warfare and production. The idea that pain can and should be managed if not elevated entirely is one of the goals of modern healthcare. It is almost presumed without question. It is so different from the concept of righteous suffering previously dominant in religious tropes that religious institutions are grappling with the role of suffering within God's plan. Designed suffering from penance to self-flagellation is seen as quaint if not bizarre practice of a bygone world and abandoned moral practice. Modernity has promised convenience and a guilt-free and pain-free existence. But for the Buddhist, this means abandoning life itself. For the Christian it means abandoning identification with Christ and His suffering. The idea that happiness is a goal in life is relatively new, an essential goal of modern positivism. Only recent Christian doctrines have argued that leading a Christian life should not necessarily lead to more suffering. To the contrary, contemporary Evangelical doctrine suggests the opposite, which an appeal of Christian conversion is the material as well as spiritual rewards God will bestow. In either case, work must be done and performance efficiency must increase. True evil is that which threatens production.

Endless work without pain is the goal. Insofar as illness and pain slow the pace of production, they must be managed. Since inherent value has become a myth, value exists only in exchange. Thus, according to use-value, we become alienated from our own bodies as useless unless they can be pressed into productive labor. Being healthy is valuable not in itself but as a precursor to being productive. Performance evaluation marks the status of the individual within administrative logic. Illness and injury no longer threaten the quality of life directly but also indirectly through career attenuation and termination. In a highly individualistic cultural environment, poverty is the "just punishment" for being unproductive. "Missing work" is a constant threat to the modern worker's very livelihood. Reliable, cheap labor and fast exchanges constitute the "good" in the industrial world. The show is alienated from the players. The show must go on even as the players falter. The show is no longer the players in a systemic coordinated process. The process of production (in a play or factory) is separated from the hands that operationalize the logistics (Horkheimer & Adorno, 1987). The producers are interchangeable with each other, and it is the production process that must not pause or cease. This is why robotics is so valued and pursued because robots are better workers. They do not complain, they do not get sick, they do not unionize, and their output is highly predictable (consistent).

Just as actors are interchangeable but the play "is the thing," so too workers have become supplemental to work. Work and worker are separated. Producer and product are separated. Profit and salary diverge. The constant threat to the worker is that they are easily replaced. They are insignificant in and of themselves. Hence the other side of the coin of modern individualism is aggregation on a mass scale. The individual is meaningless, useless, unless they can be pressed into performing the tasks assigned by the logic of the production process. Illness and injury become existential and perpetual threats. Hence, debate over healthcare policy and practice rages. Why spend a great deal to repair a broken worker when they can be easily replaced? Even when workers spend a lifetime and go into debt to educate and train themselves for the workforce, still investing in a robot is more profitable in the long run. Robots are easily reprogrammable. And fixing them is relatively simple compared with a worker healing from an injury or illness. From the perspective of profit/logic, it makes no sense to waste resources on unproductive people. Consequently, where this ideology is more pronounced, the United States, "entitlements" are constantly debated even when they are paid for by workers' taxes. In this ideological milieu, the very word "entitlement" is pejorative even when it literally means something already earned. The word itself has fallen victim to the logic of undeserved or unearned privilege. And expenditures for warehousing the unproductive in child and senior daycares are systematically repressed (Kramer, 2004).

Evaluations reduce individuals to single numbers. Resumes and vitae constitute the modern portrait. Even in an environment of near-full employment, employers are so inundated by resumes that they increasingly are turning to standardized forms and algorithms to handle the sorting. The persona with a "preexisting condition" is flagged. Life as suffering, the ultimate preexisting condition, is itself deemed untenable according to the logic of production.

Everything including health, justice, and ethics became increasingly conceived as a balance sheet in modern parlance. It may have begun with Pauline epistles to the Corinthian traders he sought to convert. Paul's language is one of business exchange. Christ pays for your sins. Balance and objectivity dominate discourse. Hence, life satisfaction must be earned, and thus the Puritan ethic of "innerworldly asceticism (*innerweltliche Askese*)" converts the soul to a record of accomplishments (Weber, 1992). Control finally wedded to the modern self, and systematic synchronicity as the binding principle of productivity gives birth to rigorous self-control and self-discipline without need for gods. Internalized governance, self-control, and conscience are the subroutines of culture. A subroutine is a set of presumed rules that govern cognition and behavior and are replicable. The "stable" "mature" person is consistent and reliable. The good person is the productive one. Work is no longer seen as a means to other ends, to leisure and the pursuit of the liberal arts (innovation), but instead as an end in itself (Hunnicutt, 2013), indeed as the only real end. Routinized patterns of thought and action are "programmed" through acculturation and enculturation (communication patterns) to assure "quality control." Feedback and control is the major type of communication between superordinate and subordinate. In fact, "personal" contact is increasingly outlawed.

According to this subroutine that justified cultural patterning itself, what one deserves is what one earns through sacrifice and self-discipline within the rationalization of administrative systemization, the organization of egoism that leads to the "iron cage" domicile of the assembly-line worker and salaryman. Modern rules of finance determine the credit rating of each person. The irony that one has what one earns, the self-made human, presumes the structures of production and administrative rationality. Agency in the making of the system is eliminated. Consequently, democratic modes of comportment and public sphere are increasingly seen as friction within the system. Education, critical assessment, and a free press are "enemies" of the system. They cause the system pain. Systems operate most efficiently without exogenous interference such as democratic institutions that may disrupt operation and reevaluate their founding purpose. Since value is no longer an inherent quality, to be of value is nothing other than a measurement of performance outcome. To be of value is to demonstrate utility within a system of production/consumption. No other value is recognized (Kramer, 2004). In fact, nothing, such as a rain forest, has value, until and unless it can be assimilated into the system, processed, and commodified. The value of the forest is calculated in board feet and current market demand (Kramer, 2004). Otherwise it is useless, valueless. Value and meaning are reduced to use: utility.

Domestication, the convergence of nature into an artifact of culture, is the first move of control (Kramer, Adkins, Kim, & Miller, 2014). The dominant ideas are the ideas of the dominant class, and it is the dominant class that establishes what counts as valid (not even valued) goals and purposes of life. Management posits a goal and since profit is actualized with each unity "moved," time becomes the dominant factor in production and the accumulation of wealth/power. Taylorism is but one expression of the modern utilitarian view with its presumption of objective rationality, but not a rationality based in a transcending principle but rooted in subjective desires and needs. Confronted with a profound expansion of empty, dead space, the modern becomes "encapsulated," isolated and must strive to be adequate. Modernity is thus characterized with endless confrontations. Encapsulated ego sees nothing but alterity and Otherness. Time is compartmentalized and schedules dominate life (Kramer, 1997a, 1997b). Time-rooms (boxes on calendars, subdivided down to minutes) dictate appropriateness. And timing "is everything." The good person is the reliable one, the one that is "just like clockwork." As time and space rigidify, the self responds, and identity becomes of paramount concern. Privacy of property and information intensifies. And increasingly production has nothing to do with democratic comportment except when regulation is suggested and then the relationship is adversarial. Thus access to healthcare is defined as a liability, especially when the worker's body is no longer necessary.

Robotics, artificial intelligence, algorithmic pattern recognition, and other innovations are meant to eliminate the worker's body and with it needs for its maintenance or nurturance. Work achieves increased efficiency by not just dissociating from the worker but by eliminating the worker's body entirely and along with it democratic institutions because without a body there is no perspective on issue including healthcare policy itself. Eliminating workers and their unions eliminates the need for regulation and social support. Thus domestication, the essence of production, reflexively applies to itself, doubling down. It thus rids itself of the last element that may resist control or offer an ulterior perspective. The worker that once conceived of the product and the mode of production is domesticated and reproduced. Mortal aspects are replaced by robotic action. The work ethic is fulfilled. Sin is eliminated with the elimination of the sinner.

References

Arkansas Department of Human Services. (2018). *Arkansas Works program*. Arkansas Department of Human Services. Retrieved from https://humanservices.arkansas.gov/images/uploads/newsroom/111518_AWreport.pdf

Arkansas Department of Human Services. (n.d.). *AR Works Information*. Retrieved from https://ardhs.sharepointsite.net/ARWorks/default.aspx

Burke, K. (1969). *A rhetoric of motives*. Berkeley, CA: University of California Press.

Centers for Medicare & Medicaid Services. (2018a, January 11). *1115 community engagement initiative*. Retrieved from https://www.medicaid.gov/medicaid/section-1115-demo/community-engagement/index.html

Centers for Medicare & Medicaid Services. (2018b). *NHE fact sheet*. Retrieved from https://www.cms.gov/research-statistics-data-and-systems/statistics-trends-and-reports/nationalhealthexpenddata/nhe-fact-sheet.html

Centers for Medicare & Medicaid Services. (n.d.-a). *Medicaid*. Retrieved from https://www.medicaid.gov/medicaid/index.html

Centers for Medicare & Medicaid Services. (n.d.-b). *November 2018 Medicaid & CHIP enrollment data highlights*. Retrieved from https://www.medicaid.gov/medicaid/program-information/medicaid-and-chip-enrollment-data/report-highlights/index.html

Cicero. (1933). *De natura deorum, Academica* (R. H. Rackham, Trans.). Cambridge, MA: Harvard University Press.

Falk, G., McCarty, M., & Aussenberg, R. A. (2016). *Work requirements, time limits, and work incentives in TANF, SNAP, and housing assistance*. (7-5700). Washington, DC: Congressional Research Service. Retrieved from https://greenbook-waysandmeans.house.gov/sites/greenbook.waysandmeans.house.gov/files/R43400%20-%20Work%20Requirements,%20Time%20Limits,%20and%20Work%20Incentives%20in%20TANF,%20SNAP,%20and%20Housing%20Assistance_0.pdf

Fisher, W. (1984). Narration as a human communication paradigm: The case of public moral argument. *Communication Monographs, 51*, 6.

Garfield, R., Rudowitz, R., & Musumeci, M. (2018). *Implications of a Medicaid work requirement: National estimates of potential coverage loss*. Kaiser Family Foundation. Retrieved from https://www.kff.org/medicaid/issue-brief/implications-of-a-medicaid-work-requirement-national-estimates-of-potential-coverage-losses/

Gebser, J. (1985). *The ever-present origin* (N. Barstad & A. Mickunas, Trans.). Athens, OH: Ohio University Press.

Greene, T. W. (2008). Three ideologies of individualism: Toward assimilating a theory of individualisms and their consequences. *Critical Sociology, 34*, 117–137.

Hahn, H. (2018). *Work requirements in safety net programs: Lessons for Medicaid from TANF and SNAP.* Retrieved from https://www.urban.org/sites/default/files/publication/98086/work_requirements_in_safety_net_programs_0.pdf

Hahn, H., Kenny, G. M., Allen, E., Burton, R., & Waxman, E. (2018, January 12). *Guidance on Medicaid work and community engagement requirements raises many important questions.* Retrieved from https://www.urban.org/sites/default/files/publication/95846/2018.1.12.questions_final_for_pdf_v1_0.pdf

Hahn, H., Pratt, E., Allen, E. H., Kenny, G. M., Levy, D. K., & Waxman, E. (2017, December 22). *Work requirements in social safety net programs: A status report of work requirements in TANF, SNAP, Housing Assistance, and Medicaid.* Retrieved from https://www.urban.org/research/publication/work-requirements-social-safety-net-programs-status-report-work-requirements-tanf-snap-housing-assistance-and-medicaid

Hardy, B. (2018, August 9). *Scrubbed from the system: Why Medicaid enrollment has dropped almost 60,000 in 18 months.* Retrieved from https://www.arktimes.com/arkansas/scrubbed-from-the-system/Content?oid=21285998

Hill, T. B. (2018). *Beduge neutrality policies for Section 1115(a) Medicaid demonstration projects.* Centers for Medicare & Medicaid Services. Retrieved from https://www.medicaid.gov/federal-policy-guidance/downloads/smd18009.pdf

Horkheimer, M., & Adorno, T. (1987). *Dialectic of enlightenment* (E. Jephcott, Trans.). Stanford, CA: Stanford University Press.

Hunnicutt, B. (2013). *Free time: The forgotten American dream.* Philidelphia, PA: Temple University Press.

Kaiser Family Foundation. (2019a). *Federal and state share of Medicaid spending.* Retrieved from https://www.kff.org/medicaid/state-indicator/federalstate-share-of-spending/

Kaiser Family Foundation. (2019b, January 23). *Medicaid waiver tracker: Approved and pending section 1115 waivers by state.* Retrieved from https://www.kff.org/medicaid/issue-brief/medicaid-waiver-tracker-approved-and-pending-section-1115-waivers-by-state/

Kauff, J., & Derr, M. K. (2008, December). *Achieving higher TANF work participation rates: Case studies from Maryland and Utah.* Retrieved from https://aspe.hhs.gov/system/files/pdf/75606/report.pdf

Kramer, E. M. (1992). Gebser and culture. In E. M. Kramer (Ed.), Consciousness and culture: An introduction to the thought of Jean Gebser (pp. 1-60). Westport, CT: Greenwood.

Kramer, E. M. (2004). Vanishing meaning, the ideology of value-addition, and the diffusion of broadband information technology. In J. M. Choi, J. W. Murphy, & M. J. Caro (Eds.). Globalization with a human face. Westport, CT: Praeger, 87-108.

Kramer, E. (2013). Dimensional accrual and dissociation: An introduction. In J. Grace & E. M. Kramer (Eds.), *Communication, comparative cultures, and civilizations* (Vol. 3, pp. 123–184). New York, NY: Hampton.

Kramer, E. (1997a). *Modern/Postmodern.* Westport, CT: Praeger.

Kramer, E. (1997b). In J. M. Choi, J. W. Murphy, & M. J. Caro (Eds.),. Globalization with a human face *Vanishing meaning, the ideology of value-addition, and the diffusion of broadband information technology* (pp. 87–108). Westport, CT: Praeger.

Kramer, E., Adkins, G., Kim, S., & Miller, G. (2014). *Environmental communication and the extinction vortex.* New York, NY: Hampton Press.

Kramer, E. M., & Hsieh, E. (2012). Anti-culture and aging. In S. L. Arxer & J. W. Murphy (Eds.), *The symbolism of globalization, development, and aging* (pp. 135–156). New York, NY: Springer.

Kramer, E. M., & Hsieh, E. (2019). Gaze as embodied ethics: Homelessness, the Other, and humanity). In M. J. Dutta & D. B. Zapata (Eds.), *Communicating for social change: Meaning, power, and resistance* (pp. 33–62). Singapore: Palgrave Macmillan.

Kramer, E. M., & Kim, T. (2009). The global network of players. In J. M. Choi & J. W. Murphy (Eds.), *Globalization and the prospects for critical reflection* (pp. 183–211). Delhi, India: Aakar.

Levine, R. (1997). A geography of time. New York: Basic Books.

Leonard, K. (2015). *Opposing Medicaid expansion*. U.S. News. Retrieved from https://www.usnews.com/news/the-report/articles/2015/12/04/opposing-medicaid-expansion

Meier, A. (2017). *Kentucky HEALTH §1115 demonstration modification request*. Retrieved from https://www.medicaid.gov/Medicaid-CHIP-Program-Information/By-Topics/Waivers/1115/downloads/ky/ky-health-pa2.pdf

Musumeci, M., Garfield, R., & Rudowitz, R. (2018). *Medicaid and work requirements: New Guidance, state waiver details, and key issues*. Kaiser Family Foundation. Retrieved from https://www.kff.org/medicaid/issue-brief/medicaid-and-work-requirements-new-guidance-state-waiver-details-and-key-issues/

Nietzsche, F. (1974). *The gay science* (W. Kaufmann, Trans.). New York: Vintage.

Rudowitz, R., & Garfield, R. (2018). *10 things to know about Medicaid: Setting the facts straight*. Kaiser Family Foundation. Retrieved from https://www.kff.org/medicaid/issue-brief/10-things-to-know-about-medicaid-setting-the-facts-straight/

Social Security Act, 42 U.S.C.A. § 1396-1 (2019).

Solomon, J. (2018). *Administration's re-approval of Kentucky's Medicaid waiver again ignores harm to beneficiaries. Center on Budget and Policy Priorities*. Retrieved from https://www.cbpp.org/blog/administrations-re-approval-of-kentuckys-medicaid-waiver-again-ignores-harm-to-beneficiaries

The Commonwealth Fund. (2019). *Status of Medicaid expansion and work requirement waivers*. Retrieved from https://www.commonwealthfund.org/publications/maps-and-interactives/2019/feb/status-medicaid-expansion-and-work-requirement-waivers

Toulmin, S. (1958). *The uses of argument*. Cambridge, UK: Cambridge University Press.

USDA Office of Inspector General. (2016, September). *FNS controls over SNAP benefits for able-bodied adults without dependents*. Retrieved from https://www.usda.gov/oig/webdocs/27601-0002-31.pdf

Weber, M. (1992). *The Protestant ethic and the spirit of capitalism* (T. Parsons, Trans.). London, UK: Routledge.

Chapter 12
Overcoming Institutional Barriers Faced by Community-Based Healthcare Institutions

Airín D. Martínez

> *However, a powerful lever has yet to be pulled: the implementation of upstream policies that change the underlying systems that promote health inequities*
>
> Alberti, Bonham, & Kirch, 2013, p. 1620.

Although the United States is the wealthiest nation, it is also a society with severe income inequality (Pickett & Wilkinson, 2015) that does not guarantee a basic standard of living, including access to medical care for all its members, not even US citizens. Through community organizing and coalition building, local communities in the United States have established grassroots community-based health centers to address the absence of clinics and healthcare providers, either in rural or low-resourced urban areas. Moreover, some of these needs have been the absence of providers that can address the unique health issues faced by members of marginalized groups such as women; lesbian, gay, bisexual, transgender, and queer (LGBTQ) persons; language minorities; and migrant communities.

The model of community-based health centers that we have in the United States has roots in South Africa. Dr. H. Jack Geiger (1926–), an internist, social activist, and health policy scholar, completed an internship in South Africa in the late 1950s. There, Dr. Geiger witnessed the first community health centers and community health workers program, which were created by Black communities in apartheid South Africa to address their exclusion from formal medical care. Specifically, in Pelola, South Africa, Dr. Geiger witnessed the transformative work of community health workers (CHWs) or lay health advisors that serve as a bridge between community members and the community health center.

A. D. Martínez (✉)
University of Massachusetts-Amherst, School of Public Health & Health Sciences, Amherst, MA, USA
e-mail: admartinez@umass.edu

S. L. Arxer, J. W. Murphy (eds.), *Community-Based Health Interventions in an Institutional Context*, International Perspectives on Social Policy, Administration, and Practice, https://doi.org/10.1007/978-3-030-24654-9_12

Upon returning to the United States in the early 1960s, Dr. Geiger became part of the Civil Rights Movement's medical arm. During his civil rights involvement, Geiger realized he did not have to go to Africa or Latin America to promote public health, human rights, and social justice. There were plenty of inequalities and public health problems in the United States. He witnessed the immense poverty that many African American sharecroppers experienced in the South and the almost complete absence of medical facilities for the African American rural community. Moreover, Dr. Geiger realized that there was a high prevalence of infectious and communicable diseases that were preventable with improved sanitation, opportunities to well-paying jobs, low-cost public health interventions like vaccinations, and community gardens (National Association for Community Health Centers [NACHC], n.d.).

Taking advantage of President Lyndon B. Johnson's War on Poverty initiatives, Dr. Geiger sought to replicate the South African model of community health centers (CHCs) in rural and urban African American communities. In collaboration with an African American physician, Dr. John Hatch, Dr. Geiger helped established a CHC in Mound Bayou, Mississippi. Meanwhile, another CHC was established in a public housing complex in Columbia Point, Boston, Massachusetts. In addition to providing medical care, these CHCs created programs that addressed the social, economic, and environmental conditions that caused ill health, trained and empowered community health workers, and most importantly, shared governance and operating ownership with community resident boards. Every African American household in poverty in northern Bolivar County, where Mound Bayou stood, had at least one adult member actively participating in decision-making, program planning, and program operation through a local health association (Geiger, 2016, p. 1739). So, one of the initial goals of the CHCs was to empower patients and community health workers to reverse the inequalities in their communities through structural intervention and political advocacy.

These two clinics were the birth of the community health centers in the United States. The initial institutionalization of the community health centers commenced with government funding from the Office of Economic Opportunity, directed by Sargent Shriver (1915–2011). Since these two CHCs were successful in improving population health outcomes, eight more opened around the country in a demonstration project to evaluate the provision of comprehensive health services to the nation's poorest populations. Today, there are more than 1600 community health centers in the United States serving more than 27 million patients (NACHC, 2018). The primary funding source for community health centers is Medicaid, the public health insurance program for very poor individuals and disabled persons in the United States (NACHC, 2018).

Present Chapter

Although CHCs in the United States have a foundational history in grassroots advocacy and community autonomy, today they face multiple barriers in promoting the community's values and addressing the community's material, political, and health needs. The goals of this chapter are to identify the institutional barriers that CHCs in the United States face to promote health in their communities and to propose solutions to overcome these institutional barriers in order to return to CHC's purpose of empowering local community members to eliminate health inequalities. This topic is significant because since the inception of the Mound Bayou and Columbia Point clinics, the policy and regulatory landscape of the publicly financed medical delivery system in the United States has become more neoliberal after the implementation of the Patient Protection and Affordable Care Act (ACA) of 2010, all while participatory discourses have become institutionalized in health policy discourse. Representation of marginalized groups has become the equivalent of transformative participation.

I argue that one of the fundamental ways that US community-based health institutions can overcome these barriers and foment the grassroots advocacy that shaped the community health center movement of the 1960s and 1970s is if the United States implemented a single-payer universal healthcare system. Given the current administration, a single-payer system may not be feasible in the near future, but there are less strident policies that can be implemented at the federal, state, and local levels to increase the political and financial autonomy of CHCs and their patients. The neoliberal marketization of publicly financed care in the United States has stymied the autonomy that CHCs have to eliminate health inequalities by having CHCs focus on financial deliverables instead of improving the social determinants of health that produce their "sicker" populations.

I will begin by providing some clarifying definitions about the types of community-based health institutions that I address in this chapter and the conceptual frameworks that I will use to guide this analysis. Then, I will identify the institutional barriers that CBHIs face to circumvent constant fiscal threat, deliver patient-centered care, and empower marginalized populations. In response to each barrier, I will propose solutions which include legislative and regulatory recommendations, organizational changes, grassroots involvement, and finally, implementing a single-payer system.

Clarifying Definitions

Institutions consist of a system of behavioral and relational patterns that are densely interwoven and enduring to function across an entire society. Institutions order and structure individuals and organizations' behavior through norms (Scott, Ruef, Mendel, & Caronna, 2000). In this chapter, community-based health institutions (CBHIs) refer to healthcare delivery organizations that deliver clinical care and health goods and services to marginalized populations. The provision of care and delivery of goods and services are not limited to consultation with healthcare providers (e.g., dentists, nurse practitioners, and physicians) or allied health professionals (e.g., chiropractors, dental hygienists, physician's assistants) but also include the receipt of prescription drugs, personalized medical technologies, health information, health promotion activities, and material necessities. CBHIs are a field that consist of privately funded CHCs, publicly funded CHCs, community-based organizations, home health agencies, tribal organizations, and hospitals. The two main archetypes of CBHIs that I will discuss in this chapter are federally qualified health centers (the current iteration of Dr. Geiger's CHCs) and specialty CHCs like Planned Parenthood Clinics because they serve the most patients and are some of the most regulated CBHIs by federal and state government agencies. Although hospitals are part of the CBHI field, the majority of community-based hospitals have been consolidated to larger hospital systems through mergers since the early 2000s (Anderson, Hussey, & Petrosyan, 2019).

Most CHCs in the United States have the designation of being federally qualified health centers (FQHCs), which receive funding from Section 330 of the Health Care Consolidation Act of 1996 (Peters & Wooley, 1996). FQHCs maintain their designation by providing comprehensive medical care (including oral health, mental health, and substance use services) to medically underserved areas and/or medically underserved populations, without refusing care to patients who do not have medical insurance and/or the ability to pay for services up front. FQHCs must also have 51% or more representation from the patient population to serve on their governing advisory boards (NACHC, 2018).

However, there are other CHCs that do not have the FQHC designation to provide specialized healthcare that is often politicized, such as family planning. For example, Planned Parenthood Federation of America (Planned Parenthood) has several programs, but one of the most important is the Planned Parenthood Clinics, which provide preventive sexual and reproductive healthcare to youth, family planning, and gynecological care to one in five patients with Medicaid in the United States. Similar to FQHCs, Planned Parenthood Clinics often serve medically underserved areas or populations and do not refuse care to patients without health insurance or the ability to pay (Guttmacher Institute, 2017).

In the last 10 years, Planned Parenthood has been threatened by conservative Republicans in state and federal legislatures to be defunded of Title X Family Planning Funds and Medicaid reimbursement on the grounds that the organization uses federal dollars to subsidize abortion. Although Planned Parenthood is the largest provider of abortions in the United States, only 2% of Planned Parenthood's care consists of abortions, and under Section 1008 of the Title X statute, Title X grantees are prohibited from recommending abortion as a method of family planning. Moreover, the Hyde Amendment of 1977 prohibits the use of Medicaid funding for abortion care, unless it is a case of life endangerment, rape, or incest (Planned Parenthood Federation of America, 2019). More recently, the Trump Administration will deny Title X funding to any clinic that provides or even provides patients information about abortion. This will go into effect on April 1, 2019, and will certainly disqualify Planned Parenthood Clinics from receiving Title X funds (Salganicoff & Rice, 2019). If Planned Parenthood Clinics were to close as a result of this exclusionary regulation, millions of low-income women who do not qualify or live in a state with expanded Medicaid would lose their only source of medical care, and FQHCs do not have the capacity to absorb these millions of patients (Guttmacher Institute, 2017). Ultimately, this institutional barrier reduces healthcare providers' ability to provide necessary medical care and denies women of their corporal liberties.

In addition to these two examples of CBHIs, FQHCs and Planned Parenthood clinics, there are more archetypes of CBHIs that do not have professional healthcare providers treating patients with biomedical approaches but rather provide health interventions that are directly developed and administered by community members. For example, Reyna Montoya's organization, *Aliento*, is an undocumented and youth-led organization committed to organize people who are directly affected by immigration enforcement policies by providing art therapy to Dreamers (undocumented youth brought to the United States as children) and children in mixed-status families, whose parents face or have experienced immigration detention and deportation. There is no clinical curriculum that is being administered, but *Aliento* provides an intervention that was developed by undocumented youth and solely supported from philanthropic grants and personal donations.

LGBTQ persons face discrimination in medical encounters and often avoid seeking care as a result. When they do receive care, studies indicate that LGBTQ persons are not treated with respect, nor do they receive quality care. Moreover, transgender and gender diverse persons face the most discrimination in the LGBTQ community, not only in healthcare but also in securing their basic needs such as completing their secondary education, obtaining state-issued identification, securing employment, and trusting local law enforcement to protect their safety (Human Rights Campaign, 2019; Stroumsa, 2014). Part of the problem lies in the fact that there is no comprehensive, federal nondiscrimination law that includes gender identity (Human Rights Campaign, 2019). Thus, CBHIs like the TransActive Gender Center in Portland, Oregon, are created to address the needs of transgender persons. The TransActive Gender Center is a nonprofit organization founded by transgender individuals in 2007 to provide healthcare and support to transgender and gender diverse children and their families (TransActive Gender Center, 2019).

A Note on Positionality

I come to this space to write about the institutional barriers that CBHIs face and their solutions as a Latina medical sociologist and public health scholar with some disillusionment in community-engaged research and advocacy approaches. I was in the final cohort of the W.K. Kellogg Health Scholars Community-Track program (2010–2012) which, among its many goals, sought to train the future generation of health disparities researchers who conduct community-based participatory research (CBPR). Briefly, CBPR is a research approach that is based on producing an equitable research collaboration that includes representatives from community organizations, with their broad experiences working in and on behalf of communities, and community members affected by the particular health issue in all aspects of the research process—from research question development, study design, and implementation to interpretation and dissemination of results.

Although I continue to appreciate the experience I gained from this program, I felt that the institutionalization of the CBPR's approach to nine principles (see Israel et al., 2005, citing W.K. Kellogg Foundation), the lack of autonomy that community members have to independently obtain or administer federal research funding, and the bureaucratic administration of academic research, often prolonged the development of interventions or policy recommendations that could reverse health inequalities. I am devoted to acknowledging the diversity within marginalized communities in order to address structural sources of health inequity, but I am cautious when dominant institutions in the civil society, such as government agencies or research universities, claim that they "engaged the community" to create a specific recommendation, product, or solution.

For Antonio Gramsci (1929/2015), one of the ways that hegemonic processes can thrive in modern capitalist societies is if the society provides the possibility of resistance through civic participation. Through ideologies and ideological practices that allow the masses to cooperate and "civilly" challenge institutional arrangements, we are led to believe that we can influence politics and make a systemic difference. Yes, small gains are made every day in the United States to reduce health disparities through CBPR, despite our vast limitations from corporate influence on health policy and healthcare delivery. Yet, it is not large enough to prevent the social and health inequities from recurring, nor does it grant authority and legitimacy to community members' grievances, recommendations, and innovative ideas for local health improvements. This is not only based on my anecdotal experience of conducting participatory research and volunteering at CBHIs, but also by how the community's health and material needs have been ignored. This is witnessed in areas with decades-long concentrated poverty, whether they be places like Appalachia, Southwestern *colonias*, or the West Baltimore.

That being said, I take the sociological conflict perspective to examine the institutional barriers that US CBHIs face because CBHIs are not meant to benefit every member of the US society. Hegemonic processes stabilize current power arrangements where only certain populations obtain the care that they need with few material or cultural barriers. The system and policies that maintain and fund CBHIs in the United States are not designed to transform the unequal social and economic arrangements, which could promote social justice and human rights for all of the country's members. Paradoxically, the proliferation of CBHIs in the last 50 years represents an overarching system that does not value all humans as deserving because it is absent of universal access to care.

Institutional Barriers that Community-Based Health Centers Face

Community health centers' ability to address the community's needs and empower local members to advocate for improving the health and living conditions of their local geographies are impeded because most community health centers are bound to regulations and deliverables that are imposed upon them by their main funding source and regulator, the Centers for Medicare and Medicaid Services (CMS). In addition, diverse state and local policies and politics exclude large segments of the population, such as unauthorized immigrants and their children, from receiving culturally-specific care (see Rodríguez et al., 2015 and Suro et al., 2015).

We cannot discuss institutional barriers that CHCs face without discussing the Patient Protection and Affordable Care Act (ACA) of 2010. The ACA was President Barack Obama's signature healthcare legislation, which, among its many policies, increased access to medical insurance for millions of uninsured and underinsured Americans. Moreover, it lifted several barriers imposed by insurance companies such as denying insurance coverage to persons with pre-existing conditions, having a lifetime cap, allowing young adults up to the age of 26 to remain on their parents' health insurance, and discriminating prices for preventive, gender-specific healthcare goods and services (Kominski, 2013). Insurance companies were also required to provide a suite of essential benefits such as comprehensive preventive care, well-woman visits, chronic disease management, emergency care, and prescription coverage (Kominski, 2013). In order to subsidize the money needed to cover sicker patients, who utilize more health services, individuals are mandated to have either public or private health insurance or pay a penalty when they file taxes with the Internal Revenue Service. To reduce total federal spending, much of the costs were passed onto individuals by increasing their premiums, deductibles, or co-pays (White, 2018). Besides these individual changes, the ACA includes several policies that are meant to increase patient engagement, increase research activity on the social determinants of health and health disparities, and create cost-savings in Medicaid and Medicare expenditures.

The challenges that FQHCs face as a result of the ACA are the budget cuts to their discretionary funding for programming, the increased patient demands given increased access to care with the expansion of Medicaid and health insurance enrollment in one of the exchanges, and more importantly, the new payment structure from a fee-for-service reimbursement to payment for value (Wright & Martin, 2014). Value-based care is the new payment structure being employed by the CMS to reduce costs and improve quality of care by bundling payments for "episodes of care" offered in medical homes and accountable care organizations (ACOs; Alberti et al., 2013), instead of paying for each service provided by a healthcare provider. ACOs consist of consolidation of independent clinics, FQHCs, hospital clinics, and specialty care facilities that are part of the same geographic area, serve the same patient population, and share savings via value-based reimbursements from the Medicare Shared Savings Program (MSSP) (Barnes, Unruh, Chukmaitov, & van Ginneken, 2014). The ACA authorized and established a "Medicare Shared Savings Program for ACOs, to take effect no later than January 2012... the law makes contracts with ACOs a permanent option under Medicare" (Merlis, Berenson, & Fisher, 2010, p. 2). The ACA also establishes a new Center for Medicare and Medicaid Innovation within CMS to test a variety of new payment and delivery models for both Medicare and Medicaid (Merlis et al., 2010).

The Integration of FQHCs into Accountable Care Organizations (ACO)

The concept of the ACO emerged from a group of health policy scholars led by John Wennberg and colleagues (The Engelberg Center for Health Care Reform & the Dartmouth Institute, 2013) at the Dartmouth Institute for Health Policy and Clinical Practice. They wrote a report indicating that healthcare costs in the United States were high because 30% of the services received by patients were due to "unnecessary care" (White, 2018). The Dartmouth team also wrote that these costs could be reduced with patient behavioral changes, reducing medical error and improving communication between providers using electronic health records. They pushed for paying for performance, not volume of care given. Overall, the cost-savings assumption behind ACOs is that if there is coordinated care and there are fewer duplicative services given to patients reducing "unnecessary costs" and, supposedly, fewer medical errors. The CMS gives a financial incentive to ACOs that save money, which is then shared among the organizations in the ACO. However, there was little procedural information on how to allocate this incentive among the organizations, and these are being developed as more CBHIs join ACOs. White (2018) observes that there were few ACOs in existence during the time when the ACA was drafted; thus, there was little evidence that ACOs could reduce costs and improve the quality of patient care. ACOs are primarily a theoretical idea, from a group of elite academics who are geographically and socioeconomically sheltered from the realities of CBHIs (White, 2018). The very workers in FQHCs are not the main catalysts for organizational or financial innovations in the delivery of care.

One of the other challenges for FQHCs has to do with the metrics used to evaluate quality care in ACOs. These metrics are an interpretation of Section 1899 of Title XVIII of the Social Security Act, which have generally included clinical processes and outcomes, patient and caregiver experiences, and utilization. Quality metrics vary by the number of Medicaid and Medicare enrollees in a state and the most pressing disparities of an ACO's patient population. Yet, most of the measures have focused on clinical processes and outcomes and utilization such as nosocomial infections, 30-day hospital readmissions, hospitalizations for chronic diseases manageable with medication adherence and behavior modification (e.g., congestive heart failure, COPD/Asthma, diabetes), preventive screenings like mammograms, and preventative services for diabetes (hemoglobin A1c, lipids panel, and retinal exams) (McWilliams, Hatfield, Chernew, Landon, & Schwartz, 2016). These quality metrics are problematic for several reasons. First, because older patients and low-income patients tend to have multiple chronic conditions, they are more difficult to medically control, and they may require hospital readmission. On the other hand, ACOs that serve affluent patient populations will skew quality results. Second, these metrics are almost exclusively clinical and based on providers' report of their own performance (Woolhandler & Himmelstein, 2017b). If they do request patients or caregivers' level of satisfaction, these measures still do not reflect the patients' interpretation of quality, including respectful encounters with staff and healthcare providers.

Third, these quality metrics may not be achievable when patients' socioeconomic conditions and their physical environments have not changed. There are social, economic, or environmental conditions that are keeping patients from managing their chronic conditions such as the lack of safe and walkable streets, healthy food access, and money for adequate housing, transportation, and out-of-pocket health expenses. The Centers for Disease Control and Prevention attribute over 75% of health disparities to the social and environmental conditions that people have encountered throughout their life course, not solely their biological or genetic precursors (National Center for HIV/AIDS, Viral Hepatitis, STD, & TB Prevention, 2014, citing Tarlov, 1999). Patients using FQHCs are usually in poor and under-resourced areas with a lack of services, dilapidated housing, with communities that have been historically deprived of economic opportunities and political participation. FQHCs could be penalized for not meeting quality benchmarks, but they serve the most vulnerable populations (Alberti et al., 2013). In turn, their ACO may not achieve savings, and at a later day, may have to assume risk, and pay back losses from not delivering "quality" of care. The new electronic health records shared between CBHIs in ACOs are supposed to capture social determinants of health such as housing, neighborhood safety, and food security, with hopes that community health workers (CHWs) including *promotores de salud* and patient navigators will put patients into contact with programs that fill their material and social needs. FQHCs (before and after the ACA) heavily rely on community health workers to connect their patients to these resources.

The ACA also sought to increase patient engagement in research, the service delivery agenda of CBHIs, and in the governance of FQHCs. For instance, the ACA requires hospitals receiving Medicaid and Medicare funding to conduct community health needs assessments of their residents in their service areas every 3 years. These community health needs assessments are not only supposed to identify needs in the community but also inform interventions based on patient participants' recommendations (Alberti, 2014). In the specific community where I live, Springfield, Massachusetts, residents of this city have claimed that they are "community-assessed to death" but are disappointed that the environmental and economic conditions of their city have yet to change for the African American and Latinx communities, whom are the racial/ethnic majority.

The implementation of ACOs is one strategy that the ACA attempts to reduce healthcare expenditures, but these controls are relegated to publicly financed community-based health institutions and the Centers of Medicare and Medicaid Services. The ACA did not contain any cost-saving measures used in other countries toward the private sector, such as provider rate-setting or the government negotiating lower prices on pharmaceuticals or the provision of high-cost technological diagnostics, such as magnetic resonance imaging, which are the primary drivers of healthcare spending in the United States (Anderson et al., 2019). Also, as Woolhandler and Himmelstein (2017a) write, the incentives created to control costs are "weak" because doctors and hospitals can still expand profit opportunities. The proliferation of ACOs has been one of the largest financial and organizational changes affecting FQHCs and other community health centers receiving Medicare and Medicaid funding.

In 2009 there were only a few ACOs being developed in the private sector (JSI & NACHC, 2013), and by the end of 2016, there were 458 ACO initiatives (Kaiser Family Foundation, 2017). Preliminary evidence suggests that incorporating quality measures were burdensome for staff, and compliance with the top-down metrics redistributed resources away from more meaningful structural changes (Blustein et al., 2011). In their early implementation, traditional ACOs (MSSP Track 1) have cost Medicare $72 million more than traditional pay-for-service payments, but the ACO systems overall have reduced Medicare spending by only $47 million (Kaiser Family Foundation, 2017).

FQHC Community Advisory Boards

The earliest iteration of FQHCs, community health centers, addressed local health issues and needs through active community participation in community advisory boards. To this day, FQHCs, under Section 330, are mandated to have governing boards that consist of 51% or more of their patients who are representing the patient population. Patient members of the governing boards should receive their primary care from the FQHC and represent the patient population in terms of race, ethnicity, and gender (Wright, 2013, citing HRSA 1998). However, studies by Wright (Wright, 2013; Wright & Martin, 2014) indicate that over 60% of patients on FQHCs community advisory boards are patients from high-status occupations, whose socioeconomic status does not reflect that of the majority of FQHC patients. He also demonstrates that representative patient trustees are less likely than higher SES members to hold a position on the executive member or serve as board chair, which limits the authority that community members have in shaping the delivery of care and programming at FQHCs (Wright, 2015). Similarly, Sharma and colleagues (2018) found in their study that most members in these community advisory boards do not engage in financial or hiring decision-making but do influence the quality improvement of materials and day-to-day operations at the clinic. Decision-making regarding the organization's operations and strategic development is often delegated to the FQHC's senior management like the CEO and CFOs. This current level of participation from the community advisory boards is far from the structural interventions that were led, developed, and executed by the patients of the Mound Bayou and Columbia Point Clinics in the 1960s. Moreover, they are not addressing social determinants of health, the way those programs did with the creation of community gardens and economic development programs.

Another issue with community advisory boards in FQHCs rests on the government-issued categories of marginalized populations. Steven Epstein (2008) wrote about the paradoxical consequences of the US federal government's attempts to institutionalize the inclusion of women, children, communities of color, and other vulnerable populations in biomedical research and randomized clinical trials. Instead of ameliorating the health inequalities produced on diverse, overlooked, or silenced populations in the United States, this *niche standardization* has circumscribed the meaning of representation and has perpetuated biological difference in biomedical and public health discourses to represent women and racial/ethnic minorities in particular. For example, by circumscribing diverse "representation" to the Office of Management and Budget Statistical Directive No. 15's one ethnic group (Hispanic/Latino) and four racial groups (Asian/Pacific Islander, Black non-Hispanic, Native American/Alaskan Native, and White, non-Hispanic), FQHCs do not receive input from people who are outside of these racial and ethnic designations and fail to create programs along other lines of difference that may be more important for delivering equitable care that represents a specific communities' needs.

The configuration of community advisory boards rests on gender, racial, and ethnic categories that are not historicized and depoliticized. When a specific marginalized group does not have a niche that is standardized by Statistical Directive No. 15, our major health agencies—the Centers for Medicare and Medicaid Services, the Centers for Disease Control and Prevention, the Health Resources and Services Administration, and the National Institutes of Health—there will be little to no federal dollars earmarked for other marginalized groups who share an identity, such as minority religious groups like Muslims. More importantly, having a member on the CAB that is one of the "designated" minorities does not guarantee representation of the patient population receiving care at the FQHC. Complying with narrow federal rules and regulations hinders the ability for community advisory boards and community liaisons in CBHIs to identify and represent the needs of heterogeneous, medically underserved populations. For example, in the Latinx community, there are intragroup heterogeneities, stratification, and discrimination along multiple dimensions (racial/ethnic, nationality, immigration, gender, and sexuality) that are silenced like that of non-Spanish-speaking indigenous Latin Americans or members of mixed-immigration status families.

The community advisory boards that emanated from Dr. Geiger's community health center demonstration project have evolved from a serious driver of programming and community asset-building to a symbolic collective that fulfills an administrative checklist. Moreover, I wondered how much influence community advisory boards had in deciding whether or not their FQHC would join an ACO. The goals behind the ACO to reduce duplicative care and increase care coordination and resource sharing are important for efficiency (Alberti et al., 2013). However, health policy analysts are still figuring out if many savings are being produced and if the quality of care is being improved (see Levinson, 2017; Schulman & Richman, 2016; Song & Fisher, 2016) and how to equitably distribute Medicare and Medicaid savings across organizations. Moreover, the measures used to assess quality lack the patient's humanity. We still need to better understand what encourages patients to return to a healthcare facility or adhere to a care plan. Also, these quality metrics may jeopardize FQHCs in an ACO agreement if they do not take into consideration the economic, environmental, and social conditions which patients are living in that exacerbate their conditions. The requirements for representation and promoting "patient-centered" input from hospital community health needs assessments or FQHC community advisory boards need to go beyond categories of difference related to race/ethnicity or gender in order to capture the material and political needs of diverse FQHC patient populations.

Recommendations to Overcome These Institutional Barriers

The solutions that will be presented in this section try to promote patient and community participation in the governance and operations of CBHIs and health equity. Health equity refers to a condition in which the nation-state provides every single person in the society the material resources and opportunities to achieve health (Braveman et al., 2011). Health inequality is a health disparity that is avoidable, unnecessary, and unjust (Whitehead, 1991). Promoting health equity requires actions from the bottom (community health workers, community residents, small business owners, local workers collectives, and youth-led groups), the middle (CBHIs and other organizations), and the top (federal and state agency policies and regulations).

The implementation of the ACO is an intervention at the clinical and organizational levels and will not address the problems emanating from the larger society and environment driving health inequalities. That is why having as much of the community involved in the process of shaping the healthcare services and programming that are delivered at FQHCs is so important. FQHCs need to be utilized as conveners for diverse community members to design, plan, and implement structural interventions that improve local social and environmental conditions. Community health centers are spaces to collaborate and incorporate multiple diverse perspectives from the side of service providers, researchers, and patients or community members. More effort is needed to improve the social and environmental conditions patients face.

Janet K. Shim (2005) demonstrates why people who are affected by a specific social or health inequality need to be a part of the decision-making processes. Shim's research investigates the lay-scientific divide in the social determinants of cardiovascular disease, in which biomedical and epidemiological researchers include race, gender, and age in their studies to capture diverse health disparities. The researchers she studies could not articulate the mechanisms by which these three structural positions can shape one's risk for cardiovascular disease and mortality. In contrast, people of color suffering from various cardiovascular diseases identify their low-paying jobs, occupational status, skin color, accents, neighborhoods, and historical trauma as drivers of their disease. Moreover, they interpret them as consequences of institutionalized racism.

The "lay" audience had a more complex understanding of the mechanisms, whereas the health researchers conflated race with culture or biological determinants. Similar to Marx, the oppressed have a more comprehensive perspective of society and social relations of production than do the privileged healthcare administrators who are limited by regulations from the Agency for Healthcare Research and Quality and their primary funder, CMS. It is also safe to say that most clinical administrators and healthcare providers are not from nor do they live in the same geographic areas as their patients. For this reason, it remains paramount for community members to have active collaborations and governance in the workings of FQHCs.

Social and health needs differ by locality because each place is shaped by a history of economic, demographic, and environmental changes. To ameliorate social determinants of health that are the cause or are strongly associated with health inequalities requires that we restructure and democratize community advisory boards (CABs), refine community health needs assessments, and provide additional financial resources for FQHCs and other CBHIs to implement structural interventions or engage in multilevel political advocacy. The restructuring of the CABs starts by changing the language at HRSA regarding the categories of patients that need to be represented in CBHI's advisory boards. Representation of women and racial and ethnic minorities needs to be interpreted by health center executives as a bare minimum. HRSA should not only include more diverse categories of marginalized and minority populations (disabled, immigrants, rural residents, sexual and gender minorities, etc.) but also provide flexible language that allows the composition of community advisory boards to represent other patient subpopulations identified from the triannual community health needs assessment and by the CAB members. Beyond representation, community advisory boards need to be democratized by being given more authority to vote and influence organizational re-structuring, hiring decisions, the use of financial resources, and the overall vision and mission of the community health center. This also means that the CAB shares ownership of data, resources, and products from programming and grant writing opportunities.

To ameliorate social determinants of health that are strongly associated with local health inequalities requires FQHCs to refine community health needs assessments (CHNAs). The ACA created three federal agencies to increase the research activity on the social determinants of health and health disparities: the Patient-Centered Outcomes Research Institute (PCORI), the Centers for Medicare and Medicaid Innovation (CMMI), and the Prevention Trust. However, these centers are meant to create evidence and recommendations that work within our existing healthcare delivery system, which favors the profits gained by managed care organizations, health insurance companies, hospitals, and pharmaceutical and biotechnology companies. They are not meant to transform the entire system to the benefit of the people.

In addition to identifying the needs and barriers that community members and patients face to access medical care, these needs assessments need to identify the community's strengths, assets, and *recommendations* for improving health promotion and their local communities. Although I am cautious about identifying a community's sources of resilience because it can minimize the community's suffering or the state's responsibility to intervene in social and political conditions, I also believe that viewing marginalized populations as solely deficient is not empowering or transformative. Knowing a community's strengths and assets facilitates the construction of interventions that leverage and promote the preservation of these assets.

Moreover, the CHNA can be used to identify and plan structural interventions that can be undertaken by community task forces in partnership with CHCs and other agencies or local businesses.

To implement structural interventions that engage in multilevel political advocacy requires that FQHCs have access to additional financial resources outside of the healthcare services and goods that they sell to patients. These financial resources can be leveraged by reviving discretionary funds given to FQHCs and CHCs prior to the implementation of the ACA or fund multisector collaborations to address a specific issue that is associated with a health inequality. For instance, the Medicaid Innovation Accelerator Program has a Medicaid Housing Agency Partnerships demonstration project in some states to ensure that patients who are unstably housed or living in poor housing conditions are placed in affordable housing (Medicaid Innovation Accelerator Program, 2017). In another example, "Live Well Springfield" is a coalition working to modify the built environment, which requires changes in zoning, land use, and resource management policies (see https://www.publichealthwm.org/what-we-do/coalition-building/live-well-springfield).

Sadly, improving the quality of care given to patients utilizing publicly funded CBHIs gained importance in the ACA as a strategy to reduce government spending and not toward actually improving quality of life for patients. Community-based health institutions, and FQHCs specifically, should continue to capture the quality of care in their patient populations to identify areas for improvement in the delivery of healthcare services in marginalized populations. Quality metrics need to go beyond clinical outcomes and reflect patients' perspectives. Their interpretation of "quality" is so important if we are to create trust between healthcare providers and patients, especially from groups that have a history of biomedical research abuse, like African Americans and the USPHS-sponsored Tuskegee Syphilis Study (Washington, 2006) and the randomized control trial of the oral contraceptive pill in Puerto Rican women on the island (Briggs, 2002).

Moreover, quality metrics collected from CBHIs need to ascertain that patients are not facing discrimination from the facility's staff or healthcare providers on the grounds of age, criminal status, gender, income, occupational status, race, and sexuality. Besides grievances reported by patients, there is little way of knowing on what grounds a provider or staff person provides unfair treatment to a patient. With feedback from diverse CABs, health services researchers examining FQHC data FQHCs need to create novel and community-specific quality indicators or construct categories of vulnerable populations not captured by government guidelines. For example, a healthcare provider denying gynecological care to a preoperative trans female-to-male because they are uncomfortable providing care to someone who presents physically as male. Another data source for CHNAs are the patient records. With feedback from diverse CABs, health services researchers examining FQHC data need to create novel and community-specific quality indicators or construct categories of vulnerable populations not captured by government guidelines.

If policy makers and economists are truly concerned about reducing federal spending and promoting health equity, there are only a few solutions in our current healthcare delivery system that could place some accountability on providers, especially medical doctors, and the private sector. First, the CMS could set prices with pharmaceutical companies, doctor's fees, and expensive medical diagnostics. Second, if the United States insists on maintaining the Medicare Shared Savings Program and Medicaid ACOs, they need to modify their quality metrics and take into consideration the social, economic, and environmental conditions of the patients utilizing FQHCs to avoid penalizing these safety-net organizations. CMS should also incentivize how ACOs develop participatory solutions with multiple sectors and diverse representation. Diverse representation on these interventions could be assessed by the number of community members serving as researchers and research assistants and on the level of shared decision-making, interpretation, and governance of those interventions. Another solution for CMS to reduce spending is for private or for-profit CBHIs to cover the risk of entering an ACO, by paying back for any losses they acquired in the process. However, these are merely marginal solutions that will not address larger ideological and structural issues in the United States and its dwindling welfare state. Surely, these propositions will be met with immense resistance from hospital systems, large pharmaceutical corporations, medical insurance lobbyists, and individual taxpayers.

In order to prevent large corporations from influencing the politics of health and eliminate the many institutional barriers that CBHIs face, the United States needs to implement a single-payer healthcare delivery system. The United States is one of the few OECD countries that does not have a single-payer system and the only country in the Americas that does not ensure health as a human right. In order to implement a single-payer system, we need to institutionalize health as a human right in our constitution and, again, in the vision of the Department of Health and Human Services (DHHS). This double commitment is so that in the event that health as a human right is overturned at the legislative or executive branches, at least health as a human right will permeate throughout all DHHS agencies. This will facilitate multisectoral collaborations between DHHS agencies to create programs that address the social determinants of health that are being promoted by the Centers for Medicare and Medicaid Innovation.

The public will face many hurdles to change a medical delivery system that is the fifth largest segment of the US gross domestic product. The fact that the single-payer option was never on the table during Barack Obama's healthcare reform negotiations (Navarro, 2010) makes it difficult to believe that there is now a possibility to reform healthcare. As I write this chapter, there is yet another attempt by President Trump to eliminate the ACA. This is not only a public health crisis with insurmountable repercussions, but it is not a reflection of what the majority in this country wants. A Reuters-Ipsos survey in 2018 indicated that 70% Americans support Medicare-for-All (Keller, 2019).

Given that people's healthcare has been constantly under threat by legislative, judicial, and executive actions since the inception of the ACA, having a single-payer Medicare-for-All entitlement program would curtail private or political action to eradicate any health protections. If voters were central to shaping the healthcare delivery system in the United States, there would be a smaller likelihood that these executive actions would be entertained. These political actions violate several government agencies' commitment to health equity. Below, I describe the ways in which a single-payer system, like Medicare-for-All, would lower many institutional barriers that CBHIs face such as financial detriment and threats to patient participatory engagement.

There are two Medicare-for-All bills that I will discuss in this final analysis: Senator Bernard Sanders (I-VT) Medicare-for-All Senate Bill (S. 1804) proposed in 2017 and, more recently, Representative Pramila Jayapal's (D-WA) Medicare-for-All House Bill (H.R. 1384). I will discuss both of them because researchers at the University of Massachusetts-Amherst Political Economy Research Institute (Pollin, Heintz, Arno, Wicks-Lim, & Ash, 2018) have conducted a very thorough economic analysis of Senator Sanders' bill, while Representative Jayapal's builds on Senator Sanders' bill by adding more patient protections.

One of the institutional barriers that was discussed in this chapter was that providers are often limited in providing certain medical goods and services that are considered controversial to conservative politicians and agency heads, with the consequence of losing their federal funding, such as Planned Parenthood Clinics losing Title X funds. There have been many court challenges to Section 1557 of the ACA, which prohibits individuals from being excluded from, denied benefits, or subject to discrimination by health providers, programs, and activities. H.R. 1384 tries to circumvent legal challenges to whom is protected under this law by "… explicitly defining sex discrimination to include sex stereotyping and discrimination based on gender identity, sexual orientation, and pregnancy and related medical conditions, including termination of pregnancy" (Keith, 2019). H.R. 1384 also ensures that providers are allowed to override national practice standards if the service is a medical necessity, appropriate, and consistent with the individual's wishes.

A more pressing institutional barrier that CBHIs face is that they have historically struggled to remain financially viable. Medicare-for-All would eliminate the complexity of value-based payment structures. Cost-savings will not be confined to the most vulnerable of healthcare organizations, like FQHCs, but will be universal across healthcare organizations. By having one payer (Medicare), the government will have the power to negotiate prices with service providers, pharmaceutical companies, and healthcare service organizations and promote universal cost-sharing (Pollin et al., 2018). The fear of unnecessary care and fraud that shaped the ACO would be greatly reduced as electronic health records will be part of a universal system across states.

The healthcare system will produce savings by eliminating much of the administrative costs associated with insurance claims (by 9%), prescription pricing (by 5.9%), and uniform Medicare rates of hospitals, clinics, and healthcare providers (by 2.8%) (Pollin et al., 2018, p. 1). Lastly, there are also broader economic implications such as the increase in job productivity (regaining lost days from illness), a reduction in income inequality due to families spending 2.6–14% less of their income on healthcare expenditures, and job creation by lowering the costs small- and medium-size businesses spend on employee health insurance (Pollin et al., 2018, p. 3).

Another institutional barrier that CBHIs face is how to democratize patient engagement in center governance and programming. Both S. 1804 and H.R. 1384 would maintain community advisory boards for community health centers, but H.R. 1384 would also create regional governance boards. However, as discussed above, we have to ensure that those board members reflect the diversity of the patient population in a specific geographic area. Medicare-for-All facilitates the creation of democratic processes in shaping the clinical practices that shape the ways that healthcare should be delivered.

Conclusion

A single-payer system like Medicare-for-All will not resolve all of the health inequalities experienced by marginalized populations in the United States, because this program alone will not automatically change social, economic, environmental, and political conditions that are responsible for health inequalities. However, Medicare-for-All would free up resources to focus on primary prevention and structural interventions. Additionally, it would eliminate politicians and healthcare lobbyists' main argument against improving quality and access to healthcare in community-based health institutions—the rising costs of healthcare. Surely, costs are rising partly because of the aging population, but more importantly, the US healthcare expenditures are far higher than any other country because we do not have policies that adequately contain costs or set the price of goods and services provided by healthcare providers and healthcare organizations (Anderson et al., 2019; Pollin et al., 2018). Piecemeal healthcare reforms are strangling patients and community engagement, giving private enterprise too much power. The very regulations (not to price-set) and political practices (legislators receiving campaign finances from health lobbies) violate the possibility for the United States to achieve health equity.

Health equity and profit cannot be in the same equation with equitable healthcare reform as the outcome. The jury is still out on ACOs ability to save CMS money and provide quality care to vulnerable populations. However, healthcare financing policies like the implementation of ACOs for the receipt of Medicare and Medicaid funds are based on neoliberal ideologies that give health insurance companies, biotechnology companies, and pharmaceuticals too much power and influence in shaping health policy, but little in institutional regulations that could shape their behavior in the healthcare delivery system. Meanwhile, we need to end symbolic participation of community members in patient advisory boards in order to increase the representation of other marginalized patient populations and gain authority over deciding the services that community-based health institutions provide. Nevertheless, we are in a critical moment in the United States with support from the public and the new politicians trying to strengthen the welfare state in an effort to reverse decades of exclusionary practices and institutional barriers that disenfranchise the public from influencing the politics and services provided in community-based health institutions.

References

Alberti, P. M. (2014). Community health needs assessments: Filling data gaps for population health research and management. *eGEMs, 2*(4), 1174.

Alberti, P. M., Bonham, A. C., & Kirch, D. G. (2013). Making equity a value in value-based health care. *Academic Medicine, 88*(11), 1619–1623.

Anderson, G. F., Hussey, P., & Petrosyan, V. (2019). It's still the prices, stupid: Why the US spends so much on health care, and a tribute to Uwe Reinhardt. *Health Affairs, 38*(1), 87–95.

Barnes, A. J., Unruh, L., Chukmaitov, A., & van Ginneken, E. (2014). Accountable care organizations in the USA: Types, developments and challenges. *Health Policy, 118*(1), 1–7.

Blustein, J., Weissman, J. S., Ryan, A. M., Doran, T., & Hasnain-Wynia, R. (2011). Analysis raises questions on whether pay-for-performance in Medicaid can efficiently reduce racial and ethnic disparities. *Health Affairs, 30*(6), 1165–1175.

Braveman, P. A., Kumanyika, S., Fielding, J., LaVeist, T., Borrell, L. N., Manderscheid, R., et al. (2011). Health disparities and health equity: The issue is justice. *American Journal of Public Health, 101*(S1), S149–S155.

Briggs, L. (2002). *Reproducing empire: Race, sex, science, and US imperialism in Puerto Rico* (Vol. 11). Berkeley, CA: University of California Press.

Epstein, S. (2008). *Inclusion: The politics of difference in medical research.* Chicago: University of Chicago Press.

Geiger, H. J. (2016). The first community health Center in Mississippi: Communities empowering themselves. *American Journal of Public Health, 106*(10), 1738–1740.

Human Rights Campaign. Understanding the transgender community. Retrieved on 15 March 2019 at https://www.hrc.org/resources/understanding-the-transgender-community

Israel, B., Eng, E., Schulz, A., & Parker, E. (Eds.). (2005). *Methods in community-based participatory research for health.* San Francisco, CA: Jossey-Bass.

Kaiser Famiy Foundation. (2017). Medicare delivery system reform: The evidence link. Retrieved from https://www.kff.org/medicare-delivery-system-reform-the-evidence-link/

Keith, K. Unpacking the House Medicare-for-All Bill. 3 March 2019. Health Affairs Blog: Following the ACA. Retrieved on 31 March 2019 at: https://www.healthaffairs.org/do/10.1377/hblog20190302.150578/full/

Keller, M. Seventy percent of Americans support 'Medicare for all' in new poll. 23 August 2019. *The Hill.* Retrieved on 30 March 2019 at: https://thehill.com/policy/healthcare/403248-poll-seventy-percent-of-americans-support-medicare-for-all

Kominski, G. F. (2013). *Changing the US health care system: Key issues in health services policy and management.* San Francisco: Wiley.

Levinson, D. (2017, August). Medicare Shared Savings Program Accountable Care Organizations have shown potential for reducing spending and improving quality. Department of Health and Human Services Office of the Inspector General. Retrieved 27 January 2019 at: https://oig.hhs.gov/oei/reports/oei-02-15-00450.asp

McWilliams, J. M., Hatfield, L. A., Chernew, M. E., Landon, B. E., & Schwartz, A. L. (2016). Early performance of accountable care organizations in Medicare. *New England Journal of Medicine, 374*(24), 2357–2366.

Medicaid Innovation Accelerator Programs. (2017, 18 May). Promoting Community integration through long-term services & supports in state medicaid-housing agency partnerships:

Program overview. Retrieved on 25 January 2019 at: https://www.medicaid.gov/state-resource-center/innovation-accelerator-program/iap-downloads/program-areas/partnerships-program-overview.pdf

Merlis, M., Berenson, R. A., & Fisher, E. S. (2010). Health policy brief: Accountable care organizations. *Health Affairs, 7*, 27.

National Association for Community Health Centers. (n.d.) Dr. H Jack Geiger and Dr. John Hatch on the earliest CHCs. Retrieved at: https://www.chcchronicles.org

National Association for Community Health Centers & John Snow, Inc. (2013). Health centers and payment reform: A primer. Emerging issues #7, October 2013. Retrieved at: http://www.nachc.org/wp-content/uploads/2015/11/Health-Centers-and-Payment-Reform.pdf

National Association for Community Health Centers. (2018). About our health centers. Retrieved from: www.nachc.org/about/about-our-health-centers/

Navarro, V. (2010). Consequences of the privatized funding of medical care and of the privatized electoral process. *American Journal of Public Health, 100*(3), 399–402.

Peters, G., & Woolley, J. T. (1996). "William J. Clinton. "Statement on Signing the Health Centers Consolidation Act of 1996," October 11, 1996". The American Presidency Project. University of California-Santa Barbara.

Pickett, K. E., & Wilkinson, R. G. (2015). Income inequality and health: A causal review. *Social Science & Medicine, 128*, 316–326.

Planned Parenthood Federation of America. "Hyde Amendment." Retrieved on 3 March 2019 at: https://www.plannedparenthoodaction.org/issues/abortion/hyde-amendment.

Pollin, R., Heintz, J., Arno, P., Wicks-Lim, J., & Ash, M. (2018). Economic analysis of Medicare for all. November. Political Economic Research Institute. University of Massachusetts-Amherst. Retrieved on 30 November 2018 at: https://www.peri.umass.edu/publication/item/1127-economic-analysis-of-medicare-for-all

Rodríguez, M. A., Young, M., & Wallace, S. P. (2015). *Creating conditions to support healthy people: State policies that affect the health of undocumented immigrants and their families*. Los Angeles, CA: University of California Global Health Institute.

Salganicoff, A. & Rice, C. (2019). Alina Salganicoff answers 3 questions on final title X regulations for family planning clinics. Kaiser Family Foundation, 27 Feb 2019. Retrieved at: https://www.kff.org/womens-health-policy/issue-brief/ask-kff-alina-salganicoff-answers-3-questions-on-final-title-x-regulations-for-family-planning-clinics/

Schulman, K. A., & Richman, B. D. (2016). Reassessing ACOs and health care reform. *JAMA, 316*(7), 707–708.

Scott, W. R., Ruef, M., Mendel, P. J., & Caronna, C. A. (2000). *Institutional change and healthcare organizations: From professional dominance to managed care*. University of Chicago Press. Chicago, IL.

Sharma, A. E., Huang, B., Knox, M., Willard-Grace, R., & Potter, M. B. (2018). PatientEngagement in community health center leadership: How does it happen? *Journal of Community Health, 43*(6), 1069–1074.

Shim, J. (2005). Constructing 'race' across the science-lay divide: Racial formation in the epidemiology and experience of cardiovascular disease. *Social Studies of Science, 35*(3), 405–436.

Song, Z., & Fisher, E. S. (2016). The ACO experiment in infancy—looking back and looking forward. *JAMA, 316*(7), 705–706.

Stroumsa, D. (2014). The state of transgender health care: Policy, law, and medical frameworks. *American Journal of Public Health, 104*(3), e31–e38.

Suro, R., Suárez-Orozco, M. M., & Canizales, S. (2015). Removing insecurity: How American children will benefit from President Obama's Executive Action on Immigration. USC Sol Price School of Public Policy, Tomas Rivera Policy Institute, April 2015, USC/UCLA. Retrieved on April 27, 2015 from: http://trpi.org/pdfs/research_report.pdf.

Tarlov, A. R. (1999). Public policy frameworks for improving population health. *Annals of the New York Academy of Sciences, 896* (Special Issue: Socioeconomic Status and Health in Industrial Nations: Social, Psychological and Biological Pathways), 281–293.

The Engelberg Center for Health Care Reform & the Dartmouth Institute. (2013, June). Opening Plenary Session of the Fourth National Accountable Care Organization Summit, Washington, D.C.

The Guttmacher Institute. "Federally Qualified Health Centers Could Not Readily Replace Planned Parenthood." 17 May 2017. https://www.guttmacher.org/news-release/2017/federally-qualified-health-centers-could-not-readily-replace-planned-parenthood

The TransActive Gender Center. (n.d.). "About Us." Retrieved on 22 March 2019 at: https://www.transactivegendercenter.org/about-us

Washington, H. A. (2006). *Medical apartheid: The dark history of medical experimentation on black Americans from colonial times to the present*. New York: Doubleday.

White, J. (2018). Hypotheses and hope: Policy analysis and cost controls (or not) in the Affordable Care Act. *Journal of Health Politics, Policy and Law, 43*(3), 455–482.

Whitehead, M. (1991). The concepts and principles of equity and health. *Health Promotion International, 6*(3), 217–228.

Woolhandler, S., & Himmelstein, D. U. (2017a). The Affordable Care Act: How Nixon's health reform proposal became Democrats' Albatross. *International Journal of Health Services, 47*(4), 612–620.

Woolhandler, S., & Himmelstein, D. U. (2017b). Single-payer reform the only way to fulfill the President's pledge of more coverage, better benefits, and lower costs. *Annals of Internal Medicine, 166*(8), 587–588.

Wright, B. (2013). Who governs federally qualified health centers? *Journal of Health Politics, Policy and Law, 38*(1), 27–55.

Wright, B. (2015). Do patients have a voice? The social stratification of health center governing boards. *Health Expectations, 18*(3), 430–437.

Wright, B., & Martin, G. P. (2014). Mission, margin, and the role of consumer governance in decision-making at community health centers. *Journal of Health Care for the Poor and Underserved, 25*(2), 930.

Chapter 13
Conclusion: A Re-evaluation of Institutionalized Health Care

Steven L. Arxer

Introduction

Community-based health care is a growing interest to academics and policymakers. As questions are raised about the status of the Affordable Care Act and rising health-care costs, scholars and practitioners are exploring the benefits that community-based models can offer healthcare delivery, service, and management. The nature of health care is thus changing, and alternative, "local," solutions are being integrated into the mainstream.

In *The New Public Health*, Baum (2016) emphasizes the growing scope of a new public health vision. Health and environment planners are faced with challenges to improving community health outcomes. In this vein, scholars have examined the link between theory and practice in community-based health care, with some providing general guidelines (Bartholomew, Parcel, Kok, Gottlieb, & Fernandez, 2016; Minkler & Wallerstein, 2008). Others have highlighted community-based theory in various professions, such as nursing (Billings & Halstead, 2016) and social work (Gould & Baldwin, 2016). Still others note the importance of community-based theory across disciplinary boundaries (Nelson & Stagger, 2018).

A trend found in the literature is the "institutionalization" of alternative health models in the professional sphere. However, investigations are lacking that have explored the theoretical and practical considerations of institutionalizing a community-based model. In other words, community-based theory is designed to overcome the limitations associated with traditional organizations of health care. In

S. L. Arxer (✉)
Department of Sociology and Psychology, University of North Texas at Dallas, Dallas, TX, USA
e-mail: steven.arxer@untdallas.edu

S. L. Arxer, J. W. Murphy (eds.), *Community-Based Health Interventions in an Institutional Context*, International Perspectives on Social Policy, Administration, and Practice, https://doi.org/10.1007/978-3-030-24654-9_13

this respect, a theory of organizations and institutions is implied by community-based theory that is often overlooked.

The aim of this volume, accordingly, is to focus on the theoretical and practical implications of institutionalizing a community-based approach to health care. Discussions of community-based work often are focused on human agency and community well-being. And these traits should not be overlooked. A problem, however, is that community-based practitioners' work in institutions is assumed to have a unique status, more significant than either individuals or communities. Nonetheless, discussions of institutional challenges to community-based work are rare. The goal of this collection has been to remedy this shortcoming and address some important institutional issues in community-based projects.

The chapters in this volume emphasize the benefits of institutionalizing community-based health projects, but in a manner different from the past. To the extent that community-based efforts are described as substantially different from conventional practices, service institutions must be conceptualized and operationalized to preserve the intention of communities. Furthermore, an entirely new ethic of health care is presumed by institutionalizing a community-based philosophy. In short, a careful examination of how community-based projects can be institutionalized has the prospect for advancing effective strategies for community health planning.

A recurring theme in this book is that planning should not be reduced to simply assisting communities or managing health services within certain locales. At the center of community-based theory is also a new image of social planning that goes beyond traditional models of leadership and management. Rather than developed and controlled by expert professionals, planning efforts emerge from below or, as Ulrich Beck (1997, p. 157) suggests, from a "sub-politics" that represents the direct action and goals of community members.

Reimagining Institutions Through Community-Based Philosophy

Clearly, community-based approaches seek a deeper involvement of community members because their biographies and contextual perspectives on community life shed important light on discussions about community well-being. However, the radical centering of community members in social planning suggests a reimagining of how these efforts are institutionalized. In short, being community-directed supplies important insight into how organizational life is transformed and a style of health organization emerges that is different from traditional health interventions. An important part of this movement toward self-directed projects is a need to reconceptualize the institutional contexts in which health projects take place.

Perhaps important to appreciate is the traditional descriptions of institutions, particularly their social imagery for the operation of organizations and the implications for the delivery of health services. Most often, institutions are understood to give stability and regularity to society. Institutions are meant to restrict idiosyncratic behavior and foster predictable interactions. As Anthony Giddens (1987, p. 11) notes, an institution represents "patterns of social activity reproduced across time and space." In short, institutions offer the continuity necessary to organize social life.

This description of institutions emerges alongside the positivist thinking of the latter half of the nineteenth and early part of the twentieth century. The continued development of industrial capitalism and the growing prestige of science led to a preference for scientific management as a means to regulate institutional behavior. In particular, specialization and technical knowledge became favored tools to guide how persons run businesses, economies, political organizations, and schools (Bentley, 1908). Using the techniques and guidelines of science to bring rationality, efficiency, and objectivity to any endeavor is thought to be a welcomed contribution to any organization.

Important for this discussion is that formalizing the practices of human organization has been presumed a positive development. By the 1930s, the Human Relations School began to argue that successful organizations train a cadre of professional managers (Whitley, 1984). For example, through principles of standardization and formalization characteristic of bureaucracies, managers can better regulate key individuals (workers) by developing discrete roles and clear lines of communication. The message becomes that human organizations simply work better when managed by an elite group of individuals who possess technical skills. These talents, moreover, allow them to think beyond their individual experience, so as to conceptualize the broader needs of the organization.

This image of human organization, nonetheless, is anathema to a community-based approach to health care. The problem is that a penchant for technical and formalized skills leads to the marginalization of the non-initiated. In the context of social research in academic and health institutions, professional researchers or health practitioners are in charge of most projects (Leitz & Zayas, 2010). Particularly insidious about this conceptualization of institutions is how the hierarchical system of authority, which situates professional experts on top of the organizational structure, means that inequality and marginalization of laypersons gain a sense of legitimacy. Because institutions and their leaders are presumed to be impersonally guided by formalized rules, they are not implicated in the process of prejudice or exclusion.

Considering the emphasis on self-direction in community-based theory, institutions and the hierarchy between professional and community members cannot be justified easily. Following the linguistic turn to knowledge, no perceptive is unbiased, even those of scientific professionals (Ugalde, 1985). The organization of institutionalized research pursued by academics and health professionals is no exception. As opposed to being objective, institutions and roles that make them up represent just one rendition of how social interaction should take place. The cultural hegemony of research is difficult to sustain, since their standardized methods are not neutral nor do they offer persons a more privileged position to judge reality.

Making Institutional Health Planning Transparent

From a community-based perspective, the institutional context where community health planning takes place needs to be made transparent. Here transparency is used in a way similar to Jean Gebser (1985, pp. 6–7), who defines this term as "everything latent behind and before the world" is revealed. Put differently, what Gebser means is that human action is recognized to pervade all that is known and thus nothing is preserved as an unbiased foundation. Thinking in terms of community-based institutions, this claim means that all persons can be legitimate participants in fomenting a vision of how social behavior should unfold.

This view of institutions is grounded in what Marx called *praxis* or human action. In this light, Tervalon and Murray-Garcia (1998, pp. 117–125) argue that from a community-based perspective, professional practitioners, researchers, and other social service agents should base their work in "cultural humility." They suggest that rather than centering the views of experts, these individuals should work toward a "lifelong commitment to self-evaluation and self-critique" so as to not obscure the views of community members through a power imbalance (Tervalon & Murray-Garcia 1998, pp. 117–125). This attitude is meant to curb the impact of professional cultures that can unnecessarily shadow the ideas and efforts of the community.

When institutions are reclaimed through collective praxis and partnership with communities, the rationale for community-based work becomes visible and a pathway is available for its actualization. Simply put, with collective praxis at the heart of institutions, the behavioral repertoire that goes along with community health research is expanded and power differentials minimized between communities and health professionals. When the deliberative process is opened in this manner, a democratic view of institutions is promoted, which is consistent with the aim of community-based social planning to have community members direct all local projects.

Instead of representing universal standards, the institutional context of community-based health care represents a human endeavor that may include competing views of need, risk, and illness. The point is that institutions are not sacrosanct; they are rooted in human actions and local language games. Institutions are thus made out of human praxis and do not represent a set of idealized traits. Treating institutions as monuments can promote the idea that certain skilled individuals best characterize the properties of institutions (formalism, standardization, technical), and thus, professionals should be granted special status.

And yet this type of hegemony is antithetical to community-based theory. What community-based strategies emphasize is that institutional arrangements are positional in nature and, thus, emerge from the outcomes of debate. As Stanley Fish (1992, p. 261) describes, institutions should be imagined to be "always emerging and re-emerging in response to historical needs and conditions." Rather than structural and mechanical, institutions are based on contingent understandings. In this way, institutions are never finalized, but always available for modification arising from local initiatives.

Issues of Power and "Community-Driven" Health Institutions

A central focus of community-based health planning is self-governance; self-regulation is the hallmark of a community-based style of institutionalization. To the extent that institutions represent human praxis, persons have nothing else to rely on but themselves for order. Institutions are thus discursive and represent the record of human activity. An important element of participatory health care is the idea that the community should drive health planning at all levels. Given the nonrealistic stance that community-based practitioners adopt, institutions and the power concealed by these entities can be examined. Subsequent to the demise of dualism, a neutral or universal standpoint is not possible to attain. Institutions are not an exception; they do not carry inherent autonomy due to their formal character. Institutional arrangements, instead, represent a set of specific assumptions made about human organization. Given the perspectival origin of institutions, these organizations should be receptive to local challenges and become polyvalent.

When community health projects unfold, however, a range of challenges often emerge. Most notably, community health initiatives "paradoxically … would not occur without the initiative of someone outside the community" (Minkler, 2005, p. ii8). And as is often noted, these individuals have the time, skills, commitment, and privilege to engage in these endeavors (Minkler, 2005, p. ii8). This reality, in turn, leads to "insider-outsider tensions," which has been discussed by community-based practitioners for some time (Ugalde, 1985). In this situation, community members remain on the periphery of the decision-making process, such as in the selection and understanding of health issues, the research process, and intervention strategies. At worst, these persons are used and exploited for information and labor, with the local communities seeing few benefits. As Wallerstein (1999) argues, community-based researchers and practitioners do not recognize the degree of power that is embedded in the privileges of professionals and other outsiders.

A key philosophical ingredient behind the insider-outsider dynamic, however, is often overlooked. The metaphysical claims that have been used to describe and justify institutions and the hierarchal relationships within them need to be exposed. To paraphrase Marx (1952), individuals create institutions but not always in terms of their own interests. More esteemed discursive formations gain power over institutions, such as those of technical experts, and may begin to inferiorize others. Here certain behaviors are institutionalized and are allowed to discriminate against community members who do not carry organizational positions or possess specific competencies. Moreover, this type of inequality carries the allure of neutrality given that they are associated with formal, institutional relationships.

But when institutions are reclaimed through human praxis and reflection, the rationale for institutional hierarchies is made visible for critique. Community-driven planning thus should include a new raison d'être for institutions, as well as for the health work accomplished within these settings. With institutions imagined to be mediated fully by human interpretation and action, these organizations should represent collective deliberations and the choices made to pursue one course of action or another. However, now these choices cannot be understood to be value-free but rather as political. In this context, political refers to the idea that human involvement and intentionality are inextricably tied institutions (Lyotard, 1993, p. 5). Community-based planning, accordingly, involves a re-evaluation of how persons and their communities have been positioned with respect to health-care institutions and the policies that emerge from these organizations.

References

Bartholomew, L. K., Parcel, G. S., Kok, G., Gottlieb, N. H., & Fernandez, M. E. (2016). *Planning health promotion programs: An intervention mapping approach*. California, USA: Jossey-Bass.

Baum, F. (2016). *The new public health*. South Melbourne, Australia: Oxford University Press.

Beck, U. (1997). *The reinvention of politics: Rethinking modernity in the global social order*. Cambridge, MA: Polity.

Bentley, A. (1908). *The process of government: A Study in social pressures*. Chicago, IL: The University of Chicago Press.

Billings, D., & Halstead, J. (2016). *Teaching in nursing: A guide for faculty*. St. Louis, MO: Elsevier.

Fish, S. (1992). The common touch, or one size fits all. In D. J. Gless & B. H. Smith (Eds.), *The politics of liberal education* (pp. 31–50). Durham, NC: Duke University Press.

Gebser, J. (1985). *The ever-present origin*. Athens, OH: Ohio University Press.

Giddens, A. (1987). *Sociology*. New York, NY: Harcourt Brace Jovanovich.

Gould, N., & Baldwin, M. (Eds.). (2016). *Social work: Critical reflection and the learning organization*. New York, NY: Routledge.

Leitz, C. A., & Zayas, L. E. (2010). Evaluating qualitative research for social work practitioners. *Advances in Social Work, 11*(2), 188–202.

Lyotard, J. F. (1993). *Libidinal economy*. Bloomington, IL: Indiana University Press.

Marx, K. (1952). The eighteenth Brumaire of Louis Napoleon. In R. C. Tucker (Ed.), *The Marx-Engels reader: A second edition*. New York, NY: Norton.

Minkler, M. (2005). Community-based research partnerships: Challenges and opportunities. *Journal of Urban Health, 82*(2), ii3–ii12.

Minkler, M., & Wallerstein, N. (Eds.). (2008). *Community-based participatory research for health: From process to outcomes*. California, USA: Jossey-Bass.

Nelson, R., & Stagger, N. (2018). *Health informatics: An interpersonal approach*. St. Louis, MO: Elsevier.

Tervalon, M., & Murray-Garcia, J. (1998). Cultural humility vs cultural competence: a critical distinction in defining physician training outcomes in medical education. *Journal of Health Care for the Poor and Underserved*, 9, 117–125.

Ugalde, A. (1985). Ideological dimensions of community participation in Latin America health programs. *Social Science & Medicine, 21*, 41–53.

Wallerstein, N. (1999). Power between evaluator and community: Research relationships within New Mexico's healthier communities. *Social Science & Medicine, 49*, 39–53.

Whitley, R. (1984). The development of management studies as a fragmented adhocracy. *Social Science Information, 23*(4–5), 775–818.

Index

S. L. Arxer, J. W. Murphy (eds.), *Community-Based Health Interventions in an Institutional Context*, International Perspectives on Social Policy, Administration, and Practice, https://doi.org/10.1007/978-3-030-24654-9

D

E

F

G

H

MIX
Papier aus verantwortungsvollen Quellen
Paper from responsible sources
FSC® C105338

If you have any concerns about our products,
you can contact us on
ProductSafety@springernature.com

In case Publisher is established outside the EU,
the EU authorized representative is:
Springer Nature Customer Service Center GmbH
Europaplatz 3, 69115 Heidelberg, Germany

Printed by Libri Plureos GmbH
in Hamburg, Germany

Magdalena Grenda-Kurmanow

Herbaria

Preservation and Conservation

Springer

Magdalena Grenda-Kurmanow
Faculty of Conservation and Restoration of Works of Art
Academy of Fine Arts in Warsaw
Warsaw, Poland

ISBN 978-3-032-21903-9 ISBN 978-3-032-21904-6 (eBook)
https://doi.org/10.1007/978-3-032-21904-6

The original submitted manuscript has been translated into English. The translation was done using artificial intelligence. A subsequent revision was performed by the author(s) to further refine the work and to ensure that the translation is appropriate concerning content and scientific correctness. It may, however, read stylistically different from a conventional translation.

Cover Illustration: Specimen from the Helwing/Boretius herbarium (1724–45), Herbarium of the Faculty of Biology, University of Warsaw (WA). Photo: M. Grenda-Kurmanow

This Springer imprint is published by the registered company Springer Nature Switzerland AG
The registered company address is: Gewerbestrasse 11, 6330 Cham, Switzerland

Preface

Herbaria containing dried botanical specimens serve as documentation of the relationships between humans and the plant world, and as such are a source of knowledge in many fields that study these interactions in various ways. As scientific tools, herbaria are currently used, among other things, in genetic analyses. The knowledge gained from research utilising plant specimens is applied in broader studies of biodiversity, species migration, climate change, environmental pollution, pharmacy, the history of diseases, and numerous other issues in the fields of ethnobotany, religious studies, sociology, and anthropology.

Modern scientific collections are required to meet several fundamental criteria: specimens should allow for species identification, be accompanied by the collector's name, and include the date and a precise description of the collection site (nowadays, the provision of exact geographical coordinates is indispensable). Historical herbaria very often lack complete scientific information: typically, only the name accompanies the specimen, while the place and date of collection are missing or the descriptions are incomplete. Nevertheless, they can still serve as valuable sources of information on the historical nomenclature and classification of species, their uses and popularity, as well as on the botanists themselves, as emphasised by the authors of monographic studies. The archival value of historical herbaria is also evident in the handwritten notes, which may constitute a valuable artefact for document analysis, and in the substrate itself, whose internal structure and fibrous composition can provide provenance information. Herbaria also continue to serve an educational function, both in school botany courses and in the educational activities of museums and herbarium institutions.

According to current knowledge, the first albums containing dried plants, intentionally created as scientific and educational aids, appeared in the sixteenth century. With the development of the natural sciences, they began to compete with herbal publications and botanical illustration, which, for a time, was considered a superior scientific resource. A turning point in the status of herbaria in science was the work of Carl Linnaeus, who not only established a system for organising the plant kingdom and the natural world as a whole but also popularised the method of mounting specimens on individual sheets—a technique still used today in the creation of herbarium collections. The standardisation of specimen collection methods increased the popularity of botanical collections among researchers. Although the history of their use as sources of scientific information has seen both periods of prominence and decline, today dried plants are the subject of numerous studies in which their DNA is analysed.

Throughout their history, herbaria have been produced, preserved, and repaired in various ways, which have led to a range of issues concerning their condition at both the macro- and microscales. The methods used to mount plants, the materials from which herbaria are constructed, the techniques for drying specimens, and the measures taken to protect them from insects have often had a significant impact on the preservation of genetic material.

Genetic studies typically utilise specimens specifically designated for this purpose, with strictly defined provenance and undamaged by biocides. However, historical herbaria, as unique collections and sources of information—sometimes incomparable to what can be obtained from more recent herbaria (e.g., regarding the oldest preserved specimens of a given species, extinct species, etc.)—may potentially become the subject of such analyses, even if they do not contain a complete set of scientific data. Advances in DNA research in the last decade of the twentieth century led to the growing popularity of genetics in taxonomic and phylogenetic analyses and to significant developments in these fields, associated, among other things, with the re-evaluation of existing taxonomic relationships. Therefore, curators of collections, regardless of the current perspective on the use of the herbarium under their care, should consider the potential future use of the collection for DNA research.

Who Is This Book For?

This publication provides information on the history of botany, the techniques and technologies used in the preparation of herbaria, the chemical composition of elements found in historical herbaria, the degradation of these elements and of genetic material, and methods for their preservation and conservation. It is primarily intended as a source of knowledge for institutional herbarium curators responsible for the care of both historical and contemporary herbarium collections. The publication will also be of use to curators of mixed collections that include herbaria, such as staff of natural history and regional museums, academic units with natural history collections, libraries, archives, and other institutions responsible for similar objects. The ethical and historical issues discussed here, along with the topics of degradation, storage, and preservation methods for collections, provide a comprehensive overview of herbaria as objects that require curatorial care. Many of the issues addressed pertain to natural history collections in general, not solely those of a botanical nature. The preservation methods described in the book are or have been used globally in collections, and thus the information presented is relevant not only to the oldest historical herbaria but also to contemporary collections. Many of these methods were used in the past and later found to be harmful, which means that current curators might sometimes be unaware of the risks associated with working with certain collections. An additional problem, encountered worldwide, is insufficient documentation of past collection care practices. Knowledge of potential hazards enables curators to conduct targeted analyses of hazardous substances and ensure safe working conditions. The same applies to conservators of natural history collections, which include herbaria. Information on degradation and conservation allows for the proper design of collection preservation policies. The historical section and the presentation of objects from Polish collections also facilitate the development and deepening of research on one's own collections.

This publication will also be useful to researchers who utilise herbarium collections or plan to conduct studies using herbaria as sources of information, including botanists, geneticists, ethnobotanists, pharmacists, students of pharmaceutical botany, anthropologists, and others. In addition to outlining the historical and technological context, the work explains the condition of the collections and their potential as scientific tools.

The interdisciplinary nature of this work makes it relevant to a broader audience. The book can serve as a resource for students of biological sciences, pharmacy, and medicine. It offers an opportunity to expand their knowledge of the origins of the natural sciences, in which botany and herbaria play a pivotal role as forms of documentation. Readers will also find information on toxic substances used to preserve collections, which can cause persistent contamination of biological information repositories such as herbaria, and are also present in other plant-related human activities, such as agriculture. The book can be successfully used as supplementary reading for botany courses, classes on the creation of herbarium collections, and issues related to the preservation of their genetic material.

This publication may also be useful for students of disciplines such as archival studies, cultural heritage protection, or conservation studies, due to the comprehensive description of selected aspects of the degradation of historic paper-based objects.

Finally, this book may prove useful to all botany enthusiasts, serving as a source of inspiration and knowledge on the conscious creation of plant catalogues and their conservation. It may also encourage the responsible documentation of the biological information that surrounds us, which future generations will value as part of their heritage.

Book Structure

The book is divided into five chapters: a historical analysis (Chap. 1), a technological analysis (Chap. 2), a review of degradation processes (Chap. 3), an overview of preventive and interventive conservation methods (Chap. 4), and a section presenting case studies of conservation treatments on three eighteenth-century herbaria (Chap. 5).

Chapter 1 presents a broad historical context for the emergence and development of botany as a scientific discipline, which directly prompted the creation of the first herbaria as scientific tools. Additionally, the earliest examples of using dried and pressed plant specimens in the field of botany are described, initially serving as aids to botanical illustration. Each chapter seeks to capture the processes that enabled the emergence of herbaria and their application in science. The technological challenges that led to herbaria being regarded as inferior sources of information are also discussed, as are the ways how these challenges contributed to the development of appropriate techniques for their preparation and preservation. The role of herbaria as artefacts—components of natural history collections associated with the phenomenon of fashionable *curiosités*—is examined, with particular emphasis on Polish collections. Ethical issues related to the creation of herbaria, which may affect the functioning of collections and, in selected cases, their conservation, are also addressed.

Chapter 2 describes various technological aspects of herbarium preparation, including their form and methods of production, as well as the physicochemical characteristics of the main components, with particular emphasis on the shared structural features of plant specimens and the paper substrate. The description of techniques includes references to historical methods of herbarium preparation. The chapter lists many techniques that are no longer in use, assuming that technological information is important not only for planning the preservation and conservation of herbarium collections but also for designing research involving herbaria.

Chapter 3 describes degradation processes occurring at the macroscale of herbarium structures and at the molecular level. Subsequent chapters are devoted to acid hydrolysis, alkaline degradation, oxidation, contamination, biodeterioration, and the destructive effects of biocidal agents. A separate section discusses known processes of genetic material degradation, citing numerous publications that demonstrate that methods of preparation, storage, and preservation significantly influence the condition of collections.

Chapter 4 addresses issues related to the preservation of herbarium specimens. The focus is on evaluating the strategic principles of Integrated Pest Management (IPM), describing the evolution of perspectives, and assessing the mixed evaluations of individual IPM components. The section also discusses challenges associated with decontamination and the preservation of genetic material.

Chapter 5 outlines the conservation-restoration methodology for historic herbaria, developed on the basis of archival queries and technical analysis conducted on three bound eighteenth-century herbaria from Polish collections: the herbarium of Izabela Czartoryska (1746), held in the collections of the National Museum in Kraków and the Czartoryski Library; the herbarium of Johann Friedrich Zeidler (1732), from the Main Library of the University of Life Sciences in Lublin; and the herbarium attributed to Helwing or Boretius, from the Herbarium of the Faculty of Biology at the University of Warsaw (1724–1745). For each object, the principles of a safe conservation methodology were defined, encompassing non-invasive or micro-destructive analytical studies and technical solutions that minimise physical intervention in the structure of the objects. The outcomes of the conservation treatments carried out are also presented.

At the very end of the work, there is an index of cited herbaria by location, as well as names and subject indexes.

The book devotes considerable attention to several aspects considered the most significant and distinctive in the context of preserving historical herbaria. The first aspect concerns the methods of mounting specimens, with particular emphasis on the adhesives used to attach plants to paper substrates. The second aspect is the presence of biocides, which have been used to poison herbaria to protect against insects since the earliest days of their creation. The presence of biocidal agents also poses a threat to the health and safety of collection users—a risk that is, unfortunately, often underestimated. For both adhesives and biocides, information is compiled regarding their impact on the condition and preservation of herbaria on various levels. Special attention is also given to the preservation of genetic material. Genetic research is a rapidly developing field, yet it remains a challenging area of study, still full of mysteries and enticing in terms of what remains to be discovered, particularly in the field of heritage conservation and preservation. It can be said that viewing collection care through the lens of genetic material preservation opens a new dimension of conservation and related competencies, while also broadening the scope of responsibility for collection curators and conservators to include the conservation of the genetic matter of the artefact.

The cross-interdisciplinary scope of this work is evident in the breadth of topics addressed: from historical aspects, through issues related to chemical degradation at various levels, to laboratory analysis and conservation practice. The study's extensive scope necessitated certain abbreviations and simplifications to maintain clarity. This applies to both the historical section and the description of chemical processes. Where information was deemed useful, references have been provided to enable the reader to explore further contexts and conduct their own analyses.

A special place in the book is given to references to Polish aspects related to herbaria. The work includes information on the development of natural history collections in Polish territories and cites a number of publications by Polish researchers that may not always be familiar to international readers.

Warsaw, Poland Magdalena Grenda-Kurmanow

Acknowledgements

The relationship between the plant world and humanity has long fascinated me, as has the remarkable world of historical documents. I chose to pursue a professional path as a conservator of heritage objects on paper, but by chance, plants would also become part of this field. This occurred through an anonymous nineteenth-century herbarium containing dried plants from the collection of the Krzysztof Kluk Museum of Agriculture in Ciechanowiec, which required conservation intervention. Working on this object proved to be both a challenging task and a captivating adventure. Since then, herbaria have regularly appeared in my professional practice. Delving into the history and preservation of historical herbaria led to a scientific project that subsequently resulted in a doctoral dissertation on the protection and conservation of these extraordinary objects. This book is based on part of that dissertation and is a revised and updated version of the Polish edition published in 2023.

The queries, research, and conservation work cited in this study were carried out as part of a research programme funded by the National Science Centre in Poland. For the English edition, I have included references to more recent publications related to herbaria.

This research would not have been possible without the encounters with remarkable people whom I have been fortunate to meet along the way. I would like to thank my doctoral supervisor, Professor Weronika Liszewska, for all the time and attention she has devoted to me as a doctoral student and for her longstanding support, as well as my co-supervisor, Dr Piotr Klepacki, for his valuable comments and inspiring meetings, and Professor Łukasz Łuczaj, who encouraged me to publish this book. I am also grateful to everyone who contributed to the research conducted as part of the scientific project, without which this book would not have come into being.

I would like to thank the collection owners for their trust and for granting access to the objects for research and conservation: the National Museum in Kraków and the Princes Czartoryski Library, the Herbarium of the Faculty of Biology at the University of Warsaw, and the Main Library of the University of Life Sciences in Lublin. I must emphasise that the decisions and the quality of collaboration are closely linked to the work and kindness of the individual people with whom I have had the good fortune to work. Therefore, I extend my sincere thanks to Dr Paulina Studzińska-Jaksim, Dr Marian Butkiewicz, Dr Maja Graniszewska, and Marta Winiarczyk. I am also grateful to all other institutions that provided images of their objects for this publication: Polish herbaria: KRAM, KRA; the Herbarium of the Natural History Museum in Wrocław; the Poznań Society for the Advancement of Arts and Sciences Library; the Herbarium of the Nicolaus Copernicus University in Toruń; the Central Archives of Modern Records in Warsaw; and herbaria outside Poland: Naturalis Biodiversity Center in Leiden, Muséum national d'Histoire naturelle, Linnaean Society, Natural History Museum in London, British Library, Burgerbibliothek in Bern, BIU Santé Médecine—Université Paris Cité, and the Bayerische Staatsbibliothek.

I would like to thank everyone who assisted me during my research visits, especially Dr Ewa Lenard from the Herbarium in Wrocław, Professor Marcin Nobis from the KRA Herbarium, and Dr Wojciech Paul from the KRAM Herbarium. I am also grateful to the curators, conservators, and staff of international institutions, particularly Gerard Thijsse and Roxali Bijmoer from the Naturalis Biodiversity Center in Leiden, as well as colleagues from SPNHC, Kew, and the Smithsonian Institution, and many others who work or have worked with natural history collections, for their support at various stages of writing my doctoral thesis, their interest, discussions, participation in the survey, and willingness to generously share their knowledge.

Finally, I would like to thank the most important and dearest people in my life—my wonderful family—for their support and understanding. Such support cannot, of course, be described in a single sentence. Without you, none of this would have been possible.

Competing Interests The author has no competing interests to declare that are relevant to the content of this manuscript.

Contents

About the Author

Magdalena Grenda-Kurmanow, PhD, is an Assistant Professor at the Faculty of Conservation and Restoration of Works of Art, Academy of Fine Arts in Warsaw, Poland. Her PhD dissertation focused on conservation and restoration of historic herbaria regarding the preservation of DNA material of herbarium specimens. She is a member of the Best Practice Committee at the Society of the Preservation of Natural History Collections (SPNHC) and Associate Editor of the *Journal of Paper Conservation*.

Chapter 1
History and Significance of Herbaria with Dried Plant Specimens

Abstract This chapter presents a broad historical context for the emergence and development of botany as a scientific discipline, which directly prompted the creation of the first herbaria as scientific tools. Additionally, the earliest examples of using dried and pressed plant specimens in the field of botany are described, initially serving as aids to botanical illustration. Each chapter seeks to capture the processes that enabled the emergence of herbaria and their application in science. The technological challenges that led to herbaria being regarded as inferior sources of information are also discussed, as are the ways how these challenges contributed to the development of appropriate techniques for their preparation and preservation. The role of herbaria as artefacts—components of natural history collections associated with the phenomenon of fashionable *curiosités* — is examined, with particular emphasis on Polish collections. Ethical issues related to the creation of herbaria, which may affect the functioning of collections and, in selected cases, their conservation, are also addressed.

Keywords History of herbaria · History of botany · Herbarium ethics · Botanical illustration

This work was written to provide a comprehensive understanding of herbaria as objects of natural heritage, with the aim of enabling informed planning for their preservation and conservation, as well as for the management of herbarium collections in ways that ensure their preservation for future generations. The information presented in this book has been selected through consultations with curators and conservators of herbarium collections, to create a practical source of knowledge on the conservation of such objects.

Textbooks such as *Herbarium Handbook* (Bridson and Forman 1999, Davies et al. 2023) and *Zielnik i zielnikoznawstwo* (Drobnik 2009) address issues related to the preservation of collections as a secondary topic, with their primary focus being the formation, development and management of new collections. However, none of

M. Grenda-Kurmanow, *Herbaria*, https://doi.org/10.1007/978-3-032-21904-6_1

them discusses, to a similar extent, the various aspects of herbarium technology, the degradation of botanical material, the history of the preservation of collections, and, at the same time, delves into source texts concerning the history of herbarium creation. This book expands the body of information in these areas, drawing on extensive literature from various fields as well as original research, and thus may serve as a supplement to the aforementioned key works on herbaria.

Texts on conservation treatments of herbaria also do not constitute a large body of sources. This category includes several articles and conference papers (Clarck 1986; Egenberg and Moe 1991; Menei 2005; Dauwalder 2013; Grenda 2013, 2015; Gersten et al. 2017; Popławska et al. 2017; Popławska and Zając 2018; Berli and Belhadj 2020), short chapters in the latest edition of the *Herbarium Handbook* (Young 2023a, b), unpublished or available to a limited extent theses (Margez 2004; Dauwalder 2012; Keijzers 2013; Popławska 2014a, b), as well as unpublished scripts or conservation reports.[1] These sources allow for the examination of contemporary conservation methodologies, though the detail they provide varies.

Herbarium collections and their conservation were also the subject of several post-conference publications held in the 1990s: *Conservation and the Herbarium*, organised by the Institute of Paper Conservation in 1994 in Leigh (UK)[2]; the *Conference on the Preservation of Botanical Collections*, with its first edition in 1993 in St Petersburg and the second edition (*Botanical Collections Throughout the World*) in 1997 in Kraków, organised in this instance by the Władysław Szafer Institute of Botany, Polish Academy of Sciences (Stuchlik 1998); and *Managing the Modern Herbarium* in 1999 in Ontario (Canada), organised by the Society for the Preservation of Natural History Collections (SPNHC).[3] However, this remarkable surge of interest in the subject over just 5 years was not followed by further post-conference monographs devoted entirely to herbarium collections. For years, individual works addressing conservation issues related to herbarium collections have been presented at conferences organised by SPNHC, the Natural Sciences Collections Association (NatSCA), and occasionally at other conference meetings,

[1] Research report: Wierda A (1994) Het gebruik van o.a. PVA-lijm ter bevestiging van gedroogd plantenmateriaal in herbaria. Een onderzoeksrapport. Met een kort overzicht van bevestiginingsmethoden van plantenmateriaal op papier. Den Haag, Algemeen Rijskarchief, research report, Naturalis Biodiversity Center, Leiden; and conservation reports: Jacobi E, Phan TL, (2012) Herbaria Restauratie-documentatie. Fase I. Nationaal Herbarium Nederland; Mertens S, Vries de H (2013) Herbaria Restauratie-documentatie. Fase II, Nationaal Herbarium Nederland; Valk de M (2010) Het Herbarium van de Stedelijke Musea Zierikzee. Beschrijving en conserveringsadvies; Vries de H (2013) Herbaria Restauratie-documentatie. Fase II. Nationaal Herbarium Nederland; Wierda A (1995) De restauratie van het Boerhave Herbarium (Rijksherbarium Leiden), Amsterdam—all stored at the Naturalis Biodiversity Center in Leiden, and were made available to the author courtesy of Gerard Thijjse.

[2] Currently the Institute of Conservation. In this work, two texts from this conference are cited: Gunn (1994) and Walker and Hughes (1994).

[3] In this work, numerous texts published in connection with this conference are cited: Down (1999), Fenn (1999), Rader and Ison (1999), Strang (1999a, b), and Townsend (1999).

followed by publications (e.g. Hawks and Bell 1999; Menei 2005; Grenda 2013; Grenda-Kurmanow 2016).

Information regarding historical herbaria is typically scattered. The associated literature centres around several main themes. It is not difficult to find a number of articles of a historical and taxonomic nature (e.g. Scott and Hewett 2008; Bertin 2016; Ossenbach 2017; van Andel and Barth 2018; Costa et al. 2018; Stech et al. 2018; Stefanaki et al. 2018; Stefanaki et al. 2019; Thijsse 2018; Thijsse and Wesseling 2021; Zych et al. 2023; Cristofolini 2024; Grenda-Kurmanow et al. 2025). In addition to a historical introduction, these texts often include a catalogue of the plant species present in a given herbarium, with current taxonomic identifications. Studies of herbaria at varying levels of detail are also published in the form of monographic books.[4] It is worth mentioning here the first history of herbaria with dried plants, authored by Saint-Lager in 1885, who reviewed the oldest herbarium collections along with an inventory description (Saint-Lager 1885). Earlier, publications on herbarium-related topics appeared only sporadically (Meyer 1857; Kessler 1870). A comprehensive modern historical study of Thijsse (2016) is the frequently cited in this chapter.[5]

In the broader context of the development of botany as a Renaissance science of description, aiding in the mastery of the natural world, elements of the history related to herbarium collections can be found, among others, in the works of Ogilvie, Egmond, Rix, Mangani and Tomasi, as well as Zemanek.[6] Numerous references also appear in studies concerning the later development of botany, closely linked to the period of rapidly expanding colonialism (e.g. Davis 2018; Harris 2018; MacGregor 2018a, b).

The most commonly encountered texts containing information on historical herbaria however, are the aforementioned monographic articles. The popularity of works in this genre has increased, particularly in recent years.[7] Many articles addressing herbarium-related topics emphasise the usefulness of herbaria for various fields of knowledge (e.g. Davis et al. 2015; Willis et al. 2017; Craine et al. 2018; Espinosa and Pinedo Castro 2018; James et al. 2018; Kiss et al. 2018; Ent et al. 2019; Gallagher et al. 2019; Meineke and Davies 2019; Pearson 2019; Burbano and Gutaker 2023 and many others).[8]

---

[4] These studies focus on various historical aspects of a given collection, prioritising either the historical context or the origin and content of its individual components (e.g. Rytz 1933; Britten et al. 1958; Lienhard and Dauwalder 2016).

[5] However, studies conducted in recent years have introduced several updates regarding attribution and dating (e.g. Stefanaki et al. 2019; Grenda-Kurmanow et al. 2025).

[6] Frequently cited in this book (Zemanek 1997, 2009; Ogilvie 2006; Egmond 2010, 2018; Kusukawa 2012; Mangani and Tomasi 2013; Rix 2013).

[7] This is evident, for example, from the references cited later in the text, indicating that the subject of herbaria has enjoyed particular popularity over the past decade.

[8] See, among others, the useful summary in Palmer et al. (2012), Nesbitt (2014), and Burbano and Gutaker (2023).

In Poland, key historical and identification-focused publications began to appear in the 1970s and 1980s. In addition to the monograph on the two oldest herbaria in the collections of the Institute of Botany at the Jagiellonian University, which was published as a book in 1981, Professor Piekiełko (later Zemanek) published a study of the herbarium belonging to Izabela Czartoryska in the form of an article (Piekiełko 1977, 1981). At the same research centre, Professor Piotr Köhler has authored numerous monographs in the form of books and articles, including a detailed study of the herbaria of Józef Jundziłł (1994, 1995) and articles on the collections of Marian Raciborski (1989), Seweryn Udziela (1996), and (Köhler 1989, 1994, 1995, 1996). Monographic publications in book form have also been devoted to the herbaria of Brother Cyprian from the Red Monastery (in Slovakia), the herbaria of Tytus Chałubiński from the Tatra Museum in Zakopane, and the herbarium of Eliza Orzeszkowa from the collections of the Poznań Society of Friends of Sciences in Poznań (Radwańska-Paryska 1991; Ochyra and Cisło 1999; Kielak 2004). Polish collections and their history are disseminated through articles by Dr Maja Graniszewska (Graniszewska et al. 2016; Graniszewska 2018; Graniszewska and Kapler 2018) and others (including Rostański 1963; Chlebicki 1991; Spalik 2014a; Pękacka-Falkowska 2018a, 2022; Zych et al. 2023; Grenda-Kurmanow et al. 2025; Grenda-Kurmanow 2026).

Herbaria, as historical objects, are also featured in exhibitions, though they rarely become the main focus. In Poland, there are known examples of presenting a herbarium as a work of artistic craftsmanship (the *#heritage* exhibition at the National Museum in Kraków in 2017) (Paś 2017), as well as the exhibition of an anonymous nineteenth-century herbarium in the Department of Herbal Traditions at the Krzysztof Kluk Museum of Agriculture in Ciechanowiec in 2014. Against this background, an exceptional example was the 2015 exhibition *The Cultural Heritage of the Warsaw Pharmacist Ferdynand Karo in the Context of the Inventory of the World* at the Museum of Pharmacy in Warsaw, which showcased Karo's scientific achievements, his working tools, and selected herbarium sheets (Arabas 2015).

It is also worth noting that the oldest herbarium specimen in Polish collections, authored by Paolo Silvio Boccone at the end of the seventeenth century, apart from a mention by Rostański (1963), has only recently been made widely known through an article (Grenda-Kurmanow et al. 2025). Similarly, until now, the history of the two-volume, originally three-volume, herbarium of Johann Friedrich Zeidler from 1732 to 1751 was completely unknown; this herbarium is now also regarded as one of the oldest and most valuable in Poland. Other herbaria from Polish collections dating from the seventeenth and eighteenth centuries have been described by researchers to varying degrees of detail and from different perspectives. Some of these publications were written several decades ago. This book serves as an introduction to a more thorough study of these collections, and to the systematisation of knowledge the oldest known herbaria.

Editorial notes

With regard to editorial remarks, it is first necessary to address a fundamental terminological issue, namely the word "herbarium", which is used here in various forms and contexts. Today, this term has several meanings. It may refer to a herbarium containing dried plants, a collection of herbaria, or an institution housing herbarium collections. Historically, the term "herbarium" was sometimes also used to describe a collection of living plants cultivated in a garden. Additionally, it could refer to herbals, that is, illustrated catalogues of plants (either manuscript or printed). The terminology applied to herbaria containing dried plants is discussed in greater detail in a separate chapter.[9]

Another issue worth addressing is the lack of an established system for describing herbaria. These objects, due to the presence of handwritten layers, are often classified as manuscripts, which is evident, for example, in institutional catalogue numbers (*Ms.* or, for example *Rkp,* in Polish). Consequently, this study adopts a citation scheme appropriate for manuscript artefacts: author, object name (title or common name given in parentheses), holding institution, reference number (if present and known), and dating. To maintain clarity, citations have been abbreviated under illustrations in the subsections of Chap. 5, which are entirely devoted to individual objects. In these cases, the full citation appears in the first footnote to the title of the relevant chapter.

Reference numbers for the majority of cited specimens are provided in the footnotes and/or in the figure captions, where known and available. Detailed data for each cited specimen are included in the herbarium index at the end of the book, organised according to the institution of deposition. The index is a proposal for a standardised compilation of identification descriptions. When citing collections belonging to registered herbarium institutions, the institution's name is followed by the *Index Herbariorum* code (Thiers 2026, continuously updated). The dates of birth and death of botanists and other historical figures are provided only at their first mention.

1.1 Natural History: From the Image of Human Dominance Over Nature to an Independent Discipline. The Evolution of Botanical Description

The origins of herbaria are closely linked to the development of botany and the broader discipline of natural history. As will be described in the following paragraphs, the emergence of natural history as a distinct scientific field occurred during the Renaissance. However, to fully understand this process, it is necessary to refer to works on nature produced in antiquity and to outline the broader historical context of human studies of the natural world.

---

[9] See Sect. 1.3.3.

The most significant and influential works concerning nature included the treatises of Aristotle, Theophrastus, Dioscorides, Pliny the Elder, and Galen.[10] A common feature of most works devoted to plants is the description of their medicinal properties, which was related to the use of plants for medical purposes and the demand for textbooks in this field. It can be said that the utilitarian aspect of plants marked the beginnings of systematic botany (Arber 1970, p. 6).

Later authors cited their predecessors, and the most widely read works were repeatedly transcribed and copied, both in text and in illustrations. However, from around the eleventh to the fifteenth century, there is a marked decline in literary activity in the field of natural history (Reeds and Kinukawa 2013, p. 570). Only a handful of works from the Middle Ages have survived that bear witness to a creative methodology in describing of the plant world. In the spirit of Aristotelian natural philosophy, and often in the form of commentaries on the work *De plantis* by Nicolaus of Damascus, the thirteenth-century authors, such as Albertus Magnus, Simon Cordo (Simon Genuensis), and Rufinus, described their own observations of nature.[11] However, these pioneers were unaware of each other's work, there was no community of naturalists to provide a space for the development of the field. No discussions concerning botanical description and observation took place during this period.[12] It was only a little over 200 years later, through the publication of several works and the emergence of the first research methodologies, that botany was born as a science. This was already the era of printed books, which enabled the dissemination of knowledge on an unprecedented scale and offered uniform copies as sources, in contrast to the individual manuscripts (Nauert 1979, pp. 76–78). The revolution brought about by the invention of printing provided the impetus for the systematic study of ancient literature and for taking a step further — towards science.

The restoration and critical analysis of ancient texts on natural history or medicine contributed to the emergence of natural history as a scientific discipline in the mid-sixteenth century (Ogilvie 2006, pp. 1–7).[13] The process of restoration involved purging the texts of errors that had accumulated during their transmission, mistakes most often attributed to Arab copyists. The creation of revised versions of classical

---

[10] Aristotle, *Peri zōōn moriōn* (Latin: *De partibus animalium*) and *Peri zōōn istorias* (*De animalium historia*); Theophrastus, *Peri phutōn istorias* (Latin: *De historia plantarum*), c. 350–287 BC, and *Peri phutōn aitōn* (*De causis plantarum*); Dioscorides, *Peri ulēs iatrikēs* (Latin: *De materia medica*), c. 65–77 AD; Pliny the Elder, *Naturalis Historia*, c. 77 AD; Galen, *De simplicium medicamentorum temperamentis et facultatibus*, second half of the second century AD.

[11] Albertus Magnus, *De vegetabilibus*, c. 1259; Simon Cordo, *Synonyma medicinae/Clavis sanationis*, c. 1292; Rufinus, *De virtutibus herbarum*, c. 1297 (Reeds and Kinukawa 2013, pp. 573–589).

[12] "The studies of nature were a literary genre, not a social activity," writes Brian W. Ogilvie (2006, p. 99) about the natural history pursuits of that period.

[13] Previously regarded as a branch of natural philosophy, natural history first appeared as a separate category in Juan Luis Vives's 1531 encyclopaedia, *De tradendis disciplinis*, although it was understood as a literary category. It emerged as an independent discipline only in the works of Francis Bacon: *The Advancement of Learning* (1605), *Novum Organum* (1620), and *De augmentis scientiarum* (1623).

texts sparked lively debates among both philologists and scholars who relied on these sources in medical and pharmaceutical practice. It was the careful reading of these works and the sense of dissatisfaction among Renaissance scholars that laid the foundations for the modern scientific description.[14]

The treatise "Natural History" (*Naturalis Historia*) by Pliny the Elder (c. 23–79 AD) was a 37-volume encyclopaedia encompassing all phenomena of the contemporary world, both natural and those resulting from human activity. Pliny's work was compiled largely on the basis of studies of Greek[15] and Roman literature, and was essentially a compilation of knowledge drawn from other sources. In his work, Pliny included within the category of natural history not only the world of plants (books XII–XIX), animals, minerals, and celestial bodies, but also anthropology, art, industry, psychology, agriculture, and medical knowledge.[16]

Pliny's descriptions of nature reveal the subordinate role of the natural world in relation to the achievements of civilisation and human activity. In describing successive groups of plants, he primarily emphasises the ways in which they can be processed in various branches of industry. The "Natural History" is thus a celebration of civilisation's dominance over nature, highlighting the utilitarian character of various elements of the natural world.[17] In his catalogue, Pliny included not only medicinal plants, but also all plants about which he found references in the literature available to him. He declared that he had studied almost all the plants described in the "Natural History" through direct observation as well.[18]

While in the Middle Ages scholars treated the text of the "Natural History" as an encyclopaedia and drew knowledge about the world from it (Nauert 1979, p. 74), for Renaissance readers an uncritical reception was no longer sufficient. As a result, detailed commentaries on Pliny's work began to be published. Careful study revealed that, in reality, his compilation contained numerous errors, the origins of

[14] At the same time, the texts of Dioscorides and Galen were held in great esteem, as evidenced by the fact that they formed part of the medical curriculum at the universities of Padua, Bologna, and Montpellier in the 1530s (Ogilvie 2006, p. 33; Reeds 1976, p. 520). Ogilvie titled her treatise on the birth of Renaissance natural history *Science of Describing* (Ogilvie 2006, pp. 7–8), in reference to the term *Art of Describing,* used as the title of a book on seventeenth-century Dutch painting. Ogilvie compares the struggles of seventeenth-century Dutch painters to the work of Renaissance naturalists.

[15] Mainly Theophrastus of Eresos (370–287 BC).

[16] The medicinal use of plants was described by Pliny in books XX–XXVII.

[17] It can, of course, be argued that the description of nature (and subsequently the collection of its products) is, in a sense, always a specific manifestation of human dominance over nature. This idea guided many authors of classification systems and naturalists collecting specimens, especially from distant parts of the world. However, what is at issue here is a time when nature was perceived instrumentally, before it began to be admired and analysed as a phenomenon in its own right.

[18] This was to take place in the garden of Antonius Castor, whom he described as "the highest botanical authority of our time" (Pliny 1966, p. 143; see also Ogilvie 2006, p. 126).

which were interpreted in various ways.[19] More lenient critics attributed the many mistakes to the degeneration of source texts and of the "Natural History" itself during repeated copying by not necessarily well-educated scribes. Opponents of this view accused Pliny of incompetence and a lack of independent observation, while simultaneously highlighting the need to produce modern encyclopaedic works.[20]

The works of Dioscorides (c. 40–90 CE) and Galen (c. 130–200 CE) did not provoke such fierce controversies as the "Natural History". Dioscorides' *De materia medica libri quinque* was regarded as the summa of ancient descriptive botany (Ogilvie 2006, p. 96).[21] In the introduction to his catalogue of plants, the author emphasised the value of observing nature in the work of a botanist, as well as the necessity of knowing a given species at all stages of its development.[22] The primacy of an empirical approach to plant analysis was the main reason for Dioscorides' growing popularity among scholars for over 1600 years (!), making *De materia*

[19] Firstly, the fact that Pliny was not a botanist and acquired his knowledge from books—sometimes read aloud to him, from which he would then dictate notes—mediated the transfer of knowledge and allowed for numerous errors to occur (Healey 1999, p. 24). Moreover, the very sources he consulted may have contained mistakes, which Pliny subsequently perpetuated (Jones 1961, p. xviii). It is a fact that in Pliny's work, some plants appear under two different names, and at times the author uses a single name to refer to two distinct species (Jones 1961, p. xviii). This may also result from inaccuracies in the translation of Greek treatises, in which certain species names sound similar, whereas their Latin equivalents differ significantly.

[20] Such theses were advanced, among others, by Ermolao Barbaro (1454–1493) in his work *Castigationes pliniane* (1492). Guided by philological purism, Barbaro sought to cleanse Pliny's text of accretions and errors that had accumulated over time during the copying and preparation of the text for print in the early modern period ((Ogilvie 2006, pp. 121–126; Cristofolini 2024); for a detailed description see Nauert (1979)). He supplemented substantive and logical deficiencies on the basis of his reading of manuscript versions of the "Natural History" as well as works by other ancient authorities such as Theophrastus and Dioscorides. Despite correcting around 5000 errors, he still considered Pliny's work to be of value. A different view was held by Barbaro's contemporary, Niccolò Leoniceno (1428–1524), who published *De Plinii et aliorum medicorum in medicina erroribus* (1493) barely a year later. Leoniceno, a professor of medicine and practising physician, accused Pliny (as well as medieval Arab physicians) of serious negligence, including ignorance of elementary natural facts and carelessness in botanical nomenclature and descriptions (Nauert 1979, pp. 81–83; Ogilvie 2006, pp. 126–133; Touwaide 2010; Kusukawa 2012, pp. 102–103; Cristofolini 2024). At the same time, he emphasised the value of the works of Galen and, above all, Dioscorides, drawing attention to the accuracy of his plant descriptions, which stemmed from direct observation. Leoniceno's attack on Pliny earned him many enemies, but it was thanks to him that attitudes towards ancient texts changed, shifting the focus from textual restoration to the real development of modern natural knowledge.

[21] The original manuscript of *De materia medica…* was not illustrated. Each substance is described in a separate chapter. Plants are presented according to the following scheme: general description, enumeration of parts useful in medicine, the initial form from which the drug is prepared, medicinal and therapeutic properties, possible side effects, methods for verifying the prepared drug, uses in crafts, cosmetics, and veterinary medicine (Touwaide 2010).

[22] His descriptions were characterised by realism, free from philosophical considerations about the causes and soul of nature, which were typical of other ancient and medieval texts. Interestingly, Dioscorides did not indicate whether the observations on which he based his descriptions were his own. Nevertheless, his work set a standard for plant researchers and established a framework for their description (Ogilvie 2006, pp. 137–138).

medica the most widely read text in the field of natural history.[23] Beginning with a careful reading of Dioscorides, early modern naturalists gradually introduced the requirement of personal observation of nature, as well as the meticulous verification of others' observations.[24] At a certain point, the need to describe new, previously unnamed plants also became evident. The shift in how ancient authors' texts were read laid the foundation for the emergence of scientific description of nature, and above all, of the plant world. The origins of the natural history are thus closely linked to botany.[25] Plants were a more abundant and accessible material for study than animals, and, moreover, a material "unable to hide from the researcher" (Ogilvie 2006, p. 49). The predominance of interest in botany over zoology was also related to the medical and pharmaceutical education of Renaissance scholars and, consequently, to the utilitarian character of works devoted to plants.

The frequently raised and vigorously debated issues concerning the imperfections of ancient descriptions of nature led to a shift in the very approach to the

---

[23] *De materia medica*, especially the edition accompanied by the commentaries of Pier Andrea Mattioli (1501–1577), became a component of the medical curriculum at universities such as Leiden at the end of the sixteenth century and Montpellier (Ogilvie 2006, pp. 37, 73, 282). Renaissance botanists placed great trust in Dioscorides, despite certain limitations of his treatise, as described, for example, by Antonius Musa Brassavola (1500–1555) (Arber 1970, p. 11). *De materia medica* inspired the publication of further commentaries, responses, and meticulous analyses by all the most renowned naturalists of the Renaissance, including Ermolao Barbaro, Niccolò Leoniceno, Euricius (1486–1535), Valerius Cordus (1515–1544), Otto Brunfels (1488–1533), Hieronymus Bock (1498–1554), Pier Andrea Mattioli, and Caspar Bauhin (1560–1624). This work continued to be published until the eighteenth century. The enduring influence of this treatise is evidenced by the fact that all historical botanical treatises are analysed in relation to *De materia medica*. This is also the case with the oldest extant illustrated herbal, from the temple at Tebtunis (Hanson 2001; see also Touwaide 2010). Dioscorides and Pliny the Elder may have drawn on the same sources when composing their treatises. It is generally accepted that their works were based on the now-lost treatise of the Greek botanist Crateuas (Kratevas, first century BC), as both authors cite him as a source of knowledge. They also refer to the expertise of Theophrastus. The use of common sources may explain certain similarities between the texts of *Naturalis Historia* and *De materia medica*. Dioscorides' text contains fewer errors than that of Pliny, which is attributed either to the absence of a language barrier for Dioscorides when consulting Greek sources, or to Pliny's reliance on Crateuas' work through intermediaries, namely Latin translators. It has also been considered whether Pliny might have used Dioscorides' treatise, which was written around the same time as the "Natural History"; however, although Pliny lists the sources he consulted in composing his treatise, he does not mention Dioscorides among them (Jones 1961, pp. xix–xx). Healey further emphasises the Roman author's declared aversion to Greek culture (Healey 1999, p. 30). In his treatises on simple and compound medicines, Galen described the medicinal properties of plants, but did not focus on their appearance; he merely listed their names and specified their medical uses. His knowledge of the medical applications of plants was based on Dioscorides (Touwaide 2010). Galen's works were strictly medical in nature. In them, he also presented his own theory concerning the mechanism of action of herbal medicines.

[24] This approach stood in contrast to the common practice of uncritical copying of botanical texts, which, as previously mentioned, became increasingly degraded over time due to successive reworkings (see also Ogilvie (2006, pp. 96–99)).

[25] Renaissance naturalists also studied the animal and mineral kingdoms, but their primary focus of research and investigation was, above all, the world of plants.

natural world. As a result of this process, there was a turn towards direct observation of nature and the development of new standards for its description.[26] The earliest Renaissance botanical works, modelled on ancient prototypes, focused on the medicinal properties of plants or their harmful effects on health, and were strictly practical in nature. “Naturalists”, as specialists in natural history began to be called during the Renaissance, sought at that time to demonstrate the relevance of ancient treatises by searching for contemporary equivalents of the plants described therein. In their treatises, they frequently cited the authority of Galen and Dioscorides. However, since the works of these authors contained descriptions of a relatively limited number of plants—covering only several hundred species—they soon proved insufficient.

In the second half of the sixteenth century, botany transformed into a systematic description of the plant world, often without accounts of the properties of individual species. This shift stemmed from the aforementioned need to catalogue plants that had not yet been scientifically described, at a stage when the species discussed in ancient treatises had already been thoroughly analysed. The growing number of newly described, previously unknown plant species, along with the realisation that countless others awaited description, prompted the first attempts to develop a botanical classification system. This became a particular focus for the last generation of Renaissance scholars and for botanists of subsequent eras. The awareness of the vast and ever-expanding body of knowledge, which seemed to increase as new aspects of botany were discovered, necessitated the creation of auxiliary scientific tools. These tools were intended to facilitate the retention of information acquired during botanical observations and to enable repeated, detailed analysis without the need for time-consuming expeditions on each occasion. In this process, horticulture and the drying of plants—used to create herbaria—were adapted for scientific purposes (Ogilvie 2006, pp. 139–208). Publications were increasingly enriched with sophisticated illustrative material, which not only made the works more visually appealing but also allowed those just beginning to explore the world of plants to access botanical knowledge. Botanical illustrations coexisted with, and often competed against, herbarium specimens for the status of the primary scientific tool among specialists, who engaged in vigorous debate regarding their role and significance in science.

[26] It was the description of nature that formed the core of the work of so-called naturalists, that is, researchers of natural history, throughout the sixteenth and the first half of the seventeenth century.

1.2 Intermediate Forms Between Botanical Illustration and the Classical Herbarium Format

The relationship between botanical illustration and herbarium activity provides the context for the emancipation of herbaria as scientific tools. The roles of botanical illustration and herbarium specimens have undergone transformations. Before herbaria gained independence as scientific instruments, they served as auxiliary resources for illustrative material. Images of plants have accompanied botanical texts since the very beginning of natural history works and, although desired by users, were also criticised by some advanced experts in the field. The gradual move away from the use of botanical illustrations resulted from ongoing technological advances in reproduction[27] and the continued practice of working with authentic dried plants. The turn towards herbaria began to manifest itself most spectacularly in the time of Linnaeus (1707–1788), who was, incidentally, a strong critic of botanical illustration (Reeds 2004).[28] In the history of plant depiction, however, drawing, artistic vision, and herbarium specimens have repeatedly served as points of reference for one another, both as models and as comparative material presented within a shared album. Given the breadth of the subject of botanical illustration, the numerous studies, and the current availability of digitised herbaria, only those phenomena considered most significant for the emergence of herbaria with dried plants are cited here.[29]

Currently, the oldest surviving illustrated herbal is considered to be the so-called Tebtunis herbal from the second century CE, which formed part of a temple library collection (Hanson 2001; Ryholt 2013; ref. P. Tebt. 0679).[30] This is a fragmentarily preserved medical treatise written in Greek. The treatises of Pliny, Dioscorides, and Galen originally did not contain plant illustrations.[31] However, they did include

[27] The most significant change occurred as early as the sixteenth century, with the widespread adoption of metal graphic techniques.

[28] Reeds attributes Linnaeus's reluctance towards illustrations to his lack of drawing skills and the resulting negative experiences in attempting to depict plants through drawing. Furthermore, he emphasised that if any of the artists involved in producing the final image of a plant—whether draughtsman, engraver, or painter—makes a mistake during the process, it will mislead the researcher (Hentschel 2014, p. 206). Nevertheless, he appreciated the artistry of Georg Dionysius Ehret (1708–1770), with whom he collaborated on the study of Georg Clifford's (1685–1760) plant collection.

[29] Currently, there is a vast array of works available on illustrated botanical treatises, including both books and articles (e.g. Arber 1970; Pacht 1950; Blunt and Stearn 1994; Collins 2000; Kusukawa 2012; Rix 2013)—to mention just a few.

[30] Photographic documentation is available in the digital repository (University of California Berkeley Library Digital Collections): https://digicoll.lib.berkeley.edu/record/231633?ln=en&v=uv#?xywh=-2051%2C-257%2C7104%2C5137 (accessed: 5.01.2026).

[31] Nevertheless, in the case of Dioscorides, it has been suggested that the original *De materia …* may indeed have included plant illustrations, as the oldest surviving copy (AD 512) contains impressive illustrations, and it has often been argued that these are copies from the original *De materia*, or even copies from the work of Crateuas (Arber 1970, pp. 9, 185; Touwaide 2010).

critical remarks regarding the usefulness of botanical illustrations. Pliny drew attention to the degeneration of illustrations through repeated copying (Pliny 1966, p. 140; see also Kusukawa 2012, pp. 20–21; Arber 1970, pp. 188, 234).[32] Dioscorides emphasised the need to understand the complete developmental cycle of a plant, although this was not directly linked to criticism of illustrations. He also stressed the importance of personal experience (Touwaide 2010; Kusukawa 2012, p. 21).[33] Galen, on the other hand, advocated focusing on the properties of the plant rather than its shape, as he believed the latter had already been so accurately described by Dioscorides that there was no need to depict plant images (Kusukawa 2012, pp. 20, 106). Nevertheless, the most renowned copies of Dioscorides are those containing illustrations, above all the oldest extant copy of *De materia medica*, a richly illustrated Byzantine manuscript from around 512 CE.[34] The plant portraits in this codex are most likely not studies from nature, but rather copies of Hellenistic representations.[35] The extraordinary popularity of this work gave rise to the phenomenon criticised by Pliny: repeated reworking of images, not based on direct observation, often led to a decline in the informational value of the illustrations, and to their misplacement. In subsequent copies, illustrations did not always correspond to the accompanying text.

At the turn of the thirteenth and fourteenth centuries, the first illustrations began to appear, the analysis of which suggests not only direct observation from nature, but even the use of pressed specimens to create a schematic, almost diagrammatic representation of the plant (Pacht 1950). An exceptional example of an illustrated manuscript containing depictions of plants produced before the heyday of woodcut botanical illustration is the herbal from Padua, belonging to the Carrara family (*Carrara Herbal*, c. 1400, Fig. 1.1) (Pacht 1950; Smith 2010).[36] The illustrations in

[32] Pacht (1950) argues that while in Pliny's time the degeneration of illustrations may have resulted from the negligence of copyists, in the Middle Ages it was also caused by an increasing tendency towards stylisation and synthesis of images, which rendered them unreliable sources of knowledge about the actual shapes and colours of plants (see also analyses of medieval herbals by Collins (2000)). Kusukawa, on the other hand, emphasises that this is the only passage in which Pliny criticises botanical illustrations, as in other sections of the "Natural History" he praises the pursuit of imitating nature (Kusukawa 2012, p. 20).

[33] Dioscorides outlined his position in the preface to *De materia medica*.

[34] Also known as the *Codex Aniciae Julianae*. The codex is held in the collections of the Austrian National Library in Vienna (*Vienna Dioscorides*). This copy of *De materia...* is described and cited in numerous publications (including Singer 1927; Wächter 1962; Arber 1970, pp. 8–10, 185, 239; Weitzmann 1979; Collins 2000; Touwaide 2010; Janick and Stolarczyk 2012).

[35] Despite the demonstration of certain individual characteristics of a given species (Arber 1970, p. 185). See also Pacht (1950).

[36] The herbal, a translation of the *Liber aggregatus in medicinis simplicibus* by the Arab author Serapion the Younger (Ibn Serapi), who lived in the ninth century CE, was once owned by Ulisse Aldrovandi (1522–1605). It is currently held in the British Library (BL), catalogue number Egerton 2020. Selected illustrations are available on the BL website (British Library, 2020). Plant images from this manuscript were later copied in the herbal of Benedetto Rinio of Venice (1419, held in the Biblioteca Nazionale Marciana), where they were already subject to a certain degree of stylisation (Pacht 1950).

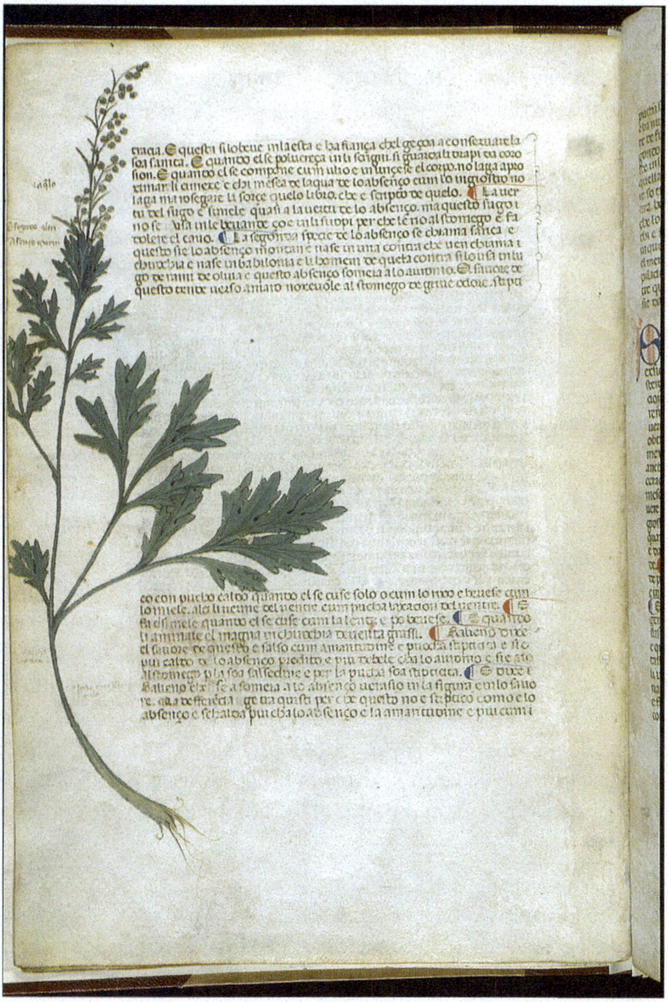

Fig. 1.1 (*Carrara Herbal*), London, British Library, folio 12v, ref. Egerton 2020, c. 1400. The depiction of *Artemisia* reveals that a dried specimen was used as the model. (© British Library Board)

this manuscript reveal meticulous observation of plant specimens, which were evidently pressed. This is evidenced by the characteristic creases in the leaves and flower petals.[37]

[37] It is possible that this practice was associated with the medical faculty of the University of Padua. However, the artistic mimesis also reflects the interests of the patron of this manuscript, Francesco II da Carrara (1390–1405), who owned many works characterised by naturalism. Francesco II da Carrara was also the patron of Cennino Cennini, author of *Il libri dell'arte* (c. 1400), in which Cennini praised the artist's pursuit of imitating nature. The Carrara family's interest in naturalism was intended to emphasise their dominance over nature and legitimise the family's rule in Padua (Smith 2010).

Images of plant specimens attached to paper appear in books of hours from the 1480s and 1490s. These are depictions of plants, most often flowers, collected during pilgrimages, intended to strengthen the pilgrim's devotion by reminding them of tangible souvenirs from their journey (Da Costa Kaufmann and Roehrig Kaumann 1991).[38]

The use of herbarium specimens as models for depicting plants is also clearly evident in Otto Brunfels's treatise, *Herbarium vivae eicones*, in illustrations by, among others, Hans Weiditz (1495–1537), a pupil of Albrecht Dürer (first edition in 1532, Fig. 1.2).[39] In Weiditz's woodcuts, the plants are portrayed as if the artist had naturalistically depicted dried specimens, flattened and broken in several places, in order to highlight all taxonomic features and to present the distinctive characteristics of each species as fully as possible to the reader (Ogilvie 2006, p. 169). Moreover, the specimens were documented with all their individual features, such as insect damage or missing parts, with some elements obscured by others, as is the case with herbarium specimen.[40]

A drawing based on the observation of a living plant was preferred. An image of a plant made from a herbarium specimen was considered an inferior form, although botanists would use it in the absence of a better alternative.[41] The development of illustration progressed towards more conventional forms, the starting point of which was the "absolute image", *pictura absolutissima*, advocated by Leonhard Fuchs (1501–1566), one of the three "fathers of German botany" (Kusukawa 2012, pp. 274–275). This also clearly signalled the divergence between the role and potential of illustration in representing real plants and the function of herbarium specimens as scientific tools.

The authors of plant depictions in sixteenth-century botanical publications, in addition to addressing the issue of realism in plant form, also drew attention to the challenge of representing plant colour. The colouring of illustrations was, in

[38] For information on the potential link between the creation of herbaria and the practice of collecting souvenirs during pilgrimages, see the Sect. 1.3.1.

[39] The attribution of the woodcuts is often limited to Weiditz's name, although there were several artists involved (Kusukawa 2012, p. 16). These illustrations displayed a much higher standard than the accompanying descriptive text, and as a result, the work was valued primarily for its iconographic content. This was a source of frustration for the author of the text, Otto Brunfels, who had not intended to collaborate with an illustrator but was persuaded to do so by his publisher, Johann Schott (Smith 2010; Touwaide 2010). The naturalism of these images marked the beginning of what is sometimes referred to as scientific illustration (Smith 2010). Weiditz's approach to depiction was not universally appreciated, as it was believed that the representation of individual specimen characteristics interfered with the perception of the image as a whole. Nevertheless, it constituted a breakthrough in the perception of plants and initiated a discussion on the appropriate form and function of botanical illustration. It also encouraged a turn towards realism and careful observation of plants and their natural environments.

[40] *Idem*, p. 194.

[41] They were valued in this way, among others, by Konrad Gessner (1516–1565) and Clusius (Charles de l'Écluse, 1526–1609) (Kusukawa 2012, pp. 143–147; Ogilvie 2006, p. 200). An example of diverse collections of teaching aids includes, among others, the watercolours from the extensive collection of Dirck Outgaertszoon Cluyt (1546–1598), pharmacist and director of the botanical garden in Leiden from 1594 to 1598, which were used at the end of the sixteenth century as teaching aids for medical students in Leiden during the winter, when it was impossible to observe living plants in the university garden. These were highly valued by students, on a par with his extensive collection of herbarium specimens (Egmond 2010, pp. 157–162; Swan 2010).

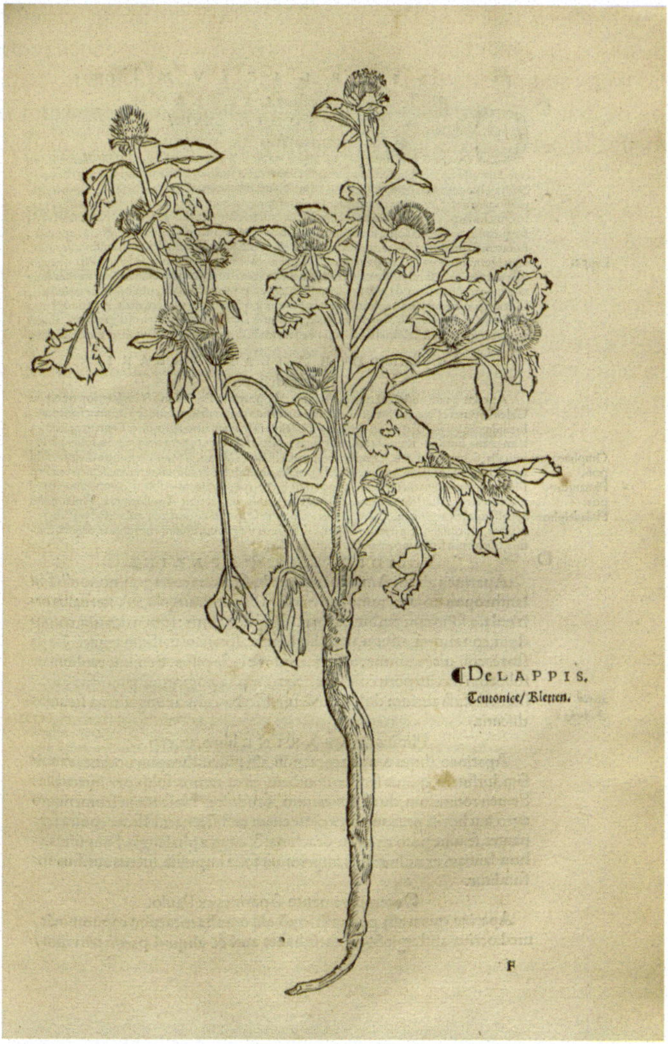

Fig. 1.2 Depiction of *Amaracus Hill*, illustration for Brunfels' *Herbarium vivae eicones*, showing the individual characteristics of the specimen used as a model for the artist. (Courtesy of the Missouri Botanical Garden Library, via Biodiversity Heritage Library)

principle, to be based on a master copy prepared under the supervision of the author.[42] However, the diversity of surviving coloured copies indicates that this rule was not always followed. Consequently, coloured illustrations were not always

[42] Drawings made prior to woodcutting also served as colour references; for example, Weiditz's coloured illustrations were used as models for hand-coloured printed editions (Arber 1940; Ogilvie 2006, p. 202).

regarded as reliable (Kusukawa 2012, pp. 69–81).[43] The main drawback of herbarium specimens, on the other hand, was their altered (most often faded) colour. Some illustrations were composed from observations *ad vivum* (that is, based on the examination of living plants), fragments of fresh plants, and herbarium specimens simultaneously, depending on the availability of the plant (Kusukawa 2012, pp. 139–161).

Herbarium specimens were also used to create nature prints, produced by using the plant as an ink stamp (Fig. 1.3).[44]

There are also known examples of combining herbarium specimens with botanical illustration. Johann Jakob Han (1656–1616) created herbaria in which plants were attached against backgrounds of "landscapes" painted by his wife Anna, presumably to compensate for the removal of the plant from its natural habitat context—a common criticism levelled at herbarium collections. He adopted this technique from his teacher, Hieronymus Harder (1523–1607) (Fig. 1.4) (Thijsse 2016).

Some naturalists also combined herbarium documentation with drawings; for example, Felix Platter (1536–1614) acquired original watercolours by Weiditz for the woodcuts in Brunfels's *Herbarium vivae eicones* and other contemporary plant illustrations, including those for Fuchs's work. He cut them out and pasted them into his own herbarium, alongside the plant specimens (Figs. 1.5 and 1.6).[45] Similarly, Caspar Bauhin used cut-out illustrations from the works of his predecessors in his own collections.[46]

Illustrations ceased to be a sufficient scientific aid in the second half of the sixteenth century, giving way to herbaria containing only dried plants, despite the critical attitude of contemporary botanists.[47] The vast and ever-increasing body of

[43] Fuchs and Clusius frequently included remarks on colours in their texts, assuming that the reader would be viewing a coloured edition (Ogilvie 2006, pp. 202–206). However, this was rare, as coloured copies of herbals significantly increased the cost of publication. As a result, partially coloured copies were also produced, while fully coloured volumes were commissioned as luxury items by wealthy representatives of secular and ecclesiastical authorities. Different authors estimate the scale of this cost increase differently, but in any case, the difference was dramatic: Kusukawa states that the cost of colouring accounted for 76% of the price (Kusukawa 2012, pp. 53, 60), while Ogilvie gives as much as 90% (Ogilvie 2006, p. 202). This was due to the fact that increasingly sophisticated botanical publications could contain over 2000 plant illustrations, which meant months of work for the painters.

[44] Such objects were held in the collections of the Renaissance botanist Konrad Gessner. The nature print method was also employed by other naturalists, including the Italian botanist Paolo Silvio Boccone (1633–1704). An example of a "herbarium" containing nature prints is the manuscript from Chantilly, shown in fig. 3; see also (Costa et al. 2018). The technique of nature printing was certainly in use in the second half of the sixteenth century. In 1554, Girolamo Cardano in *De subtilitate* described a method for portraying a plant *ad vivum* by pressing it onto paper, leaving an "architectural drawing" of the plant (*ichnographia*).

[45] Numerous examples can be found in Dauwalder (2012) and Rytz (1933); see also Ogilvie (2006, p. 175).

[46] Among the illustrations, one can find images cut out from the works of Fuchs, Matthioli, Dodoens (1517–1585), de l'Obel (1538–1616), and Clusius (Saint-Lager 1885, pp. 95–96).

[47] Illustrations aided the memory of botanists, who had to rapidly assimilate discoveries of new plant species. Ogilvie cites the assertion that a person can memorise approximately 500 species without the need for classification. He also emphasises that this level of knowledge was reflected in the works of

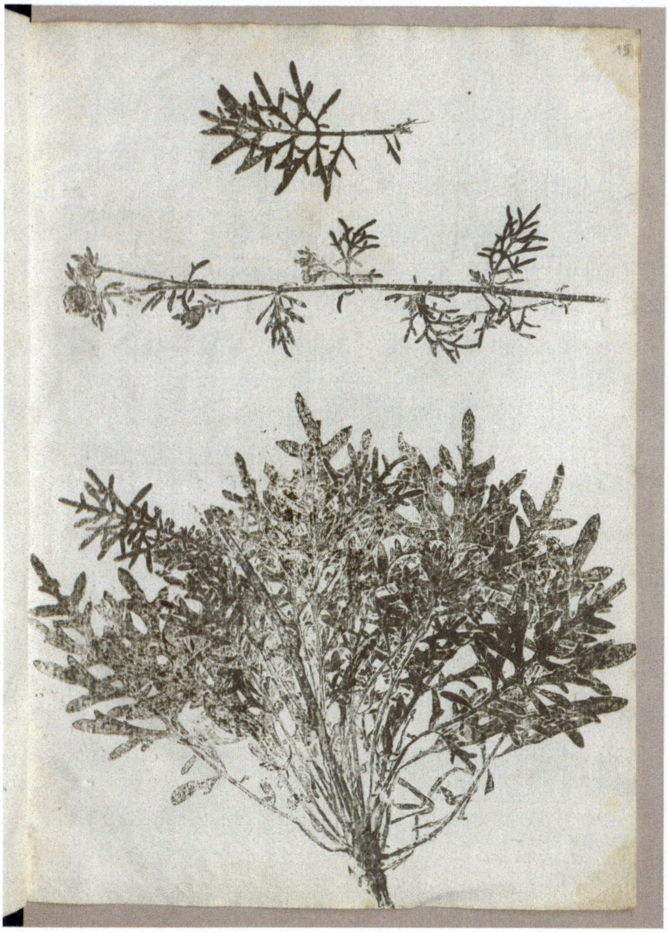

Fig. 1.3 Images of plants obtained using the imprint method, employing botanical specimens as stamps. Paolo Silvio Boccone, (*Herbier*), Chantilly, Interuniversity Library of Medicine and Dentistry (BIU), ref. ms. 2039, 1671 (BIU Santé médecine—Université Paris Cité)

information accompanying the development of botany could no longer be adequately described using illustrations alone.[48]

Fuchs and Bock, and had already been surpassed by around 1570. By 1620, Caspar Bauhin had described 6000 species (Zemanek 1997; Ogilvie 2006, p. 208). In 1823, in the work *Prodromus Systematis Naturalis Regni Vegetabilis* initiated by Augustin-Pyramus de Candolle (1778–1841), 200 years after Bauhin's *Pinax*, 59,000 plant species were described, focusing solely on dicotyledons. The work was concluded after 50 years by de Candolle's successors (Mägdefrau 2004, p. 83).

[48] For students, the key aspect was to learn about plants through "botanising" or "herborising", that is, botanical excursions incorporated into the medical curriculum. The final works of Caspar Bauhin, *Catalogus* and *Pinax Theatri Botanici* (1623), were published without illustrations. By the seventeenth century, it was already widely accepted that publications intended for scholarly naturalists did not need to include iconographic material, as the target audience was expected to possess a basic knowledge of botany. This tendency remains current to this day (Ford 2003).

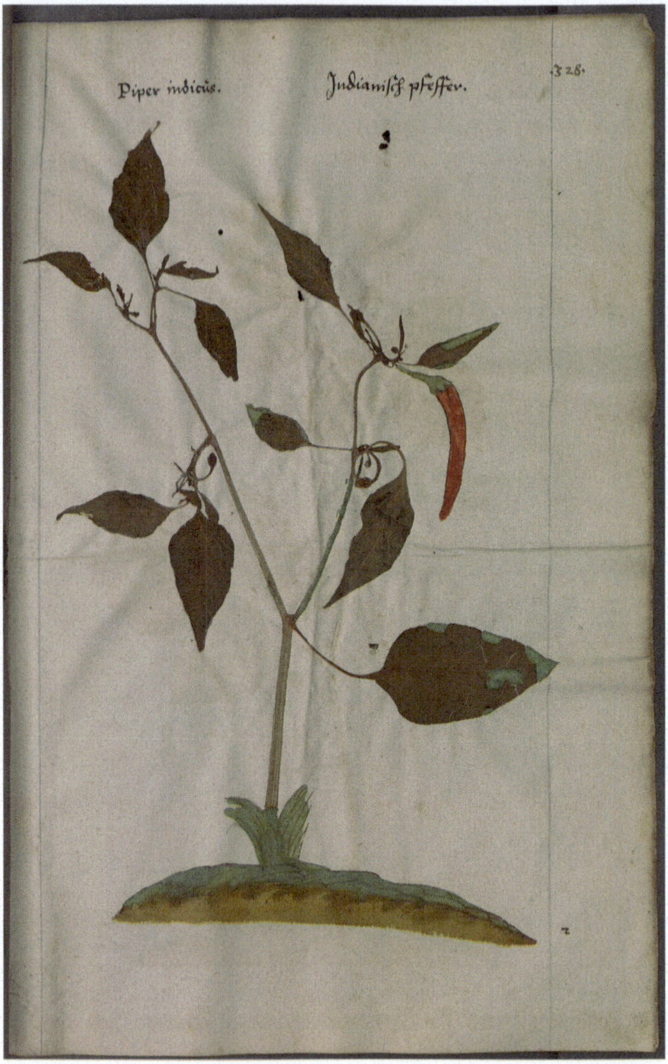

Fig. 1.4 The herbarium of Hieronymus Harder, (Hieronymus Harder, *Kreuterbuch* (*Herbarium Vivum*), Munich, Bayerische Staatsbibliothek, ref. BSB-Hss Cod.icon. 3. 1576–1600). Sheet no. 328, depiction of *Piper indicus—Capsicum annuum* L. (Bayerische Staatsbibliothek München)

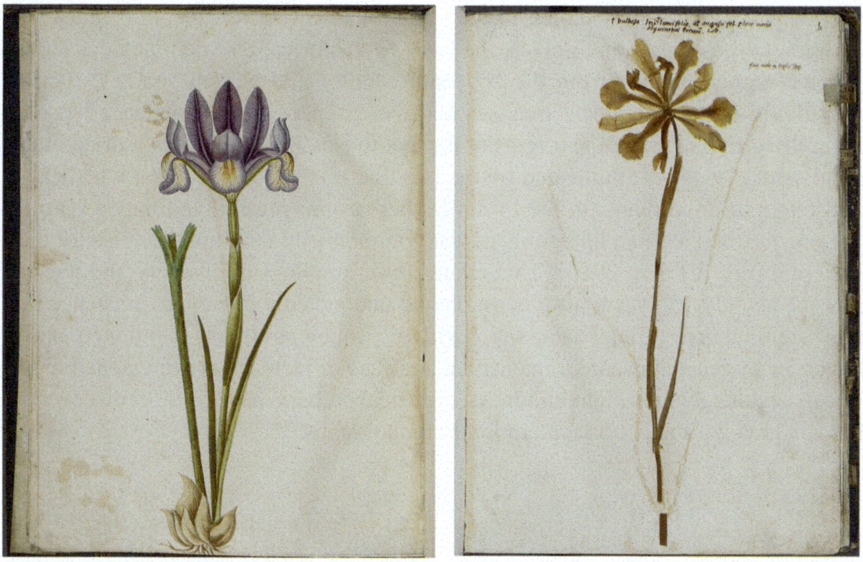

Figs. 1.5 and 1.6 Fragments (adjacent pages) from the herbarium of Felix Platter (Platter F., (*Platter Herbarium*), Bern, Burgerbibliothek Bern, ref. ES 70.2). On the left an illustration (f. 2), on the right a specimen of *Iris graminea* (f. 3), (Burgerbibliothek Bern)

1.3 Herbaria with Dried Plants

Herbarium praestat omni iconae, necessarium omni Botanico

(A herbarium is more important than any illustration; it is essential for every botanist)

Linnaeus[49]

Although the method of creating herbaria containing dried plant specimens has remained largely unchanged since the Renaissance, their status and form have evolved over the centuries. Herbaria owe their formal and official recognition as legitimate scientific tools to Linnaeus, although as early as the beginning of the seventeenth century, Bauhin, while working on the *Pinax theatri botanici* (1623), relied primarily on his extensive collection of dried specimens. Despite the widespread use of herbaria in the eighteenth century, especially for documenting exotic flora species, and their collection, study, and admiration by scientists, their history

[49] This sentence, originating from Linnaeus's *Philosophia Botanica* (Linnaeus 1751, p. 7), has become a frequently repeated maxim, often cited in abbreviated form: *Herbarium, omni botanico necessarium* (Saint-Lager 1885, p. 2).

was only systematically studied in the second half of the nineteenth century.[50] In addition to the objects themselves, the basis for historical research includes iconographic representations from the sixteenth century and written sources, such as remarks in printed botanical treatises and the extensive correspondence between naturalists. Investigating the origins of the method and the collection of dried plants from source texts is complicated by the fact that it is not always clear whether the text refers to dried plants in the form of a herbarium (pressed and flattened) or to specimens dried without flattening, as was commonly done by apothecaries for their own purposes (Thijsse 2016). This relates to terminological diversity and the fact that it was only 150 years after herbaria had undoubtedly come into existence that they acquired their official name (*herbarium*).[51] Today, as already mentioned, due to advances in genetic research, intensified analyses of increasingly threatened biodiversity and heightened plant blindness, historical herbaria have been "rediscovered" and are now the subject of contemporary monographs.[52]

[50] The first monograph on the history of herbaria is *Histoire des herbiers* by Jean Saint-Lager, published in 1885. In the very first sentence of his treatise, the author writes, "Until now, the history of herbaria has been neglected" (Saint-Lager 1885, p. 1). In his work, he describes historical herbaria not only in terms of their botanical content, but also in terms of the types of binding and the use of biocidal agents. Prior to Saint-Lager's publication, there had been more general works containing chapters on herbaria, such as *Geschichte der Botanik* by Ernst H.F. Meyer (1857), or monographs devoted to individual herbaria, for example, *Das älteste und erste Herbarium Deutschlands im Jahr 1592, von Caspar Ratzenberger angelegt gegenwärtig noch im Königlichen Museum zu Cassel* (Kessler 1870).

[51] Despite the use of the term *herbarium*, for the century following Tournefort's work, various terms related to the concept of a garden continued to be used as titles for collections of dried plants. More about the different terms applied to herbaria can be found in the Sect. 1.3.3.

[52] Only in the last decade has a significant number of such works been published in the form of books and articles (including: Spalik 2014a; Graniszewska et al. 2016; Lienhard and Dauwalder 2016; Thijsse 2016, 2018; van Andel and Barth 2018; Costa et al. 2018; Graniszewska 2018; Graniszewska and Kapler 2018; Pękacka-Falkowska 2018a; Stefanaki et al. 2018; Stefanaki et al. 2019; Thijsse and Wesseling 2021, Zych et al. 2023; Grenda-Kurmanow et al. 2025, Grenda-Kurmanow 2026). Previously, herbaria were also described in the following publications: (Rytz 1933; Britten et al. 1958; Piekiełko 1977, 1981; Köhler 1989, 1994, 1995, 1996; Chlebicki 1991; Radwańska-Paryska 1991; Ochyra and Cisło 1999; Kielak 2004). Some of the authors of these publications are long-standing researchers and curators of herbarium collections, who have been engaged in the study of historical collections for many years. Clearly, however, recent years have provided fertile ground for the publication of research on herbaria and studies based on herbaria as archival sources. Another broad group of publications comprises genetic studies conducted using herbarium material. See also the Sect. 1.3.6.

1.3.1 The Oldest Preserved Herbaria in the World and in Poland

The exact date of the creation of the first herbarium is not defined. The practice of pressing plants as flat specimens must have been known long before the Renaissance; however, it cannot be determined whether systematic attempts to create herbaria were made before the sixteenth century.[53] In efforts to identify the historical context for plant pressing, reference is often made to the medieval custom of collecting souvenirs, including naturalia, during pilgrimages. Pilgrims in the late fourteenth and fifteenth centuries, gathering mementoes from various stages of their journeys to the Holy Land, collected, among other things, plants, which they pressed and placed in prayer books. Souvenirs from pilgrimages held exceptional symbolic value, just as the pilgrimage itself had symbolic significance.[54]

The investigation into the origins of the systematic practice of plant drying remains, to some extent, a subject of speculation.[55] The oldest extant herbaria date back to the sixteenth century (Table 1.1, Figs. 1.5, 1.6, and 1.7).[56]

The examples described in the previous chapter demonstrate that dried plant specimens were used as iconographic models or even as stamps to aid in creating of graphic representations. Specimens were also adhered to the margins of herbals, and sometimes incorporated into the composition of illustrated images, thereby

[53] In his search for the origins of herbaria, Saint-Lager traces them back even to Greek mythology, writing about Flora, the Boeotian princess who, wishing to preserve the bouquets of flowers brought to her daily by the enamoured Zephyrus, would wrap them in cloth and dry them. "Thus, inspired by love, the first herbaria were created," comments Saint-Lager (Saint-Lager 1885, pp. 14–15). The goddess Flora is also featured in the illustrations on the opening pages of the herbaria of Georg Andreas Helwing (1666–1748), held in the National Library in Warsaw (Spalik 2014a, b).

[54] A reminiscence of this custom was the painted depictions of small objects, including dried plants, found in prayer books. These representations of naturalia were intended to serve the same function as the collected specimens themselves, with the added advantage of not deteriorating as real plants would. What in the fifteenth century had been a physical reminder of a journey was, over time, replaced by naturalistic reproductions (Da Costa Kaufmann and Roehrig Kaumann 1991; Ogilvie 2006, pp. 114, 168–169). According to Ogilvie, the Kaufmanns' study of illusionistic illustration in early modern manuscripts suggests that the art of creating herbaria was adapted from the surrounding material culture. The transition from personal mementos to scientific tools was made possible by the refined illustrations of Brunfels and Fuchs (Ogilvie 2006, p. 169). It is also worth noting that Saint-Lager posits that the earliest herbaria had a sentimental value, arguing in a manner consistent (albeit secular) with the Kaufmanns' theory (Saint-Lager 1885, p. 29). The mnemonic function is a motif that recurs throughout the later history of herbaria.

[55] Meyer traces the origins of drying plants back to antiquity (Meyer 1857, p. 266). Saint-Lager links the history of herbaria to the spread of paper production in Europe, arguing that fabrics, papyrus, and parchment were unsuitable for drying plants (Saint-Lager 1885, pp. 23–30). Arber, however, contends that materials other than paper (thin wooden sheets, fabric) could also have been used for this purpose (Arber 1970, p. 139). This discussion is also cited by Ogilvie (2006, p. 168).

[56] Toresella and Battini, however, cite (with photographs) two objects from the fifteenth century (N.n, untitled, Florence, Biblioteca Nazionale di Firenze, Ms. B. V.24, fifteenth c., and N.n, untitled, Brescia, Biblioteca Queriniana, Ms. B. V.24, fifteenth c.), in which a few plants or traces of their attachment are preserved (Toresella and Battini 1988). Olariu also cites them (Olariu 2014). No other work on herbaria references these objects.

Table 1.1 The oldest surviving herbaria in the world, sixteenth century

Author and/or first owner of the herbarium/name	Dating	Current location
Michele Merini	1540–1545	Museum of Natural History, University of Florence (FI)
Francesco Petrollini	(? (Herbarium A), 1550–1553 (Herbarium B))	Rome, Biblioteca Angelica
Ulisse Aldrovandi	1551–1605	Bologna, University of Bologna
Felix Platter	1552	Bern, Burgerbibliothek Bern
Andrea Cesalpino	1555–1563	Florence, Museum of Natural History, University of Florence (FI)
Caspar Ratzenberger	1556–1592, 1598	Kassel, Natural History Museum (KASSEL) and Gotha, Gotha Research Library
Jehan Girault	1558	Paris, Muséum national d'Histoire naturelle (P)
Francesco Petrollini *En Tibi Perpetuis Ridentum Floribus Hortum*	1558	Leiden, Naturalis Biodiversity Center (L)
Erbario Ducale Estense	1560?	Modena, Biblioteca Estense Universitaria
Leonhard Rauwolf	1560–1577	Leiden, Naturalis Biodiversity Center (L)
Hieronymus Harder[a]	1562–1594	Institutions in Munich, Ulm, Salzburg, Rome, Vienna, Linz, Uberlingen, London?, Lindau
Petrus Cadé	1566	Leiden, Naturalis Biodiversity Center (L)
Georg Forster	1570–1575	Nuremberg, Nürnberger Stadtbibliothek
Joachim Gagelmann	1571–1577	Wolfenbüttel, Herzog August Library
Caspar Bauhin	1577–1624	Basel, Herbaria Basel, Institute of Botany/University of Basel (BAS)
Johann Jakob Han	1578–1594	Überlingen, Municipal Museum Überlingen
unknown	1585	Bologna, University of Bologna
unknown	1596	Bologna, University of Bologna
Ferrante Imperato[b] (1550–1631)	Undetermined	Naples, Biblioteca Nazionale di Napoli

Based on Thijsse (2016) and Stefanaki et al. (2019)
[a]For Harder's herbarium, only the cities where the collections are located are provided to maintain the clarity of the table
[b]For Ferrante Imperato, due to the absence of herbarium dating, the dates of his life are provided
A detailed list of the volumes of all the herbaria mentioned can be found in Thijsse (2016). See also Cristofolini (2024).

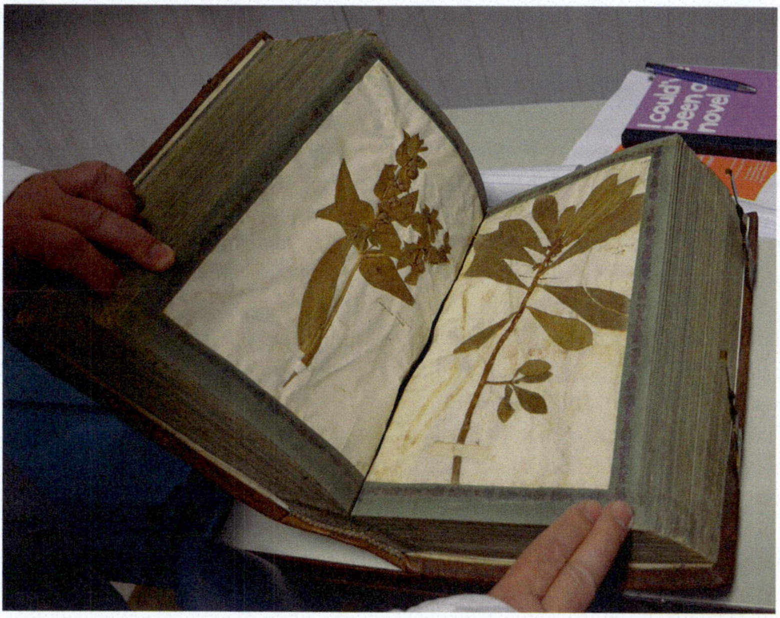

Fig. 1.7 One of the oldest surviving herbaria in the world: the herbarium of Leonhard Rauwolf (Rauwolf L., Leiden, Naturalis Biodiversity Center in Leiden (L), ref. L.2077653, 1560–1577). (Photo: M. Grenda-Kurmanow)

adding a sense of realism (Olariu 2014).[57] On the other hand, there are known cases of herbaria in which the illustrative layer served to compensate for missing parts of the botanical specimen and provided context by depicting the environment in which the plant naturally grows.[58] What, then, caused plant specimens—and subsequently entire herbaria—to move from a subordinate role to illustration in the sixteenth century, to "surpass" any form of illustration and become an indispensable tool for every botanist?

Undoubtedly, the popularisation of the practice of plant drying is attributed to Luca Ghini (1490–1556), professor of botany in Bologna from 1534 to 1544, and later director and founder of one of the world's first botanical gardens in Pisa (1544–1556).[59] The origins of herbarium creation are traditionally associated with

[57] According to Olariu, this is evidence of the artist's awareness of the limitations of botanical illustration at that time (in this case, the early sixteenth century). Anna Vasa also attached plants to the margins of her copy of Szymon Syreniusz's Herbarium, as described later in this chapter (Zemanek 1996).

[58] This refers to the herbaria of Hieronymus Harder and Johann Jakob Han, already mentioned in the Sect. 1.2.

[59] At the same time, the botanical garden in Padua was established (1545). These gardens served as scientific facilities, initially as resources for medical sciences and pharmacy, and later for botanical research (Zemanek 1997).

him (Saint-Lager 1885, pp. 15–17; Ogilvie 2006, pp. 35, 165; Arber 1970, p. 139; Cristofolini 2024).[60] Ghini himself did not publish any botanical treatise; however, he was a distinguished teacher, and his students and correspondents were among the leading figures in the natural sciences of the late sixteenth century.[61] None of his herbaria have survived, although it is known that by the mid-sixteenth century, he possessed around 300 herbarium specimens.[62] It is also known that Ghini sent dried plants from Pisa to Siena, to Pier Andrea Mattioli.[63] Mattioli, to better reproduce the plant in his drawings, would soak it in cold water, attempting to restore its appearance before the drying process.[64] Ghini taught botany students through botanical excursions (herborisation), during which specimens were collected. From the outset, herbarium collections were a natural component of academic infrastructure, and later of private botanical gardens, complementing the inventory of living plants with a "dead garden". This tradition continues to the present day.

The first printed reference to herbaria appeared in the commentaries of Amatus Lusitanus (1511–1568) on Dioscorides, published in 1553, and concerned the herbarium collections of John Falconer (dates of birth and death unknown), which have also not survived to the present day. In "Narrative (*enarratio*) 78" of Book III, Lusitanus writes[65]: "(…) For when I happened to be in Ferrara, searching for plants with certain very learned men and the most diligent investigators of natural matters,

---

[60] Ogilvie suggests that, knowing that the drying of flowers was an old technique familiar to medieval pilgrims to the Holy Land, it should rather be assumed that Ghini systematised the practice and popularised it among his students ((Ogilvie 2006, pp. 280–281); see also previous footnotes, with references to Toresella and Battini (1988) and Olariu (2014)).

[61] Among Ghini's students were, among others: Ulisse Aldrovandi, Gherardo Cibo (1512–1600), Andrea Cesalpino (1519–1603), William Turner (1509–1568), Michele Merini (dates of birth and death unknown), and Francesco Petrollini (dates of birth and death unknown). The attribution of the invention of the herbarium method to Ghini was made by Ernst H.F. Meyer (1857), who drew his conclusions from the correspondence of sixteenth-century botanists. Thijsse cites Aldrovandi's claims, in which he praised the effectiveness of his own herbarium technique and styled himself as its inventor. However, it is unclear whether this refers to the invention of the method itself or to its refinement (Thijsse 2016).

[62] Arber states that this collection must have been created much earlier, due to the existence of a herbarium preserved in the Biblioteca Angelica in Rome, formerly attributed to Gherardo Cibo and dated to around 1532 (Arber 1970, p. 139). However, the dating and attribution of the herbarium have since been questioned, and authorship has ultimately been assigned to Francesco Petrollini (Stefanaki et al. 2019).

[63] They were intended to serve as models for the plant illustrations in his commentaries on Dioscorides. In one of his letters to Bartolomeo Maranta, Mattioli admits that many of the illustrations published in the commentaries (on Dioscorides) were made based on dried plant specimens.

[64] Mattioli did not create his own herbarium and regarded dried plants merely as an aid for making drawings. He admitted his lack of expertise in this area in letters to Aldrovandi (Saint-Lager 1885, pp. 15–17).

[65] Amatus Lusitanus (João Rodrigues de Castelo Branco), *In Dioscoridis Anazarbei de medica materia libros quinque enarrationes eruditissimae doctoris Amati Lusitani, medici ac philosophi celeberrimi, quibus non solum officinarum seplasiariis, sed bonarum etiam literarum studiosis utilitas adfertur, quum passim simplicia Graece, Latine, Italice, Hispanice, Germanice, & Gallice proponantur*, 1553, *Liber III, Enarratio 78*; fragment also cited by Saint-Lager (1885, p. 18).

among whom worthy of mention are John Falconer, an Englishman, a man whom in my opinion should be compared with any most learned botanist,[66] and who, in order to study plants, travelled through various parts of the world, from which he brought back many very diverse specimens, inserted ('sown') with extraordinary skill and glued into a certain codex (…)".[67]

During the journeys mentioned by Lusitanus, Falconer became acquainted with Ghini, Aldrovandi, Cesalpino, and many other prominent botanists. Saint-Lager speculates that Falconer may have been preparing herbaria before Ghini, but there is no definitive evidence for this (Saint-Lager 1885, pp. 19–23, see also Thijsse 2016). It is a fact, however, that the earliest documented herbaria date back to the 1540s, and in the following decade, the technique of plant pressing and drying was already known and practised by numerous botanists. The herbaria of Ghini's students—Ulisse Aldrovandi, Andrea Cesalpino, Michele Merini, and Petrollini—are among the oldest surviving examples of this kind (see Table 1.1).

The technique of creating herbaria subsequently spread from Pisa throughout Europe via Ghini's students, particularly owing to Aldrovandi's contacts with Guillaume Rondelet (1506–1566), who introduced "herbarium-making" in Montpellier (Thiers 2020). Rondelet's foreign students in Montpellier—Caspar Ratzenberger (1533–1603), Leonhard Rauwolf (1535–1596), Caspar Bauhin, and Felix Platter—initiated the first such collections in Germany and Switzerland. As a result of the dissemination of this new scientific tool, more than 20 significant herbarium collections were established in the sixteenth century (Ogilvie 2006, p. 165; Drobnik 2009, p. 7; Thijsse 2016; Cristofolini 2024).[68] However, the adoption of herbaria was uneven: while in some regions the practice was well known, in others it did become widespread until the second half of the seventeenth century. Almost all of the oldest surviving herbaria were created by medical students[69]: Aldrovandi completed his medical studies in 1553, having begun collecting plants as early as

[66] Herbārius—Latin: *botanist.*

[67] Original text: *Nam quum Ferrariae mihi contigerit herbatum ire, cum nonnullis viris doctissimis & rerum naturalium diligentissimis inquisitoribus, inter quos, mihi nominandi veniunt, Ioannes Falconerius Anglus, vir mea sententia, cum quovis doctissimo herbario conferendus, & qui pro dignoscendis herbis, varias orbis partes perlustraverat, quarum plures & varias, miro artificio, codici cuidam consitas, ac agluttinandas afferebat (…)* (Amatus Lusitanus 1553, p. 322). Literal translations of certain terms are given in square brackets.

[68] Many collections have not survived to the present day, among them the herbaria of Francesco Calzolari (1522–1609), William Turner, John Falconer, Jean Bauhin (1541–1612), Paul Contant (1562–1629), and the vast majority of Ferrante Imperato's herbarium (1550–1631).

[69] An exception would be Gherardo Cibo, who was both an artist and a botanist, and a student of Ghini. Cibo was the author of botanical illustrations depicting plants painted against landscape backgrounds, which earned the recognition of contemporary botanists. For a long time, there were heated debates among researchers, whether Cibo was indeed the author of the herbarium preserved in the Biblioteca Angelica in Rome (Mangani and Tomasi 2013, pp. 17–21; Thijsse 2016; Stefanaki et al. 2019). As already mentioned, the herbarium was ultimately attributed to Francesco Petrollini (Stefanaki et al. 2019). The herbarium in question is held at the Biblioteca Angelica in Rome: Petrollini F., Erbario A, Rome, Biblioteca Angelica, ref. ms. 2344,?; Petrollini F., Erbario B, vol. I–IV, Rome, Biblioteca Angelica, ref. ms. 2345–2348, c. 1550–1553.

1551; the earliest sheets of Felix Platter, dating from his student years, are from 1552 (Lienhard and Dauwalder 2016, p. 13). Around the same time, Caspar Ratzenberger's collection was being assembled while he was a student in Wittenberg, as was that of Jehan Girault (1538?–1608), whose herbarium dates to 1558. Leonhard Rauwolf also studied in Wittenberg at the same time as Ratzenberger, but his oldest surviving specimens date from 1560 to 1562 (Fig. 1.7). Cesalpino and Bauhin were likewise students of *materia medica*; Cadé (dates unknown) was most likely a pharmacist, but it is not certain whether their collections were created during or after their studies (Ogilvie 2006, p. 172).

Polish collections

In Poland, the oldest preserved herbaria date back to the late seventeenth and early eighteenth centuries. A list of the oldest known artefacts of this type is provided in Table 1.2. This is not a particularly extensive resource, which is understandable given the history of the natural sciences in the Polish territories and the history of the country itself.[70] There are instances where, during international archival research, herbaria created by naturalists active in what is now Poland are discovered, as in the case of Jakub Breyn's (1637–1697) collection (Pękacka-Falkowska 2018a, b). Conversely, there are cases where objects are found in Polish collections that were acquired from other institutions after the war, such as the Helwing and Boretius herbaria from the Stadtbibliothek in Königsberg,[71] the Schaffgotsch collections,[72] or from the Westpreußische Provinzial—Museum Danzig.[73]

The list opens with the herbarium of Paolo Silvio Boccone, from the collections of the Herbarium of the Museum of Natural History in Wrocław (WRSL), dated to 1689–1695 (Grenda-Kurmanow et al. 2025).[74] It was brought to Wrocław by Boccone himself, who visited the city in 1695. This is the only known herbarium preserved in Poland that can be definitively dated to the seventeenth century.[75] Were it not for a certain coincidence, which, although motivated by noble intentions, had detrimental consequences, there would be another seventeenth-century herbarium present in Polish collections, predating Boccone's and of particular value. This con-

[70] Issues related to herbaria as collectible objects and components of natural history collections are discussed in the Sect. 1.3.5.

[71] Herbaria held in the collections of the National Library and the Herbarium of the Faculty of Biology, University of Warsaw (WA).

[72] With the stamp of the Majoratsbibliothek zu Warmbrunn (Cieplice), now the site of the Museum of Natural History in Cieplice.

[73] Present in the collections of the Herbarium of Nicolaus Copernicus University in Toruń (TRN) and the Rev. Krzysztof Kluk Museum of Agriculture in Ciechanowiec.

[74] In Poland during the 17th and 18th centuries, there were significantly more herbaria, which often formed part of extensive natural history collections. The earliest records of herbaria in Poland date back to the sixteenth century. The history of Polish collections containing herbaria is discussed in the Sect. 1.3.5.

[75] The history was described by Prof. Alicja Zemanek (1996), who, during her research on the preserved Polish copies of Syreniusz's *Herbarium*, also worked on the specimen from the PTPN collection, ref. 5162.III.

Table 1.2 List of the oldest pre-Linnaean herbaria preserved in Poland, from the seventeenth and eighteenth centuries

Author and/or herbarium owner	Collection years	Number of volumes	Current location
Paolo Boccone (author)	c. 1689–1695	1	Wrocław, Natural History Museum (WRSL)
Jerzy Andrzej Helwing (author)	1695–1705	2	Warsaw, National Library
Jan Antoni Camelin (author) or Jan Szaster (owner)	First half of the eighteenth century	1	Kraków, Institute of Botany, Jagiellonian University (KRA)
Maciej Ernest Borecki (Boretius, author)	1712–1738	4 (volume III missing)	Warsaw, Herbarium of the Faculty of Biology, University of Warsaw (WA)
Jerzy Andrzej Helwing and/or Maciej Ernest Borecki (Boretius) (author)	Before 1738	1	Warsaw, Herbarium of the Faculty of Biology, University of Warsaw (WA)
Jerzy Andrzej Helwing and/or Maciej Ernest Borecki (Boretius) (author)	1724–1745	2	Warsaw, Herbarium of the Faculty of Biology, University of Warsaw (WA)
Johann Friedrich Zeidler (author)	1732 (Vol. I); 1734 (Vol. II); 1751 (Vol. III)	2 (Vol. II missing)	Lublin, Main Library of the University of Life Sciences
Izabela Czartoryska (owner)	1746	1	Kraków, National Museum in Kraków
Jędrzej Badurski (owner)	Second half of the eighteenth century	4	Kraków, Institute of Botany, Jagiellonian University (KRA)

cerns the presumed herbarium of Princess Anna Vasa of Sweden (1568–1625), prepared from a copy of Szymon Syreniusz's *Herbarium* from 1613.[76] In the Library of the Poznań Society for the Advancement of Arts and Sciences, there is a copy of Syreniusz's *Herbarium*, fragments of which evidently once belonged to the Princess (Figs. 1.8, 1.9, and 1.10).

Ludwik Bierkowski (1801–1860), Professor of surgery at the Jagiellonian University and owner of the herbarium since 1830, undertook the effort to trace and subsequently describe the provenance details of these particular fragments. A document bearing his handwritten notes is attached to the block of the early printed book.[77] In this document, Bierkowski describes that the sheets ("a very incomplete

[76] Following the professor's manuscript, a second manuscript is also attached, authored by his son, Kazimierz Bierkowski, which serves as the deed of transfer of the *Herbarium* to the Poznań Society for the Advancement of Arts and Sciences. Quotations from the manuscripts can be found in Zemanek (1996).

[77] Quotation from the original text by Bierkowski.

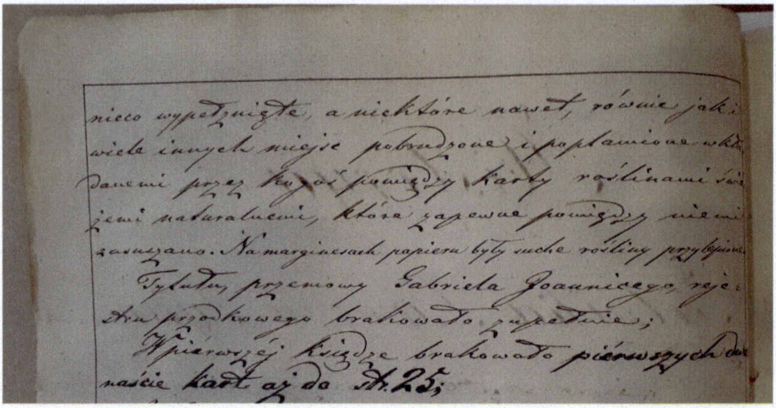
nieco wypętznięte, a niektóre nawet, również jak i
wiele innych miejsc pobrudzone i poplamione wkła-
danemi przez kogoś pomiędzy karty roślinami świe-
żemi naturalnemi, które zapewne pomiędzy niemi
zasuszano. Na marginesach papieru były suche rośliny przylepione.
Tytułu, przemowy Gabriela Joannickiego, reje-
stru przodkowego brakowało zupełnie;
W pierwszej księdze brakowało pierwszych
naście kart aż do str. 25;

Fig. 1.8 A fragment of Ludwik Bierkowski's manuscript attached to Syreniusz's *Herbarium*, Poznań Society for the Advancement of Arts and Sciences Library, ref. 5162.III. In the first five lines, Bierkowski writes about the pages that were "soiled and stained by someone placing fresh, natural plants between the sheets, which were presumably pressed and dried there." Additionally, "dried plants were affixed to the paper margins." (Photo: M. Grenda-Kurmanow)

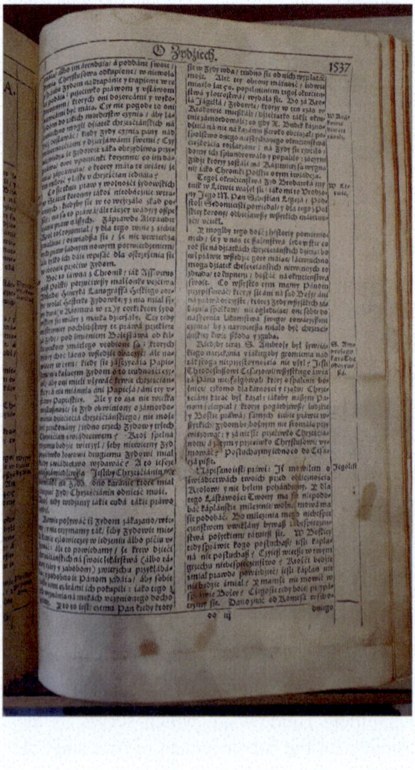

Fig. 1.9 Fragment of Syreniusz's *Herbarium*, Poznań Society for the Advancement of Arts and Sciences Library, ref. 5162.III. Visible deposits; it is possible that these are traces of the mounting of Anna Vasa's dried plants, which the conservator was unable to remove. (Photo: M. Grenda-Kurmanow)

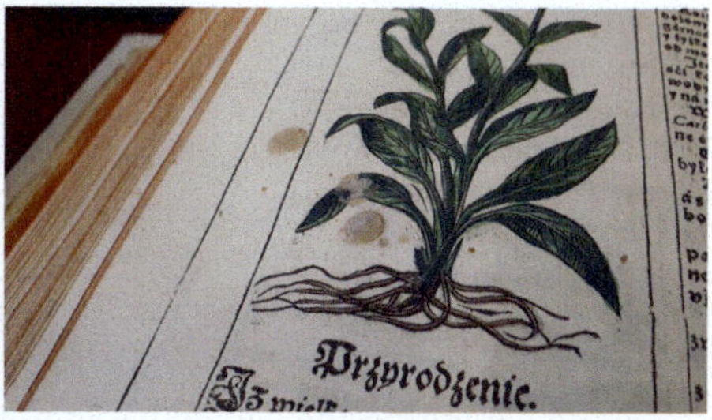

Fig. 1.10 Fragment of Syreniusz's *Herbarium*, Poznań Society for the Advancement of Arts and Sciences Library, ref. 5162.III. Visible discolourations. (Photo: M. Grenda-Kurmanow)

copy of Syreniusz's Herbarium"),[78] which he purchased in Vilnius in 1830, were not bound, but interleaved with blank sheets and used both for pressing plants and for mounting plant specimens on the margins (Fig. 1.8). Bierkowski, who sought to reconstruct and complete the valuable early printed work, describes how he compiled it using other partially preserved copies of Syreniusz's work, as well as how he restored it by removing the remnants of Anna Vasa's herbarium through cleaning, stain removal, and "refreshing." Currently, a few sheets display discolourations and accretions that may indicate the former presence of plant material in this copy (Figs. 1.9 and 1.10).

The following examples include the herbarium of the Prussian botanist and Evangelical pastor Georg Andreas Helwing (1666–1748) from the turn of the 17th and 18th centuries (c. 1695–1705), held in the collections of the National Library (Fig. 1.11) (Spalik 2014a, b), as well as herbaria of uncertain attribution, prepared either also by Helwing or by Maciej Ernest Borecki (Boretius, 1694–1738), from the first half of the eighteenth century, preserved in the Herbarium of the Faculty of Biology, University of Warsaw (WA) (Fig. 1.12). Most of these are volumes bound in parchment, with plants mounted directly onto the paper.[79] The volumes from the National Library collections are richly decorated and represent a unique example of ornamental herbarium binding (Spalik 2014a; Popławska 2014a, 2018).[80] These herbaria, now housed in various institutions, once formed a single collection, as evidenced by preserved handwritten reference numbers and stamps from the Municipal Library in Königsberg.

One of the most valuable eighteenth-century Polish herbaria is the 1746 herbarium belonging to Princess Izabela Czartoryska, which was once part of the collections of the Gothic House in Puławy and is now held by the National Museum in Kraków. This is a rather small notebook containing specimens, in which Princess Czartoryska placed her autograph (Piekiełko 1977).[81] In addition, the collections of

[78] One of the albums from this collection, bound in paper, is described in greater detail in Chap. 5, which concerns the conservation process.

[79] The digitised object can be studied in its entirety on the Polona portal: https://polona.pl/item/herbarium-vivum-plantarum-sponte-in-prussia-nascentium-t-1,Nzk3MTEwOA/3/#info:metadata (accessed: 13.01.2026).

[80] See also the chapter on conservation treatment in Chap. 5.

[81] The object is described in greater detail in Chap. 5, which concerns the conservation treatment.

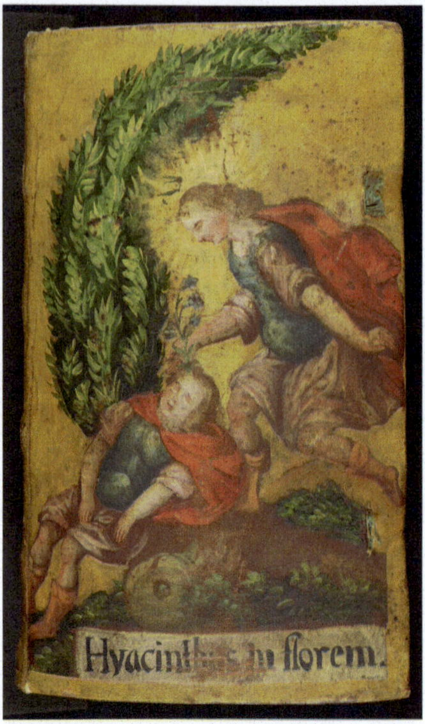

Fig. 1.11 Helwing's Herbarium, front cover, and title page of volume I. Helwing, J.A., *Herbarium Vivum*... (vol. I); *Florae Napeisque*... (vol. II), Warsaw, National Library, ref. Rps akc. 200/1–2, c. 1695–1705. (Source: Polona)

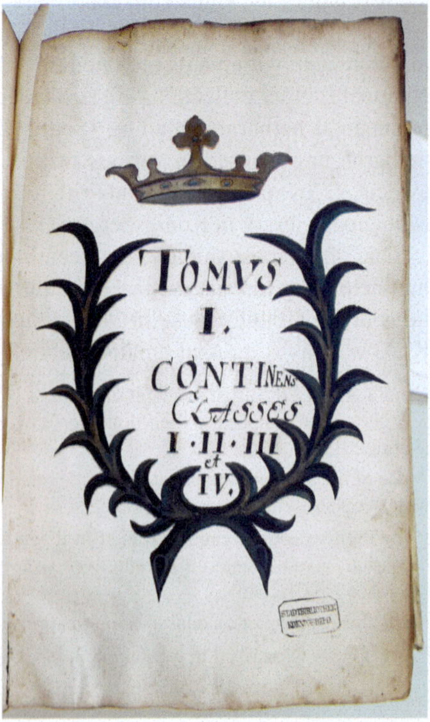

Fig. 1.12 Boretius's Herbarium, title page of volume I. Borecki, M. A., *Matth. Ern. Boretii Herbarium vivum*, Warsaw, Herbarium of the Faculty of Biology, University of Warsaw (WA), ref. WA-KH-13.1.1, 1712–1738. (Photo: M. Grenda-Kurmanow)

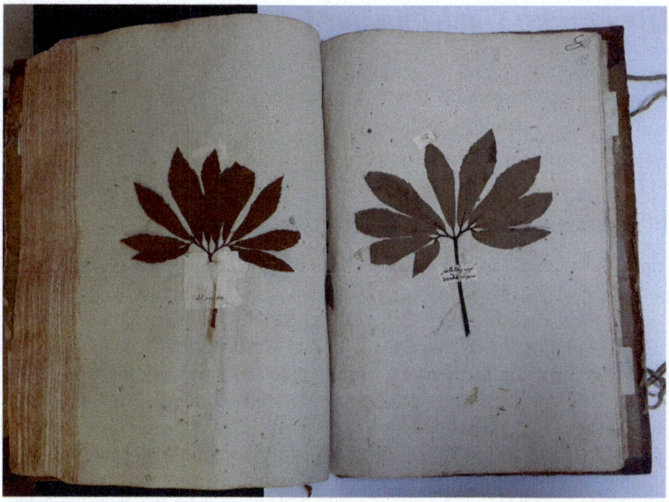

Fig. 1.13 Herbarium sheet of Jędrzej Badurski (Badurski A., untitled, Kraków, Herbarium of the Institute of Botany, Jagiellonian University in Kraków (KRA), without ref. no., first half of the eighteenth century). (Photo: M. Grenda-Kurmanow)

the Institute of Botany at the Jagiellonian University (KRA) also preserve two eighteenth-century herbaria: one attributed to lecturers in medical botany at the Jagiellonian University, Jan Antoni Camelin (d. 1774) or Jan Szaster (1741–1793), and the other belonging to Jędrzej Badurski (1740–1789), professor of medicine at the Kraków Academy (Fig. 1.13) (Piekiełko 1981; Köhler 1999). These herbaria remain a testament to the activities and interests of the medical community in Kraków.

The corpus of eighteenth-century Polish herbarium monuments is complemented by previously unstudied herbaria compiled by the Silesian pharmacist Johann Friedrich Zeidler between 1732 and 1751. These herbaria are currently held in the Main Library of the University of Life Sciences in Lublin and originate from the collection of Count Johann Anton Schaffgotsch, which was initially deposited in Sobieszów (Hermsdorf) and later in Cieplice (Warmbrunn).[82]

Many native collections have been destroyed, dispersed, or lost.[83] From time to time, traces of specimens that once left the present-day Polish territories are rediscovered. It should be noted, however, that some of the oldest herbaria currently in Poland are in fact foreign collections that were incorporated into Polish holdings after the Second World War.[84]

[82] See the Sect. 1.3.5.

[83] See the Sect. 1.3.5.

[84] Some of them bear traces of dramatic wartime events; for example, all the herbaria of Helwing and Boretius from the Municipal Library in Königsberg show damage resulting from fire.

1.3.2 *The Earliest Guidelines for Creating Herbaria*

The method of preparing herbaria was first described in 1606 by the Flemish physician Adriaan van der Spiegel (1578–1625) in *Isagoges in rem herbariam libri duo*, the first textbook of botany in history (van der Spiegel 1606, *Liber I, Caput 58*, pp. 79–81). At the end of the first book, in chapter 58, the author describes the "Method of creating winter gardens" (*Hortos Hyemales conficiendi ratio*):

> Indeed, the effort devoted to the creation of winter gardens is more praiseworthy, for it is lesser and more useful; since many things depicted in illustrations, which pertain to form—namely colour, and certain other features—cannot be rendered with such accuracy in advance. Moreover, the preliminary effort with large, rough, thorny, and very hard plants is often futile. Therefore, the method of attaching plants to sheets should be as follows: The plant of your choice, or its green stem (branch) with flower, leaves, and, if possible, seeds, in its entirety, should be placed between two sheets of clean (white) paper. For the more common sheet, which leaks, although hitherto used by everyone for this purpose, is by no means suitable, as I have found through experience that plants placed between such sheets dry with difficulty and often wither in places soiled in this way. The leaves, therefore, as I have mentioned, should be placed in a thick book with very many pages, so that it is appropriate to the size of the leaves to be placed within. A weight should be placed on this book, so that the plants are gradually pressed down, as if under a press. However, one should avoid using a heavy weight until most of the moisture has been absorbed from the plant. Therefore, the weight should be increased gradually: at first lighter, until the plants wilt (which in summer usually occurs within three or four hours), then heavier, and finally the heaviest, when the plants contain little moisture and are almost dry. Care should also be taken to inspect these plants daily, to open the sheets, straighten any folds that may be seen, and arrange the flowers and leaves so that they can be viewed from both sides, and to change the sheet until the plant is completely dry. The dried plant should be stored in a dry place between sheets until more plants have been dried in the same way and it is worthwhile to proceed with mounting. Then the following procedure should be adopted. Brushes of various sizes (for plants with large leaves require larger brushes, those with smaller leaves—smaller ones) should be dipped in the adhesive described below, with which the side of the plant to be attached to the sheet should be coated. This adhesive consists of one ounce of clear animal glue, which the people of Padua call Tedescho glue, that is, German glue, which should be dissolved overnight in six ounces of very strong vinegar; then it should be placed over a gentle fire to dissolve. After removing from the fire, when it has gradually cooled, half a drachm[85] of hepatic aloe and one scruple of clove powder should be added, and the mixture stirred. The plant to be mounted should then be placed on a common sheet, coated with the adhesive, then removed and placed on a clean (white) sheet, and, after placing a sheet, handkerchief, or linen cloth on top, it should be rubbed firmly and evenly wherever the plant adheres to the sheet. It should then be closed between two pages in another book and a good weight placed on top until the adhesive dries (which occurs after one or two hours), after which it should be removed at once. It should also be noted that not all plants should be treated in this way. There are certain plants that do not dry easily due to the abundance of liquid sap, such as houseleek, stonecrop,[86] and certain other types. For these wither, rot, lose their leaves, or retain them, but with a colour different from the natural one, and very wrinkled. These plants are better mounted while still green, but first they should be placed in a book between two sheets, one on top of the other, and gently pressed

[85] Drachma—1/8 of an ounce; the scruple mentioned later—1/24 of an ounce.

[86] Possibly *Telephium*.

> with a light weight until they wilt, become creased, and take shape, so that they can then be properly attached. In this way, I have also mounted other plants, while green, in the mountains, and exposed them to the sun or in another warm place until they dried, and this effort was successful (…).

Another description of the technique for preparing a herbarium can be found in Joseph Pitton de Tournefort's *Élemens de botanique ou methode pour connoître les plantes* (1694):

> (…) The best way to prepare a Herbarium is to cut the plants so that they do not contain water, arrange them appropriately in old books or between sheets of grey paper, above all in such a manner that there are many layers of paper between two plants; (they should be) pressed (weighted) not too heavily, and the (paper) should be changed two or three times, depending on whether the plants are more or less moist: and to ensure they are well dried, they should be stored individually between sheets, and all the sheets packed in boxes where air penetrates as little as possible and which can be opened from the top and the front and closed with hinges, so that the sheets can be easily removed whenever one wishes to study the plants. Plants are usually glued to paper, but apart from the fact that this allows the plant to be viewed only from one side, either from above or below, it also attracts moths, which destroy the plants and spoil everything. The best adhesive I have found is glove glue[87] to which calomel[88] or mercury sublimate[89] may be added, as preferred: calomel and mercury sublimate are powerful enemies of insects; nevertheless, the glue must be carefully mixed with a brush during use, as the mercury easily settles at the bottom of the pot. Glove glue made with a decoction of wormseed (*Semen contra*), wormwood (*Absinthe commune*), and aloe or similar herbs did not work well. A thin layer of such varnish may be applied to the glued plants to protect them from the effects of air and insects; but this always changes the colour of the plant, and this alteration is not appreciated by those who wish to preserve the plants for comparison with the descriptions of the authors who collected them. To dry plants in the countryside, where there are no old books or where there is often no time to change them, one may use a heated iron, such as is used by laundresses for ironing linen. It should be gently heated and used to press through two or three layers of grey paper, between which the plant to be dried is placed, carefully straightening its edges and arranging the leaves properly (…). (de Tournefort 1694, pp. 547–548)

The above descriptions, as can be seen, are precise recipes and instructions, supported by extensive practical experience derived from the authors' own observations.[90] They attest to the inclusion of herbaria among the standard tools of the botanist's work no later than the seventeenth century.

---

[87] Glue made from lambskin trimmings.

[88] Fr. *mercure doux.*

[89] Fr. *Sublimé corrosif.*

[90] An overview of the techniques and materials used in the preparation of herbaria is presented in the Sect. 2.1 in Chap. 2.

1.3.3 Terms Used for Herbaria Containing Dried Plant Specimens

When writing about herbaria, it is essential to consider the terminology used to refer to albums containing dried plants. The word "herbarium" has been employed with various meanings. Although Lusitanus uses the term *herbario* in a passage describing Falconer's activities, in this context it is most likely a variant of the word *herbārius*, meaning a botanist (an expert in plants),[91] rather than *herbarium*. Furthermore, in his text, Lusitanus refers to printed herbals (including those by Fuchs and Brunfels) and physic gardens as herbaria. The term herbarium also denoted medieval monastic rooms for drying herbs or monastic gardens.[92]

In *Isagoges…*, Spiegel uses the term *hortus hyemalis*, meaning "winter garden". This term referred to the function that herbaria undoubtedly served from their inception—the opportunity to study the plant world during the "dead season", the winter period.

It is generally accepted that the term *herbarium* was first used in its modern sense by Tournefort in his already cited *Élemens de botanique…* (1694). In the dictionary of botanical terms (*Dictionnaire ou explications de termes de botanique et des quelques autres qui peuvent servir pour l'intelligence de cet ouvrage*), which forms part of the *Élemens…* ((de Tournefort 1694, pp. 515–562), entry *Herbier* (Herbarium) on pp. 547–548),[93] the herbarium is defined as follows: "(…) Herbarium. This is essentially a collection of dried plants, which are kept in boxes or in books, so that they may be carefully studied at any time of the year; in Latin it is called *Herbarium*, or *Hortus siccus* (…)".[94] Other terms used for herbaria included *hortus mortus* ("dead garden"), *Hortus perennis* ("everlasting garden"),[95] *Giardino di cella*

[91] *Herbariō* is the ablative form of the word *herbārius* (Latin case *ablativus*).

[92] Other names include *herbularium* and *hortus medicus*.

[93] He uses the term *Herbarium* in the same sense when referring to Gesner's lost herbarium collection. Its uniqueness was said to be demonstrated by the excellence of the illustrations, created on the basis of the plants (de Tournefort 1694, p. 17).

[94] Original text: *C'est proprement un amas de plantes sèches que l'on conserve dans des boites ou dans des livres, afin de les pouvoir examiner avec soin dans toutes les saisons de l'année: on l'apelle en Latin* Herbarium, *ou* Hortus siccus (de Tournefort 1694, p. 547). This is followed by instructions for preparing herbaria, cited in the previous section.

[95] Title used in the herbaria of Johann Friedrich Zeidler from 1732 and 1751 [title of Volume I: *Hortus Perennis/Immer grünendes/Gewachs-Hautz/das ist:/Aller au(s)s dem hoch Reich graffs Schaff-/gotschitschischen Territorio mais-/tenden Kräutern und Blu-/men/Erster Theil/zu/ Betrachtung der mannigfaltigen Natur/Belustigung des curieusen Gemüthes/Preitz(?) des allermeistesten Shönsters/veröffnet/von/Johann Friedrich Zeidler/Medicinae Practico/in/Petersdorff/ Anno* (Zeidler J.F., *Hortus Perennis* …, Lublin, Main Library of the University of Life Sciences, Special Collections and Old Prints 14, D. 104.57.646, 1732)]. The title of Volume III begins with the same phrase: *Hortus Perennis/ das ist/Immer Grunendes GewachsHaus/Betrachtung der mannigfaltigen* (Zeidler J.F., Hortus Perennis…, vol. III, Lublin, Main Library of the University of Life Sciences, ref. Zb. Specj. Starodruki XVIII.14; D. 104.57.646, 1751).

("garden in a monk's cell"),[96] *Herbarium vivum*,[97] *theatrum vegetabilium* (Kessler 1870, pp. 14–15),[98] and *regnum vegetabile*. Occasionally, a herbarium might be referred to by a highly poetic phrase, as in the case of one of the oldest herbaria in the world, preserved at the Naturalis Biodiversity Center in Leiden: *En Tibi Perpetuis Ridentum Floribus Hortum* (Latin: "for you, this smiling garden of everlasting flowers") (Stefanaki et al. 2018). The terminology relating to herbaria was not always used consistently; for example, *herbarium vivum* could also refer to an album of illustrations (Kessler 1870, p. 14).

The same terms were used in Poland as in other parts of Europe, as exemplified by *Herbarium vivum* as the title of the herbaria of Helwing and Czartoryska. In the catalogue of the Duchess's collections from 1828, the herbarium is referred to as a "natural herbarium" (Czartoryska 1828, p. 99). In the nineteenth century, the collection of Camelin (or Szaster) from the eighteenth century was also designated as a "herbarium" (Piekiełko 1981, p. 9).[99] The terms "herbarium" and "herbal", were used until the end of the seventeenth century to describe a catalogue of plants, with descriptions of their properties and uses (Zemanek 1997).[100]

Today, the Latin term *herbarium* refers not only to a publication serving as a catalogue of plants with descriptions of their properties, but also to a collection of dried plants—on a global scale, as a collection (for example, the entire collection of a single author), and on an individual scale, as a single set (such as a volume or a series of herbarium sheets), as well as to the institution that houses herbarium collections.

---

[96] A term used by the Italian Capuchin Fra Gregorio da Reggio (d. c. 1618) (Egmond 2010, pp. 93–94, *eadem* 2018).

[97] This is the title of one of the oldest herbaria in Poland, authored by Jerzy Andrzej Helwing (Helwing J.A., *Herbarium Vivum …*, Warsaw, National Library, ref. Rkps akc. 200, 1695–1705): *Herbarium Vivum Plantarum sponte in Prussia nascentium, Herculeo labore comparatum M. Georgii Andreae Helwingii Pastoris Angerburgensium. et Reg. Societ. Scient. Brand. Membrii*; as well as the herbarium of Izabela Czartoryska (n.n., *Herbarium Vivum …* (Herbarium of Izabela Czartoryska), Kraków, National Museum in Kraków, Czartoryski Library, ref. Rkps 2782, 1746).

[98] Kessler suggests that Ratzenberger was among the first to use this term.

[99] Many herbaria do not include a similar designation in their titles, and their titles are more characteristic of catalogues, defining the specificity of the collected species—for example, Breyne's *Plantae rariores Borussicae et Cassubicae* (Pękacka-Falkowska 2018a).

[100] This is evidenced for example by some of the earliest Polish publications on herbal medicine: *Herbarz to iest Ziół tutecznych, postronnych y zamorskich opisanie* ("This Herbal is a description of local, foreign, and overseas herbs) by Marcin Siennik (1568), *Herbarz Polski* ("Polish Herball") by Marcin of Urzędów (1595), and the work of Szymon Syreniusz from 1613, *Zielnik herbarzem z łacińskiego języka zowion* ("Herbarium, known as herbal in Latin"). Similarly to many herbaria containing dried specimens, the earliest herbal publications do not include a term defining a catalogue in their titles, but are rather descriptive, for example, Stefan Falimirz's *O ziołach i o mocy ich…* ("On Herbs and Their Properties…" 1534).

1.3.4 The Earliest Representations of Herbaria

The herbarium as an iconographic motif appears for the first time in 1562, in the portrait of the renowned Parisian apothecary Pierre Quthe (1519–1590), painted by François Clouet (1510–1572) (Fig. 1.14).[101] As an attribute, it likely attests to the

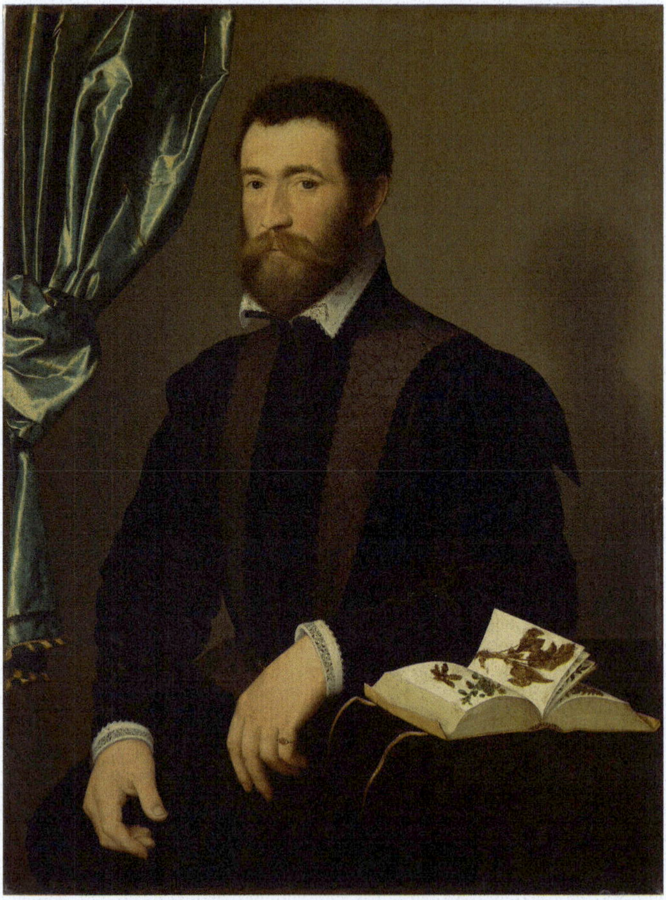

Fig. 1.14 Portrait of the apothecary Pierre Quthe (1562), painted by François Clouet (Musée du Louvre). (Photo © GrandPalaisRmn (musée du Louvre) / Tony Querrec / RMN GP/ BE&W)

[101] The painting is held in the collection of the Louvre. It depicts Pierre Quthe at the age of 43. Quthe also maintained a medicinal garden in the heart of Paris. The man is shown seated, with an open herbarium lying on the table beside him. Thijsse emphasises that this is one of the few pieces of evidence for the existence of herbarium collections in France, alongside the herbarium of Girault (1558) and an engraving depicting the collections of Paul Contant (Thijsse 2016, see also Arber 1970, p. 143).

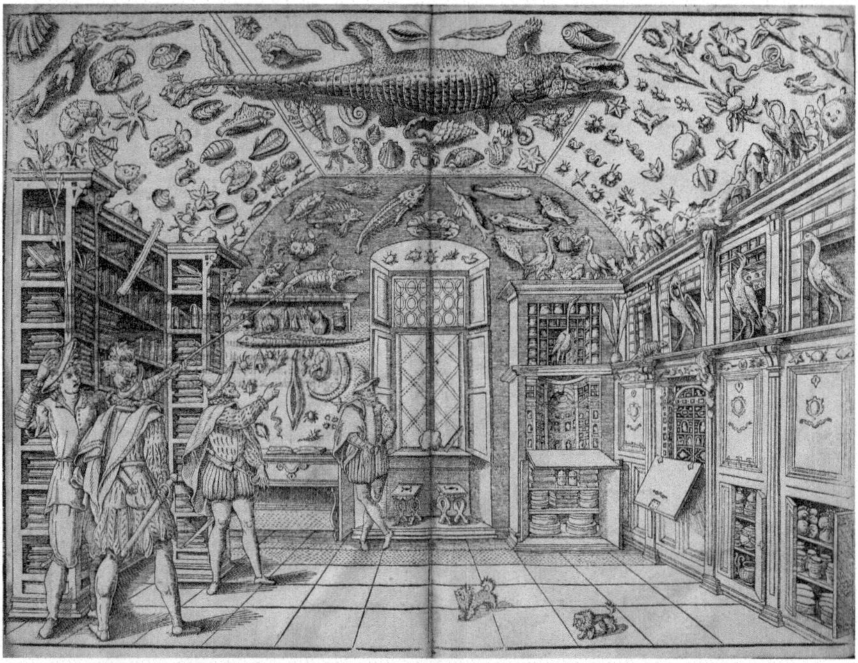

Fig. 1.15 Ferrante Imperato, *Dell'historia Naturale*, 1599, frontispiece. (Courtesy of the Smithsonian Libraries and Archives via Biodiversity Heritage Library)

pharmacist's established knowledge and expertise. Subsequently, herbaria begin to appear as elements of natural history collections, depicted as tightly packed books alongside other naturalia. The first representation of a herbarium collection is an engraving depicting the museum of Ferrante Imperato (c. 1525–c. 1615) from 1599 (Fig. 1.15).[102] The engraving shows visitors to the Neapolitan apothecary's cabinet, guided by a host, most likely the owner himself. Among the many natural specimens on the right, books with plants protruding from their pages can be seen on the shelves. This refers to Imperato's vast, for its time, 80-volume herbarium collection. Shortly afterwards, a section of the collection belonging to Paul Contant (1562–1629), a wealthy apothecary, poet, and collector from Poitiers, was immortalised in the catalogue of his holdings (Fig. 1.16). The engraving illustrates the organisation of the collection, which comprised 15 herbaria containing around 3000 specimens of both local and exotic plants (Egmond 2010, p. 127).[103]

[102] The illustration is taken from the catalogue of his own collection, *Dell'historia Naturale*, published by Imperato in 1599; see also the following section.

[103] The volumes are arranged in alphabetical order, with the exception of the legume (*Legumes*) and bulbous plant (*Bulbes*) volumes. The books are housed in an ornately decorated cabinet with 32 small drawers in the upper section and on three shelves in the lower section. Above the drawers is the inscription *Capsulae 32 Varia Naturae Mirabilia*, and above the herbarium volumes, the inscription *Libri 15 De Indigenis et Exoticis Plantis*.

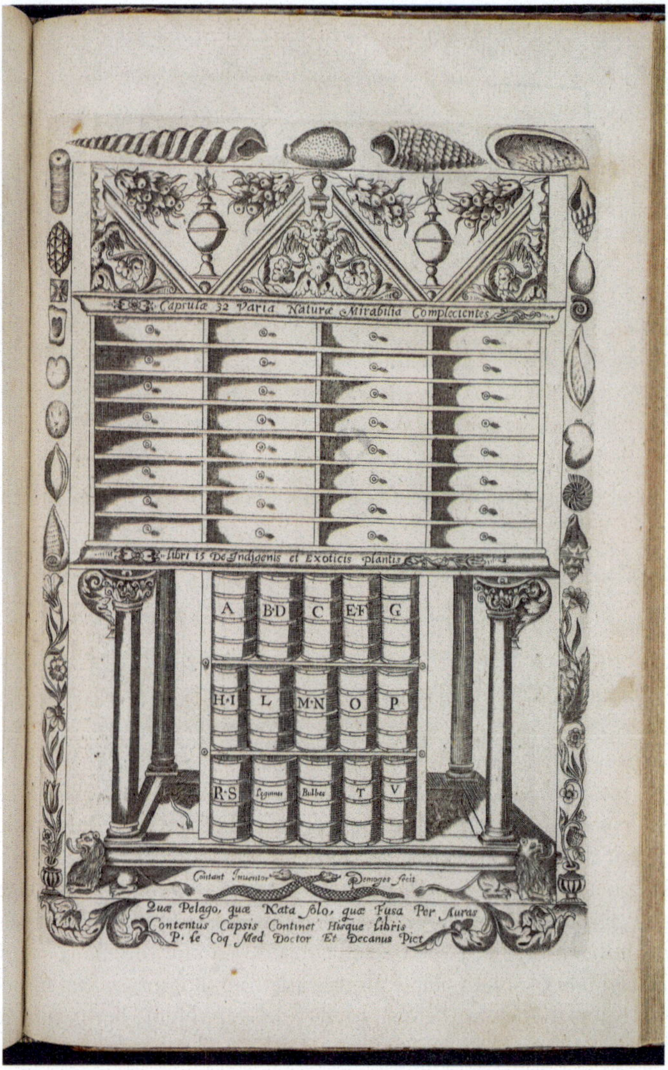

Fig. 1.16 Illustration depicting the herbarium collections of Paul Contant, from *Les œuvres de Jacques et Paul Contant* (1628) (Bibliothèque nationale de France, BnF)

1.3.5 Herbaria as Collectible Phenomena and Components of Natural History Collections

In the second half of the sixteenth century, when natural history had already become a distinctly separate field supported by specialised publications, its ties with medicine began to loosen. On the one hand, an increasing number of physicians were studying botany; on the other, new descriptions of plants were being compiled not for their medicinal properties, but with a focus on morphology. The generation of medical students at the turn of the sixteenth and seventeenth centuries had already become a group regularly engaged in botanical pursuits, and botanical walks introduced by Felix Platter and Theodor Zwinger (1533–1588) in Basel formed part of the medical curriculum (Ogilvie 2006, p. 38). At the same time, among the enthusiasts of the young and appealing discipline of natural history, one could find representatives of various professions and social standings, from apothecaries and gardeners to nobles and emperors. What united them was a passion for collecting.[104]

Natural specimens had attracted interest long before the sixteenth century, but it was in the latter half of the sixteenth century that collecting developed into an intellectual pursuit, taking on a systematic and knowledge-based form. At that time, it became customary for collectors to possess detailed information about their collections in order to truly "own" them.[105] Rare naturalia were especially prized, as they combined scientific value with a fascination for that which lay beyond the everyday and served as nourishment for the flourishing *curiosité* of the period (Egmond 2010, p. 42).[106] Owners often acted as guides, leading visitors through their collections. They consistently included specialist publications that explained the contents of their collections (Ogilvie 2006, pp. 38–46).

Large collections of natural specimens were destinations for visits and subjects of study for naturalists, contributing to the development of the field of science. In

---

[104] Already at that time, one can speak of the beginnings of a split between natural history as a strictly scientific discipline and the hobby of collecting of impressive curiosities. This growing divergence was evident in the emergence of publications intended for amateurs, rather than scientific works (Ogilvie 2006, p. 46).

[105] The irresistible urge to create a synthesis of the world within the lens of a collection was the driving force for collectors from the sixteenth to the late seventeenth century. The new perspective on the natural world and its analysis, which resonated in Bacon's *Novum Organum* (see the Sect. 1.1), provided the impetus for the creation of collections known as *Kunst- und Wunderkammern*. In these collections, the worlds of art and nature intersected in various ways. Many of these collections were not scientific in character, yet without their emergence, the development of science would not have been possible. Renaissance and Baroque scientists were motivated by different factors than collectors of curiosities, although it should be remembered that many of the figures mentioned here combined the traits of both scientist and collector of *curiositas*. For members of the highest social strata, collections served a prestigious and political function, attesting to their power over the world, as represented by their rich and diverse holdings. Scientists, faced with the rapid accumulation of information accompanying the discovery of new species, were compelled to undertake meticulous and laborious comparative studies. The evolution of collecting practices occurred in the eighteenth century, as the status of the kunstkammer as a collection of diversity shifted towards specialised collections with a narrower thematic focus. As Mauriès writes: "(...) the idea of the cabinet of curiosities changed when differences began to dominate over similarities. Those belonging to the world of art formed gallery collections, while naturalia became the holdings of natural history museums (...)" (Mauriès 2015, p. 185). Many authors have written about the processes associated with these transformations, also analysing individual collections (see, among others, Findlen 1994; Pomian 1996; Mencfel 2010; Mauriès 2015).

[106] Curiosity, which, as Pomian writes, "(...) prevailed during the interregnum between the age of theology and the age of science (...)" (Pomian 1996, p. 84).

cabinets of curiosities, herbaria occupied a position between being natural objects in their own right and serving as specialised scientific resources; their role thus extended beyond mere adornment of an intriguing collection. Some herbaria belonging to the Kunstkammer even "travelled" between cabinets.[107]

Many Renaissance naturalists possessed their own extensive collections of naturalia, more or less reflecting the trend of cabinets of curiosities, among which herbaria were included. The most renowned (and recognised) botanist-collectors include Luca Ghini, Ulisse Aldrovandi, Felix Platter, Jacob Zwinger, and Caspar Bauhin. Remarkable collections were also held in the sixteenth century by other naturalists who never became established scientists, such as the Italian apothecaries Ferrante Imperato and Francesco Calzolari, or the papal physician Michele Mercati (1541–1593) (Findlen 1994, p. 31; Egmond 2010; Cristofolini 2024).[108] The largest of these collections was in Naples, belonging to Imperato (the previously cited 1559 illustration, Fig. 1.15), which, according to accounts, comprised over 80 volumes of herbaria (Mauriès 2015; Jaussaud 2003; Egmond 2010, p. 99; Cristofolini 2024).[109] His museum functioned simultaneously as a "library" of naturalia and a research laboratory (Egmond 2010, p. 98). Both public and private collections were made accessible and used for educational purposes.[110] Bauhin primarily used his herbarium as a scientific tool, yet in his *Pinax theatri botanici* he announced that it was open to visitors.[111] Linnaeus also established a private natural history museum in Hammarby in 1769 (Frey 2010, p. 51). Naturalists often collected specimens to exchange them with their correspondents.[112] Acquired specimens were incorporated

[107] The Rauwolf herbaria and the *En Tibi* herbarium, now housed in Leiden, were once part of Emperor Rudolf II's (1552–1612) collections in Prague. These herbaria were removed during the Thirty Years' War and taken to Munich, to the Kunstkammer of Maximilian I (1573–1651), Elector of Bavaria. Subsequently, after being looted by Swedish troops in 1632, they were transported to Sweden and incorporated into the collections of Queen Christina of Sweden (1626–1689) (Ogilvie 2006, pp. 38–46). An example of a herbarium specifically created as part of a Kunstkammer collection is the Harder herbarium, held in the collection of Johann Egolf van Knöringen (1537–1575), Bishop of Augsburg (Thijsse 2016).

[108] Many of these collections were of a prestigious nature and were intended to secure fame and status for their founders.

[109] Imperato was also regarded as an expert in the field of drying herbarium specimens. Sixty years after the establishment of the herbarium, the specimens remained in excellent condition. One volume, containing 442 specimens, has been preserved in the Biblioteca Nazionale di Napoli (Thijsse 2016). Thijsse estimated that Imperato's collection may have comprised as many as 35,000 specimens and was most likely the largest collection of its kind in Europe at the time.

[110] For example, by Cluyt, Bauhin and Platter.

[111] Clusius represented a different approach, focusing on the possession of knowledge rather than objects. However, this did not mean that he did not collect dried plants or make use of them—he maintained active contacts with many botanists, through the exchange of specimens. Nevertheless, he became known as a critic of the herbarium technique (Ogilvie 2006, pp. 38–46).

[112] The earliest examples of specimen dispatch and exchange include correspondence between Ghini and Mattioli as early as 1551 (Arber 1970, p. 139), as well as Platter, Zwinger, and Bauhin (Ogilvie 2006, p. 43), and also Clusius and Fra Gregorio (Egmond 2010, p. 94). Carefully packed living plants, bulbs, and seeds were also exchanged (Ogilvie 2006, pp. 61, 151–164). Herbaria

into their own collections.[113] Many herbaria were also created as gifts (*En Tibi* herbarium) or dedicated to members of the clergy and aristocracy (Thijsse 2016; Cook 2007). Boccone, travelling throughout Europe, "left behind" herbaria, presenting them to successive hosts and patrons.[114]

Since the eighteenth century, alongside the dynamic development of botany, there has been a fashion for herbarium-making, botanical excursions, amateur collections of dried specimens, and a general interest in botany (Drobnik 2009, p. 10). This was facilitated by Linnaeus's clear systematics and by the fact that, thanks to his work, he permanently changed the way the plant world was perceived.[115]

The drive to collect was further stimulated by expeditions to previously unknown regions of the world, from which travellers brought back or sent previously unrecorded botanical specimens. The first herbarium containing non-European plants was compiled in 1573 by Rauwolf during his stay in Tripoli (Thijsse 2016). In 1577, Francisco Hernández, returning from a research expedition to Mexico, brought back 38 volumes of herbarium material along with notes and illustrations of the local flora, which were deposited in the Escorial Library (Thijsse 2016). Clusius, who did not himself participate in expeditions, commissioned travellers to collect specimens along with descriptions and drawings, providing instructions regarding collection methods, drying, and transportation of the specimens (Egmond 2010, pp. 82–83; MacGregor 2018a). At this time, the scientist-naturalist became an indispensable member of expeditions to distant parts of the world, tasked with enriching the wealth of the sponsoring country with new collections and discoveries. Tournefort (1656–1708), sent in 1700 by Louis XIV on a scientific journey to the Levant, brought the king a herbarium containing 1400 species (Vadon 2013).[116] In subsequent centuries, the significance and productivity of such expeditions did not diminish: Sir Joseph Banks and Daniel Solander (1733–1782), from the 1768 voyage with James Cook on the *Endeavour* to Brazil, Tahiti, Australia, New Zealand, and Indonesia, collected 30,000 specimens, including 1400 new species; Alexander von Humboldt and Aimé Bonpland (1773–1858), from their expedition to South

played an important role in the "economy of exchange" of early modern natural history and fostered the integration of the scientific community (*idem*, pp. 171–172). See the Sect. 1.3.6.

[113] Therefore, in the collections of an experienced botanist-collector, one may find specimens originating from other renowned botanists. Among domestic examples of scientific collections containing specimens gathered by other botanists, one can cite the herbarium of Józef Jundziłł, assembled in the 1820s, which includes specimens collected by Johann Reinhold Forster (1754–1794) and his son Johann Georg Forster (1754–1794) during Cook's expedition of 1772–1775, as well as specimens gathered by Jean Emmanuel Gilibert (1741–1814) (Köhler 1995, p. 9).

[114] These included Archduke Ferdinand Charles (1628–1622), Louis II de Bourbon, Prince of Condé (1621–1686), Hieronymus van Beverningh (1614–1690), and Charles Montagu, Earl of Manchester (1656–1722) (Pulvirenti et al. 2017a).

[115] As Krzysztof Pomian put it: "(...) in the eighteenth century, botany thus plays the role of a kind of general propaedeutic to the natural sciences, and numerous naturalists begin their interests with plants, only to turn subsequently in another direction (...)" (Pomian 1996, p. 276).

[116] Tournefort also had his own collection, which he bequeathed to the King of France. Today, these are among the oldest collections in the Muséum national d'Histoire naturelle in Paris.

America, returned with 4500 new species; and another renowned botanist-explorer, Sir Joseph Dalton Hooker, brought back specimens of 1500 new species from the Antarctic expedition of 1839–1843, as well as thousands of specimens from the Himalayas in 1847 (Rix 2013, pp. 92, 194; Vadon 2013).[117] At the same time, in the sixteenth and seventeenth centuries, numerous collections of local floras were also established (Mägdefrau 2004, p. 61).[118]

Herbarium collections, in the form in which they are most commonly found today, are grouped within institutions. The earliest collections that served as the foundations of institutional herbaria, such as the herbaria of the botanical garden and university in Padua, or the herbarium in Leiden, were established as early as the sixteenth century.[119] In the following centuries, a number of the most important herbarium institutions were founded: in the seventeenth and eighteenth centuries, the herbarium in Paris (now the Muséum national d'Histoire naturelle in Paris), the Royal Botanic Gardens at Kew, as well as herbaria in Edinburgh, Oxford, Berlin, Munich, Vienna, and many other cities; in the nineteenth century, in the USA (including New York and Philadelphia) (Drobnik 2009, p. 10).[120] The eighteenth century also marked the emergence of the first public museum institutions, initiated by the opening of the British Museum in 1759. The British Museum's collections were based on the extensive collection of Sir Hans Sloane (1660–1753), which included, among other items, 337 herbaria from his own collections in Jamaica as well as entire collections acquired from other botanists and collectors.[121] Another extremely valuable collection is also housed in London: the Linnaean collections, begun during his botanical expedition to Lapland in 1732, which were put up for sale after the death of his son in 1783 and purchased 4 years later by James Edward Smith (1759–1828).[122] In 1828, after Smith's death, the collections were acquired

[117] These are merely a few significant examples from some of the most renowned expeditions.

[118] The majority of such studies have been conducted in Germany.

[119] The herbarium in Leiden has undergone numerous transformations and is now part of the Naturalis Biodiversity Center, a centralised collection of herbaria formerly housed in Leiden, Utrecht, and Wageningen, as well as other natural history collections.

[120] According to Thiers (2020), by 1900 there were 250 herbaria operating in Europe, and a further 368 were established from then until the early twenty-first century. Currently, approximately 45% are university collections, while 38% are herbaria associated with botanical gardens and museums. The remaining collections are attributed to museum and research institutions (Thiers 2020). However, historical herbaria may also be found in other types of institutions, such as libraries or archives.

[121] These included the collections of Herman Boerhaave (1710–1738), Leonard Plukenet (1641–1706), and James Petiver (1658–1718), as well as those of Uvedale, Courten, Merrett, the Duchess of Beaufort, Buddle, Kigallaer, and many other smaller ones (Britten et al. 1958). Currently, various sources report different numbers of volumes. In 1881, the Natural History Museum was established in London as a branch of the British Museum, to which Sloane's collection was eventually transferred and where it remains to this day.

[122] Linnaeus appointed his student, Daniel Solander, as the curator of the collection. However, due to his work for the British Museum, Solander was unable to accept the offer. Initially, Linnaeus's son, Carl (1741–1783), was to take care of the collection, but it was deemed that he was not sufficiently committed to science to properly oversee it. Consequently, decisions regarding the collec-

by the Linnaean Society of London, which he had founded in 1788.[123] The collection, comprising 14,300 specimens, including 4000 so-called types (reference specimens on which scientific descriptions of a given species are based), has been preserved in its original order.[124] Although in the eighteenth century the circle of natural history collectors increasingly included representatives of social and professional groups other than those previously involved—so, in addition to rulers, aristocrats, botanists, physicians, and pharmacists, more and more collectors were wealthy merchants, members of the clergy, teachers, and officials—their collections were often dispersed or incorporated into institutional holdings. From the moment natural history collections became institutionalised, this has remained the dominant form of their existence. Furthermore, the method of creating herbaria popularised by Linnaeus, namely in the form of individual herbarium sheets, has facilitated the dispersal of collections. With the exception of selected named collections, botanical collections are often organised by species classification, and distributed throughout the general herbarium collection (*Herbarium Generale*).

Natural history collections in Poland

The first natural history collections in Poland appeared in the seventeenth century.[125] The oldest such collection was probably the Gdańsk natural history cabinet of Marcin Bernhardi-Bernitz (c. 1625–1682), court physician to King John II Casimir Vasa. His cabinet of curiosities was described by Bernard O'Connor (c. 1666–1698), court physician to John III Sobieski, in his work *The History of Poland* from 1698.[126]

---

tion were made by Linnaeus's wife. After Linnaeus's death, due to the family's strained financial situation (the need to provide dowries for Linnaeus's four daughters), his widow set a high sale price of 1000 guineas. The University of Uppsala and the King of Sweden delayed their decision. As a result, despite attempts to keep the collection in Sweden, it was purchased by the British naturalist and collector James Edward Smith. According to anecdote, King Gustav III, upon learning of the loss of the herbarium, sent a war frigate in pursuit of the Englishmen (Frey 2010, pp. 75–78).

[123] Smith's collections remained his private property throughout his life. Linnaeus's herbarium was purchased from his widow for the then astronomical sum of £3000, plunging the institution into financial difficulties that were not resolved until 1861 (Frey 2010, p. 76).

[124] Smaller Linnaean herbarium collections are also held at the Swedish Museum of Natural History (Naturhistoriska riksmuseet) (4000 specimens), as well as in the herbarium in Helsinki, the Bergius Foundation in Stockholm, and at Uppsala University (Frey 2010, p. 78).

[125] The term "Poland" is used here in a broad sense and, regardless of the historical period referenced, encompasses both the present-day territory of the country and, in some instances, the Eastern Borderlands.

[126] The full title of O'Connor's work is: *The History of POLAND, IN Several LETTERS to Persons of Quality. Giving an Account of the Antient and Present State of that Kingdom, Historical, Geographical, Physical, Political, and Ecclesiastical; V i Z. Its Origin and Extent, with a Description of its Towns and Provinces, the Succession and remarkable Actions of all Kings, and of the Great Dukes of Lithuania: Th e Election, Power, and Coronation of the King: Th e Senate, or House of Lords: Th e Diet and Form of Government: The Privileges of the Gentry; their Religion, Learning, Language, Customs, Habits, Manners, Riches, Trade, and Military Aff airs; together with the State of Physick and Natural Knowledg; as also an Account of the Teutonick Order, and of the Duke of Curland, his Family and Territories. With Sculptures, and a new Map after the best Geographers. With several Letters relating to Physick.*

Among the various natural specimens, "(...) All sorts of plants also were there, well preserv'd and pasted upon Paper (...)" (O'Connor 1698, p. 88). After Bernitz's death, his collection was purchased by the Grand Hetman of Lithuania, Prince Dominik Radziwiłł (1643–1697). Radziwiłł transferred the collection to Warsaw, which was most likely the first cabinet of curiosities in the city open to visitors (Pawęski 1970, p. 20). Before his death, the collection was moved to Nieśwież. Subsequently, the Nieśwież collection was either confiscated by the Russians in 1772 and 1813, or in the meantime, transported between Kraków, Warsaw, and Nieborów. In later years, the collection was transferred to Vilnius, where it became further dispersed or was destroyed in a fire during the Second World War.[127]

At the turn of the seventeenth and eighteenth centuries, extensive natural history collections including herbaria and plant specimens could be found in Gdańsk, which, owing to its location, was at the forefront of acquiring rare and exotic natural specimens. The collections of Gdańsk naturalists were renowned across Europe and were frequently visited.[128] Among the most highly valued were three collections in particular, all containing botanical specimens: those of the Gottwald brothers, Jakub and Philippe Breyne, and Theodor Klein. The first of these most likely did not include herbarium specimens mounted on paper.[129] The other two—the extensive natural history museum of the botanists Jacob Breyne (1637–1697) and his son Johann Philipp Breyne (1680–1764), who expanded the collection after his father's death—were of a distinctly scientific character. In addition to a large library, the collections included herbaria, which the Breynes compiled both independently and through numerous scientific contacts and exchanges. The herbaria contained specimens from India, the Americas, Africa, as well as France, Italy, the Netherlands, Siberia, and, in part, from the vicinity of Gdańsk (Schwarz 1986; Arabas 2009a; Pękacka-Falkowska 2022).[130] The collections, put up for sale in 1766, were purchased by Catherine the Great (Pawęski 1970).

The next remarkable and highly valued collection belonged to the naturalist and lawyer Jakob Theodor Klein (1685–1759), known as the "Pliny of Gdańsk." Klein

---

[127] See, among others, Jankowski (2014). Among the treasures of the Nieśwież collection was the aforementioned herbarium of Anna Vasa, prepared from a copy of Szymon Syreniusz's *Herbarium*. Considered lost, it was identified by Prof. Alicja Zemanek in a copy of Syreniusz's work held in the collections of the Poznań Society for the Advancement of Arts and Sciences (PTPN) (Zemanek 1996).

[128] For example, Klein's natural history cabinet was visited by rulers and dignitaries: Stanisław Leszczyński, Augustus II, Peter I, and Frederick William I (Schwarz 1986).

[129] The collections of Christoph (1636–1700) and Jan (1670–1713) Gottwald undoubtedly included medicinal plants, stored in bulk. These collections functioned as cabinets of curiosities, showcasing specimens of various natural objects and artistic works. In 1716, following the collectors' deaths, the collections were put up for sale and purchased by Tsar Peter the Great (Pękacka-Falkowska 2018b).

[130] Pękacka-Falkowska describes two herbaria compiled by Jacob Breyne in 1659 and 1673, which are held in the herbarium collections in Leiden and were gifted to Hieronymus van Beverningk (1614–1690) by Breyne. These herbaria contain specimens of the flora of Kashubia and the Gdańsk region (Pękacka-Falkowska 2018a).

donated his herbarium to the *Naturforschenden Gesellschaft* (Natural Science Society of Gdańsk), which he founded in 1743 together with his son-in-law, Daniel Gralath (1708–1767), the mayor of Gdańsk (Conwentz 1911).[131] The remainder of his collections was purchased, among others, by Augustus II the Strong and transported to Dresden (Conwentz 1911). The activities of the *Naturforschenden Gesellschaft* fostered the development of botany and inspired naturalists in Gdańsk to create herbarium collections (Schwarz 1986).[132] These often became part of the society's holdings, among them the herbaria of Nathanael Mattheus von Wolf (1724–1784) (a herbarium in 40 volumes) and Ernst Ferdinand Klinsmann (1794–1865), curator of the society's botanical collections. Others were transferred to the Westpreußisches Provinzial Museum in Gdańsk (West Prussian Provincial Museum)[133]: the herbaria of Carl Julius von Klingräff (1808–1879) and his brother Hugo Ernst von Klingräff (1820–1902); or to the botanical garden in Königsberg, such as the collections of Otto Ohlert (1816–1875) (Conwentz 1911).

Georg Andreas Helwing (1666–1748), known as the Prussian Pliny, maintained close contacts with the Gdańsk scientific community at the turn of the seventeenth and eighteenth centuries. He owned a collection of naturalia, including herbaria he created himself, which were primarily studies of the local flora. He also produced herbaria that he presented to prominent individuals, such as Augustus II the Strong and renowned scientists like Jakob Klein (Schwarz 1986).[134] Some of these herbaria were prepared with the assistance of Matthias Ernst Boretius (1694–1738), which today complicates the unequivocal attribution of the collections (Spalik 2014a; Graniszewska 2018). It is most likely that they jointly compiled multi-volume sets of herbarium specimens, which were sent to the Stadtbibliothek in Königsberg and to St Petersburg. While the fate of the St Petersburg collection and the herbarium recovered by Conwentz remains unknown, the series of Königsberg herbaria was transferred after the Second World War to the Herbarium of the Faculty of Biology at the University of Warsaw. The herbarium that Helwing is known to have compiled independently is a two-volume work held in the collections of the National Library in Warsaw.[135]

---

[131] *Naturforschenden Gesellschaft* ceased operations in 1936. Daniel Gralath also possessed natural history collections, but there is no information as to whether these included herbaria.

[132] The association operated until 1936. The collections were destroyed and dispersed after the Second World War.

[133] The museum operated from 1880 to 1945. After the war, the collections were dispersed. Specimens from one crate that survived the evacuation of the collections are preserved in the herbarium of Nicolaus Copernicus University in Toruń (TRN). One bound herbarium is also held in the collections of the Rev. Krzysztof Kluk Museum of Agriculture in Ciechanowiec.

[134] Klein sold his copy of Helwing's herbarium, which was kept in Erlangen and was later retrieved by Hugo Conwentz through an inter-institutional exchange for the Westpreußisches Provinzial Museum.

[135] Helwing A.J., *Herbarium Vivum …*, Warsaw, National Library, ref. Rps akc. 200/1–2, ca. 1695–1705. It is speculated that they may have been kept in the castle library in Königsberg, but the sources are inconclusive.

During the Enlightenment, numerous private collections belonging to the nobility were established, and among the enthusiasts of natural history were, among others, King Stanisław August Poniatowski, Prince Józef Poniatowski, Aleksander Lubomirski, the Radziwiłł family, Prince Michał Ogiński, Adam Kazimierz Czartoryski, and Antoni Tyzenhauz (Maroszek 2011, Pawęski 1970). However, it is difficult to determine whether these collections included herbaria. It is known that the natural history cabinet of Stanisław August Poniatowski at the castle, which functioned as a *Wunderkammer*, contained plant specimens and botanical preparations, but there is no explicit mention of herbaria (Zawartko-Laskowska 2008).

Between the mid-seventeenth and mid-eighteenth centuries, natural history collecting also flourished in the Silesian region (Mencfel 2010, p. 17). The owners of these collections, which included botanical specimens, were[136]: Leonard David Hermann (1670–1736), Carl Heinrich Börner (1745–1807), Johann Christian Glaser (c. 1700–1753), Conrad Ernst Maximilian Graf von Hochberg (1682–1752), Johann Christian Kundmann (1684–1751), Johann von Mattuschka; Christian Stieff; Christian Ulrich von Württemberg-Oels (1652–1704) (Mencfel 2010, pp. 259–289)[137] and Count Johann Anton Schaffgotsch (1675–1742). Unfortunately, there is currently a lack of precise information regarding the specific items that comprised these botanical collections. The exception is the Schaffgotsch collection, which is known to have included herbaria.[138] As with the previously mentioned collections,

[136] This does not necessarily mean, however, that they contained herbaria (see Sect. 1.3). Similarly, the fact that contemporary sources do not mention herbaria does not imply that they were not part of a given collection. This has been demonstrated by the author's own research—the identification of Zeidler's herbaria as part of the Schaffgotsch natural history collection and the chracterisation of his activities as those of a botanist and collector. Eighteenth-century interests often revolved around mineralogy and fossils, and in descriptions of collections, greater attention was frequently paid to zoological specimens, with botany listed at the end of inventories or omitted altogether. This is also the case with the collections of Jan Anton Schaffgotsch and his heirs, whose collection, although published in various printed inventories before its dispersal, has never been comprehensively studied. At present, the catalogues of this collection are also scattered across different parts of Poland.

[137] Mencfel also lists a number of other owners of seventeenth-century natural history collections, in which it is possible that herbaria were also included. These owners include: Johann Friedrich Zeidler, Gottfried Alde, Georg Moritz von Hoffmannswalda, Sebastian Alischer, Daniel Gottlieb von Buchs, Hans Heinrich von Hochberg auf Rohnstock, Friedrich Kaltschmied, Christian Ernst Kopisch, Otto von Nostitz, Georg Christoph Graf von Proskau, Friedrich Maximilian von Rethel und Hennersdorf, Philip Jacob Sachs von Loewenheim, Caspar Schwenckfeld, Albrecht von Sebisch, Gottfried Seydel, Johann Christoph Stettinsky, Georg Anton Volkmann, Carl Friedrich von Wehner.

[138] This information was reconstructed as a result of queries related to the present work. In the handwritten catalogues of the collections of the Library in Sobieszów and the Majorate Library in Cieplice (Majoratsbibliothek zu Warmbrunn), held in the collections of the National Library in Warsaw and the University Library in Wrocław, a register was found listing several herbaria (three boxes with sheets and a three-volume herbarium from the years 1732–1751 by Johann Friedrich Zeidler, of which volumes I and III have survived, from the already cited collections of the Main Library of the University of Life Sciences in Lublin, shelf marks: Vol. I: ref. Zb. Specj. I Starodruki 14, D. 104.57.646; Vol. III: ref. Zb. Specj. Starodruki XVIII.14; D. 104.57.646). In 2019, several

most of these collections have been dispersed or their current whereabouts are unknown. The fate of the Schaffgotsch collection appears particularly interesting and especially regrettable in this context. A significant portion of this collection survived the Second World War and was most likely deliberately dispersed by museum curators in the 1950s (Firszt 2009, 2016 and numerous other works by this author).[139]

The largest historical natural history collections in the Polish lands were located in Siemiatycze and were the work of Princess Anna Jabłonowska (1728–1800).[140] The Princess assembled her collection in the second half of the eighteenth century. In addition to numerous visitors representing all social classes,[141] the resources of the Princess were also used by Fr. Krzysztof Kluk from Ciechanowiec, who was a frequent guest in nearby Siemiatycze. Kluk, essentially a self-taught botanist, was highly active scientifically, conducting morphological observations of plants and publishing numerous works on natural history. He also created a herbarium in the form of loose sheets, most of which he donated to the Princess's "natural cabinet", which then became part of the Siemiatycze natural history collections (Lewandowska and Wójcik 2012). Jabłonowska's cabinet consisted of five rooms, the last of which contained "native and foreign plants, originating from five parts of the world, preserved in various ways" (Maroszek 2011).[142] In 1788, Princess Jabłonowska wished to donate her collections to the nation and house them in the Jabłonowski Palace in Warsaw, so that they would form the foundation of a National Museum of Natural History. However, the government decided that, given the country's difficult situation, such initiatives were of lesser importance.[143] Consequently, after the Princess's death in 1800, the Siemiatycze collections shared the fate of many earlier ones: they were sold to Tsar Alexander I and transported to Moscow. Most of them were probably destroyed by fire during the Napoleonic Wars in 1812, although individual objects from the Princess's collection have occasionally been identified in Russian institutions.[144]

The initiative of Princess Anna Jabłonowska was, in a sense, a response to the patriotic appeal of Michał Jerzy Mniszech to establish the *Musæum Polonicum* in

herbaria belonging to the Schaffgotsch family were also identified in the collections of the Herbarium of the Faculty of Biology, University of Warsaw (WA). The multi-volume catalogues of the Schaffgotsch collections also contain an extensive register of other naturalia.

139 Currently, the former monastery buildings, which once housed the Schaffgotsch Majorate Library, are home to the Museum of Natural History in Cieplice.

140 The Siemiatycze collections have been discussed multiple times by Professor Iwona Arabas (2009a, b, 2012a, b, 2013), as well as by Wójcik (2001), Maroszek (2011), and Pawęski (1970).

141 The variety of visitors to Princess Jabłonowska's cabinet is described in detail by Maroszek (2011). The princess kept a register of visitors, recording both the king and the baker.

142 The quotation is taken from Paulina Wilkońska's 1859 description (*Księżna Jabłonowska wojewodzina bracławska*, Czas 1859, no. 232, p. 1), cited here after Maroszek.

143 The response stated that the country "(...) does not need peculiarities now, only money and weapons (...)", quoted in Arabas (2012a).

144 Pawęski reports that Rostafiński came across herbarium sheets of Father Krzysztof Kluk in St Petersburg (Pawęski 1970, p. 27).

1775.[145] Her collections included many exotic specimens, but the intended purpose of the collection was national in character. The idea of creating such a museum was also advocated by Stefan de Rieul in 1766 in his *Projet pour rassembler sans aucune depense toutes les richesses naturelles de la Pologne*, proposing the gathering of Poland's natural resources without expense, with the assistance of its citizens (Pawęski 1970; Arabas 2009a).

Another great collector, Izabella Czartoryska née Flemming (1746–1835), assembled and displayed various objects in the Gothic House in Puławy, a branch of the first national museum in Poland, which can be classified as naturalia, but selected in the spirit of a Romantic wunderkammer (or even a reliquary), including a herbarium from 1746, which is still preserved in the collections of the National Museum in Kraków.[146] In the second half of the eighteenth century, magnates such as the Dzieduszycki and Branicki families created private collections or acted as patrons of already existing museum institutions.

Thanks to the activities of Father Stanisław Konarski, Sch.P., founder of the Collegium Nobilium (in 1740), and the work of the Commission of National Education, natural history collections began to be established in schools as well (Pawęski 1970, p. 32). In the nineteenth century, as elsewhere in the world, herbarium collections came to be represented primarily by institutional collections. The period of the partitions did not completely destroy the natural history activities of Polish institutions, as cabinets established at higher education institutions in Vilnius, Kraków, and Warsaw continued to operate. At the University of Warsaw, opened in 1816, the herbarium collections formed part of the mineralogical cabinet, having been transferred from the private collection of Professor Jakub Fryderyk Hoffmann (1758–1830). The chair of botany was entrusted to Michał Szubert (1787–1860), who had become acquainted with herbarium specimens while studying in Paris,

[145] Mniszech, in his proposal for the establishment of the *Musæum Polonicum* (*Myśli względem założenia* Musæum Polonicum, 1775), advocated presenting national natural resources, and provided detailed guidelines for the elements of the exhibition. Among the exhibits, he also listed herbaria: Regnum Vegetale *may be collected in three ways: herbs, plants, and trees may be classified as wild or cultivated, as useful or merely interesting, and in a designated area may be planted, maintained, and propagated; or alternatively, only the fruits of trees,* in spiritu vini, *or dried herbs* in herbario vivo *may be assembled and preserved. The third method involves collections that are engraved, coloured, and systematically arranged. I continue to emphasise that since these efforts and expenditures are undertaken for the common benefit of the country, it is of great importance that the methods of sowing or planting, the necessary precautions for further supervision, and the benefits of herbs and plants are adequately described and made available to the public* (Mniszech 1775).

[146] The method of selecting exhibits and the rather emotional, rather than scientific, attitude towards them is illustrated, for example, by the way in which the owner named the elements of her collection in the 1828 catalogue, e.g.: *Grasses from the northern English province, from the site of an ancient Roman camp under the command of Agricola* (item 294) or *A dried plant from Selwood Hill in Somerset, where King Alfred planted his standard after achieving a great victory over the Danes. Sent by Mr Strongways from England* (item 559) (Czartoryska 1828, pp. 30, 52). N.n., *Herbarium Vivum...*, (*Izabela Czartoryska's Herbarium*), Kraków, National Museum in Kraków, Czartoryski Library, ref. Rkps 2782, 1746.

then a leading centre of the natural sciences.[147] Szubert's collection became the nucleus of today's Herbarium of the Faculty of Biology at the University of Warsaw. His assistants, Wojciech Jastrzębowski (1799–1882), later a lecturer at the Agronomic Institute, and Jakub Waga (1800–1872) (Majewski 2016, p. 61), also amassed herbarium collections. An important artefact originating from the University of Vilnius, now preserved in Kraków, is the more than 40-volume herbarium of Józef Jundziłł (1794–1877), compiled from the 1820s onwards. The herbarium contains specimens from many botanists, including former lecturers at the university such as Jean Emmanuel Gilibert and Johann Georg Forster (Köhler 1994, 1995).[148] At this point, it is worth mentioning several other valuable collections held in Kraków: the herbarium of Józef Rostafiński (1850–1919), which includes the collections of Willibald Besser, Antoni Andrzejowski (1785–1868), and Wojciech Jastrzębowski (Köhler 1999), as well as two herbaria begun at the University of Lviv. The first of these is the herbarium of Marian Raciborski (1863–1917), professor at the University of Lviv, founder of the Botanical Institute of the Jagiellonian University, and its first director (1913–1917) (Köhler 1989).[149] The second is the herbarium of Józef Mądalski (1902–1995), which was started in the 1920s. In addition to Mądalski's own collections, this collection contains specimens from many other botanists, including older specimens dating back to the 1870s (Chlebicki 1991).[150] The collections of Szubert, Jastrzębowski, Rostafiński, Raciborski, and Mądalski were initially private scientific collections of these botanists, later transferred to institutions at the end of the owner's life or by bequest.[151] The record-holder for herbarium collections was Ferdynand Karo (1845–1927), a Warsaw pharmacist and tireless researcher of the Siberian flora. His herbarium collections, estimated at over 80,000 sheets (sometimes with two or three specimens per sheet),

---

[147] The Szubert Herbarium is housed in the collections of the Herbarium of the Faculty of Biology at the University of Warsaw. Szubert studied under Desfontaines and Jussieu (Majewski 2016, p. 53). The Muséum national d'Histoire Naturelle was regarded as a model institution in the nineteenth century (Cornish and Nesbitt 2014).

[148] Jundziłł J., (*Herbarium of Józef Jundziłł*), Kraków, Herbarium of the Institute of Botany, Polish Academy of Sciences in Kraków (KRAM), without catalogue number, 1820s, with specimens dated from the eighteenth century to 1876.

[149] Raciborski M., (*Herbarium of Marian Raciborski*), Kraków, Herbarium of the Institute of Botany, Jagiellonian University (KRA), without reference number, 1896–1900. The herbarium is housed in the collections of the Institute of Botany, Jagiellonian University (KRA). Additionally, Raciborski's collections are also present in the Mądalski collection and in the Herbarium of the Faculty of Biology, University of Warsaw (WA).

[150] The herbarium is housed in the collections of the W. Szafer Institute of Botany, Polish Academy of Sciences (KRAM). The collection is separated from the main herbarium collection (Mądalski J., untitled, Kraków, Herbarium of the Institute of Botany PAS in Kraków (KRAM), separate reference numbers for individual sheets, twentieth century, with specimens from the nineteenth century).

[151] Of course, only selected scientific collections housed in institutional herbaria are listed here. Efforts have been made to mention only the most emblematic collections. Much more information on Polish herbarium collections and the biographies of Polish botanists can be found in numerous publications by Professor Piotr Köhler (Institute of Botany, Jagiellonian University).

are now found in herbaria around the world, incorporated into the Herbarium Generale (Arabas 2015).[152]

In the Russian partition, many natural history collections were transported to Russia. Scientific societies in all three partitions initiated the establishment of museums with natural history departments (e.g. the Physiographic Museum in Kraków, the Mielżyński Museum in Poznań).[153] It was during this period that the oldest institutional herbaria in Poland were founded: the herbarium of the Institute of Botany at the Jagiellonian University (1780) and the herbarium of the Faculty of Biology at the State University in Lviv (1783, today the oldest herbarium in Ukraine). Subsequent institutional herbaria included the herbarium of the Natural History Museum at the University of Wrocław (1821) and the herbarium of the Institute of Botany of the Polish Academy of Sciences in Kraków (1867) (Drobnik 2009, pp. 10–12). In 1880, Włodzimierz Dzieduszycki opened a natural history museum in Lviv (the Dzieduszycki Museum), whose core comprised zoological collections, but which also housed the herbaria of professors from the University of Lviv, among them the herbarium of Jacek Łobarzewski (1814–1871), consisting of 70 fascicles containing 10,000 sheets representing more than 2000 species (Tabor 2013).

In the second half of the nineteenth and the first half of the twentieth century, many herbarium collections were compiled by amateur botanists, often regional patriots and ethnographers who documented the flora of their local areas. They came from various professional backgrounds (pharmacists, priests, teachers) (Drobnik 2009, p. 9), and their herbaria now constitute an invaluable ethnobotanical resource. Herbaria belonging to this group include the collections of Michał Fedorowski (1853–1923) from the 1880s (Graniszewska et al. 2016),[154] the herbarium of Seweryn Udziela (1857–1937),[155] and the herbaria of Eliza Orzeszkowa (1841–1910).[156]

At the beginning of the twentieth century, numerous regional museums were established,[157] each with dedicated natural history departments, and these continued

---

[152] The largest collection of plants gathered by Karo is held by the Herbarium of the Faculty of Biology at the University of Warsaw (WA).

[153] Pawęski provides an account of the history of natural history museology in each of the three partitions (Pawęski 1970, pp. 38–54), followed by the interwar period and after the Second World War (pp. 55–110).

[154] Fedorowski's herbarium specimens are held in the collections of the Herbarium of the Faculty of Biology, University of Warsaw, ref. WA-KH-1.1–5.10; and in the Library of the University of Warsaw, ref. Rkp. 445.

[155] Udziela S., (*Herbarium of Seweryn Udziela*), Kraków, Institute of Botany of the Polish Academy of Sciences in Kraków (KRAM), separate barcodes for individual sheets, 1890s; see also Köhler (1996).

[156] In particular, the herbarium of Eliza Orzeszkowa (Orzeszkowa E., (*Herbarium of Eliza Orzeszkowa*), Poznań, Poznań Society for the Advancement of Arts and Sciences Library, ref. Rkp. 880, 1887–1898); see also the monograph Kielak (2004).

[157] The pioneer in this field is the oldest regional museum, the Tytus Chałubiński Tatra Museum in Zakopane, established in 1888, which preserves, among other things, Chałubiński's herbarium collections (Ochyra and Cisło 1999).

to operate during the interwar period. During this time, several publications once again called for the creation of a national natural history museum.[158] As Pawęski emphasises, the greatest challenge concerned botanical collections, as evidenced by Hanna Czeczottowa's 1937 article, *On the Need to Establish a Central Botanical Museum in Warsaw* (Czeczottowa 1937). The author proposes gathering the dispersed herbaria from across the country into a single collection belonging to the proposed Central Botanical Museum. During the Second World War, almost all museums, including those devoted to natural history, suffered severe losses.[159] Many museums and private collections were further damaged after the war due to poor management and a tendency towards centralisation, which often treated smaller institutions harshly and led to the dispersal of historical collections.[160]

Currently, herbaria can be found in collections of entirely different types. Both historical and modern herbaria may be located in institutional herbaria, which aim to incorporate collections into their *Herbarium Generale* (maintaining an arrangement by species names if the collection is in the form of individual sheets and there is no explicit requirement for the collection to be kept separately); as well as in museums, not always of a natural history profile (including the National Museum in Kraków, the National Museum in Warsaw, the Tatra Museum in Zakopane); and in libraries (such as the National Library in Warsaw, the Main Library of the University of Life Sciences in Lublin). At present, there is still no national natural history museum in Poland. Natural history exhibitions, including botanical ones, are mainly part of regional natural history departments, which may be integrated into the educational centres of national parks and the State Forests. Additionally, fragments of aristocratic collections can be found in palaces, castles, and regional museums.

[158] These include the 1911 collective work *Guidelines for Establishing Natural History and Regional Museums* (*Wskazówki dla zakładających muzea przyrodniczo-krajoznawcze*), edited by M. Raciborski, as well as the 1912 brochure by S. Stobiecki published in Kraków, *On the Matter of the National Natural History Museum* (*W sprawie Krajowego Muzeum Przyrodniczego*), and Kulwieć's 1912 article *On the Matter of the National Natural History Museum* (*W sprawie krajowego muzeum przyrodniczego*) in the journal "Ziemia" (cited in Pawęski 1970, p. 54).

[159] Aside from the natural history departments of the museums in Zakopane and Płock. Moreover, many museums have ceased to exist altogether (Pawęski 1970).

[160] An example already mentioned of a collection that fell victim to such practices is the Schaffgotsch collection. However, it should not be forgotten that the reverse mechanism also occurred: under rather unclear circumstances, various institutions acquired collections that, before the war, had been part of aristocratic or institutional holdings. In this way, the Schaffgotsch collection, the Stadtbibliothek in Königsberg, and the Westpreußisches Provinzial Museum found their way into the National Library, the Herbarium of the University of Warsaw (WA), the Library of the University of Life Sciences in Lublin, the Herbarium of the Nicolaus Copernicus University in Toruń (TRN), and probably many other locations.

1.3.6 Herbaria as Scientific Tools

The remarkable popularity of the natural sciences during the Renaissance provided fertile ground for the development of botany as a distinct discipline and enabled the recognition, and at times the employment, of experts in this emerging field, who became academic teachers (Egmond 2010, p. 44).[161] During this period, a scientific community of botanical researchers began to form, initially closely linked to the medical and allied sciences. This community, established with a clear awareness of the need for collective endeavour, was centred mainly around universities and botanical gardens, although natural history research was also conducted at courts and through private scientific and educational activities. Herbaria thus became one of the fundamental tools and scientific exercises, alongside botanical excursions for specimen collection, field research and the preparation of descriptions, as well as the establishment of gardens, which enabled rapid access to the observation of living species without the need for travel.

Herbaria have served as tools for structuring researchers' experience since the early development of botany as an independent science (Ogilvie 2006 pp. 70, 141).[162] They were also widely used as teaching aids, notably by Rondelet, Bauhin, Cluyt, and Linnaeus. Naturalists were often employed by wealthy collectors of plants and other naturalia as curators of their collections and gardens, one of the most renowned examples being the collaboration between Carl Linnaeus and the banker and director of the Dutch East India Company, George Clifford III. This partnership resulted in the publication of *Hortus Cliffortianus* (1738), one of the primary sources for Linnaeus's later work *Species Plantarum* (1753), with the frequency of description and citation of particular species closely linked to their presence in Clifford's herbarium (Thijsse 2018).[163] Many collectors, even if they did not themselves possess extensive botanical knowledge, were aware of the scientific value of their collections (Maroszek 2011). In the second half of the seventeenth century, the first microscopic observations were also conducted, revealing the

[161] An example is Clusius (1526–1609), who during his career was both a teacher for children from merchant families, an advisor to aristocrats, the director of the Vienna Botanical Garden, employed by Emperor Maximilian II of Habsburg, and later, the director of the university botanical garden in Leiden.

[162] The origins of herbarium collection and the fieldwork methods of early botanists are the subject of a separate study by Florike Egmond (2018).

[163] Today, Clifford's herbarium is held partly in the collections of the Natural History Museum (BM) in London, and partly in the Naturalis Biodiversity Center (L).

complex internal structure of plants, which transformed perspectives on them and initiated research into the structure and function of plant tissues.[164]

The first leading herbarium-based scientific centre in the world was Italy, which can be attributed to the opportunity to compare the contemporary local flora with the works of ancient authors. Only later did other centres gain prominence, as the demand grew for the description of new plants beyond the ancient catalogues and local floras—a process that, in the case of European local floras, took place in the seventeenth and eighteenth centuries. Countries that established colonies simultaneously became pioneers in the creation of collections of exotic plants. Likewise, cities with access to the sea, and thus to new specimens brought back from expeditions, could take the lead in scientific activity related to natural history.

Before the era of instantaneous mass reproduction brought about by photography, the label of "winter garden" was both an advantage and a limitation for botanical researchers, although it certainly enabled work outside the growing season. Some leading botanists, such as Clusius and Matthioli, although they made intensive use of herbarium methods, were highly critical of them and did not believe they could compare to the analysis of living plants (Ogilvie 2006, p. 43).[165] For Gessner as well, the herbarium, though a fundamental tool, was considered imperfect (Kusukawa 2012, p. 279). Platter also regarded it as a flawed instrument, and therefore employed a practice that would be unacceptable from today's scientific perspective—manipulating specimens in selected cases to make them more closely "resemble" the living plant.[166] Ratzenberger likewise combined several specimens into a single "complete" specimen (Thijsse 2016). Missing parts of a specimen were

[164] In the field of microscopy, a significant milestone was the improvement of the world's first microscope, created around 1590 (known as the "flea glass", Latin *vitrum pulicare*) by Johannes and Zacharias Janssen, by Robert Hooke (1635–1703), who also described the use of the device for botanical specimen observation in his work *Micrographia: or Some Physiological Descriptions of Minute Bodies Made by Magnifying Glasses. With Observations and Inquiries Thereupon* (1665). In *Micrographia*, Hooke, among other achievements, was the first to define the concept of the cell. Scientists who further advanced microscopic botanical observations included Marcello Malpighi (1628–1694), who published his research findings in 1671 and later in *Anatome plantarum. Cui subjungitur appendix iteratas & auctas ejusdem authoris de ovo incubato observationes continens* (1675); Nehemiah Grew (1628–1711), who, like Malpighi, made his research public in 1671 and published it in *The Anatomy of plants: with an idea of a philosophical history of plants, and several other lectures read before the Royal Society* (1681); and Anton van Leeuwenhoek (1632–1723) (Mägdefrau 2004, pp. 95–102). The development of scientific instruments enabled the study of cryptogams (Thiers 2020).

[165] Clusius, employed at the botanical garden in Leiden, wished to conduct botany classes there only during the summer, as he saw no possibility for meaningful study of plant species in winter (Swan 2010). He preferred living specimens and encouraged others to send him freshly collected plants rather than herbarium specimens. While travelling in Spain, he tried every method to preserve and record newly acquired knowledge, including drying plants. In 1584 and 1605, he complained that it was impossible to work solely with dried specimens if one had not previously seen the living plant (Ogilvie 2006, pp. 170–171).

[166] For example, he used petals of *Delphinium*, which are notable for retaining their intense blue colour, to "compose" a specimen of *Campanula*, whose flowers turn brown upon drying (Rytz 1933, p. 7–8; Ogilvie 2006, p. 212). See also Benkert (2016).

sometimes painted in, and colours were "preserved" by applying a layer of paint to the surface of the specimens.[167] Herbaria undoubtedly enabled repeated study of plants regardless of the season, but they had obvious limitations. Herbarium specimens were, in a sense, removed from their context, from their natural habitat.[168] On the other hand, reliance on observations of plants artificially introduced into botanical gardens was not free of error.[169] Changes in living conditions could alter the appearance of plants and disrupt their natural vegetative cycle, leading to mistakes in their description and study.[170] The instructions for preparing herbaria by Spiegel in 1606 in *Isagoges…*, and later by Tournefort in 1694 in *Élemens de botanique…*, demonstrate that in the seventeenth century, the technique of preparing herbaria was already well established and supported by experience, on the basis of which an appropriate methodology had been developed.[171]

As previously mentioned, herbarium sheets also served to integrate the scientific community, acting as objects of exchange and loan between botanists. This network of contacts enabled the scientific development of individual researchers, who, even if unable to undertake or repeat costly expeditions, could supplement their collections with additional specimens.[172] At the same time, the great geographical discoveries and the colonisation of many regions of the world by Europeans provided new research material, stimulated interest in exotic flora, and allowed for the expansion of scientific tools as well as methodologies for preparing and transporting specimens in the form of dried plants, already at the turn of the sixteenth and seventeenth

[167] The method was applied, for example, in the herbaria of Johann Friedrich Zeidler from 1732 and 1751, as well as in the herbaria of Agostino Coltellini, from the collections of the Museo di Storia Naturale dell'Università di Firenze (see the Sect. 2.1.3; and the chapter dedicated to the conservation of Zeidler's herbarium in Part V; Coltellini's herbaria can be found in Nepi (2008)). The instrumental approach to specimens and their "consumption" was also, as mentioned earlier, a characteristic phenomenon among the first generations of modern naturalists: Clusius and Mattioli regularly soaked previously dried specimens in order to examine them again in their "natural" colour and size, so if they received specimens from others for their collections, they would often "use them up".

[168] According to Ogilvie, this was the reason for the change in the way species were described, as the use of herbaria led to the loss of locational context, which was still emphasised in the descriptions by Clusius (Ogilvie 2006, pp. 213–214).

[169] Such attempts were undertaken in many gardens as early as the Renaissance, primarily in Padua and Leiden, as well as in Poland. This contributed to the introduction of numerous species from newly discovered regions of the world (Zemanek 1997; Ogilvie 2006, p. 163, Pękacka-Falkowska 2022).

[170] Ogilvie refers here to Clusius's experiment with alpine plants introduced into the garden in Leiden, where the botanist observed a shift in flowering time (Ogilvie 2006, p. 163).

[171] See the Sect. 1.3.2. As Egmond writes, the first botany textbook, *Isagoges*, demonstrates the standardisation of methods across the entire field of botany (Egmond 2018).

[172] Since the eighteenth century, herbaria also become objects of trade, enabling botanists to cover the costs of their travels. Subscribers would order specific species or sets of plants, and collections of specimens were prepared on commission for individual collectors (Harris 2018).

centuries.[173] This was significant for ongoing research and the accurate identification of species. Expedition floristic documentation enabled many botanists to study newly discovered vegetation, for example, the *Flora Brasiliensis* initiated by Carl von Martius in 1840; the flora of the southern polar region, India, and the Himalayas, documented in the mid-nineteenth century by Joseph Dalton Hooker; or the flora of Japan collected in the 1820s by Philipp Franz Siebold (1796–1866) (Mägdefrau 2004, pp. 126–135; Thiers 2020).[174] Specimens also served to verify earlier descriptions and illustrations of exotic flora, which were often produced indirectly and thus prone to inaccuracies, which were in turn published and disseminated (Ogilvie 2006, pp. 252–254). The lending, sending, and exchange of specimens, as a form of contact with other research centres, continues to this day and constitutes one of the fundamental activities associated with the management of herbarium collections. In addition, the preparation of supplementary material for specimens, such as photographs, microscope slides, fragments of living tissue, and, until recently, also wet collections in alcohol- and formalin-based preservatives, remains current practice (Drobnik 2009, pp. 13–14, 28–33).

With the development of botany, the demand for scientific publications concerning the plant world increased. The increasingly specialised nature of botanical studies and the decline in the illustration in plant catalogues at the turn of the sixteenth and seventeenth centuries created the need for dedicated scientific tools to aid in memorising and distinguishing the growing volume of data. Plants began to be described and compared with one another not in terms of their medicinal properties, but on the basis of morphological differences.[175] The last generation of Renaissance naturalists faced the necessity of constructing systems of classification and taxonomy, as simple descriptions of plants were no longer sufficient. Among the pre-Linnaean systematists, Andrea Cesalpino, Caspar Bauhin, Joseph Pitton de Tournefort, Johann Jacob Dillenius (1648–1747), and Pier Antonio Micheli

[173] This was related to numerous failures during the initial attempts to create and transport herbaria from distant lands. Clusius, despite criticism of working with herbarium specimens, ordered exotic samples from expeditions organised by the Dutch East India Company, for example from Willem Marquisius and Coolmans in 1599. Coolmans did not return alive from the journey, and his collections, although promised to Clusius, ended up with Pieter Paaw, a professor of medicine in Leiden. Paaw lent the collections to Clusius. Coolmans did not mount his specimens, which resulted in disorder within the assembled plant collection. Consequently, for the next expedition in 1602, Clusius and Paaw drew up guidelines that required not only the collection of plants, but also the preparation of detailed drawings and field notes, including a verbal description of the plant's appearance, the site where it was collected, and any information relevant to the species in question (Ogilvie 2006, pp. 169–171, 254–256; Thijsse 2016).

[174] Siebold, von F., Ito, K., Leiden, Naturalis Biodiversity Center (L), ref. L. 2077627–207730, 2078204–207812, 211011, 1823–1830.

[175] Nevertheless, botanical knowledge remained primarily the domain of practitioners of medicine and related fields, and the predominance of representatives from these disciplines in botany was still evident in the eighteenth century. Linnaeus himself also worked as a royal court physician at some point of his career.

(1679–1737) used herbaria as fundamental research tools.[176] By the mid-eighteenth century, the use of herbaria had become so widespread that Linnaeus wrote that "every botanist should possess a herbarium".[177] His publications and teaching activities marked a turning point for both botany and herbaria, as a unified and convenient system of classification was universally adopted throughout the scientific botanical community. Herbaria ultimately owe their "ennoblement" to Linnaeus, who made them an indispensable tool in the botanist's repertoire. Linnaeus's profound influence on the perception of nature inspired many naturalists, including amateurs, to work with herbaria. As mentioned earlier, the fact that the Linnaean system originated in botany meant that it became, in a sense, a propaedeutic for other natural sciences, and many researchers engaged in botany as a model of systematic science before moving on to other natural specialisations (Pomian 1996, p. 276). Herbaria, as tools used in the creation of classification systems, could thus serve as model aids for comparative research in other fields of natural history.[178] The creators of natural classification systems also made use of herbaria in their work, for example, Antoine Laurent de Jussieu (1748–1836), Augustin-Pyramus de Candolle (1778–1841), and Robert Brown (1773–1858).

As previously mentioned, herbaria have contributed to the advancement of floristic research by serving as documentation of the studied vegetation. These studies, in turn, led to pioneering work in the emerging and developing fields of the nineteenth century: plant geography, notably through the works of Alexander von Humboldt (1769–1859) and August Grisebach (1814–1879); ecology, through the research of Eugenius Warming (1841–1924) and Andreas Schimper (1856–1901); palaeobotany, thanks to the investigations of, among others, Kaspar Maria von Sternberg (1761–1838) and Franz Unger (1800–1870), which developed rapidly from the early nineteenth century; and phylogenetics in the second half of the nineteenth century, defined by Ernst Haeckel (1834–1919) on the basis of the work of Charles Darwin (1809–1882).

---

[176] It is also worth mentioning the meticulous observations of Conrad Gessner (1516–1565), whose scientific work was published only 200 years after his premature death.

[177] Already cited *Herbarium praestat omni iconae, necessarium omni Botanico* (Linnaeus 1751, p. 7), literally "a herbarium surpasses any illustration, it is indispensable to every botanist"; this phrase has been repeatedly quoted and paraphrased in subsequent works on herbaria, including by Saint-Lager (Saint-Lager 1885, p. 2). Although Linnaeus is credited with popularising the use of herbaria, not only his supporters but also his opponents based their observations on herbaria, among them Albrecht von Haller (1708–1777), whose herbarium is preserved at the Muséum national d'Histoire Naturelle in Paris (P) (Haller, von A., (*Herbier Haller*), Paris, Muséum national d'Histoire Naturelle (P), without ref. no., before 1768).

[178] A literal, technological adaptation of the technique for creating herbarium specimens to another field of natural history occurred in the case of preparing specimens of snake and fish skins, as well as insects, at the turn of the eighteenth and nineteenth centuries. Snake skins prepared by Patrick Russell (1726–1805) and William Burchell (1782–1863), insects prepared by Burchell, and fish skins prepared by Richard Parnell (1810–1882) were dried between sheets of paper (MacGregor 2018a; Davis 2018; Nowak-Kemp 2018). Furthermore, the classification system developed with significant support from herbarium material led to changes in the design of gardens, with plants arranged according to taxonomic order.

Herbaria have also documented research that would today be classified within the field of ethnobotany. Ethnobotany as a distinct scientific discipline was defined in 1895 by John William Harshberger (1869–1929) (Klepacki 2007; Kujawska 2008; Kowalska-Lewicka 1964),[179] although ethnobotanical activities and research had been conducted much earlier. As early as the Renaissance, naturalists collecting plants for herbaria relied on the knowledge of local inhabitants—often uneducated individuals who were not members of the *studiosi* community, but who possessed considerable experience in identifying and using plants (Ogilvie 2006, p. 71; Kusukawa 2012, pp. 154–159; MacGregor 2018a).[180] They were also interested in traditional knowledge (in addition to the classical knowledge contained in ancient texts) concerning the use of plants.[181] Over time, as a result of geographical discoveries, economic and industrial factors became significant motivations for studying the uses of plants unknown on the old continent. The greatest economic growth occurred in countries with colonies, which therefore had unlimited access to natural resources and cheap labour. Economic development prior to the era of synthetic materials fuelled interest in and research on the utilisation of plants (Cornish and Nesbitt 2014). In both main branches of ethnobotany—economic botany and the humanistic study of human–plant relationships—herbarium specimens are used as one of the fundamental forms of documentation (Nesbitt 2014).[182]

The popularity of herbaria as scientific tools and the ways they were managed often led to adverse effects on their preservation and brought to light the first ethical issues associated with their use. Saint-Lager, the author of the first monograph on the history of herbaria (1885), lamented the disgraceful practices among researchers who, driven by an uncontrollable desire to possess a particular specimen or

[179] Ethnobotany is often considered within the context of Western culture, although in other cultural areas, compendia of useful plants were also compiled during the European Renaissance (Cornish and Nesbitt 2014). Initially defined as the study of plants used by various communities, over time it came to encompass folk knowledge, religious and magical practices associated with plants, and today—all relationships between humans and the plant world, both in traditional and contemporary cultures (Klepacki 2007).

[180] Among the better-known Renaissance authors of herbals, Spiegel and Aldrovandi drew on the knowledge of local inhabitants.

[181] For example, Boccone (Pulvirenti et al. 2017a).

[182] The term "economic botany" appears as early as 1748 in the works of Linnaeus (Cornish and Nesbitt 2014).

collection, committed acts of vandalism and theft. He also noted, even at that time, that the use of historical herbaria requires appropriate caution (Saint-Lager 1885, p. 43).[183]

At the beginning of the twentieth century, there was a certain decline in the use of herbarium material (Cornish and Nesbitt 2014). With the advent of mass production based on synthetic materials and a relatively well-developed plant taxonomy, botanical collections, like all natural history collections, were no longer as popular as research objects and tools as they had been a century earlier. Research interests were pursued in scientific institutes rather than in institutions housing collections. However, in the second half of the twentieth century, a gradual shift occurred, and in addition to research related to trade and industry, there was a growing interest in the cultural aspects of natural history collections (Cornish and Nesbitt 2014). A breakthrough, marking a significant return to research involving biocultural collections, took place at the end of the twentieth century with the development of genetic studies.[184] Since the publication of the DNA double helix model by James Watson

[183] Saint-Lager emphasises that nothing is as detrimental to them as improper handling and frequent changes of location. He describes the case of Aldrovandi's herbarium, which suffered as a result of being moved from the University Library in Bologna in 1796 to the Museum of Natural History in Paris, then returned to Bologna in 1815, and subsequently relocated within Bologna in 1875. The changes in location and manner of use led to "(...) significant losses, to which must be added damage caused by insects and, most regrettably, thefts committed by individuals who examined the herbarium (...)". Lager quotes a letter from a certain Dr Giovannini, inspector of the Bologna Botanical Garden: "(...) It is with great regret that I note that entire sheets have been torn out by shameless collectors, in order to satisfy the whim of possessing a plant collected by the famous naturalist, who did not hesitate to mutilate one of the most revered relics of botanical science (...)". The author further writes that some researchers limited themselves to detaching a specimen and leaving their description, while others cut out a fragment of the specimen. To make matters worse, the staff member responsible for chemically treating the specimens with mercuric chloride seriously damaged the specimens in volumes I and II, using a brush "with such force as if he were grooming a horse". In the author's opinion, the manner in which this procedure was carried out caused more destruction to the valuable herbarium than the insects from which it was intended to protect it.

[184] Awareness of issues related to the preservation of genetic material is relatively recent, as the first successes in recovering historical DNA date back to the 1980s. Today, genetics is among the most dynamic scientific disciplines, yielding new discoveries almost daily. Genetics textbooks are among the fastest to become outdated. Deoxyribonucleic acid (DNA) was first identified in 1869 by Johann Friedrich Miescher, a Swiss scientist. In his quest to understand the chemical composition of the cell, he studied pus on surgical bandages and isolated a substance he called "nuclein," as it originated from the cell nucleus (Latin *nucleus*—core, kernel). He published his discovery along with descriptions of his research protocol in 1871 (Dahm 2005). His findings were preceded by observations from other scientists concerning cell division (Louis Pasteur and Rudolf Virchow in 1855) and inheritance (Charles R. Darwin and Alfred R. Wallace in 1858 and subsequent years, as well as Gregor Mendel in 1866, whose work was "rediscovered" by Carl Correns, Hugo de Vries, and Erich von Tschermak in 1900). In 1929, Phoebus Levene identified the basic structural units of DNA, including the bases: adenine, cytosine, guanine, and thymine. In 1944, Oswald T. Avery, Colin MacLeod, and Maclyn McCarty announced that DNA is the *transforming principle*, and not, as previously thought, protein. Between 1949 and 1950, Erwin ChargaffS observed the equivalence in the number of adenine and thymine bases, and guanine and cytosine bases, as well as the species-specific variation in their quantities. The culmination of these discoveries was the publication in 1953 by James Watson and Francis Crick of the model of DNA as a double helix.

and Francis Crick in 1953 (Watson and Crick 1953), there has been ongoing revision in light of subsequent discoveries and continued work to understand genetic mechanisms and to sequence entire genomes. By the mid-1990s, the information obtainable from genetic research began to surpass that gained from morphological studies and became the primary source for phylogenetic research, sometimes in combination with morphological analysis, and at times without it (Rapini 2014). This was made possible by advances in genetics, particularly in DNA sequencing. Genetic studies have helped resolve interspecies relationships, contributing to the development of systematics. Nucleotide sequences are published in electronic gene databases such as GenBank or Whole Genome Shotgun, which contain an ever-expanding library of DNA sequences.

Thanks to improvements of analytical methods, herbarium specimens, including historical ones, have been incorporated into research. Advances in DNA studies in the last decade of the twentieth century led to the growing popularity of genetics in taxonomic and phylogenetic analyses, as well as significant development in these fields, associated, among other things, with the re-evaluation of existing taxonomic relationships (Rapini 2014). Herbaria are still used in education, both in school botany curricula and as part of museum education and activities conducted by herbarium institutions (Cornish and Nesbitt 2014; Adams and Fritz 2014; Drobnik 2009, p. 18).[185]

Currently, research using herbarium specimens continues across all the aforementioned fields. Today, for a herbarium to be classified as a scientific collection, it must meet strictly defined criteria: specimens should be collected in an undamaged state, allow for species identification, be complete, labelled with the collector's name, and include a precise description of the collection site (including exact GPS data) (Drobnik 2009, pp. 15–17; Moat and Bachman 2023).

Although historical herbaria often lack the complete information required of modern collections, they can still serve as valuable sources of knowledge and research material. In historical herbarium specimens, labels are frequently limited to a modest inscription, which from today's perspective is incomplete or overly general. It is rare to find information regarding the collection date of a specific specimen, especially in the oldest herbaria. More commonly, dating may refer to the entire volume, providing only a general indication of when the specimens were collected. The specimens themselves may have been prepared earlier and only later incorporated into a specially prepared codex, sometimes many years afterwards.[186] Nevertheless, if descriptions are present in a historical collection, they can consti-

[185] See also the chapter *The herbarium in a wider context* in (in:) *The Herbarium Handbook*, eds: N. M. J. Davies, C. Drinkell, T. M. A. Utteridge, Kew Publishing, pp. 213–249.

[186] Examples include the herbaria of Helwing or Boretius from the herbarium of the Faculty of Biology at the University of Warsaw, which have survived in various forms: "working" codices used for storing loose specimens, "final" codices that were never filled with plants and thus remain empty, as well as codices that are partially empty or completely filled. The dating of a codex is usually made possible by analysing the internal structure of the paper sheets in transmitted light. However, this does not determine the date of collection.

tute a valuable source of information on the contemporary state of knowledge and scientific practice, historical nomenclature and classification of species, as well as the use and popularity of selected plant species (Köhler 1995, 1996; Piekiełko 1981). Notes accompanying certain specimens often contain ethnobotanical information. In addition to the plants themselves, other elements of herbaria are also valuable sources of knowledge and key to the identification and attribution of particularly significant objects (e.g. Pulvirenti et al. 2017b; Stefanaki et al. 2018). Among these, the most important are the manuscript layer, which serves as a valuable graphological document, and the paper's internal structure observed in transmitted light, which, especially in historical papers, can be decisive for dating the object and defining its provenance. Further information may be provided by analysis of the paper fibre composition and, in the case of bound volumes, by codicological analysis.

The defined scientific functions of herbaria include: preserving evidence of the current and historical flora present in a given area; providing information on the present and historical: biodiversity, distribution, and evolution of species; their migrations and interrelationships; preserving nomenclatural types, which serve as reference standards for defined taxa; providing material for comparative studies in taxonomy, morphology, anatomy, palaeobotany, archaeobotany, ethnobotany, phylogenetics, ecology, biogeography, phytochemistry, and pharmacognosy; enabling the assessment of species' threat levels and verification of both historical and recent localities of species occurrence; facilitating the evaluation of environmental pollution, including in the past; enabling research into the history of insect migration and the spread of phytopathogens; preserving an archival source on scientific methodology: specimen preparation, collection methods, curation, nomenclature, classification, and the use of plants in a given region, as well as the work of botanists and the creators of the collection; preserving biocultural information, that is, concerning the mutual relationships between human civilisation and the natural world, through cataloguing plants of religious, medicinal, or economic significance (Bridson and Forman 1999, pp. 277–278; Köhler 1995, 1996; Piekiełko 1981; Drobnik 2009, pp. 15–17, 110–128; James et al. 2018).[187] Herbarium data also enable the creation of population maps, especially with current geolocation capabilities, thereby enriching knowledge of species distribution and environmental threats. Information obtained from herbarium collections can also support seemingly unrelated fields, for example, providing a basis for the responsible development of plant-based pharmaceuticals (Bridson and Forman 1999, pp. 277–278).

[187] Examples of the use of herbarium specimens in recent years include the following articles: Ames and Spooner 2008; Lehtonen and Christenhusz 2010; Yoshida et al. 2014; Davis et al. 2015; Xu et al. 2015; Kuzmina et al. 2017; Willis et al. 2017; Craine et al. 2018; Espinosa and Pinedo Castro 2018; Kiss et al. 2018; Chomicki and Renner 2019; Ent et al. 2019; Gallagher et al. 2019; Lang et al. 2019; Meineke and Davies 2019; Pearson 2019; Kistler et al. 2020; Willems et al. 2022; Campos et al. 2023; Grasso et al. 2025 and many others.

1.3.7 *Special Examples of Herbaria: Artistic and Symbolic Herbaria*

In addition to scientific herbaria, there are also album-style collections in which dried plants or their fragments are used in symbolic and artistic compositions, often incorporating patriotic themes. In such herbaria, the structure and binding can be highly unconventional,[188] and the objects themselves are sometimes associated with remarkable circumstances.

In Poland, examples include the herbaria of Eliza Orzeszkowa (1841–1910), whose structure was modelled on nineteenth-century photographic albums. Each of her herbaria was created for a specific purpose, either charitable or as a gift for friends.[189] Another example of an artistic herbarium in Polish collections is the herbarium of Janina Jenko-Sokołowska (dates of birth and death unknown) from around 1900 (Figs. 2.46 and 2.47 in Chap. 2), which was exhibited as a work of applied art. This herbarium features elements of patriotic iconography, such as an anchor or shackles (Kiljańska 2005; Paś 2017).

More modest in form, yet exceptionally powerful in its message, is the French herbarium created by Louise Gailleton (1861–1934) between 1914 and 1918 in Guiche, a small town in Burgundy (Fig. 2.48 in Chap. 2). Gailleton began acquiring plants from battlefields and nearby abandoned gardens through convalescent soldiers who had participated in the Great War. From the specimens she collected in this way, she assembled the so-called trench herbarium (Fr. *l'herbier des tranchées*), in which groups of specimens on each sheet are labelled with the soldier's name and the names of the battlefield locations. In its symbolism, this object harks back to medieval herbaria compiled during pilgrimages, in wich each specimen served as a memento of a sacred place. It also strikingly contrasts the world of nature and the romantic custom of collecting botanical souvenirs while travelling with the brutality of war. From a research perspective, such an object can provide information about the specific locations represented by the herbarium specimens or about the individuals who collected them.

Additionally, various institutions hold individual historical objects featuring compositions of dried plants, which are sometimes used to decorate letters and diaries to which they are attached. Many books and albums contain fragments of dried plants. Some herbaria are of particularly significant because of the individuals who created them. An example of such a herbarium is that of Rosa Luxemburg (1871–1919), compiled between 1913 and 1918 (Zych et al. 2023). This herbarium

[188] The technological aspects of such objects are described in the Sect. 2.1.6.3 in Chap. 2.

[189] Such was the purpose of the herbarium prepared for a charity auction in Lviv in 1890, in aid of the starving inhabitants of Galicia. In 1894, Orzeszkowa was awarded a gold medal for this herbarium at the National Exhibition in Lviv. The item is currently held in the collections of the Ossoliński National Institute, ref. 13967/II Pal. 1890. Orzeszkowa's botanical interests and ethnobotanical activities bore a patriotic character and were intended to preserve traditional knowledge and local culture.

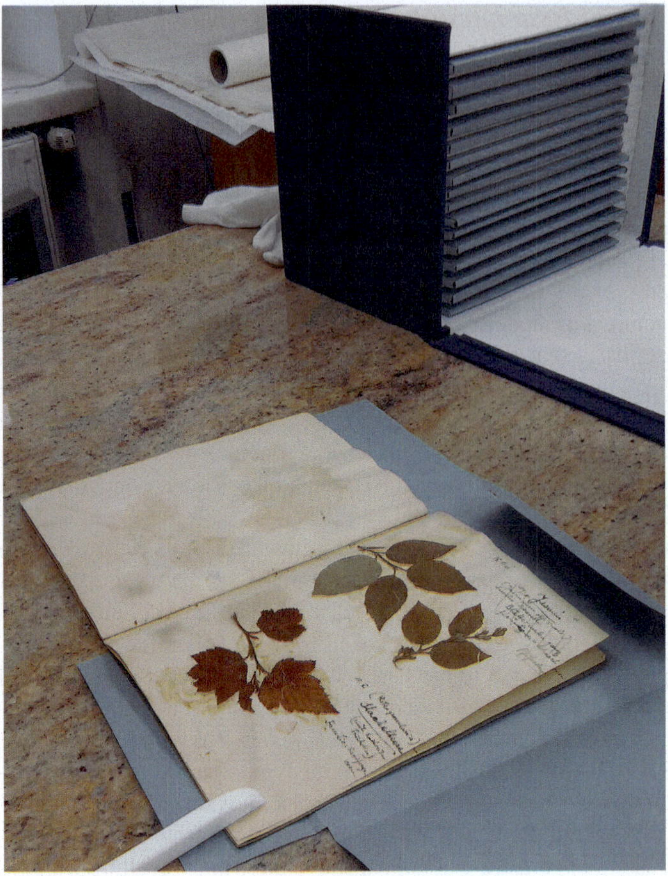

Fig. 1.17 One of Rosa Luxemburg's herbarium notebooks, (Luxemburg R., (*Rosa Luxemburg's Herbarium*), Warsaw, Central Archives of Modern Records, ref. 63/III/2, 1913–1918. In the background, a box containing the remaining herbarium notebooks is visible. (Photo: M. Grenda-Kurmanow)

is part of the collection of the Central Archives of Modern Records in Warsaw (Fig. 1.17). Herbaria also serve as inspiration for many artists, who, by referencing the technique of plant pressing, explore themes of memory, collecting, transience, and personal experience (Grenda-Kurmanow 2026). From a research perspective, such herbaria can also provide information about their creators.

1.3.8 *Ethical and Legal Issues Related to Herbarium Collections*

Currently, institutional scientific herbaria are regarded as part of the national heritage, as evidenced by the use of the terms "national" and "state" in the names of herbaria and natural history museums (e.g. National United States Herbarium at the Smithsonian Institution) (Drobnik 2009, p. 14).

The collection of plants and the management of collections by institutional staff should comply with national regulations and be accompanied by support for, or the signing of, international conventions aimed at ensuring fair and responsible use of natural resources, as well as the management of information arising from these practices. In addition, familiarity with lists of threatened plant species is essential.[190] Specimens obtained illegally should not be accepted into collections.

According to Bridson and Forman, in an ideal situation, a herbarium should contain a comprehensive cross-section of the species present in the area it represents, and its contents should reflect the distribution of species within that region (Bridson and Forman 1999, p. 277). This enables the observation of changes in the region's natural environment and the planning of conservation measures. On the other hand, plant collection should not contribute to the extinction of rare and endangered species,[191] which may result from irresponsible depletion of populations driven by an uncontrolled desire to expand collections.[192] Collections that do not take into account the conservation status of a given plant population have repeatedly led to the extinction of species (Mądalski 1955, pp. 84–85; Bridson and Forman 1999, p. 277; Drobnik 2009, pp. 18, 25–27, 34–36, 190–191).[193] For these and other reasons, such as environmental pollution and habitat loss due to human pressure, as well as climate change or shifts in species' distribution ranges, herbaria serve as repositories of specimens of species extinct in the wild or no longer present in a given area.

International documents that may influence the management of herbarium collections and their accessibility include the *Convention on International Trade in Endangered Species of Wild Fauna and Flora* (CITES) and the *Convention on Biological Diversity* (CBD) (Bridson and Forman 1999, pp. 279–286; McManis and Pelletire 2014; Dhanda 2023; Williams 2023).

---

[190] For example, the *Polish Red Data Book of Plants* (Drobnik 2009, p. 35). However, not all rare plants are classified as protected species.

[191] For example, lichens, which are becoming extinct due to the loss of natural habitats and environmental pollution (Drobnik 2009, p. 190).

[192] The phenomenon of unrestrained collection of natural resources has existed since the inception of collecting and, unfortunately, persists to this day, including among scientists working in systematics. Excessive specimen collection may be motivated, among other reasons, by the desire to obtain material for exchange with other institutions or by the wish to possess rare specimens.

[193] The latter author cites, as examples from Poland, the case of the long-flowered primrose (*Primula halleri*) and the wild onion (*Allium strictum*).

CITES, which came into force in 1975 and is currently ratified by 184 countries and the European Union (CITES 1973), appears to have little direct connection with the activities of herbaria. The Convention regulates the trade in plant and animal materials, the list of which is included in the appendices to the main text of the Convention. Countries that have ratified the Convention are required to establish a *Management Authority* and a *Scientific Authority*, which are responsible for granting trade licences and certificates. In the case of trade in plants, herbaria may serve as expert institutions and issue binding opinions. Herbaria should also refrain from accepting specimens into their collections that do not meet the criteria set out in CITES. Some countries have additional lists of species subject to similar restrictions (Bridson and Forman 1999, pp. 279–286; Dhanda 2023). The Convention also provides for special exemptions for the scientific exchange and loan of herbarium specimens, provided that the exchange or loan occurs between registered institutions and the specimens are appropriately labelled.

The CBD, established in 1992 at the initiative of the United Nations, entered into force a year later and is currently ratified by 196 signatories (CBD 1992). Its objective is the conservation of biodiversity, which has been identified as particularly threatened in contemporary times due to the destructive impact of human activity on ecosystems. The preservation of biodiversity is linked to the sustainable use of natural resources and the regulation of access to, and utilisation of, genetic resources contained within collections. The effective implementation of these principles is supported by a legal instrument, the *Nagoya Protocol*,[194] which entered into force in 2014. These regulations directly concern herbarium collections as repositories of genetic material and the rules governing their accessibility. The Convention is associated with *Access and Benefit Sharing* (ABS), which aims to ensure that the inhabitants of the host country have access to information and potential benefits arising from research conducted on their resources by external researchers. ABS may also influence the management of historical collections, as it imposes an obligation on collection managers to provide data regarding these collections (Bridson and Forman 1999, p. 283; Williams 2023). A scientifically valuable consequence of ABS is the widespread dissemination of herbarium resources through digitisation. The initial purpose of herbarium digitisation was to fulfil the ethical priority of repatriating collections. This was related to the fact that major herbaria, located in former colonial powers, held specimens collected centuries ago from various distant parts of the world. Researchers from these regions often lacked access to archives of their own country's flora (Drobnik 2009, p. 14). The availability of images in online databases now enables numerous queries to be conducted without travel.

The issues of ABS and respect for the cultures of other regions of the world are also addressed in ethical codes developed by ethnobiological associations, including the International Society of Ethnobiology (ISE). These codes are based on the concepts of *mindfulness* and respect, emphasising the undeniable link between

[194] Full name: *Nagoya Protocol on Access to Genetic Resources and the Fair and Equitable Sharing of Benefits Arising from their Utilization (ABS) to the Convention on Biological Diversity* (Secretariat of the Convention on Biological Diversity 2011).

biological and cultural diversity, the inevitable impact of research on local communities—even in the case of non-commercial studies—and the responsibility associated with the trust placed in researchers who obtain information during interviews (Salick et al. 2014). They also address the issue of intellectual property related to the knowledge shared, which affects the methods of its dissemination, as well as the necessity to respect and preserve intangible aspects of heritage, such as local knowledge, customs, and values.[195] The ISE document also marks the origin of the very concept of biocultural diversity, which has since evolved into the notion of biocultural heritage and subsequently biocultural collections (Loh and Harmon 2005; Salick et al. 2014). Biodiversity as a culture-forming factor and a value to be protected has also become the subject of locally oriented documents, such as the Oaxaca Declaration (The Oaxaca Declaration 1993).

Another problematic aspect of repatriation is the contamination of collections with biocides, many of which belong either to highly persistent inorganic compounds (e.g. arsenic, mercuric chloride) or to so-called persistent organic pollutants (POPs).[196] The repatriation and, more broadly, the accessibility of collections that have at some stage been contaminated raise questions about whether prioritising the fundamental ethical principle of accessibility may put human health and life at risk. The contamination of collections is also a concern for individuals who work daily in institutions that house such hazardous material.[197] Repeated attempts to develop methods for the decontamination of collections have achieved, at best, a success rate of approximately 80–90%, and thus the reversibility of biocidal treatments cannot be claimed.[198] Moreover, it is only in recent years that biocidal agents, originally adopted in museums and herbaria from industrial agriculture, have begun to be evaluated and studied for their potential to cause persistent environmental pollution and carcinogenic effects.

Another group of ethical issues from the perspective of collection care concerns the use of herbarium material for genetic research. To date, the vast majority of genetic analyses are destructive, meaning that each study results in the irreversible loss of unique source material (Nesbitt 2014). Consequently, over the years, protocols have been developed for requesting material for research purposes, and collection curators must assess each application for partial destruction of a specimen (Canales et al. 2022). The evaluation of such a request must take into account the significance of the research project, while also requiring a difficult judgment as to whether it is justified to sacrifice collection material for a given scientific study.

---

[195] The ISE Code of Ethics (International Society of Ethnobiology 1988) was established at the founding congress in 1988 and is known as the *Declaration of Belém*.

[196] For information on biocides, see the Sect. 3.9 in Chap. 3.

[197] The approach to the issue of collection contamination has evolved alongside growing awareness of the associated risks. Townsend cites a different attitude in the 1990s, when staff resisted the withdrawal of mercuric chloride (long recognised as hazardous), willing to sacrifice their own comfort for the protection of collections (Townsend 1999). This was likely due to a lack of awareness of the real dangers posed by the use of biocidal agents.

[198] Decontamination methods are described in the Sect. 4.2 in Chap. 4.

Currently, separate specimens are specifically collected for destructive analyses. However, in the case of historical specimens, there is no surplus material available for research, making curatorial decisions about releasing specimens extremely problematic and most often resulting in a negative outcome. In recent years, attempts have been made to develop non-destructive methods for obtaining genetic material from various types of objects (e.g. Rohland et al. 2004; Gilbert et al. 2007; Thomsen et al. 2009; Teasdale et al. 2015; Shepherd 2017).[199]

Codes of conservation ethics typically do not address such specific issues as the preservation of genetic material contained within heritage objects or the defined methodology for the conservation of scientific instruments. While there is no doubt that historical herbaria are considered heritage objects, the concepts of their conservation and preservation elude basic definitions. The points of intersection between codes of conservation ethics and those related to the management of natural resources (including natural history collections) concern the preservation of natural heritage, which is listed alongside cultural heritage, as well as the respect for biodiversity.

Over the years, numerous documents addressing these issues have been issued by UNESCO. The *World Heritage Convention* (*Convention Concerning the Protection of the World Cultural and Natural Heritage*), adopted in 1972, defines cultural heritage as "monuments", which include works of painting, sculpture, architecture, and archaeological objects; as well as architectural ensembles within their surrounding landscape and historic sites (UNESCO 1972). Natural heritage is understood as natural monuments, geological formations, and natural areas of particular aesthetic and scientific value. Although the convention does not explicitly mention paper-based artefacts, the definition allows for the inclusion of herbaria in an intermediate category as both cultural and natural heritage. The convention imposes an obligation on each signatory to further specify the definitions, while also requiring the integration of the preservation of natural and cultural heritage into general policy frameworks. Preservation also encompasses the necessity of scientific activity, conservation, education in the field of cultural and natural heritage conservation, and the promotion of scientific research. In 2001, the *Universal Declaration on Cultural Diversity* was adopted in Paris (UNESCO 2001). It refers to the concepts of cultural pluralism, as established by the Nara Document on Authenticity (1994) (ICCROM 1994), and to their protection as an ethical imperative. In the main lines of the declaration's implementation plan, point 13 emphasises the need to develop strategies for the protection and revitalisation of cultural and natural heritage, while point 14 highlights the need to recognise traditional knowledge, especially in the context of environmental conservation and natural resource management. The plan also addresses the need to preserve intangible heritage, respect for traditional knowledge, and the importance of considering the values present in other cultures in activities that draw upon their intellectual resources.

[199] Attempts at non-destructive analysis of genetic material from such objects mainly involve extraction by passing an eluent through the structure of the object or by sampling with an eraser (Shepherd 2017).

In 2015, in the *Recommendation concerning the protection and promotion of museums and collections, their diversity and their role in society* by UNESCO, (2015a) a collection was defined as an *assemblage of natural and cultural properties, tangible and intangible, past and present.*[200] In the same year, UNESCO also issued the *Recommendation concerning the preservation of, and access to, documentary heritage including in digital form*, which introduced an additional category—documentary heritage, encompassing both historical and contemporary herbaria (UNESCO 2015b). According to the text of the *Recommendation*, *documentary heritage comprises those single documents—or groups of documents—of significant and enduring value to a community, a culture, a country or to humanity generally, and whose deterioration or loss would be a harmful impoverishment. Significance of this heritage may become clear only with the passage of time. The world's documentary heritage is of global importance and responsibility to all, and should be fully preserved and protected for all, with due respect to and recognition of cultural mores and practicalities. It should be permanently accessible and re-usable by all without hindrance. It provides the means for understanding social, political, collective as well as personal history. It can help to underpin good governance and sustainable development. For each State, its documentary heritage reflects its memory and identity, and thus contributes to determine its place in the global community.* The *Recommendation* lists not only archives, museums, and libraries as so-called memory institutions, but also, among others, research organizations. The principle for the preservation of documentary heritage is to be *integrity, authenticity and reliability*. Once again, detailed definitions should be established at the national level.[201]

The ethical codes of the International Council of Museums (ICOM) also include the concept of natural heritage. The first edition of the document (ICOM 1986) defines cultural heritage as any concepts or objects, natural or man-made, of aesthetic, historical, scientific, or spiritual significance. In the subsequent sections of the document, the established terms natural and cultural heritage, as known from UNESCO documents, are used. In later editions (ICOM 2004, 2017), the term natural heritage (in this case *natural inheritance*) is already employed. ICOM documents are likely the first ethical codes on such a scale to recognise natural specimens as a specific element of collections, which may be subject to conservation and destructive analysis (ICOM 2017). The title of the first chapter of the code states: *Museums preserve, interpret and promote the natural and cultural inheritance of humanity.*[202] According to the document, museums are obliged to protect both the tangible and intangible natural and cultural heritage. The second chapter of the code also addresses the issue of biological specimens, which should be acquired in accordance with the law and environmental protection principles, as well as their inclusion in collections used by external researchers (working collection). The primary

[200] At the same time, the *Recommendation* imposes an obligation on signatories to specify the definitions individually.

[201] The documentary nature of herbarium collections is also emphasised by the authors of an article on the practice and ethics of working with herbaria (Rabeler et al. 2019).

[202] ICOM (2017).

aim of conservation is the stabilisation of the object or specimen. All conservation activities should be thoroughly documented and as reversible as possible, with any changes introduced being easily distinguishable from the original structure. In the case of destructive analysis, detailed documentation of the object or specimen prior to examination is required. Subsequent editions reveal an interesting difference: the 1986 code mentions that *recognition and respect for the cultural and physical integrity and authenticity of individual objects, specimens or collections are fundamental values in conservation work* and notes that an object or specimen may require interventive conservation. Later editions (from 2004 and 2017) are more concise on this matter, not defining the issue of authenticity, but instead suggesting that conservation procedures should be "as reversible as possible", rather than simply "reversible" as in the 1986 code, reflecting the relative nature of the concept of reversibility in such procedures.

In all editions of the document, collections are defined as *primary evidence*, underscoring their uniqueness and scientific value. Cultural heritage is defined as *any thing or concept considered of aesthetic, historical, scientific or spiritual significance;* and natural heritage as *any natural thing, phenomenon or concept, considered to be of scientific significance or to be a spiritual manifestation.*[203]

In 2013, ICOM also published a code for natural history museums, which describes natural history collections in museums as a *three-dimensional archive of the natural world and relationships of societies with their environment.*[204] The code addresses issues of storage and display, but does not provide any definitions for the conservation treatment of objects such as herbaria.[205]

Herbaria, which are not merely collections of individual specimens and often also possess aesthetic value, may be regarded as objects of both cultural and natural heritage. Due to their function as repositories of biological information, they can also be considered elements of documentary heritage. In this context, the concept of herbarium restoration may refer to the mounting and fixing elements, which should be characterised by minimal intervention. Given the nature of such collections, the methods employed in conservation and potential restoration should primarily take into account the scientific use of the object. Owing to the current rapid advancement of analytical techniques and genetic research, regardless of the present assessment of the condition, completeness of the collection, or any exclusion of the object from genetic analyses and other studies, it is essential to assume that this artefact may nevertheless be utilised in future scientific research.

[203] ICOM (2017).

[204] ICOM (2013).

[205] General guidelines are provided: *Objects should be stored and cared for according to best practice guidelines (…) displayed in appropriate environmental conditions, (…) adequately supported and protected from human interference, e.g. unwanted handling or theft* (ICOM 2013).

References

Adams CT, Fritz GJ (2014) Using biocultural collections for education. In: Salick J, Konchar K, Nesbitt M (eds) Curating biocultural collections: a handbook. Royal Botanic Gardens, Kew, pp 347–366

Ames M, Spooner DM (2008) DNA from herbarium specimens settles a controversy about origins of the European potato. Am J Bot 95:252–257. https://doi.org/10.3732/ajb.95.2.252

Arabas I (2009a) Przyrodnicy, kolekcjonerzy, muzealnicy i teoretycy muzealnictwa. Kwart Nauki Hist Tech 54(1):115–130

Arabas I (2009b) Losy kolekcji księżnej Anny Jabłonowskiej na podstawie dokumentów z Archiwum Rosyjskiej Akademii Nauk w St. Petersburgu. Kwart Nauki Hist Tech 54(2):95–108

Arabas I (2012a) Niezrealizowany projekt Narodowego Muzeum Historii Naturalnej księżnej Anny Jabłonowskiej. Kwart Nauki Hist Tech 57(3–4):167–180

Arabas I (2012b) Petersburskie ślady kolekcji Anny ks. Jabłonowskiej z Siemiatycz. In: Anna ks. Jabłonowska i ks. Krzysztof Kluk – ludzie, którzy wyprzedzili swoją epokę. Materiały sesji naukowej 30.09–01.10.2011. Muzeum Rolnictwa w Ciechanowcu, Towarzystwo Naukowe Societas Scientarum Klukoviana et Jablonovianae w Ciechanowcu, Ciechanowiec, pp 10–27

Arabas I (2013) Ocalałe z moskiewskiej pożogi. Materialne ślady kolekcji przyrodniczej księżnej Anny Jabłonowskiej. Cenne, bezcenne utracone 1(74)–4(77):52–57

Arabas I (2015) Dziedzictwo kulturowe warszawskiego farmaceuty Ferdynanda Karo na tle inwentaryzacji świata. Muzeum Warszawy, Warszawa

Arber A (1940) The colouring of sixteenth-century herbals. Nature 145:803–804. https://doi.org/10.1038/145803a0

Arber A (1970) Herbals. Their origin and evolution, 2nd edn. Hafner Publishing Co., Darien, Connecticut

Benkert (2016) 8 The 'Hortus Siccus' as a focal point: knowledge, environment, and image in Felix Platter's and Caspar Bauhin's Herbaria. In: Göttler C, Burkart L, Burghartz S (eds) Sites of mediation. Connected histories of places, processes, and objects in Europe and beyond, 1450–1650, Series intersections, vol 47. Brill, pp 211–239

Berli J, Belhadj O (2020) Consolidating herbarium specimens using two-sided hydroxylpropylcellulose pre-coated paper. J Pap Conserv 21(1):31–34. https://doi.org/10.1080/18680860.2020.1835112

Bertin A (2016) The historic herbarium of Simone D'Oignies (1780) and its current scientific importance. Dissertation, Leiden University

Blunt W, Stearn WT (1994) The art of botanical illustration. An illustrated history. Dover Publications, New York

Bridson D, Forman L (1999) The Herbarium Handbook. Royal Botanic Gardens, Kew

Britten J, Savage S, Dandy JE (1958) The Sloane herbarium: an annotated list of the Horti sicci composing it; with biographical details of the principal contributors. Trustees of the British Museum, London

Burbano HA, Gutaker R (2023) Ancient DNA genomics and the renaissance of herbaria. Science 382:59–63. https://doi.org/10.1126/science.adi1180

Campos PE, Pruvost O, Boyer K, Chiroleu F, Cao TT, Gaudeul M, Baider C, Utteridge TMA, Becker N, Rieux A, Gagnevin L (2023) Herbarium specimen sequencing allows precise dating of Xanthomonas citri pv. citri diversification history. Nat Commun 14(1):4306. https://doi.org/10.1038/s41467-023-39950-z

Canales NA, Clarke AC, Nesbitt M, Gutaker R (2022) Chapter 2. DNA from museum collections. In: de Boer H, Rydmark MO, Verstraete B, Gravendeel B (eds) Molecular identification of plants: from sequence to species. Advanced books. https://doi.org/10.3897/ab.e68634

Chlebicki A (1991) Zielnik prof. Dr Józefa Mądalskiego. Wiad Bot 35(3–4):90–93

Chomicki G, Renner SS (2019) Climate and symbioses with ants modulate leaf/stem scaling in epiphytes. Sci Rep 9:2624. https://doi.org/10.1038/s41598-019-39853-4

Clarck S (1986) Preservation of herbarium specimens: an archive conservator's approach. Taxon 35(4):675–682. https://doi.org/10.2307/1221610

Collins M (2000) Medieval herbals: the illustrative traditions. British Museum and University of Toronto Press

Convention on Biological Diversity (CBD) (1992). www.cbd.int. Accessed 21 Jan 2026

Conwentz H (1911) Westpreussische Botaniker der Vergangenheit. Begrüssungsrede. Berichte d Deutschen Botanischen Gesellschaft 29:6–15

Cook A (2007) Botanical exchanges: Jean-Jacques Rousseau and the Duchess of Portland. Hist Eur Ideas 33:142–156. https://doi.org/10.1016/j.histeuroideas.2006.08.010

Cornish C, Nesbitt M (2014) Historical perspectives on western ethnobotanical collections. In: Salick J, Konchar K, Nesbitt M (eds) Curating biocultural collections: a handbook. Royal Botanic Gardens, Kew, pp 271–293

Costa RMS, van Andel T, Pavonea P, Pulvirenti S (2018) The pre-Linnaean herbarium of Paolo Boccone (1633–1704) kept in Leiden (the Netherlands) and its connections with the imprinted one in Paris. Plant Biosyst 152(3):489–500. https://doi.org/10.1080/11263504.2018.1445132

Craine JM, Elmore AJ, Wang L, Aranibar J, Bauters M, Boeckx P, Crowley BE, Dawes MA, Delzon S, Fajardo A, Fang Y, Fujiyoshi L, Gray A, Guerrieri R, Gundale MJ, Hawke DJ, Hietz P, Jonard M, Kearsley E, Kenzo T, Makarov M, Marañón-Jiménez S, McGlynn TP, McNeil BE, Mosher SG, Nelson DM, Peri PL, Roggy J, Sanders-DeMott R, Song M, Szpak P, Templer PH, Van der Colff D, Werner C, Xu X, Yang Y, Yu G, Zmudczyńska-Skarbek K (2018) Isotopic evidence for oligotrophication of terrestrial ecosystems. Nat Ecol Evol 2(11):1735–1744. https://doi.org/10.1038/s41559-018-0694-0

Cristofolini G (2024) Origin and evolution of herbaria in the sixteenth century. Rend Fis Acc Lincei 35:63–75. https://doi.org/10.1007/s12210-024-01232-1

Czartoryska IE (1828) Poczet pamiątek zachowanych w Domu Gotyckim w Puławach. Drukarnia Banku Polskiego, Warsaw

Czeczottowa H (1937) O potrzebie utworzenie Centralnego Muzeum Botanicznego w Warszawie. Nauka Polska 23:178–181

Da Costa Kaufmann T, Roehrig Kaumann V (1991) Sanctification of nature: observations of the origins of Trompe l'oeil in Netherlandish book painting of the fifteenth and sixteenth centuries. J Paul Getty Mus J 19:43–64

Dahm R (2005) Friedrich Miescher and the discovery of DNA. Dev Biol 278(2):274–288. https://doi.org/10.1016/j.ydbio.2004.11.028

Dauwalder L (2012) Das Herbarium des Felix Platter. Die Erhaltung eines historischen Buch-Herbariums. Dissertation, Fachochshule Bern

Dauwalder L (2013) Felix Platter's Herbarium: the preservation of a historical 'Bound Herbarium'. J Pap Conserv 14(3):26–32

Davies NMJ, Drinkell C, Utteridge TMA (2023) The herbarium handbook. Kew Publishing, Kew

Davis P (2018) Collecting and preserving fishes: a historical perspective. In: MacGregor A (ed) Naturalists in the field. Collecting, recording and preserving the natural world from the fifteenth to the twenty-first century. Brill, Leiden, Boston, pp 149–165

Davis CC, Willis CG, Connolly B, Kelly C, Ellison AM (2015) Herbarium records are reliable sources of phenological change driven by climate and provide novel insights into species' phenological cueing mechanisms. Am J Bot 102:1599–1609

de Tournefort JP (1694) Élémens de botanique: ou Méthode pour connoître les plantes, vol 1. Imprimerie Royale, Paris

Dhanda (2023) Convention on international trade in endagered species of wild fauna and flora (CITES). In: Davies NMJ, Drinkell C, Utteridge TMA (eds) The herbarium handbook. Kew Publishing, Kew, pp 104–105

Down J (1999) Adhesive research at the Canadian Conservation Institute as it relates to herbarium collections. In: Metsger DA, Byers SC (eds) Managing the modern herbarium – an interdisciplinary approach. SPNHC, Ontario, pp 205–223

Drobnik J (2009) Zielnik i zielnikoznawstwo. Wydawnictwo Naukowe PWN, Warszawa

Egenberg IM, Moe D (1991) A "stop-press" announcement. Damage caused by a widely used herbarium mounting technique. Taxon 40(4):601–604. https://doi.org/10.2307/1222768

Egmond F (2010) The world of Carolus Clusius: natural history in the making, 1550–1610. Pickering & Chatto, London

Egmond F (2018) Into the wild: botanical fieldwork in the sixteenth century. In: MacGregor A (ed) Naturalists in the field. Collecting, recording and preserving the natural world from the fifteenth to the twenty-first century. Brill, Leiden, Boston, pp 166–211

Ent AV, Echevarría G, Pollard AJ, Erskine PD (2019) X-Ray fluorescence ionomics of herbarium collections. Sci Rep 9:4746. https://doi.org/10.1038/s41598-019-40050-6

Espinosa F, Pinedo Castro M (2018) On the use of herbarium specimens for morphological and anatomical research. Bot Lett 165(3–4):361–367. https://doi.org/10.1080/23818107.2018.1451775

Fenn J (1999) Plastic materials used in the herbarium. In: Metsger DA, Byers SC (eds) Managing the modern herbarium – an interdisciplinary approach. SPNHC, Ontario, pp 235–259

Findlen P (1994) Possessing nature: museums, collecting, and scientific culture in early modern Italy. California University Press, Berkeley, Los Angeles, London

Firszt S (2009) Co się stało z cieplickimi zbiorami. Pamiętny rok 1952, vol 5. Muzeum w Cieplicach, Jelenia Góra–Cieplice

Firszt S (2016) Wyniki wstępnej kwerendy w sprawie rozproszonych zbiorów Schaffgotschów. Rocz Jeleniogór 18:199–210

Ford BJ (2003) Scientific illustration in the eighteenth century. In: Porter R (ed) The Cambridge history of science. Cambridge University Press, Cambridge, pp 561–583. https://doi.org/10.1017/CHOL9780521572439.025

Frey L (2010) Karol Linneusz. Książę botaników, profesor profesorów. Instytut Botaniki im. W. Szafera, Polska Akademia nauk w Krakowie, Kraków

Gallagher RV, Allen S, Wright IJ (2019) Safety margins and adaptive capacity of vegetation to climate change. Sci Rep 9:8241. https://doi.org/10.1038/s41598-019-44483-x

Gersten T, Michineau M, Paternotre A, Thys N (2017) Herbarii Bruxellenses, le projet de conservation des herbiers de la Bibliothèque Royale de Belgique. Monte Artium 10:83–101. https://doi.org/10.1484/J.IMA.5.114683

Gilbert MT, Moore W, Melchior L, Worobey M (2007) DNA extraction from dry museum beetles without conferring external morphological damage. PLoS One 2:e272

Graniszewska M (2018) Drzewa i krzewy w zielniku pruskiego lekarza Matthiasa Ernesta Boretiusa (1694–1738). Rocznik Polskiego Towarzystwa Dendrologicznego 66:59–83

Graniszewska M, Kapler A (2018) Herbaria of the Prussian physician Boretius (1694–1738) in the Herbarium WA. Biodiv Res Conserv 52:1–6. https://doi.org/10.2478/biorc-2018-0012

Graniszewska M, Leśniewska H, Galera H (2016) Zielnik Zioła lecznicze... Michała Fedorowskiego jako dokumentacja badań etnograficznych. Etnobiol Polska 6:191–251

Grasso G, Debruyne R, Adamo M, Rué O, Lejzerowicz F, Bittner L, Bianciotto V, Marmeisse R (2025) Ancient microbiomes as mirrored by DNA extracted from century-old herbarium plants and associated soil. Mol Ecol Resour 25:e14122. https://doi.org/10.1111/1755-0998.14122

Grenda M (2013) Ethical considerations concerning the restoration of a herbarium from the 19th century. In: ICOM-CC graphic documents working group interim meeting | Vienna 17–19 April 2013. ICOM-CC, Vienna, pp 93–96

Grenda M (2015) Remedial conservation of a severely deteriorated 19th century bound herbarium. J Nat Sci Collect 2:54–59

Grenda-Kurmanow M (2016) Challenges of conservation treatment of historic herbaria. In: Green Museum – how to practice what we preach: 31th annual meeting of the society for the preservation of natural history collections. Botanic Garden and Botanical Museum Berlin, Freie Universitat Berlin, Berlin, pp 117–119. https://doi.org/10.3372/SPNHC2016

Grenda-Kurmanow M (2026) Pośmiertne życie zielnika Róży Luksemburg. Medycyna Nowożytna 31(Suplement I):571–592. https://doi.org/10.4467/12311960MN.25.053.22740

Grenda-Kurmanow M, Drobnik J, Stebel A, Alziar G (2025) The pre-Linnaean herbarium of Paolo Boccone (1633–1704) in Wrocław, Poland: its history, description, its purpose, and its usefulness for historians of science. J Hist Biol. https://doi.org/10.1007/s10739-025-09841-8
Gunn A (1994) Past and current practice: the botanist view. In: Child RE (ed) Conservation and the herbarium. The Institute of Paper Conservation, Leigh, pp 11–14
Hanson AE (2001) Text & context for the illustrated herbal from tebtunis. In: Atti del XXII Congresso di Papirologia, Firenze, pp 585–604
Harris SA (2018) Snapshots of tropical diversity: collecting plants in colonial and imperial Brazil. In: MacGregor A (ed) Naturalists in the field. Collecting, recording and preserving the natural world from the fifteenth to the twenty-first century. Brill, Leiden, Boston, pp 550–557
Hawks C, Bell D (1999) Removal of stains caused by mercuric chloride treatments from herbarium sheet labels. In: Bridgeland J (ed) BidICOM Committee for conservation preprints, vol II, 12th Triennial Meeting Lyon, 29 August–3 September. James and James, London, pp 723–727
Healey JF (1999) Pliny the elder on science and technology. University Press, Oxford
Hentschel K (2014) Visual cultures in science and technology a comparative history. Oxford University Press, Oxford
ICCROM (1994) The Nara Document on Authenticity. https://www.iccrom.org/sites/default/files/publications/2020-05/convern8_06_thenaradocu_ing.pdf. Accessed 19 Jan 2026
ICOM (International Council of Museums) (1986) ICOM Code of Ethics for Museums. https://www.schielemuseum.org/wp-content/uploads/2019/11/ICOM_Code_of_Ethics_Sec_10_-_ICOM_Code_of_Professional_Ethics.pdf. Accessed 10 Jan 2026
ICOM (International Council of Museums) (2004) ICOM Code of Ethics for Museums. https://www.wipo.int/tk/en/databases/creative_heritage/codes/link0007.html. Accessed 10 Jan 2026
ICOM (International Council of Museums) (2013) ICOM Code of Ethics for Natural History Museums. https://icom.museum/wp-content/uploads/2018/07/nathcode_ethics_en.pdf. Acessed 27 Jan 2026
ICOM (International Council of Museums) (2017) ICOM Code of Ethics for Museums. https://icom.museum/wp-content/uploads/2018/07/ICOM-code-En-web.pdf. Accessed 27 Jan 2026
ISE (International Society of Ethnobiology) (1988) Declaration of Belém. http://www.ethnobiology.net/what-we-do/core-programs/global-coalition-2/declaration-of-belem/. Accessed 27 Jan 2026
James SA, Soltis PS, Belbin L, Chapman AD, Nelson G, Paul DL, Collins M (2018) Herbarium data: global biodiversity and societal botanical needs for novel research. Appl Plant Sci 6(2):e1024. https://doi.org/10.1002/aps3.1024
Janick J, Stolarczyk J (2012) Ancient Greek illustrated dioscoridean herbals: origins and impact of the Juliana Anicia Codex and the Codex Neopolitanus. Not Bot Horti Agrobot 40(1):9–17
Jankowski R (2014) Opis Archiwum nieświeskiego Radziwiłłów z 1957 roku. Miscellanea Historico-Archivistica 21:309–340
Jaussaud P (2003) Les curiosités des trois apothicaires. Rev Hist Pharm 91(340):603–610. https://doi.org/10.3406/pharm.2003.5556
Jones WHS (1961) Introduction. In: Jones WHS (ed) Pliny. Natural history with an English translation in ten volumes, vol VI. Harvard University Press/William Heinemann, Cambridge, Massachussets/London, pp ix–xxvi
Keijzers V (2013) Historische herbaria: inzicht in de conservatie problematiek en een aanzet tot een leidraad voor de conservering en restauratie van gedroogd plantenmateriaal. Dissertation, Artesis Hogeschool Antwerpen
Kessler HF (1870) Das älteste und erste Herbarium Deutschlands, im Jahre 1592 von Dr. Caspar Ratzenberger angelegt, gegenwärtig noch im Königlichen Museum zu Cassel. Verlag von August Freyscmidt, Cassel
Kielak AM (2004) Zielnik Elizy Orzeszkowej. Nieznany zabytek botaniczny przechowywany w zbiorach PTPN. Wydawnictwo Kontekst, Poznań
Kiljańska A (2005) Album – zielnik w kasecie. In: Leszczyńska-Cyganik B (ed) Fin de siècle w Krakowie. Grafika użytkowa, tkaniny, rzemiosło artystyczne ze zbiorów Muzeum Narodowego

w Krakowie, exhibition catalogue. Muzeum Narodowe w Krakowie, Kraków, reg. 181, pp 108–110

Kiss L, Kovács GM, Bóka K, Bohár G, Bohárné KV, Németh MZ, Takamatsu S, Shin H-D, Hayova V, Nischwitz C, Seier MK, Evans HC, Cannon PF, Ash GJ, Shivas RG, Müller-Schärer H (2018) Deciphering the biology of Cryptophyllachora eurasiatica gen. et sp. nov., an often-cryptic pathogen of an allergenic weed, Ambrosia artemisiifolia. Sci Rep 8:10806. https://doi.org/10.1038/s41598-018-29102-5

Kistler L, Bieker VC, Martin MD, Pedersen MW, Madrigal JR, Wales N (2020) Ancient plant genomics in archaeology, herbaria, and the environment. Annu Rev Plant Biol 71(1). https://doi.org/10.1146/annurev-arplant-081519-035837

Klepacki P (2007) Etnobotanika w Polsce–przeszłość i teraźniejszość. Analecta 16(1–2)(31–32):191–245

Köhler P (1989) The Javanese Pteridophyta collected by Marian Raciborski housed in the Herbarium of the Jagiellonian University (KRA). Zesz Nauk Univ Jagiellon Prace Bot 18:127–133

Köhler P (1994) Rośliny z terenu Białorusi w zielniku Józefa Jundziłła. Kwart Hist Nauki Tech 39(3–4):93–102

Köhler P (1995) Zielnik Józefa Jundziłła. Polish Botanical Studies Guidebook Series No. 13, Szafer Institute of Botany, Polish Academy of Sciences, Kraków

Köhler P (1996) Zielnik Seweryna Udzieli – dokumentacja pracy Rośliny w wierzeniach ludu krakowskiego. Lud 80:179–186

Köhler P (1999) Historia Zielnika Instytutu Botaniki Uniwersytetu Jagiellońskiego (KRA) w latach 1780–1910. Kwart Hist Nauki Tech 44(2):7–60

Kowalska-Lewicka A (1964) Etnobotanika. Etnografia Polska 8:207–214

Kujawska M (2008) Etnobotanika. Op. Cit 4(41):58–62

Kusukawa S (2012) Picturing the book of nature: image, text, and argument in sixteenth-century human anatomy and medical botany. The University of Chicago Press, Chicago

Kuzmina ML, Braukmann TWA, Fazekas AJ, Graham SW, Dewaard SL, Rodrigues A, Bennett BA, Dickinson TA, Saarela JM, Catling PM, Newmaster SG, Percy DM, Fenneman E, Lauron-Moreau A, Ford B, Gillespie L, Subramanyam R, Whitton J, Jennings L, Metsger D, Warne CP, Brown A, Sears E, Dewaard JR, Zakharov EV, Hebert PDN (2017) Using herbarium-derived DNAs to assemble a large-scale DNA barcode library for the vascular-plants of Canada. Appl Plant Sci 5:1700079. https://doi.org/10.3732/apps.1700079

Lang PLM, Willems FM, Scheepens JF, Burbano HA, Bossdorf O (2019) Using herbaria to study global environmental change. New Phytol 221(1):110–122. https://doi.org/10.1111/nph.15401

Lehtonen S, Christenhusz MJM (2010) Historical herbarium specimens in plant molecular systematics – an example from the fern genus Lindsaea (Lindsaeaceae). Biologia 65(2):204–208. https://doi.org/10.2478/s11756-010-0008-8

Lewandowska E, Wójcik Z (2012) Ks. Jan Krzysztof Kluk i Siemiatycze. In: Anna ks. Jabłonowska i ks. Krzysztof Kluk – ludzie, którzy wyprzedzili swoją epokę. Materiały sesji naukowej 30.09–01.10.2011. Muzeum Rolnictwa w Ciechanowcu, Towarzystwo Naukowe Societas Scientarum Klukoviana et Jablonovianae w Ciechanowcu, Ciechanowiec, pp 127–137

Lienhard L, Dauwalder L (2016) Das Herbarium des Felix Platter. Burgerbibliothek Bern, Haupt Verlag, Bern

Linnaeus C (1751) Philosophia Botanica in qua explicantur fundamenta botanica cum definitionibus partium, exemplis terminorum, observationibus rariorum adjectis figuris aeneis. Godofr. Kiesewetter, Stockholm

Loh J, Harmon D (2005) A global index of biocultural diversity. Ecol Indic 5:231–241

Lusitanus A (1553) In Dioscoridis Anazarbei de medica materia libros quinque enarrationes eruditissimae doctoris Amati Lusitani medici ac philosophi celeberrimi, quibus non solum officinarum seplasiariis, sed bonarum etiam literarum studiosis utilitas adfertur, quum passim simplicia Graece, Latine, Italice, Hispanice, Germanice, & Gallice proponantur. Gualtero Scoto, Wenecja

MacGregor A (2018a) Introduction. In: MacGregor A (ed) Naturalists in the field. Collecting, recording and preserving the natural world from the fifteenth to the twenty-first century. Brill, Leiden, Boston, pp 1–39

MacGregor A (2018b) European enlightenment in India: an episode of Anglo-German collaboration in the natural sciences on the Coromandel Coast, late 1700s–Early 1800s. In: MacGregor A (ed) Naturalists in the field. Collecting, recording and preserving the natural world from the fifteenth to the twenty-first century. Brill, Leiden, Boston, pp 365–392
Mądalski J (1955) Jak należy zbierać i konserwować rośliny do celów naukowych. PWN, Warszawa
Mägdefrau K (2004) Historia botaniki. Życie i dokonania wielkich badaczy. In: Prace Ogrodu Botanicznego Uniwersytetu Wrocławskiego, vol 7, issue 1. Wydawnictwo Uniwersytetu Wrocławskiego, Wrocław
Majewski T (2016) Nauki biologiczne. In: Nauki ścisłe i przyrodnicze na Uniwersytecie Warszawskim, seria Monumenta Universitatis Varsoviensis 1816–2016. Wydawnictwa Uniwersytetu Warszawskiego, Warszawa, pp 51–197
Mangani G, Tomasi LT (2013) Gherardo Cibo. Dilettante di botanica e pittore di 'paesi'. Arte, scienzia e ilustrazione botanica nel XVI secolo. Il Lavoro Editoriale, Ancona
Margez M (2004) L'herbier Haller du Muséum national d'Histoire naturelle: un objet d'intérêt historique et scientifique. Dissertation, Institut national du patrimoine, Departement des restaurateurs, Paris
Maroszek J (2011) Gabinet siemiatycki i zbiory księżnej Anny z Sapiehów Jabłonowskiej. In: Anna ks. Jabłonowska i ks. Krzysztof Kluk – ludzie, którzy wyprzedzili swoją epokę. Materiały sesji naukowej 30.09–01.10.2011. Muzeum Rolnictwa w Ciechanowcu, Towarzystwo Naukowe Societas Scientarum Klukoviana et Jablonovianae w Ciechanowcu, Ciechanowiec, pp 140–157
Mauriès P (2015) Cabinets of curiosities. Thames and Hudson, London
McManis CR, Pelletire JS (2014) Legal aspects of biocultural collections. In: Salick J, Konchar K, Nesbitt M (eds) Curating biocultural collections: a handbook. Royal Botanic Gardens, Kew, pp 229–241
Meineke EK, Davies TJ (2019) Museum specimens provide novel insights into changing plant–herbivore interactions. Philos Trans R Soc B 374:20170393. https://doi.org/10.1098/rstb.2017.0393
Mencfel M (2010) Skarbce natury i sztuki. Prywatne gabinety osobliwości, kolekcje sztuki i naturaliów na Śląsku w wiekach XVII i XVIII. Wydawnictwo DiG, Warszawa
Menei E (2005) Conservation et restauration d'herbiers: un cas exemplaire à la Bibliothèque de l'Institut de France. In: Actes du colloque Voyages en botanique, Besançon 16–17 juin 2005. ACCOLAD, Agence régionale de cooperation de Franche-Comte, Besançon. https://papyrusetpapierconservation.com/wp-content/uploads/2020/08/2005-Actes-Colloque-Voyages-en-botanique-Menei.pdf. Accessed 21 Jan 2026
Meyer EHF (1857) Geschichte der Botanik, Vierter Band. Verlag der Gebrüder Bornträger, Königsberg
Mniszech MJ (1775) Myśli względem założenia Musaeum Polonicum. In: Zabawy przyiemne i pozyteczne z rożnych Autorow zebrane XI, (2). M Gröl J. K. Mci Kommisarza i Bibliopoli w Marywilu, Warszawa, pp 211–226
Moat J, Bachman S (2023) Field notes. In: Davies NMJ, Drinkell C, Utteridge TMA (eds) The herbarium handbook. Kew Publishing, Kew, pp 24–31
Nauert CG (1979) Humanists, scientists, and pliny: changing approaches to a classical author. Am Hist Rev 84(1):72–85
Nepi C (2008) L'erbario Coltellini della Sezione Botanica del Museo di Storia Naturale. In: Nepi C, Gusmeroli E (eds) Gli erbari aretini da Andrea Cesalpino ai giorni nostri, Firenze University Press, Firenze, pp 23–28
Nesbitt M (2014) Use of herbarium specimen in ethnobotany. In: Salick J, Konchar K, Nesbitt M (eds) Curating biocultural collections: a handbook. Royal Botanic Gardens, Kew, pp 313–328
Nowak-Kemp M (2018) William Burchell in Southern Africa, 1811–1815. In: MacGregor A (ed) Naturalists in the field. Collecting, recording and preserving the natural world from the fifteenth to the twenty-first century. Brill, Leiden, Boston, pp 500–549
O'Connor B (1698) The history of Poland, in several letters to persons of quality. Giving an account of the antient and present state of that kingdom, historical, geographical, physical, political, and ecclesiastical; viz. Its origin and extent, with a description of its towns and provinces, the succession and remarkable actions of all kings, and of the Great Dukes of Lithuania:

the election, power, and coronation of the king: the senate, or house of lords: the diet and form of government: the privileges of the gentry; their religion, learning, language, customs, habits, manners, riches, trade, and military affairs; together with the state of physick and natural knowledge; as also an account of the teutonick order, and of the duke of Curland, his family and territories. With sculptures, and a new map after the best geographers. With several letters relating to physick, vol II. Dan Brown and T Leigh, London

Ochyra R, Cisło G (1999) Mchy w zielniku Tytusa Chałubińskiego w Muzeum Tatrzańskim w Zakopanem, Polish Botanical Studies 1999, Guidebook series no. 22. Muzeum Tatrzańskie im. Dr. Tytusa Chałubińskiego, Polska Akademia Nauk–Instytut Botaniki im. W. Szafera, Zakopane–Kraków

Ogilvie BW (2006) The science of describing. Natural history in Renaissance Europe. The University of Chicago Press, Chicago and London

Olariu D (2014) The misfortune of Philippus de Lignamine's Herbal, or new research perspectives in herbal illustrations from an iconological point of view. In: Kiedroń S, Rimm AM (eds) Early modern print culture in Central Europe. Proceedings of the young scholar section of the Wrocław seminars. September 2013. Wydawnictwo Uniwersytetu Wrocławskiego, Wrocław, pp 39–62

Ossenbach C (2017) Precursors of the botanical exploration of South America. Willem Piso (1611–1678) and Georg Marcgrave (1610–1644). Lankesteriana 17(1). https://doi.org/10.15517/LANK.V17I1.28527

Pacht O (1950) Early Italian nature studies and the early calendar landscape. J Warburg Courtauld Inst 13(1/2):13–47

Palmer SA, Smith O, Allaby RG (2012) The blossoming of plant archaeogenetics. Ann Anat 194:146–156. https://doi.org/10.1016/j.aanat.2011.03.012

Paś M (2017) Album–zielnik w kasecie, #dziedzictwo, exhibition catalogue. Muzeum Narodowe w Krakowie, Kraków: reg 210, pp 554–555

Pawęski F (1970) Polskie Muzealnictwo Przyrodnicze. Państwowe Wydawnictwo Naukowe – Oddział w Poznaniu, Poznań

Pearson KD (2019) A new method and insights for estimating phenological events from herbarium specimens. Appl Plant Sci 7(3):e01224. https://doi.org/10.1002/aps3.1224

Pękacka-Falkowska K (2018a) Horti sicci Jacoba Breyne'a z 1659 i 1673 roku. Zeszyty Historyczne 83(2):47–83. https://doi.org/10.15762/ZH.2018.23

Pękacka-Falkowska K (2018b) Wokół kolekcji przyrodniczych w Rzeczpospolitej Obojga Narodów. Cz. 1. Christoph i Johann Christoph Gottwaldowie oraz ich gdańskie muzeum. Kwart Hist Nauki Tech 63(2):51–97

Pękacka-Falkowska K (2022) Jacob Breyne, jego przyjaciele i rośliny: Uwagi na marginesie Breyne'owskich exsiccatae z kolekcji Jamesa Petivera. Kwart Hist Kult Mater 70(3):287–331. https://doi.org/10.23858/KHKM70.2022.3.002

Piekiełko A (1977) Osiemnastowieczny zielnik ze zbiorów Izabeli Czartoryskiej. Stud Mater Dziej Nauk Pol Ser B 27:157–174

Piekiełko A (1981) Dwa osiemnastowieczne zielniki ze zbiorów Instytutu Botaniki Uniwersytetu Jagiellońskiego. Ossolineum, Wrocław

Pliny (1966) Natural history with an English translation in ten volumes. In: Jones WHS (ed) vol VII. Harvard University Press/William Heinemann, Cambridge, Massachussets/London

Pomian K (1996) Zbieracze i osobliwości, Paryż–Wenecja XVI–XVIII wiek. Państwowy Instytut Wydawniczy, Warszawa

Popławska S (2014a) Gdy suszone rośliny stają się zabytkiem. Historia, technologia, problem konserwacji i przechowywania zielników, Dissertation, Akademia Sztuk Pięknych w Warszawie

Popławska S (2014b) Problematyka Konserwacji Artystycznego Zielnika i papeterii autorstwa Elizy Orzeszkowej podarowanych Leopoldowi Méyetowi, przechowywanych w Muzeum Narodowym w Warszawie, Dissertation, Akademia Sztuk Pięknych w Warszawie

Popławska S, Zając I (2018) Artystyczne i naukowe zielniki z zasuszonymi roślinami. Problematyka konserwacji zielników w formie kodeksu. Toruńskie Studia Bibliologiczne 1(20):67–87. https://doi.org/10.12775/TSB.2018.004

Popławska S, Sobucki W, Zając I (2017) Zastosowanie Aquazolu 500 i środka odkwaszającego Bookkeeper podczas konserwacji artystycznego zielnika Elizy Orzeszkowej ze zbiorów Muzeum Narodowego w Warszawie. Notes Konserwatorski 19:61–84

Pulvirenti S, Pavone P, Carbonaro RA, Costa RMS (2017a) The controversial biography of Paolo Boccone (1633–1704) and his "Grand Tour" from the Mediterranean to northern Europe. Plant Biosyst 151(3):377–380. https://doi.org/10.1080/11263504.2017.1302515

Pulvirenti S, Pavone P, Carbonaro RA, Costa RMS (2017b) Taxonomic study of the plants to be found in the only herbarium of Paolo Boccone (1633–1704) at present existing in Italy. Plant Biosyst 151(4):745–759. https://doi.org/10.1080/11263504.2017.1320317

Rabeler RK, Svoboda HT, Thiers B, Prather LA, Macklin JA, Lagomarsino LP, Majure LC, Ferguson CI (2019) Herbarium practices and ethics III. Syst Bot 44(1):7–13. https://doi.org/10.1600/036364419X697840

Rader L, Ison C (1999) Legacy of mercuric chloride. In: Metsger DA, Byers SC (eds) Managing the modern herbarium – an interdisciplinary approach. SPNHC, Ontario, pp 353–354

Radwańska-Paryska Z (1991) Zielnik Brata Cypriana z Czerwonego Klasztoru. Polish Botanical Studies, Guidebook series no. 5. Polska Akademia Nauk – Instytut Botaniki im. W. Szafera, Kraków

Rapini A (2014) Introduction to botanical taxonomy. In: Methods and techniques in ethnobiology and ethnoecology. Springer, New York, pp 123–139

Reeds KM (1976) Renaissance humanism and botany. Ann Sci 33(6):519–542. https://doi.org/10.1080/00033797600200481

Reeds K (2004) When the botanist can't draw: the case of Linnaeus. Interdiscip Sci Rev 29(3):248–258. https://doi.org/10.1179/030801804225018882

Reeds K, Kinukawa T (2013) Medieval natural history. In: Lindberg D, Shank M (eds) The Cambridge history of science. Cambridge University Press, Cambridge, pp 569–589. https://doi.org/10.1017/CHO9780511974007.026

Rix M (2013) The golden age of botanical art. University of Chicago Press, Kew

Rohland N, Siedel HA, Hofreiter M (2004) Nondestructive DNA extraction method for mitochondrial DNA analyses of museum specimens. BioTechniques 36:814–816, 818–821

Rostański K (1963) Historia Zielnika Instytutu Botanicznego Uniwersytetu Wrocławskiego. Acta Univ Wratislav Prace Bot I:283–304

Ryholt K (2013) The illustrated herbal from Tebtunis: new fragments and archeaeological context. Z Papyrol Epigr 187:233–238

Rytz W (1933) Das Herbarium Felix Platters. Ein Beitrag zur Geschichte der Botanik des XVI. Jahrhunderts. Separatabdruck aus den Verhandlungen der Naturforschenden Gesselschaft in Basel. Band XLIV, 1, Teil Basel. BuchdruckereiEmil Birkhäuser & Cie, Basel

Saint-Lager J (1885) Histoire des herbiers. J.-B, Baillère et fils, Paris

Salick J, Konchar K, Nesbitt M (2014) Biocultural collections: needs, ethics and goals. In: Salick J, Konchar K, Nesbitt M (eds) Curating biocultural collections: a handbook. Royal Botanic Gardens, Kew, pp 1–13

Schwarz Z (1986) Prywatne ogrody botaniczne a rozwój nauk przyrodniczych w ośrodku gdańskim w XVI–XVII wiekach. Kwart Hist Nauki Tech 31:411–444

Scott G, Hewett ML (2008) Pioneers in ethnopharmacology: the Dutch East India Company (VOC) at the Cape from 1650 to 1800. J Ethnopharmacol 115(3):339–360. https://doi.org/10.1016/j.jep.2007.10.020

Secretariat of the Convention on Biological Diversity (2011) Nagoya protocol on access to genetic resources and the fair and equitable sharing of benefits arising from their utilization (ABS) to the convention on biological diversity. https://www.cbd.int/abs/doc/protocol/nagoya-protocol-en.pdf. Accessed 5 Jan 2026

Shepherd LD (2017) A non-destructive DNA sampling technique for herbarium specimens. PLOS ONE 12(8):e0183555. https://doi.org/10.1371/journal.pone.0183555

Singer C (1927) The herbal in antiquity and its transmission to later ages. J Hell Stud 47:1–52. https://doi.org/10.2307/625251

Smith PH (2010) Artisanal knowledge and the representation of nature in sixteenth-century Germany. In: O'Malley T, Meyers ARW (eds) The art of natural history. Illustrated treatises and botanical paintings, 1400–1850. National Gallery of Arts, Washington, pp 15–31

Spalik K (2014a) Pre-Linnean herbaria viva of Helwing in the collections of the National Library of Poland and the University of Warsaw. Acta Soc Bot Pol 83(1):13–16. https://doi.org/10.5586/asbp.2014.008

Spalik K (2014b) Zielnik Georga Andreasa Helwinga, Part I and II. http://blog.polona.pl/2014/10/zielnik-helwinga-i/ oraz http://blog.polona.pl/2014/11/zielnik-helwinga-ii/. Accessed 21 Jan 2026

Stech M, van Andel T, Aptroot A, Bertin A, Stefanaki A (2018) Bryophytes and lichens in 16th-century herbaria. J Bryol 40(2):99–106. https://doi.org/10.1080/03736687.2018.1447304

Stefanaki A, Thijsse G, Uffelen, van GA, Eurlings MCM, Andel van T (2018) The En Tibi herbarium, a 16th century Italian treasure. Bot J Linn Soc 20:1–31

Stefanaki A, Porck H, Grimaldi IM, Thurn N, Pugliano V, Kardinaal A (2019) Breaking the silence of the 500-year-old smiling garden of everlasting flowers: the En Tibi book herbarium. PLoS One 14(6):e0217779. https://doi.org/10.1371/journal.pone.0217779

Strang TJK (1999a) A healthy dose of the past: a future direction in herbarium pest control? In: Metsger DA, Byers SC (eds) Managing the modern herbarium – an interdisciplinary approach. SPNHC, Ontario, pp 59–80

Strang TJK (1999b) Sensitivity of seeds in herbarium collections to storage conditions, and implications for thermal insect pest control methods. In: Metsger DA, Byers SC (eds) Managing the modern herbarium – an interdisciplinary approach. SPNHC, Ontario, pp 81–102

Stuchlik L (ed) (1998) Botanical collections throughout the world. Proceedings of the second international conference on the Preservation of Botanical Collections. Cracow, June 26–29, 1997. Instytut Botaniki Polskiej Akademii Nauk im. Władysława Szafera, Kraków

Swan C (2010) The uses of botanical treatises in the Netherlands, c. 1600. In: O'Malley T, Meyers ARW (eds) The art of natural history. Illustrated treatises and botanical paintings, 1400–1850. National Gallery of Arts, Washington, pp 63–81

Tabor A (2013) Geneza i dzieje Muzeum Przyrodniczego im. Dzieduszyckich we Lwowie. Opusc Musealia 21:189–207. https://doi.org/10.4467/20843852.OM.13.015.2925

Teasdale MD, van Doorn NL, Fiddyment S, Webb CC, O'Connor T, Hofreiter M, Collins MJ, Bradley DG (2015) Paging through history: parchment as a reservoir of ancient DNA for next generation sequencing. Philos Trans R Soc B 370(1660):20130379. https://doi.org/10.1098/rstb.2013.0379

Tebtunis Herbal (2026) University of California Berkeley Library Digital Collections. https://digicoll.lib.berkeley.edu/record/231633?ln=en&v=uv#?xywh=-2051%2C-257%2C7104%2C5137. Accessed 5 Jan 2026

The Oaxaca Declaration (1993). http://www.conabio.gob.mx/remib_ingles/doctos/declaracion_ing.html. Accessed 21 Jan 2026

Thiers B (2020) Herbarium: the quest to preserve & classify the world's plants. Timber Press, Portland

Thiers B (continuously updated) Index Herbariorum: a global directory of public herbaria and associated staff. New York Botanical Garden's Virtual Herbarium. http://sweetgum.nybg.org/science/ih/. Accessed 25 Jan 2026

Thijsse G (2016) Tusschen pampier geleyt, ontstaan, verspreiding en gebruik van de vroegste herbaria. In: IJapelaar I, Chavannes-Mazel LCA (eds) De gorene middeleeuwen. Duizend jaar gebruik van planten (600–1600). Lecturis B.V., Eindhoven, pp 64–93

Thijsse G (2018) A contribution to the history of the herbaria of George Clifford III (1685–1760). Arch Nat Hist 45(1):134–148. https://doi.org/10.3366/anh.2018.0489

Thijsse G, Wesseling M (2021) Herman Boerhaave: a search for his herbarium collections. Taxon 70(1):170–181. https://doi.org/10.1002/tax.12368

Thomsen PF, Elias S, Gilbert MT, Haile J, Munch K, Kuzmina S, Froese DG, Sher A, Holdaway RN, Willerslev E (2009) Nondestructive sampling of ancient insect DNA. PLoS One 4:e5048

Toresella S, Battini M (1988) Gli erbari a impressione e l'origine del disegno scientifico. Le Scienze 239:64–78

Touwaide A (2010) Botany and humanism in the renaissance: background, interaction, contradictions. In: O'Malley T, Meyers ARW (eds) The art of natural history. illustrated treatises and botanical paintings, 1400–1850. National Gallery of Arts, Washington, pp 33–61

Townsend J (1999) Preventive conservation: concept and strategy for long-term preservation. In: Metsger DA, Byers SC (eds) Managing the modern herbarium – an interdisciplinary approach. SPNHC, Ontario, pp 23–35

UNESCO (1972) World Heritage Convention. https://whc.unesco.org/en/conventiontext/. Accessed 25 Jan 2026

UNESCO (2001) UNESCO Universal Declaration on Cultural Diversity. https://www.unesco.org/en/legal-affairs/unesco-universal-declaration-cultural-diversity. Accessed 27 Jan 2026

UNESCO (2015a) Recommendation of concerning the protection and promotion of museums and collections, their diversity and their role in society. https://www.unesco.org/en/legal-affairs/recommendation-concerning-protection-and-promotion-museums-and-collections-their-diversity-and-their. Accessed 27 Jan 2026

UNESCO (2015b) Recommendation concerning the preservation of, and access to, documentary heritage including in digital form. https://www.unesco.org/en/legal-affairs/recommendation-concerning-preservation-and-access-documentary-heritage-including-digital-form. Accessed 27 Jan 2026

Vadon C (2013) Portraits de botanistes. In: Versini AR (ed) L'Herbier du Museum. L'aventure d'une collection. Muséum national d'Histoire naturelle, Paris

van Andel T, Barth N (2018) Paul Hermann's Ceylon Herbarium (1672–1679) at Leiden, the Netherlands. Taxon 67:977–988. https://doi.org/10.12705/675.8

van der Spiegel A (1606) Isagoges in rem herbariam libri duo. Paulus Meiettus, Padua (Patavia)

Wächter O (1962) The restoration of the 'Vienna Dioscorides'. Stud Conserv 7(1):22–26

Walker N, Hughes D (1994) Conservation and the herbarium: the Royle Herbarium – a conservation approach. In: Child RE (ed) Conservation and the herbarium. The Institute of Paper Conservation, Leigh, pp 35–41

Watson JD, Crick FHC (1953) A structure for deoxyribose nucleic acid. Nature 171:737–738. https://doi.org/10.1038/171737a0

Weitzmann K (ed) (1979) Age of spirituality. Late antique and early christian art. Third to seventh century. Princeton University Press, New York, pp 205–208

Willems FM, Scheepens JF, Bossdorf O (2022) Forest wildflowers bloom earlier as Europe warms: lessons from herbaria and spatial modelling. New Phytol 235(1):52–65. https://doi.org/10.1111/nph.18124

Williams C (2023) Access and benefit sharing legislation. In: Davies NMJ, Drinkell C, Utteridge TMA (eds) The herbarium handbook. Kew Publishing, Kew, pp 104–105

Willis CG, Ellwood E, Primack RB, Davis CC, Pearson KD, Gallinat AS, Yost J, Nelson G, Mazer S, Rossington N, Sparks T, Soltis P (2017) Old plants, new tricks: phenological research using herbarium specimens. Trends in Ecology and Evolution 32(7):531–546. https://doi.org/10.1016/j.tree.2017.03.015

Wójcik Z (2001) Siemiatycki Gabinet Historii Naturalnej Anny Jabłonowskiej. In: Księżna Anna z Sapiehów Jabłonowska. W dwusetną rocznicę zgonu, praca zbiorowa pod redakcją A. Wołek, Z.J. Wójcik. Towarzystwo Przyjaciół Siemiatycz, Urząd Miasta Siemiatycze, Siemiatycki Ośrodek Kultury, Siemiatycze, pp 104–105

Xu C, Dong W, Shi S, Cheng T, Li C, Liu Y, Wu P, Wu H, Gao P, Zhou S (2015) Accelerating plant DNA barcode reference library construction using herbarium specimens: improved experimental techniques. Mol Ecol Res 15:1366–1374. https://doi.org/10.1111/1755-0998.12413

Yoshida K, Burbano HA, Krause J, Thines M, Weigel D, Kamoun (2014) Mining herbaria for plant pathogen genomes: back to the future. PLoS Pathog 10(4):e1004028. https://doi.org/10.1371/journal.ppat.1004028

Young D (2023a) Repairing and cleaning. In: Davies NMJ, Drinkell C, Utteridge TMA (eds) The herbarium handbook. Kew Publishing, Kew, pp 150–151
Young D (2023b) Remounting specimens. In: Davies NMJ, Drinkell C, Utteridge TMA (eds) The herbarium handbook. Kew Publishing, Kew, pp 152–153
Zawartko-Laskowska M (2008) Mecenat naukowy Stanisława Augusta i jego przyrodnicze pasje. Kron Zamk 1–2(55–56):66–112
Zemanek A (1996) Odnalezienie prawdopodobnych śladów pierwszego polskiego zielnika królewny Anny Wazówny. Kwart Hist Nauki Tech 41(3–4):197–205
Zemanek A (1997) Botanika renesansu w świetle współczesnej nauki. Wiad Bot 41(1):7–19
Zemanek A (2009) O symbiozie nauki i sztuki w czasach Renesansu–kolekcja obrazów roślin ze zbioru "Libri picturati" A. 18–30. Prace Komisji Historii Nauki Polskiej Akademii Umiejętności 9:181–207
Zych M, Dolatowski J, Kirpluk I, Werblan-Jakubiec H (2023) A "plant love story": the lost (and found) private herbarium of the radical socialist revolutionary Rosa Luxemburg. Plants People Planet 5(6):852–858. https://doi.org/10.1002/ppp3.10396

Chapter 2
Techniques and Technology of Herbarium Preparation and Structure

Abstract This chapter describes various technological aspects of herbarium preparation, including their form and methods of production, as well as the physicochemical characteristics of the main components, with particular emphasis on the shared structural features of plant specimens and the paper substrate. The description of techniques includes references to historical methods of herbarium preparation. The chapter lists many techniques that are no longer in use, assuming that technological information is important not only for planning the preservation and conservation of herbarium collections, but also for designing research involving herbaria.

Keywords Herbarium techniques · Herbarium structure · Herbarium preparation · Herbarium adhesives · Specimen structure

Publications addressing technological aspects that serve as sources of information on materials present in herbarium collections predominantly concern the creation of new collections and their management, as well as methods for their preservation. These texts, in addition to describing contemporary practices related to the creation of herbaria, also refer to historical methods of their production.[1] They also provide valuable insights into the history of herbarium collections, as many old publications mention outdated preservation methods. Some of these works are focused on

[1] In addition to conference proceedings and publications specifically focused on conservation, these also include, among others, historical works containing technological information: (Spiegel 1606; Tournefort 1694; Linnaeus 1751); contemporary textbooks: (Bridson and Forman 1999; Drobnik 2009; Davies et al. 2023); and articles: (Robinson 1903; Merrill 1926, 1948; Archer 1952; Fassett 1952; Rollins 1955; Gates 2009; Eusebio and Stern 1964; Sharp 1964; Whitmore and Fosberg 1965; Lundell and Kirkham 1966; DeWolf 1968; Stern et al. 1968; Lellinger 1972; Croat 1978; Tillet 1979, 1989; Schofield and Crisafulli 1980; Briggs et al. 1983; Hill 1983; Hall 1988; Purewal 1999, 2001; Purewal et al. 2008; Shchepanek 2001; Hawks et al. 2004; Oyarzun et al. 2007; Kataeva et al. 2008; Yesilyurt 2009; Webber et al. 2011; Havermans et al. 2015; Fallon et al. 2016; Kaczkowski et al. 2017; Yesilyurt et al. 2025)—to mention only those publications cited in the present work.

M. Grenda-Kurmanow, *Herbaria*, https://doi.org/10.1007/978-3-032-21904-6_2

specific technological topics, such as the use of biocidal agents and various adhesives for mounting specimens.

The fundamental techniques for preparing herbaria have changed little since the sixteenth century. The main differences concern the development of methods for drying fungi and mosses, the availability of professional equipment for drying and pressing specimens, and the materials used for their mounting. Nevertheless, as other authors have noted, a sixteenth-century botanist would have no difficulty using a twenty-first-century herbarium (Ogilvie 2006, p. 165; Drobnik 2009, p. 7). This chapter focuses on the diversity of techniques and materials found in herbaria, which may be of key importance for those involved in the preservation and conservation of collections.

The first herbarium preparation instruction cited in the chapter *The Earliest Guidelines for Creating Herbaria* is highly detailed: Spiegel recommends gradually drying plants between sheets of absorbent paper, replacing the paper as needed, and storing the specimens in this manner until a larger collection has been assembled.[2] He then describes mounting the specimens onto paper using hide glue with the addition of clove oil and aloe extract. The adhered plant should be manually pressed into the sheet and any excess glue blotted with another piece of paper or cloth. The specimen should be left sandwiched between absorbent layers of paper or fabric under pressure until completely dry.[3]

The method of drying specimens between the pages of books, as described by him, appears to be the most natural and probably the earliest way of drying plants for herbarium purposes. However, in the process of refining herbarium techniques, many practices were employed that would no longer be considered acceptable today, such as the previously mentioned ironing of specimens, assembling a single specimen from several different individuals of the same or other species, stylising an "ideal" image of the plant, and painting in missing parts. Another practice, also previously mentioned, was the "preservation" of the plant's natural colours using a layer of paint.[4]

Although plants were most commonly adhered to paper substrates, this was not the only method used for storing dried specimens. Plants could also be stored loose or sewn onto paper. These approaches entailed various challenges related to the long-term preservation of such collections. Additionally, plants were protected against insect and microbial infestation using a range of biocidal agents, which were either added to the adhesives used to mount specimens (as in the case of Spiegel,

[2] As previously mentioned, according to Saint-Lager, the development of herbarium techniques is linked to the spread of paper production in Europe (Saint-Lager 1885, pp. 23–30). By the end of the sixteenth century, European papermaking, which can be traced back at least to the twelfth century, was already a highly developed craft, and paper mills were operating in most European countries (Dąbrowski and Siniarska-Czaplicka 1991, pp. 69–88).

[3] (Spiegel 1606, pp. 79–81), full translation of Spiegel's text in the section *The Earliest Guidelines for Creating Herbaria* in Chap. 1.

[4] Described further in the section *Additional Procedures Used in the Preparation and Examination of Specimens* in Chap. 2.

who used clove oil for this purpose) or applied directly to the specimens by various methods.[5] This also significantly impacts on their condition. It should also be noted that herbaria, in addition to their obvious botanical content, are to a large extent, from a technological perspective, also classified as manuscripts and are catalogued as such in libraries and archives.

The following chapters describe various technological aspects of herbarium specimen preparation,[6] as well as the physicochemical characteristics of the main components of herbaria, with particular emphasis on the similarities and differences between the properties of plant specimens and the paper substrate.

2.1 Techniques and Technology of Herbarium Preparation[7]

2.1.1 Specimen Collection

Until around the mid-twentieth century, plants were collected in the field using a cylindrical metal container (Latin *vasculum*, "a small vessel") (Allen 1965; Thiers 2020). Storing plants in a *vasculum* was intended to prevent them from wilting. Other containers used included bags made of leather or waterproofed canvas, and from the mid-twentieth century, plastic bags (Drobnik 2009, pp. 9–10). Plants could also be collected into envelopes carried in a plastic bag, after preliminary flattening (Drobnik 2009, pp. 59–60), interleaved with newspapers and wrapped in plastic, or placed directly in thin packets between mesh frames for drying.[8] Detailed collection procedures depend on the species and the purpose of the collection.[9] Some of the

[5] A discussion of biocidal agents and their methods of application is provided in Chap. 3, dedicated to degradation processes, section *Damage Caused by the Use of Biocidal Agents* in Chap. 3.

[6] The description of the technology omits, among others, microalgae herbaria, which are prepared and preserved on glass substrates in a specific manner, as well as seed collections and carpological herbaria, which are stored in various types of containers. The descriptions focus on herbarium specimens mounted on paper sheets.

[7] The sections *Specimen Collection*, *Drying of Specimens*, and *Additional Procedures Used in the Preparation and Examination of Specimens* in Chap. 2 are based primarily on information from comprehensive manuals on herbarium preparation (Bridson and Forman 1999; Drobnik 2009; Davies et al. 2023). The authors of these publications provide numerous references to additional sources, including older manuals. In selected cases, additional publications are cited, taking into account historical techniques of herbarium preparation. As previously mentioned, knowledge of herbarium preparation techniques and technologies may be crucial for those involved in their preservation and conservation. Technological information is also important for designing research utilising herbarium collections.

[8] A technique still in use today; see the description in the following subsection.

[9] The principles of collecting individual plant species have been described in detail, among others, in the aforementioned comprehensive textbook publications on herbaria (Bridson and Forman 1999; Drobnik 2009; Davies et al. 2023). In this work, herbarium preparation techniques are described, with particular attention to the potential physical conditions and the chemical substances used, both currently and in the past, as part of the process of preparing a plant as a herbarium specimen.

basic principles state that collection should not be carried out during rain, and that small, delicate specimens should not be transported or field-dried together with large, bulky ones (Drobnik 2009, p. 60). The highest-quality specimens can be obtained using a field mesh press, while lower-quality results from transporting specimens loosely in a plastic bag.

Before drying, the collected plant should be cleaned of soil clumps, cobwebs, insects, remnants of other plants, silt, and deposits. For aquatic plants, this can be achieved by rinsing the specimen (Drobnik 2009, p. 78). Nevertheless, in some collections, one may encounter specimens that have not been thoroughly cleaned, and thus bear accumulations such as soil clumps or traces of insect activity.

2.1.2 Drying of Specimens

The drying process for specimens may vary depending on the plant species collected, the climatic conditions on the day of collection, the type of materials used for drying, and the quantity of collected material. Drying conditions (currently within the range of 20–40 °C) ensure that a slight amount of water remains in the plant tissues, which depends on the prevailing climatic conditions (Drobnik 2009, p. 65).

The earliest texts on herbarium preparation recommend drying specimens between absorbent papers in loose sheets or in thick books, weighted down with other books (Spiegel 1606, p. 81; Tournefort 1694, pp. 547–548).[10] For rapid drying of specimens, ironing through layers of grey paper was also employed. Tournefort describes this as a method suitable for rural conditions, where books may be less readily available (Tournefort 1694, p. 548; see also Linnaeus 1751, p. 7).

Preliminary drying was often carried out in the field, using additional treatments[11] and field presses. Currently, after collection, following initial shaping and arrangement into the desired form, specimens are placed between layers of newspaper or blotting paper. After covering with another layer of newspaper, blotting paper, a board or piece of cardboard, followed by further layers of absorbent paper or blotting paper, are placed on top with the specimen in the centre. Smaller pieces of paper may be inserted between overlapping plant parts. The layers of newspaper or blotting paper should be changed more frequently at first (once a day), and less often later. For specimens with large leaves, more frequent changes of blotting paper ensure a better specimen shape (improved flattening) and better colour retention. Maintaining tissue continuity, in turn, provides greater durability of the specimen after drying. Individual, more hydrated or mucilage-rich parts of the specimen could be dried on separate pieces of blotting paper, to which they would adhere

[10] According to this principle, plants from the oldest known Polish herbarium, prepared by Anna Vasa (1568–1625), were dried on separate sheets of paper, including uncut sheets from the printed *Herbarium* by Szymon Syreniusz from 1613 (Zemanek 1996).

[11] Described in the following section.

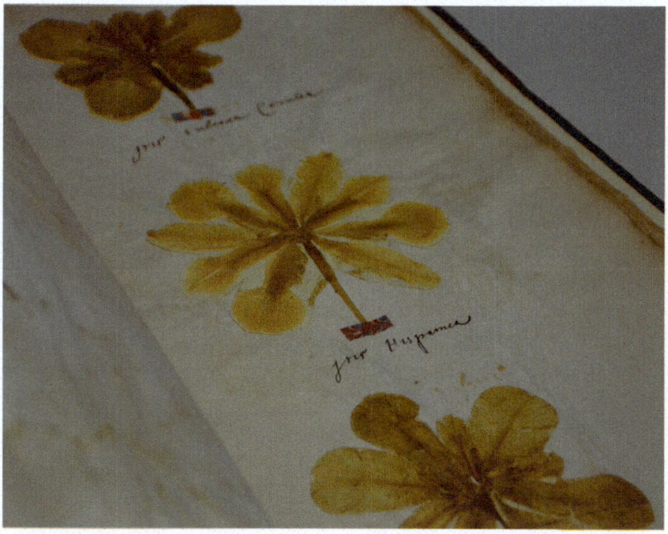

Fig. 2.1 Irises dried on additional layers of paper, cut to the shape of the specimens and mounted together with them. Boerhaave Herbarium, [Boerhaave H., (*Boerhaave Herbarium*, Leiden, Naturalis Biodiversity Center (L), ref. L.2077675, eighteenth century]. (Photo: M. Grenda-Kurmanow)

naturally and be mounted together with them on the final herbarium sheet (Fig. 2.1) (Drobnik 2009, pp. 71–72; Wilbraham 2023).

Thick parts of the specimen, such as roots, shoots, bulbs and tubers, as well as fleshy fruits and fungi, may be cut open before drying or sliced, and after drying, attached to the herbarium sheet (Drobnik 2009, pp. 75–78). The weight applied to the stack of flattened specimens should not be excessive, as this helps to prevent damage to the specimens and allows for better air circulation. Interleaving papers are often reused. They may also have been soaked in a weak solution of table salt to better preserve the colours of the specimens.[12]

In the 1950s, Józef Mądalski developed an original drying model involving the use of wire grids (meshes) placed at the beginning and end of the stack instead of boards (Mądalski 1951, 1955, 1958).[13] The bundle, enclosed with meshes, is then tied with string or compressed using clips or clamps. The use of meshes allows for rapid air circulation and, in some cases, enables drying without the need to replace papers, particularly when specimens are dried in small, manageable bundles (7–10 cm). This method is still widely used for drying specimens, especially in the field and under tropical conditions where humidity is high. The described press is known as the *Madalski press* or *Polish press* (Bridson and Forman 1999,

[12] A method used, for example, at the Department of Botany, University of Rzeszów, as reported by Professor Krzysztof Oklejewicz in 2015.

[13] The Mądalski method has gained great popularity and is cited by many authors, including many textbooks and manuals on herbarium preparation.

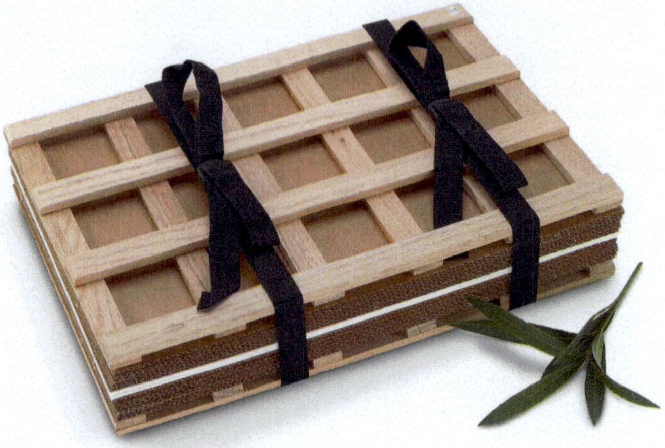

Fig. 2.2 Classic field botanical press

pp. 222–223). The prototype for the wire mesh was the botanical press in the form of frame-grids made from wooden, rattan, or bamboo slats, bound with straps or buckles (Fig. 2.2). The bundle could also be enclosed with plywood or thick cardboard, although this did not provide as effective air circulation as the grids. All of the mentioned types of presses are still in use today. A modification of the Mądalski press involves drying large stacks between grids and tying them with a string. Using grids in this way enables a clamping method of drying instead of pressing the stack from above (Fig. 2.3).

During field drying, specimen bundles compressed in botanical presses were exposed to temperatures of approximately 35–45 °C (Bridson and Forman 1999, pp. 221–222), while current recommendations advise not exceeding 50–60 °C (Briggs and Damas 2023a). Drying methods include the use of gas or electric heaters, or placing the press (or individual specimens, e.g. in the case of fungi) near a campfire. Presses filled with specimens were dried using any available field methods, including exposure to sunlight, and even by transporting them on a car roof rack (Bridson and Forman 1999, pp. 221–222). Fungal specimens could be dried in a desiccator in the presence of calcium chloride (Bridson and Forman 1999, p. 244).

Drying can also be carried out in specialised drying ovens, which is used when the relative humidity after collection exceeds 65% (for example, on rainy days). The drying ovens served as containers that provided circulation of warm air at 30–40 °C, achieved in various ways: of convection currents, blowers, gas heating, and infrared lamps. Specimens were placed inside in batches wrapped in mesh. Drying lasted 1–2 days, and in the case of succulents, several days (Drobnik 2009, pp. 83–85). Briggs and Damas (2023a), recommend a drying temperature in the range of 40–60 °C.

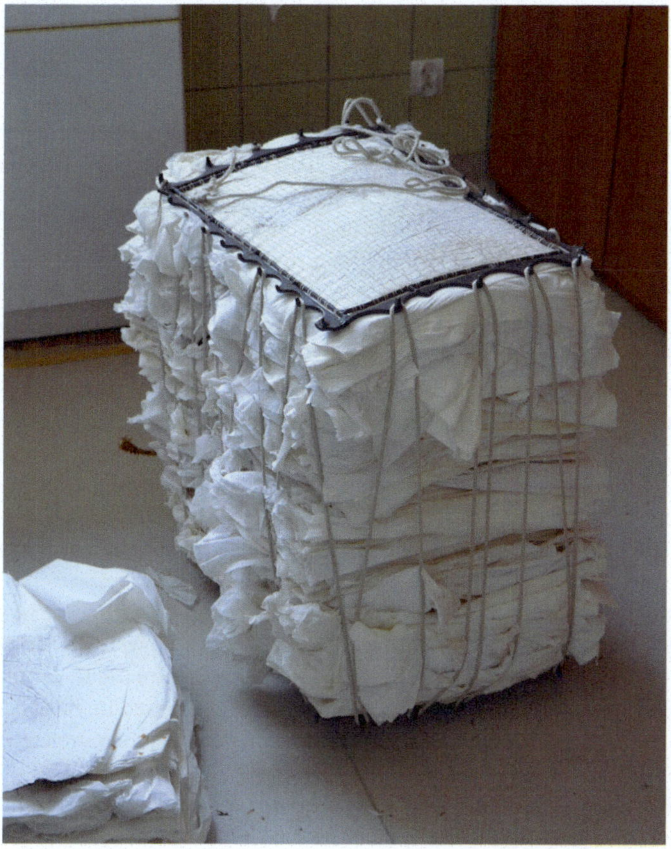

Fig. 2.3 Modification of the Mądalski press. Drying in large batches requires changing the blotting papers, but does not require top pressure and allows for stacking in high piles. Laboratory at the Department of Botany, University of Rzeszów, 2015. (Photo: M. Grenda-Kurmanow)

Studies on the durability of herbarium specimens have shown that high temperatures accelerate the degradation of dried plants, citing drying temperatures as high as 60 °C as examples (e.g. Lindahl and Nyberg 1972; Kumar et al. 2000; Marota et al. 2002; Staats et al. 2011).[14]

[14] For information on the detrimental effects of temperature on herbarium specimens, see the sections *Thermal Degradation*, *Degradation of Genetic Material* in Chap. 3 and *Integrated Pest Management (IPM) for Herbarium Collections* in Chap. 4.

2.1.3 *Additional Procedures Used in the Preparation and Examination of Specimens*

Specimens that wilted during collection were soaked in water to flatten them or stored in a refrigerator at approximately 10 °C in plastic bags (Drobnik 2009, pp. 67–68; Bridson and Forman 1999, p. 233).[15]

Plants that could not be completely dried immediately after collection could be stored between sheets soaked in 60–95% ethyl alcohol, wrapped in plastic bags ("Schweinfurth method"). The sheets or entire bundles of compressed plants were also sometimes soaked in formaldehyde, paraformaldehyde, or pentachlorophenol in alcohol (Coradin and Giannasi 1980). Such prepared bundles could be kept for up to six weeks before final drying.[16]

For succulents and fleshy plants (for example, from the families *Cactaceae, Aloaceae, Euphorbiaceae*), tissue was killed using various methods, such as putting in hot water, boiling, prolonged freezing, or storage in alcohol, petrol, or a microwave oven.[17] The cut tissue parts were also sprinkled with salt, which was removed from the specimen after the water had been extracted (Bridson and Forman 1999, p. 196; Drobnik 2009, p. 85).

For many plants, flowers (including those of *Aristolochiaceae*, *Balsaminaceae*) or entire plants (such as *Balanophoraceae*, *Burmanniaceae*) were preserved in spirit immediately after collection, until final drying (Bridson and Forman 1999, pp. 197–203).[18] Conifer specimens were sometimes immersed in 70% alcohol, followed by a 50% aqueous solution of glycerol, to prevent disintegration (Bridson and Forman 1999, pp. 197–203).

Marine plants may be rinsed for several hours prior to drying in order to remove salts. To eliminate bacteria from plants washed ashore, hot water with soap was used, sometimes with the addition of sodium hypochlorite (NaClO) or copper(II) sulfate.

[15] There are historical records confirming that soaking dried plants was frequently practised by early naturalists, for example by Mattioli, in order to "revive the plant" (Saint-Lager 1885, pp. 15–17). William Burchell (1781–1863) soaked his specimens eight years after collection to incorporate them into his herbarium. Previously, they had been stored in bundles of specific dimensions, which were dried collectively between sheets of paper (Nowak-Kemp 2018).

[16] See also Briggs and Damas (2023b). Most authors consider alcohol and the use of preservative fluids containing alcohol to be detrimental to the preservation of genetic material in botanical specimens (Bridson and Forman 1999, p. 292–293; Salick and Solomon 2014; Briggs and Damas 2023b). See the section *The Impact of Storage Conditions and Historical Preservation Methods on DNA* in Chap. 3. Furthermore, Coradin and Giannasi demonstrated that storing specimens in preservative fluids within sealed plastic packaging results in the chromatographic extraction of flavonoids from the specimens onto adjacent newspapers, leading to the loss of the so-called chemotaxonomic profile characteristic of a given species, as well as colour changes in the specimens (Coradin and Giannasi 1980).

[17] The destructive effects of microwaves are described in the section *Microwaves* in Chap. 4.

[18] See also Davies et al. (2023, pp. 40–43).

Specimens from the *Asteraceae* family may contain insects or their eggs within the flower heads. For this reason, they may be subjected to prophylactic freezing at approximately −20 °C prior to incorporation into the herbarium (Bridson and Forman 1999, p. 77).[19]

To preserve the colours of specimens and prevent them from blackening, at the beginning of the twentieth century it was recommended to expose fresh specimens to sulphur fumes for one hour. Soaking flower corollas in petrol was also practised (Bridson and Forman 1999, p. 87). Aquatic plants were sometimes soaked in a solution that helped maintain their natural colour. For this purpose, copper(II) sulphate $CuSO_4$ was used at a concentration of 2–5%. A precipitate forms from the solution, which should be removed while wet, after which the specimen could be dried between sheets of paper or blotting paper (Drobnik 2009, p. 80).

An unusual and rarely practised technique was to paint over specimens after mounting them on a sheet, in order to "preserve" or rather "commemorate" their colour. A remarkable example of this is found in the herbaria of Johann Friedrich Zeidler from the first half of the eighteenth century, in which four different colouring substances have so far been identified (Figs. 2.4–2.6).[20] A similar case was discovered in a herbarium from the second half of the eighteenth century, compiled by Agostino Coltellini, held in the collections of the Museo di Storia Naturale dell'Università di Firenze (FI) (Nepi 2008) and in the collections of the Natural History Museum in London, also dated c. 1750.

Herbarium specimens have been, and continue to be, subjected to treatments that facilitate the examination of their morphology, after which they are returned to the herbarium collection. As with wilted plants after collection, specimens were

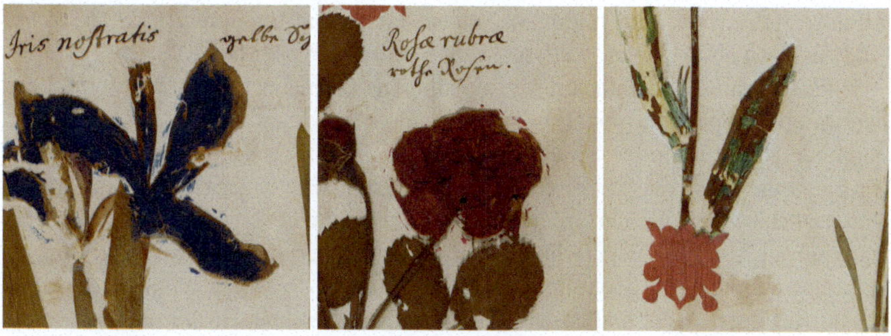

Figs. 2.4–2.6 Examples of the use of pigments and dyes to "preserve" the colours of specimens in Johann Friedrich Zeidler's herbarium (Zeidler J. F., *Hortus Perennis...*, Lublin, Main Library of the University of Life Sciences, Vol. I, ref. Zb. Specj. I Starodruki 14, D. 104.57.646, 1732). (Photo: T. Rizov-Ciechański)

[19] See also the section *Freezing* in Chap. 4.

[20] See also the section *Conservation Objectives* in Chap. 5, concerning the technology and preservation state of the Zeidler herbarium.

rehydrated in water. Additionally, softening procedures were employed, such as immersing the specimen in boiling water—sometimes with the addition of ammonia—or boiling a fragment of the plant in water for 1–2 min, or using Pohl's solution: a 1% aqueous-alcoholic (3:1) solution of the detergent sodium 1,4-bis-(2-ethylhexyl)-sulfosuccinate (Drobnik 2009, p. 22; King 2023).[21] After treatment and drying, the specimen was returned to the herbarium. Putting in hot water was also used to improve the appearance of poorly flattened specimens (Drobnik, p. 90).

2.1.4 *Mounting Specimens on Sheets*

After drying the specimen, which typically takes several days with successive replacement of blotting paper or other interleaving materials, the plant is mounted onto the herbarium sheet. Until the mid-eighteenth century, these were mainly pages from codices—bound volumes produced according to the papermaking and bookbinding techniques of the time.[22] Consequently, the paper used in bound herbaria is often high-quality laid paper, made from rags and long-fibre plant material. After the mid-eighteenth century, herbarium collections in the form of codex continued to be produced, but they became less common. The materials used for these were generally of poor quality, reflecting changes in papermaking technology introduced in the mid-nineteenth century. As a result, machine-made papers from wood pulp, characterised by high brittleness and low mechanical strength, were used as a substrate for specimens.[23] Current recommendations are to use wood-free, acid-free, and sulphur-free or even buffered papers, made from cotton fibres or high-quality cellulose pulp, for sheets (mounts), covers, labels, and mounting strips (DeWolf 1968; Bridson and Forman 1999, p. 31; Drobnik 2009, pp. 106–107).

Since the mid-eighteenth century, a method that remains popular today has been increasingly employed: mounting specimens on individual sheets of heavy paper, which are stored in protective covers or folders, usually made from thinner paper. The paper used for covers is often semi-translucent, allowing for convenient organisation of the sheets without frequently opening of the cover. Sheets within covers can be grouped into folders, which in turn are collected in fascicles, depending on the policy adopted by a given institution.[24]

The specimens were and are stored on sheets in various ways. Frequently, they were not attached to the sheets at all, lying loose between the pages of a bound

[21] The author provides several of the many trade names for the detergent: AOT, Aerosol OT, Docusate sodium.

[22] See the section *Forms of Appearance and Storage of Herbarium Sheets* in Chap. 2.

[23] The processes of paper and botanical specimen degradation are described in Chap. 3.

[24] See the section *Forms of Appearance and Storage of Herbarium Sheets* in Chap. 2.

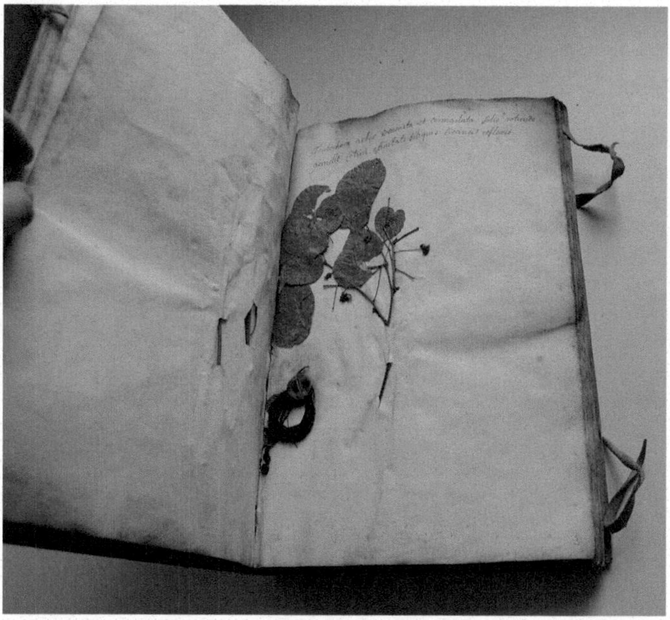

Fig. 2.7 Mounting by incising the sheet and threading the specimen through. Begon M., *Herbier Begon*, Paris, Muséum national d'Histoire naturelle (P), without ref. no., second half of the seventeenth century. (Photo: M. Grenda-Kurmanow)

volume, in individual gatherings, or in herbarium folders.[25] Such collections are often interpreted as working material, which was yet to be organised and processed into a developed herbarium.

Mounting could also be performed without adhesives. The simplest adhesive--free method involved making a slit in the sheet across the axis of the herbarium specimen and threading the specimen through the incisions (Fig. 2.7).

Another method utilising only paper material entailed making slits parallel to the axis of the specimen and threading paper strips through these slits (Fig. 2.8).[26]

[25] An example of this is, for instance, the herbarium of Caspar Bauhin (Saint-Lager 1885, pp. 50–51), as well as the herbaria of Boretius, e.g. Helwing A.J. or Boretius M., untitled, Warsaw, Herbarium of the Faculty of Biology, University of Warsaw (WA), ref. WA-KH-13.2.2, 1724–1745; "Treviranus Herbarium": N.n., (*Treviranus Herbarium*), Wrocław, Herbarium of the Museum of Natural History in Wrocław (WRSL), no reference number, undated; the herbarium of Józef Jundziłł: Jundziłł J., (*Herbarium of Józef Jundziłł*), Kraków, Herbarium of the Institute of Botany, Polish Academy of Sciences in Kraków (KRAM), no reference number, 1820s, with specimens dated from the eighteenth century to 1876; or the herbarium of Marian Raciborski: Raciborski M., (*Herbarium of Marian Raciborski*), Kraków, Herbarium of the Institute of Botany, Jagiellonian University (KRA), reference numbers for individual sheets, 1896–1900. Some researchers suggest that, in the case of early naturalists, this was a deliberate practice, allowing for subsequent soaking of the specimen, as described in the previous chapter (Ogilvie 2006, p. 212).

[26] See also the section about the conservation treatment of the Helwing/Boretius herbarium in Chap. 5.

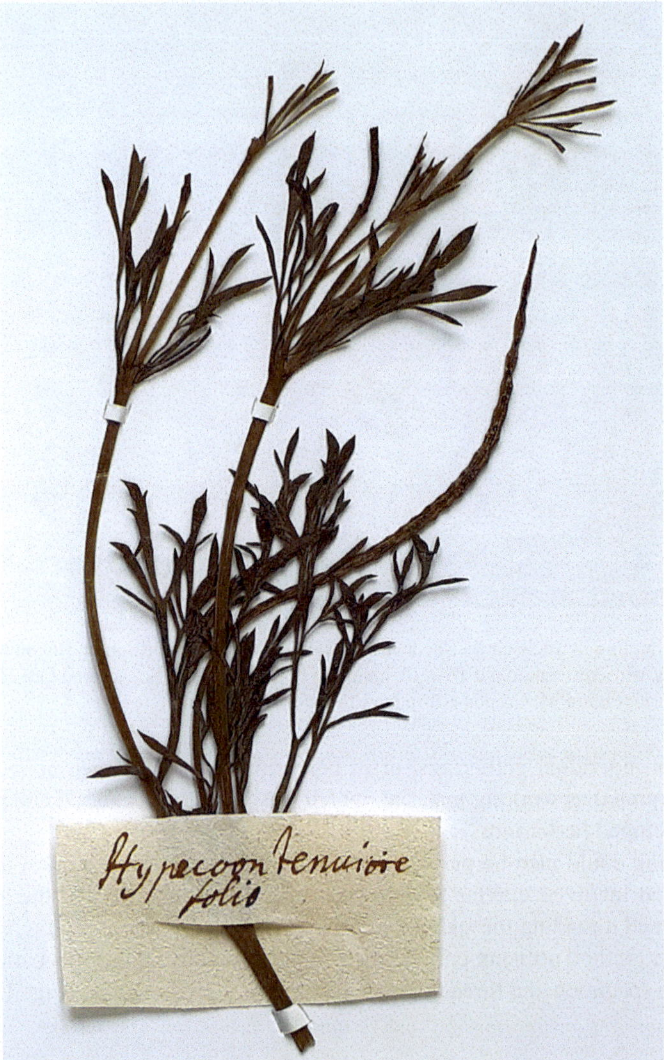

Fig. 2.8 Contemporary adhesive-free mounting of a historical specimen by threading paper strips through incisions in the sheet. Specimen from the Helwing/Boretius herbarium [Helwing A.J. or Boretius M., untitled, Warsaw, Herbarium of the Faculty of Biology, University of Warsaw (WA), ref. WA-KH-13.2.2, 1724–1745 (modern backing)]. (Photo: M. Grenda-Kurmanow)

In a modification involving adhesive, the threaded ends of the strips could be adhered to the *recto* of the sheet. Incisions could also be made in the centre of a large leaf (Fig. 2.9).

Further adhesive-free methods included securing the specimen with a pin, often piercing a paper strip (Fig. 2.10), as well as using staples, paper clips, and other similar metal elements.

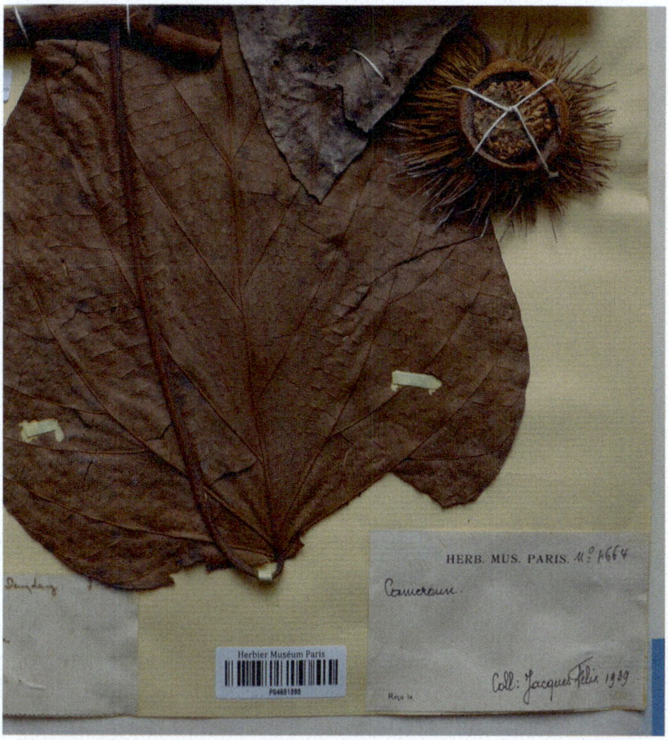

Fig. 2.9 Strips threaded through a slit leaf of the specimen and secured by stitching. Felix J., untitled, Paris, Muséum national d'Histoire naturelle (P), ref. MNHN-P-P04691898, 1939. (Photo: M. Grenda-Kurmanow)

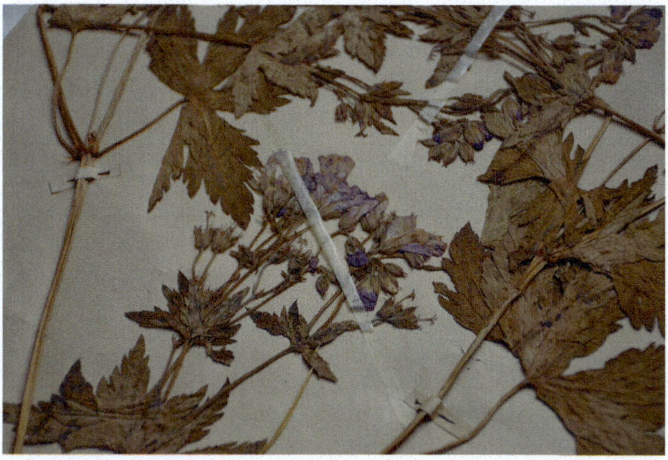

Fig. 2.10 Mounting using pins and straps. Retz, de B., untitled, Paris, Muséum national d'Histoire naturelle (P), ref. MNHN-P-P04892559, 1936. (Photo: M. Grenda-Kurmanow)

Fig. 2.11 Mounting by stitching. N.n., *Herbarium Vivum…*, [Izabela Czartoryska Herbarium], Kraków, National Museum in Kraków, Czartoryski Princes Library, ref. Rkps 2782, 1746. (Photo: M. Grenda-Kurmanow)

A fairly common and still used adhesive-free method is to sew specimens onto the sheet (Figs. 2.11 and 2.12).[27] This technique is particularly useful for bulky specimens. The ends of the thread were sometimes secured on the *verso* of the sheet with paper or textile tape.

The most common method of mounting specimens has been, and still remains, the use of paper, thread, or textile straps attached with various types of adhesives.[28] Mounting with paper straps is among the oldest techniques, although early herbarium authors considered it less durable and useful than adhering the entire surface of the plant to the substrate.[29] The strips could be glued along their entire length or just at the edges, in such a way that the specimen did not come into direct contact with the adhesive. From the eighteenth century onwards, decorative vase-shaped labels, attached at the base of the specimen (see Figs. 2.13 and 2.14), were used as a complement to strip mounting.

Mounting with straps was often combined with the equally common method, already mentioned, of attaching specimens directly to the substrate *recto* (Yesilyurt et al. 2025). These are, in fact, the two oldest mounting techniques, and they remain

[27] The oldest known surviving herbarium in which specimens are sewn onto paper is a French herbarium from 1558, created by Jehan Girault (Thijsse 2016); Girault J., untitled, Paris, Muséum national d'histoire naturelle (P), without ref. number, 1558.

[28] See the list of adhesives in the following section.

[29] As Thijsse reports, in the preface to one of his herbaria, currently held in the Bibliotheca Apostolica Vaticana in Rome, Hieronymus Harder (Harder H., untitled, Rome, Bibliotheca Apostolica Vaticana, ref. Pal. Lat. 1276, 1574) refers to foreign herbaria as "(…) of inferior quality, because the plants are mounted with strips rather than glued to the paper (…)" (Thijsse 2016).

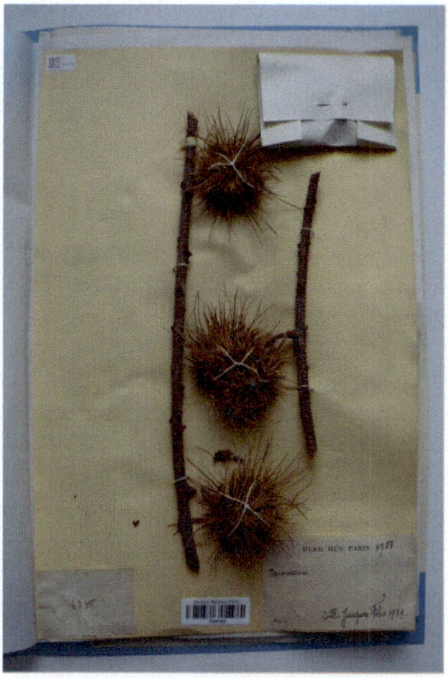

Fig. 2.12 Attachment by stitching. Felix J., untitled, Paris, Muséum national d'Histoire naturelle (P), ref. MNHN-P-P04691899, 1939. (Photo: M. Grenda-Kurmanow)

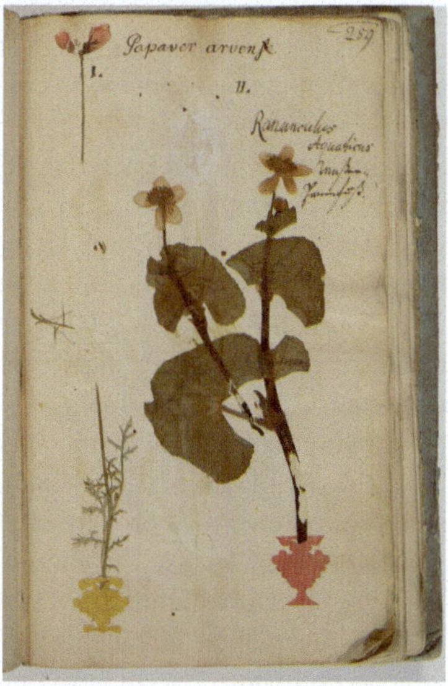

Fig. 2.13 Herbarium sheet of Johann Friedrich Zeidler (Zeidler J.F., *Hortus Perennis*…, Lublin, Main Library of the University of Life Sciences, Vol. I, ref. Special Collections and Early Printed Books 14, D. 104.57.646, 1732. Decorative labels are visible at the base of the specimens, cut from ornamental paper. (Photo: T. Rizov-Ciechański)

widely used. Direct application of the adhesive can be performed either at specific points or across the entire surface (coating the entire specimen). Various types of glue have been used for this purpose.[30] The adhesive could be applied with a brush,

---

[30] See the next section.

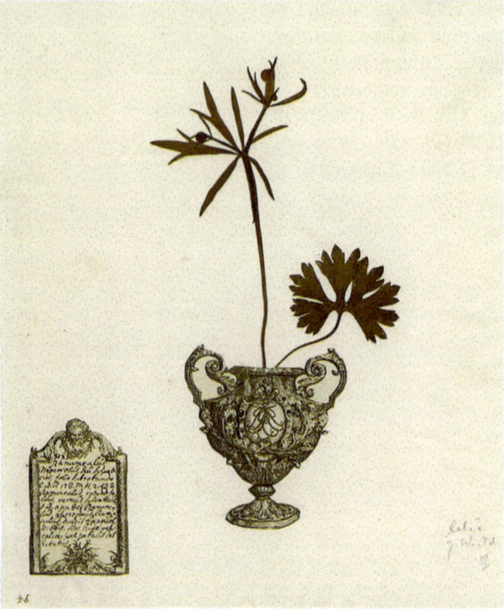

Fig. 2.14 Sheet from the herbarium of George Clifford III: Clifford III G., (*Clifford Herbarium*), Leiden, Naturalis Biodiversity Center (L), ref. WAG0271984, first half of the eighteenth century. A vase cut out from a graphic print is visible

an applicator, or spread onto a glass, ceramic, or foil surface, onto which the specimen was then placed. For selected small and delicate parts of the specimen, glue was applied using a paper strip coated with adhesive or the edge of a knife (Bridson and Forman 1999, pp. 76–77; Drobnik 2009, pp. 98–100). A modification of the strap mounting method was the Archer method, used in the 1950s–1980s, in which segments of synthetic "Archer glue" thread replaced paper straps.[31] This adhesive was also used for both overall and spot adhesion of specimens. However, it was highly toxic and was unequivocally recognised as hazardous (Down 1999; Croat 1978; Grenda-Kurmanow 2021).[32] Other materials used for strap mounting included fragments of adhesive tape, which over time often underwent detrimental degradation.

In many cases, more than one type of mounting was used simultaneously in herbaria (Yesilyurt et al. 2025), which has a significant impact on the preservation state and physico-chemical properties of historical herbaria.

If adhesive was used to mount the specimen, the sheet was then stacked with other sheets and weighted down. Along with the herbarium specimen, a label containing information about the specimen was usually attached to the sheet, sometimes accompanied by an envelope with specimen fragments, and nowadays also a barcode. Finally, a cover or sheet wrapper is attached (glued) to the sheet.

[31] The method was first described by Archer (1950) and later cited by numerous authors (see Table 2.1). The composition of the adhesive has undergone modifications (see the following section). Thick *hot-melt glues* have also been used in a similar manner.

[32] See also the following section.

2.1.4.1 Materials Used for Mounting Herbarium Specimens

Almost all of the previously mentioned mounting methods are still in use today, with the exception of discredited metal elements and industrial adhesive tapes, as well as certain adhesives. The discontinuation of these materials is widely attributed to their recognised detrimental effects on herbarium specimens and the unfavourable ageing of mounting materials (such as metal corrosion, detachment of mounts, yellowing of adhesives, and adverse health effects associated with mounting materials), as well as the disappearance of some glues or their components from the market.

2.1.4.1.1 Threads

Linen and cotton threads have been and continue to be used for mounting. Bridson and Forman recommend smooth-finished linen threads and suggest reinforcing cotton threads with beeswax (Massey 1974; DeWolf 1968; Bridson and Forman 1999, p. 41).

2.1.4.1.2 Strips, Other Paper-Based Components, Adhesive Tapes

For mounting with strips, both historically and currently, strips of paper or textile tape coated with adhesive have been used. Historically, the strips were typically made from paper offcuts and could vary in width. In conservation practice, they are often made from Japanese paper (Dauwalder 2013; Grenda 2013, 2015a, b). The adhesive may be applied to the strip immediately before mounting, or as a layer activated by water, alcohol, or another solvent. Strips may be adhered using starch paste, animal glue, gum, or synthetic adhesive. Textile tapes as a strapping material became popular in the early twentieth century and were often coated with gelatine (Down 1999). For ready-made products intended for use in herbarium collections, manufacturers often do not specify the type of adhesive used to coat the tape. This may, for example, be gelatine mixed with starch adhesive, which provides weaker adhesion than tapes coated with pure gelatine (Down 1999). Bridson and Forman cite an example of an archival-quality tape coated with acrylic adhesive (Bridson and Forman 1999, p. 41).

Many conservators emphasise the need to avoid direct contact between adhesive and plant material, which is characteristic of direct adhesive mounting (described in the following section), and recommend the use of mounting strips (Grenda-Kurmanow 2021). However, since most commercially available tapes are coated with adhesive over their entire surface, the issue of direct adhesive contact with plant material also arises with this mounting method. Although the adhesive is intended to be activated only at the edges of the tape, there is always a risk that temporarily elevated relative humidity (during mounting, handling, or storage) may also activate the adhesive on the remaining part of the tape. Another factor to consider in this context is the emission of volatile organic compounds, typical of PVA adhesives, which may contribute to cellulose degradation (Grenda-Kurmanow 2021).

Decorative mounts in the shape of vases and ribbons were also made of paper and could have been either cut from graphic prints or from sheets of coloured decorative paper (Figs. 2.13 and 2.14).

Archer's adhesive, used as the material for the "strips" to which specimens were mounted, had a variable composition depending on the availability of individual components. Originally, it consisted of ethyl cellulose, a mixture of methanol and toluene, and Dow Resin 276-V2 [poly(α-methyl)styrene resin] (Archer 1950). The composition of the adhesive changed over time, mainly through the use of alternative resins: Amoco Resin 18–210 and Hercules Piccolastic™ A5/A25 (hydrocarbon resin, styrene monomer). These resins are now either unavailable on the market (as with Dow and Amoco resins) or inaccessible to individual buyers (Piccolastic™). The original formulation was criticised for its persistent tackiness, which led to specimens sticking together and becoming damaged (Croat 1978). As previously mentioned, the adhesive posed a health risk to users because it contained toxic volatile organic compounds (VOCs) such as methanol and toluene, resulting in a range of side effects among those who used it (Croat 1978; Bridson and Forman 1999, p. 39; Down 1999, pp. 207–208; Grenda-Kurmanow 2021). Among the side effects experienced by herbarium technical staff working with Archer's adhesive were nausea and dizziness; however, the long-term emission of VOCs and the toxicity of Archer's adhesive have not been studied, and the current health risks associated with working with collections mounted using this adhesive remain unknown.

Industrial adhesive tapes used for mounting specimens were selected from commonly available products. These were typically standard office supplies (e.g. Sellotape or Scotch tape), as well as medical adhesive plasters. Thus, among the tapes used for mounting specimens, one can find products comprising various film coatings with adhesives of diverse compositions, made from a wide range of manufacturing ingredients (Croat 1978; Bridson and Forman 1999, pp. 41, 62; Down 1999).[33] Sealing waxes of various colours were also used for mounting specimens (Figs. 2.15 and 2.16) (Piekiełko 1981; Margez 2004).[34]

[33] The earliest type of adhesive tapes were surgical tapes, consisting of a piece of cloth and a rubber-based adhesive. The first official surgical tape, using an adhesive made from Indian and pine rubber, turpentine, and red lead (lead oxide), was patented in 1845 (US 3965, 1845). Film-based adhesive tapes entered industrial production in the USA in the 1920s as masking tools in the automotive industry. The formulation of tapes was developed and diversified over the following decades. The earliest backing material for film tapes was cellophane, later replaced by cellulose acetate, which is still in use today, followed by poly(vinyl chloride) (PVC) and polypropylene and polyethylene compounds. Among the elastomers found in tape adhesives are natural and synthetic polydiene rubbers; styrene block copolymers; acrylic copolymers; polyisobutylene and butyl rubbers; ethylene-vinyl acetate copolymers; and silicone elastomers. The adhesives also contain terpene and hydrocarbon resins; plasticisers, including mineral oils and alkyl esters; fillers, mainly inorganic; and stabilisers. Additionally, tapes may be reinforced with glass, polyester, or polyamide fibres (Karmann and Kummer 2000).

[34] Sealing wax may contain shellac, turpentine, resins, chalk or gypsum, as well as colouring additives, including cinnabar and red lead for a red colour, soot for black, and verdigris for green.

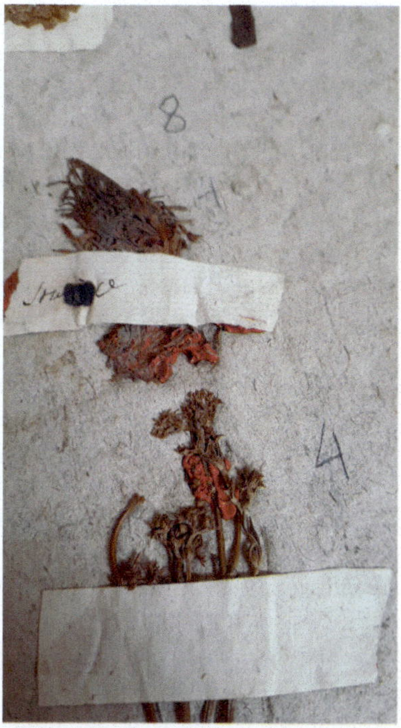

Fig. 2.15 Mounting of the specimen using red and black sealing wax. Fragment of the Camelin or Szaster herbarium [Camelin A. or Szaster J., *Herbarium, probably…*, Kraków, Institute of Botany, Polish Academy of Sciences (KRAM), without ref. no, first half of the eighteenth century]. (Photo: M. Grenda-Kurmanow)

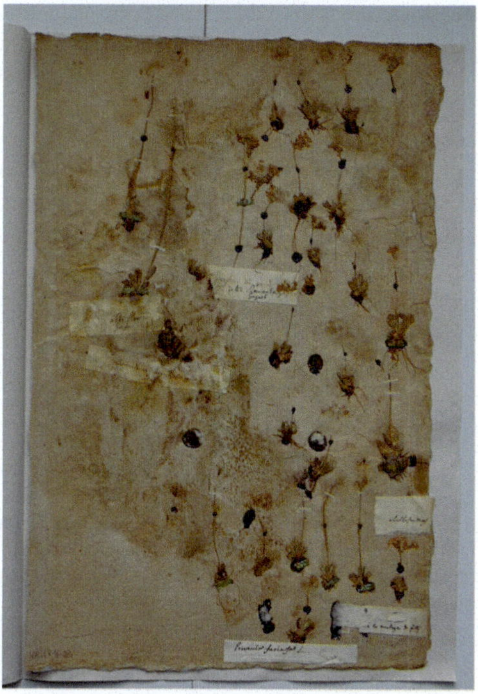

Fig. 2.16 Herbarium sheet of Albrecht von Haller, [Haller, von A., (*Herbier Haller*), Paris, Muséum national d'histoire naturelle (P), without ref. no., before 1768. (Photo: M. Grenda-Kurmanow)

2.1.4.1.3 Adhesives Used Historically and in Contemporary Practice

For point and overall mounting (adhering the entire surface of the specimen to the substrate), various adhesives have been and continue to be used. Historically, these were exclusively natural adhesives, primarily of animal origin (hide glue, isinglass) (Tournefort 1694; Spiegel 1606; Linnaeus 1751, p. 7), but plant-based adhesives were also employed (gum arabic, various types of starch pastes). Biocidal agents were sometimes added to the adhesives to protect specimens from insects and microorganisms.[35] Table 2.1 presents a compilation of adhesives mentioned in the literature from 1606–2025, used for mounting specimens, together with their application methods and solution concentrations. The adhesives have been categorised by their chemical structure. The "other" group includes adhesives that could not be assigned to the previously listed groups, primarily because these materials are now generally unavailable and/or known only by their trade names.

An international survey, published in 2021, revealed that a limited range of adhesives is currently used for mounting (Table 2.2) (Grenda-Kurmanow 2021).

According to the survey results, the choice of adhesive for mounting depends on the individual performing the procedure on the herbarium specimen and the policies of the respective institution. In some institutions, more recent collections and those of lesser significance are often handled by technical staff, whereas collections considered valuable or historical are entrusted to a specialist with conservation training. Respondents emphasised that mounting a specimen by gluing it to a substrate hinders its study. It was also highlighted that every specimen should be regarded as part of the heritage. For this reason, the valuation of individual objects should not be differentiated, and mounting materials should be approved by a conservator and regularly evaluated. Nevertheless, in many institutions, there are specimens of varying status requiring minor repairs, which are carried out by available staff without conservation training, using methods they are accustomed to in their daily work, rather than those recommended by conservators.

The most popular adhesive among mounters is poly(vinyl acetate)-based glue, although it is also occasionally used by conservators (Grenda-Kurmanow 2021).[36] In current conservation practice, the most commonly used mounting adhesive is methylcellulose. Adhesives recommended by conservators often require preparation

[35] For example, the previously mentioned clove oil in Spiegel's work, or mercuric chloride added to animal glue by Tournefort (Tournefort 1694, pp. 547–548). See also the section *Damage Caused by the Use of Biocidal Agents* in Chap. 3.

[36] The survey responses clearly indicate that conservators and technical staff in herbaria adopt different approaches to specimen mounting. Conservators are expected to assess the materials used in treatments for their chemical stability, whereas technicians are generally instructed to carry out tasks using approved materials. There is no doubt that working within an institution requires methods that are time- and cost-efficient, easy to apply, and that prioritise mounting a specified number of specimens each year. Technical staff are therefore required to meet certain expectations, and their working comfort is closely linked to time efficiency. Consequently, respondents who were conservators frequently reported (and criticised) the use of PVA adhesives, commonly employed by technical staff, which facilitate a quick, easy working style.

Table 2.1 Adhesives used in herbarium work, based on publications from 1606–2025, unpublished master's theses, and conservation reports

Adhesive name	Solution concentration (if specified)	Mounting method (if specified)	References
Cellulose ethers and their mixtures with other types of adhesives			
Methylcellulose in water or ethyl alcohol	4%; 7.5%; 10%	Spot adhesion; adhering the specimen to the substrate over the entire surface; as a coating on the mounting strip	Bedford (1999), Bridson and Forman (1999), Collins (2000), Clarck (1986), Dauwalder (2012), Down (1999), Gunn (1994), Popławska (2014a, b), Tillet (1979), Wierda (1994), Wierda (1995) and Yesilyurt et al. (2025)
Sodium carboxymethyl cellulose	2%	Adhesion of the specimen to the substrate over the entire surface	Bridson and Forman (1999), Collins (2000), Dauwalder (2012), Walker and Hughes (1994) and Wierda (1994)
Methylcellulose mixed with wheat starch paste	7.5% MC, 7.5% wheat starch paste, 1:1	As a coating on a paper mounting strip	Keijzers (2013)
Klucel E (hydroxypropylcellulose)	25%		Dauwalder (2012, 2013) and Fuchs (2008)
Klucel G (hydroxypropylcellulose)	2% in ethanol; 8%; 10%	Spot adhesion; "consolidation" by attaching a fragment of the specimen with Japanese paper coated with adhesive	Gersten et al. (2017), Keijzers (2013) and Berli and Belhadj (2020)
Cellulose esters			
Acetylcellulose			Fassett (1952)
Nitrocellulose			Yesilyurt (2009)
Starches (pastes)			
Starch pastes (in general)		Adhering the specimen to the substrate over its entire surface, spotadhesion of the specimen, as a coating on the mounting strip	Lecky (1972), Grenda--Kurmanow (2017) and Wierda (1994)
Wheat starch paste	10%	Adhering the specimen to the substrate over its entire surface, spot adhesion the specimen, as a coating on the mounting strip	Bridson and Forman (1999), Collins (2000), Dauwalder (2012), Jacobi and Phan Tan Luu (2012), Keijzers (2013), Margez (2004), Menei (2005), Mertens and Vries (2013), Popławska (2014a, b), Vries (2013) and Wierda (1995)

(continued)

Table 2.1 (continued)

Adhesive name	Solution concentration (if specified)	Mounting method (if specified)	References
Rice starch paste	10%	Spot adhesion of the specimen	Bridson and Forman (1999), Grenda (2013, 2015a) and Keijzers (2013)
Corn starch paste			Keijzers (2013)
Potato starch paste			Keijzers (2013)
Dextrin		Adhesion of the specimen with its entire surface to the substrate, as a coating on the mounting strip	Keijzers (2013)
Paste made from arrowroot starch			Collins (2000)
Gums			
Gum arabic		As a coating on the fastening strip	Bridson and Forman (1999), Keijzers (2013), Merrill (1926), Poncy et al. (2012) and Popławska (2014a, b)
Tragacanth gum		Adhering the specimen to the substrate with its entire surface	Bridson and Forman (1999) and Merrill (1926)
Protein adhesive and their mixtures with other types of adhesives			
Hide glue, bone glue		Adhering the specimen to the substrate with its entire surface	Bedford (1999), Bridson and Forman (1999), de Vries et al. (2025), Keijzers (2013), Popławska (2014a), Spiegel (1606) and Tournefort (1694)
Fish glue		Adhering the specimen to the substrate with its entire surface	Bridson and Forman (1999), Dauwalder (2012), DeWolf (1968), Down (1999), Grenda--Kurmanow (2017), Gunn (1994), Keijzers (2013), Merrill (1926), Popławska (2014a) and Rytz (1933)
Gelatine		Adhering the specimen to the substrate with its entire surface; spot-mounting of the specimen; as a coating on the mounting strip	Bridson and Forman (1999), Collins (2000), Down (1999), Grenda--Kurmanow (2017), Popławska (2014a, b), Vries (2013) and Wierda (1994, 1995)

(continued)

Table 2.1 (continued)

Adhesive name	Solution concentration (if specified)	Mounting method (if specified)	References
Gelatine mixed with starch paste (unspecified)		As a coating on a textile mounting strip	Down (1999)
Isinglass		Attachment of the specimen to the substrate with its entire surface	Bridson and Forman (1999), Grenda--Kurmanow (2017) Linnaeus (1751)[b]
Isinglass mixed with wheat starch paste		Spot reinforcement of the specimen	Dauwalder (2012, 2013)
Adhesives from the poly(vinyl acetate) group—PVA (PVA, PVAc, VAE, others) and their mixtures with other types of adhesives			
PVA (unspecified)			Bedford (1999), Bridson and Forman (1999), Collins (2000), Dauwalder (2012), Grenda-Kurmanow (2017), Keijzers (2013), Popławska (2014a), Smith (2010), Wierda (1994), Yesilyurt (2009) and Yesilyurt et al. (2025)
PVA (unspecified) mixed with methylcellulose in ethanol			Gunn (1994)
Jade 403			Down (1999)
Hewit Mi55			Wierda (1994)
Weldbond®		Spot mounting of the specimen	Down (1999) and Shchepanek (2001)
Elmer's® Glue-All		Adhering the specimen to the substrate with its entire surface, used as a coating on the mounting strip	Croat (1978), DeWolf (1968), Down (1999) and Yesilyurt (2009)
Gaylord Magic Mend			Croat (1978) and Down (1999)
Vinibond			Wierda (1994)
Mowilith DMC2			Suggested by Down (1999) and Keijzers (2013)
DM2			Wierda (1994)
Planatol			Wierda (1994)
Evacon-R™		Full-surface adhesion of the specimen to the substrate, spot adhesion of the specimen, repairs within the specimen	Collins (2000), Dauwalder (2012), Popławska (2014a), Purewal et al. (2008) and Yesilyurt (2009)

(continued)

Table 2.1 (continued)

Adhesive name	Solution concentration (if specified)	Mounting method (if specified)	References
Evacon-R™ mixed with methylcellulose	MC 5% in water, 1:1; MC 7.5%, 1:1	Adhering the specimen to the substrate over the entire surface, spot adhesion of the specimen, repairs within the specimen	Mertens and Vries (2013), Valk (2010) and Vries (2013)
Evacon-R™ mixed with starch paste (unspecified)	Paste (from unspecified type of starch) 7.5%, 1:1	Repairs within the specimen	Keijzers (2013)
Evostick Resin W			Bridson and Forman (1999), Clark (1986), Gunn (1994) and Wierda (1994)
Bulldog Grip 20 min or 2311			Down (1999)
Bondfast			Down (1999)
Polyvinyl Acetate Beads dissolved in alcohol	1:3 PVA: alcohol		Croat (1978)
Poly(vinyl alcohols) (PVAL)			
Mowiol 48-6, 4-88			Keijzers (2013) and Wierda (1994)
Mowiol + Planatol			Wierda (1994)
Mowiol + DM2			Wierda (1994)
Latex adhesives			
Latex adhesives (unspecified)		Mounting the specimen with its entire surface adhered to the substrate	Bridson and Forman (1999), Grenda--Kurmanow (2017), Wierda (1994) and Yesilyurt (2009)
Latex III 6022			Wierda (1994)
Latex-based “Multilock”			Wierda (1994)
Acrylic adhesives			
Paraloid B-72 in acetone	5%		Popławska (2014b)
Rhoplex AC-33 (acrylic resin)	25%	Adhering the specimen to the substrate with its entire surface—lichen specimens	Gates (2009)

(continued)

Table 2.1 (continued)

Adhesive name	Solution concentration (if specified)	Mounting method (if specified)	References
Other			
Archer's adhesive Ethocel™ (ethyl cellulose) + toluene + methanol + Dow Resin 276 V2 (methylstyrene) (alternatively: Amoco 18-210 resin; Hercules Piccolastic A5 or A25)		Mounting on threads of dried Archer's adhesive, adhering the specimen with its entire surface to the substrate, spot-gluing the specimen	Archer (1950), Bridson and Forman (1999), Clarck (1986), Croat (1978), DeWolf (1968), Down (1999), Grenda-Kurmanow (2017), Gunn (1994), Rollins (1955) and Sharp (1964)
Bexol SR 101			Clarck (1986), Bridson and Forman (1999) and Wierda (1994)
Hot-melt glue		Attaching the specimen to the substrate with its entire surface; mounting analogous to the "Archer method"	Gunn (1994), Poncy et al. (2012), Tillet (1979) and Wierda (1994)
Swift Adhesives 5032, 1452, 41452		Attachment of the specimen to the substrate over its entire surface, mounting using strips	Croat (1978)
Nicobond B		Attachment of the specimen to the substrate over its entire surface, mounting using strips	Croat (1978)
Wilhold Glue		Attachment of the specimen to the substrate with its entire surface, mounting using strips	Croat (1978)
H. B. Fuller Adhesive #3957 (Library Paste) + a few drops of Tergitol Anionic		Adhering the specimen to the substrate with its entire surface	Croat (1978)
Alling and Corey Padding Compound		Adhering the specimen to the substrate with its entire surface	Croat (1978)
National Resyn 33-2041 and 35-6262		Adhesion of the specimen to the substrate over its entire surface	Croat (1978)
Lepages #135 glue		Attachment of the specimen to the substrate over its entire surface	Croat (1978)

(continued)

Table 2.1 (continued)

Adhesive name	Solution concentration (if specified)	Mounting method (if specified)	References
IPI Makeready Paste		Adhering the specimen to the substrate over its entire surface	Croat (1978)
Duco Cement		Mounting lichen specimens onto cardboard	Croat (1978) and Gates (2009)
Improved Process Glue			Merrill (1926)
'Mikah' remoistenable adhesive			Merrill and Wyman (1939)
Cow gum rubber solution			Bridson and Forman (1999) and Wierda (1994)
Stephens Gripfix			Wierda (1994)
Stephens Trufix			Wierda (1994)
Gloy Glue			Wierda (1994)
Special A Tin Paste		Adhering the specimen to the substrate with its entire surface	Croat (1978) and Merrill (1926)
Supercel Wallpaper Paste		Adhering the specimen to the substrate over its entire surface	Croat (1978)
Prittstick			Bridson and Forman (1999)
Aquazol 500 in ethanol	2%	Specimen consolidation	Popławska (2014a, b)

[a]This table mentions published and unpublished sources, including research report: Wierda A (1994) Het gebruik van o.a. PVA-lijm ter bevestiging van gedroogd plantenmateriaal in herbaria. Een onderzoeksrapport. Met een kort overzicht van bevestiginingsmethoden van plantenmateriaal op papier. Den Haag, Algemeen Rijskarchief, research report, Naturalis Biodiversity Center, Leiden; and conservation reports: Jacobi E, Phan TL, (2012) Herbaria Restauratie-documentatie. Fase I. Nationaal Herbarium Nederland; Mertens S, Vries de H (2013) Herbaria Restauratie--documentatie. Fase II, Nationaal Herbarium Nederland; Valk de M (2010) Het Herbarium van de Stedelijke Musea Zierikzee. Beschrijving en conserveringsadvies; Vries de H (2013) Herbaria Restauratie-documentatie. Fase II. Nationaal Herbarium Nederland; Wierda A (1995) De restauratie van het Boerhave Herbarium (Rijksherbarium Leiden), Amsterdam; Lecky M (1972) Hortus Siccus. Gaevmans (Antonio) Volume I. Property of University of California, Los Angeles—all stored at the Naturalis Biodiversity Center in Leiden, and were made available to the author courtesy of Gerard Thijjse

[b]In the case of Linnaeus, it is not clear whether he used fish glue or isinglass. Based on a source from Linnaeus's time (Valmont de Bomare 1775, p. 583), the author assumes that in Linnaeus's work *ichtyocolla* refers to isinglass, although publications mentioning the technique used by Linnaeus usually suggest that he used fish glue. This is probably a matter of literal translation of the Latin term (*ichtys*—fish, *colla*—glue)

Table 2.2 Adhesives currently used in herbaria, recommended by survey respondents, or mentioned as being used in their institutions

Material name	Company (if provided)	Concentration/ratio/preparation method
Methylcellulose (MC)	Lineco; Talas	2.5%; 3% 4% spot consolidation 7.5%
Wheat paste	La Route du Papier	
Methylcellulose + wheat starch paste		12% starch paste +3% MC, 1:1 Wheat starch paste (unspecified viscosity) + 7.5% methylcellulose, 1:1
Charlock		5%, on moistened filter paper
Gelatine		On a cloth tape
Klucel® E		25+%
PVA (PVA, PVAc, EVA) and acrylic adhesives		
Hewit M218 PVA	Hewit and Sons	8:1 (adhesive: Water)
Unspecified PVA		
2% Ethulose mixed with Jade 403	Blade	1:1 (Ethulose: Jade 403)
Evacon R™		
Lascaux 498 HV and Lascaux 360 HV (currently 303 HV)		498 HV: 303 HV in a 1:1 ratio, used as a coating layer on Japanese kozo paper, reactivated with ethanol
Polyethylene adhesive		Adhesive-coated, thermally activated tape
Adhesives of unspecified composition	Lineco, Herbarium Supply	'Neutral pH adhesives', on paper and textile tapes
Other adhesives/materials for assembly listed as not recommended, but used currently or in the past		
Weldbond® PVA	Currently in use	
Hot-melt adhesive	Currently in use	
Tape coated with gum arabic	Previously used	
Archer's glue	Previously used	

Based on Grenda-Kurmanow (2021)

according to a specific protocol, familiar to conservators but not necessarily obvious to other users (non-conservators). Individual respondents developed complex formulations for various purposes: some for "ordinary" specimens, others for bulky specimens with complex three-dimensional structures, and still others for paper mounting strips.

The diverse utilisation of plant material across various scientific disciplines, along with advances in DNA analysis methods, has led to a shift in approaches to the preparation and preservation of herbaria. The choice of adhesive is determined not only by its working properties, but also by its long-term chemical stability and compatibility with plant material. Current discussions regarding adhesives address issues such as the accelerated degradation of cellulose-based materials and the contamination of herbaria with irreversible, or rather irremovable, substances.[37] Only curatorial awareness can ensure the implementation of conservation standards in the daily, "technical" work within herbaria. Among the adhesives identified in the survey, several groups can be distinguished, as described below.[38]

2.1.4.1.3.1 Cellulose Ethers

The use of methylcellulose (MC), a cellulose ether, is well established in the field of conservation (Down 2015, p. 53). Methylcellulose is available in various types, grades, and molecular weights, which influence its properties such as viscosity and flexibility. In many European countries, conservators frequently use Tylose MH. This product is commonly referred to as methylcellulose or "cellulose glue", although chemically it belongs to the related group of cellulose ethers, methylhydroxyethylcelluloses (MHEC or HEMC). MHEC is produced by introducing a methoxyl group into the cellulose chain and generally exhibits similar properties to MC. However, it is more hydrophilic and its gelation temperature is higher than that of MC (Yoo and Um 2013). Both MC and MHEC are known to form stable and flexible films and are resistant to biodeterioration (Down 2015, p. 53). MC and MHEC form weaker bonds than starch paste and gelatine, but retain their strength better after ageing (Down 2015, p. 56). Methylcellulose is a mild ("weak") adhesive that is highly hydrophilic (retains water) and dries slowly (Nasatto et al. 2015). For this reason, attention is drawn to the risk of staining in historic papers when using methylcellulose. Therefore, it is sometimes mixed with other adhesives, such as wheat starch paste or PVA, to obtain stronger and faster-drying bonds (Feller and Wilt 1990, p. 101; Down 2015, p. 56). It also does not cause discolouration or lose viscosity upon ageing (Feller and Wilt 1990, p. 101).

Another cellulose ether belonging to the group of hydroxypropylcelluloses (HPC), Klucel E, is characterised by its flexibility and good ageing behaviour. It belongs to the group of low molecular weight (80,000) HPCs, which are considered to possess better properties than high molecular weight Klucels (up to 1,150,000): it is more stable, exhibits less discolouration, and shows lower molecular mass loss during ageing (Feller and Wilt 1990, pp. 63–73). In contrast to methylcellulose, HPCs are susceptible to biodeterioration. In general, Klucels are reversible and retain their solubility during ageing (Down 2015, pp. 54–56). However, some studies have reported pronounced substrate discolouration caused by Klucel E (Geiger

[37] See the section *Physical Degradation of Plant Material* in Chap. 3, as well as *Preservation of Genetic Material in Collections—Studies on the Impact of Preservation and Conservation Methods on aDNA* in Chap. 4.

[38] See the section *Physical Degradation of Plant Material* in Chap. 3, as well as *Preservation of Genetic Material in Collections—Studies on the Impact of Preservation and Conservation Methods on aDNA* in Chap. 4.

and Michel 2005; Michel 2011). Klucel E has not been studied with regard to its ageing properties in the context of conservation purposes.[39]

2.1.4.1.3.2 *Starch Adhesives (Pastes)*

Wheat starch paste is another adhesive widely used in paper conservation and has a long history of use. Starch paste is a relatively stable adhesive, but in its pure form, it is susceptible to microbial attack and becomes brittle with age (Down 2015, pp. 48–49). It forms strong bonds; however, films of wheat starch paste are less flexible than those of methylcellulose. The "reversibility" attributed to starch pastes may in fact be related to their removability.[40] Although dry films of wheat starch paste do not dissolve in water, they can be removed after swelling in water or with the use of enzymes (Down 2015, pp. 50–51).

2.1.4.1.3.3 *Animal Glues*

Animal glues (gelatines and isinglass) exhibit good flexibility and excellent ageing properties, as evidenced by the well-preserved condition of historical specimens mounted with this type of adhesive (Grenda-Kurmanow 2021).[41] However, it should be noted that gelatines are available in a wide range of types, and their chemical properties depend on the collagen source and processing method, which determine the key characteristics influencing their performance: molecular weight and its distribution (Schellmann 2007). Isinglass is a form of pure gelatine extracted from the inner lining of the swim bladders of certain fish species. Traditionally, it is prepared from the swim bladders of sturgeon. Depending on the species and preparation method, these adhesives may differ. It should not be confused with fish glue, which is produced from the skins and bones of non-oily fish species (Schellmann 2007). Currently, isinglass may be obtained from the swim bladders of other fish species due to the decline in sturgeon populations (Schellmann 2007; Down 2015, p. 38). The molecular weight of mammalian gelatines ranges from 110,000 to 168,000, whereas for isinglass it starts at 150,000 and can reach up to 300,000, making this adhesive highly viscous yet also penetrating. Its gel temperature is significantly lower than that of other animal glues, allowing for prolonged penetration. Due to

[39] See also the section *Preservation of Genetic Material in Collections—Studies on the Impact of Preservation and Conservation Methods on aDNA* in Chap. 4.

[40] The removability of an adhesive is not synonymous with reversibility, a term, that is currently complex and ambiguous in the field of conservation. At present, it most often refers not only to the removal of the material added during conservation, but also to the reversal of all effects associated with its use. Horie distinguishes four levels of reversibility, ranging from irreversibility, through a stage in which the object appears as it did prior to treatment; a further stage in which actions to remove the effects of treatment do not interfere with subsequent conservation interventions; to the highest degree of reversibility, where the treatment can be undone without leaving any trace or contamination in the object (Horie 2010). See discussions (Horie 2010, pp. 6–8; Down 2015, p. 27). In the case of porous materials such as paper, this is virtually unattainable.

[41] Isinglass demonstrates greater flexibility and higher stability during ageing than gelatine.

these unique properties, the setting time and viscosity development are longer than in the case of gelatine (Schellmann 2007). However, animal glues are quite susceptible to microbial attack, making their use inadvisable in tropical climates and posing a risk of pest infestation in the event of accidental increases in relative humidity (Schellmann 2007).

2.1.4.1.3.4 Poly(vinyl Acetate)

PVA adhesives, which are critically assessed by conservators, come in a wide variety, which may result in inconsistent overall evaluations of this group of adhesives. It is important to remember that the same abbreviation (PVA) may refer to both poly(vinyl alcohol) and poly(vinyl acetate) (Down 2015, p. 65). Among poly(vinyl acetates), there are subgroups of copolymers: EVA, which is a copolymer of ethylene and vinyl acetate (VAC) (with a higher proportion of ethylene than VAC); VAE, which is a copolymer of VAC and ethylene (with a higher proportion of VAC than ethylene); VADBM, which is a copolymer of VAC and di-butyl maleate; and others. Similarly, within this group, for copolymers of VAC and ethylene (regardless of the ratio of the two components), the most common abbreviation is EVA (Scheper 2005). Long-term studies by the Canadian Conservation Institute (CCI) on adhesives, including natural ageing processes, have provided data on the chemical stability and ageing of several poly(vinyl acetates) and acrylic adhesives (Down et al. 1996; Down 2015, pp. 81–91; 2016). Analyses of volatile organic compounds emitted by poly(vinyl acetates) have shown that dry PVA films tend to release volatile acetic acid, with the highest emission rate occurring within the first three months after application, decreasing to almost zero over the following two years (Down et al. 1996, with updated results in Down 2014, 2015, p. 69). Most of the acetic acid is released during setting and drying, and the effect is intensified in the presence of pure acetic acid, which is sometimes added by manufacturers to stabilise the dispersion (Down 2014). Another acid identified in these studies was formic acid, emitted only by Elmers Glue-All PVA (Down et al. 1996). Tests conducted at the British Library confirmed that Evacon-R (not tested by CCI) produces volatile organic acids under Oddy test conditions and during ageing (the study included artificial ageing tests) (Stevens et al. 2011). The same result was obtained for Hewit M218 PVA adhesive during internal tests at the British Museum (British Museum 2014–2018). Acetic and formic acids contribute to lowering the pH and accelerating the acid hydrolysis of cellulose,[42] especially if the object (e.g. a herbarium sheet) is enclosed in protective packaging (Dupont and Tétreault 2000). In CCI tests, acetic acid emission was generally associated with the acidity of the adhesive itself (the lower the pH, the higher the emission).[43] Many polyvinyl acetate adhesives, both as dispersions and as dry films, are indeed acidic, e.g. Bulldog Grip 20 Minute, Elmer's

[42] See the section *Acid Hydrolysis* in Chap. 3.

[43] Weldbond PVA is an example of an adhesive with low pH and high acetic acid emission (Down et al. 1996; Down 2014).

Glue-All, Gaylord Magic Mend and Weldbond (Down 2014). Dispersions become more acidic during storage, which is why it is not recommended to store large quantities of PVA for more than one year (Down et al. 1996; Down 2014, 2015, p. 69). However, an increase in the acidity of dry layers after ageing (as suggested in the survey) does not occur in most adhesives studied by CCI. For many products, the pH remained stable even after 27 years of ageing, and in some cases, it increased slightly over time. A notable exception is Jade 403 adhesive, which is acidic as a dispersion (pH = 5.8 before ageing and 5.62 after ageing), but neutral as a dry film, even after ageing (Down 2014).

The CCI tests did not take into account the reversibility factor of poly(vinyl acetate)s, but earlier studies by Baer, Phelan, and Indictor examined solubility and swelling as factors enabling adhesive removal (Phelan et al. 1971). The study demonstrated that none of the tested products is completely reversible and, for this reason, they are not recommended for the conservation of paper as a porous material (Baer et al. 1978). There are no more recent studies on the removability of PVA adhesives that examine products currently available on the market. Nevertheless, despite manufacturers' claims of reversibility, this group of adhesives is considered, in conservation practice, to be non-removable from cellulosic substrates and thus constitutes a contaminant.[44]

2.1.4.1.3.5 Acrylic Adhesives

The acrylic adhesives mentioned in the query (Lascaux HV498 and HV360,[45] i.e. copolymers of butyl acrylate and methyl methacrylate) are characterised by high bond strength (Lascaux HV498), high flexibility, and retention of tack even after drying (Kite and Thomson 2006). Lascaux HV360 and Rhoplex 235, which has a composition similar to Lascaux HV498, were included in CCI testing (Down et al. 1996). Although acrylic adhesives are considered lightfast, they tend to yellow upon light ageing. In CCI tests, HV360 was the only acrylic adhesive to emit a small amount of acetic acid (Down 2014). In internal material tests at the British Museum, HV303 successfully passed Oddy tests[46] (British Museum 2014–2018). CCI also investigated the removability of certain acrylic adhesives as part of a project on pressure-sensitive and heat-set tapes (Down et al. 2011). Tapes coated with Lascaux HV498 and HV360 adhesives were found to be removable both mechanically and with water or organic solvents (e.g. ethanol or acetone). However, removal of HV360 required soaking the sample in solvent, which is not always feasible in conservation practice. Overall removability of the adhesives was assessed by the ease

[44] See also the section *Preservation of Genetic Material in Collections—Studies on the Impact of Preservation and Conservation Methods on aDNA* in Chap. 4.

[45] In 2012, the adhesive manufacturer Lascaux replaced the HV360 adhesive with another product, HV303, a copolymer of 2-ethylhexyl acrylate/ethyl acrylate that remains permanently tacky (Down 2015, p. 85).

[46] This is the so-called accelerated corrosion test used to identify emitted volatile organic compounds, introduced in 1973 at the British Museum by Andrew Oddy (Green and Thickett 1995).

of tape layer removal, but the cleanliness of paper fibres after this process was not analysed. The studies also showed that removability depends on the type of paper to which the tape was applied, and may decrease with ageing. Therefore, the reversibility of this group of adhesives is questionable and would require further research.

2.1.5 Descriptive Layer

Historical herbaria typically feature a descriptive layer in the form of handwritten species names. These notes are most often made in ink, less frequently in pencil or crayon, and frequently refer solely to the names of the specimens. The description may appear directly on the sheet to which the specimen is attached, on an adjacent sheet, on a mounting strip, on a specially designated label, or on an additional sheet inserted into the block (Figs. 2.17, 2.18; Figs. 2.19 and 2.20; Figs. 2.21 and 2.22; Figs. 2.23, 2.24, 2.25 and 2.26). In addition to specimen names, herbaria may also contain supplementary information, such as details regarding the properties of a given plant.

In the oldest herbaria, metal-tannin inks were very often used for descriptions. These inks were commonly employed as writing materials until the nineteenth century, when a range of inks containing newly invented synthetic dyes began to be produced (Reissland et al. 2017). Metal-gall inks, of which iron-gall inks are the most well-known, had a variable composition. The ingredients included an extract from oak galls, pathological growths on tree leaves (most often oaks), which are induced by insects of the family Cynipidae as a habitat for their larvae; vitriol, that is, hydrated iron or copper sulphate; gum, most commonly gum arabic; water,

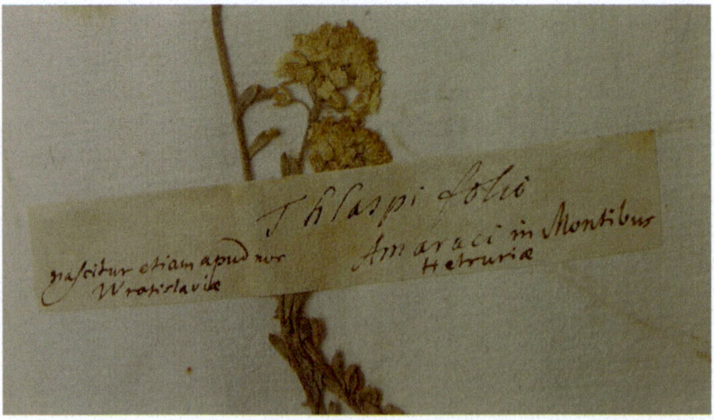

Fig. 2.17 Silvio Boccone P.S., [*Herbarium of Paolo Silvio Boccone*], Wrocław, Herbarium of the Museum of Natural History in Wrocław (WRSL), without ref. no., 1689–1695. Example of the presence of two types of handwriting on a single label (and simultaneous mounting) of a plant specimen. In addition to Boccone's own signature, the note *Nascitur etiam apud nos/nur? Wratislavia* ("also grows near Wrocław") was added later by another researcher. (Photo: E. Lenard)

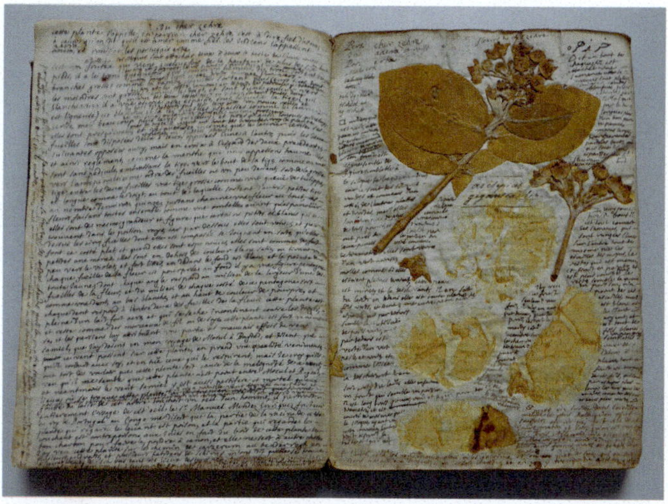

Fig. 2.18 Herbarium of Jean de Thévenot, Thévenot, de J., untitled, Paris, Muséum national d'Histoire naturelle (P), without ref. no., 1664–1666. On the left, a page densely covered with notes closely surrounding the botanical specimens. (Photo: M. Grenda-Kurmanow)

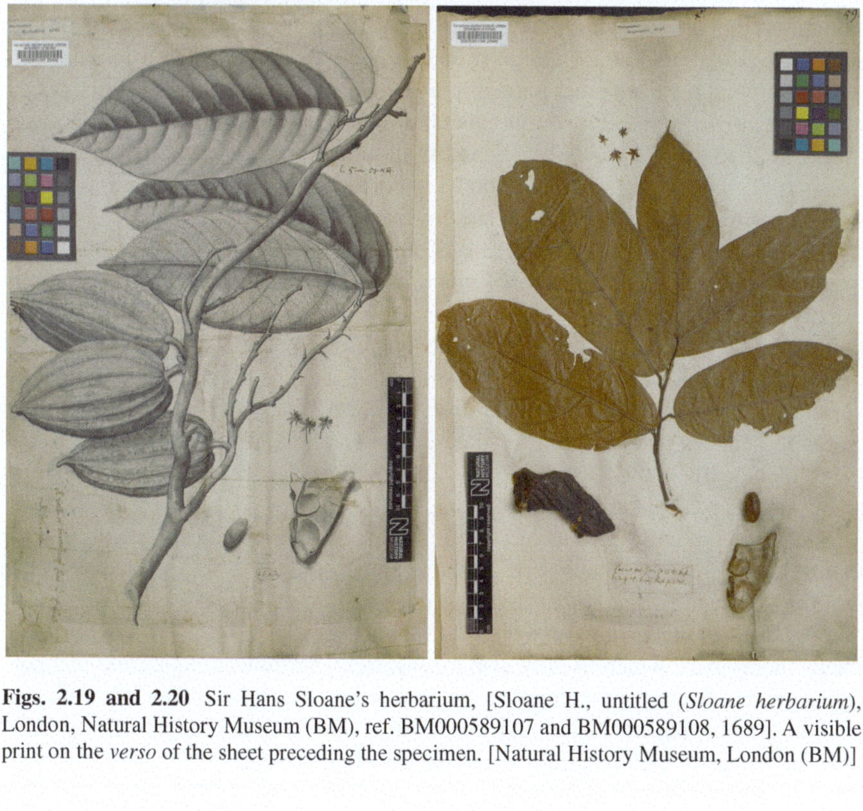

Figs. 2.19 and 2.20 Sir Hans Sloane's herbarium, [Sloane H., untitled (*Sloane herbarium*), London, Natural History Museum (BM), ref. BM000589107 and BM000589108, 1689]. A visible print on the *verso* of the sheet preceding the specimen. [Natural History Museum, London (BM)]

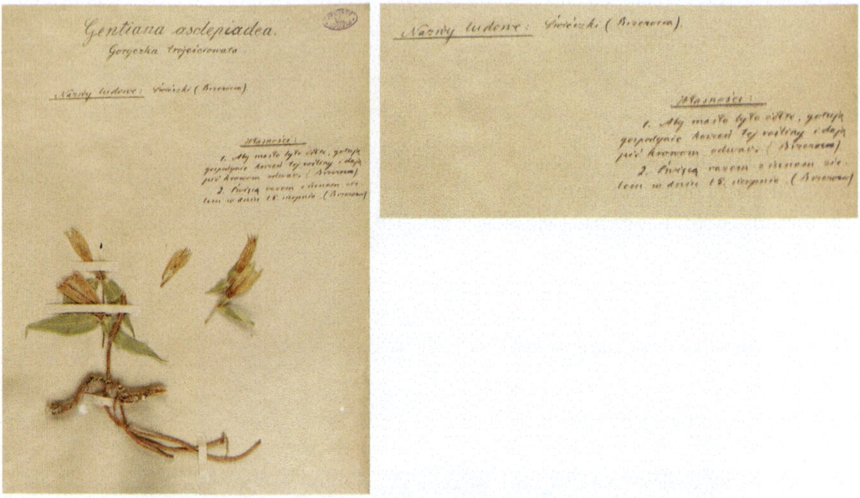

Figs. 2.21 and 2.22 Seweryn Udziela's Herbarium [Udziela S., (*Seweryn Udziela's Herbarium*), Kraków, Herbarium of the Władysław Szafer Institute of Botany, Polish Academy of Sciences (KRAM), without ref. no., barcode: KRAM00030598-V, 1890s. (Photo: Władysław Szafer Institute of Botany, Polish Academy of Sciences)

sometimes replaced by wine, vodka, beer, urine, or vinegar; and colouring additives such as logwood, aniline, or indigo (Sobucki 2013, pp. 74–80). Occasionally, tannins were obtained from other parts of plants, tree bark, or tannin-rich fruits. Metal ions were also introduced by boiling metal filings, nails, etc., in the oak gall extract (Sobucki 2013, pp. 74–80). The variability in ink composition was determined by the recipe, and by the fact that natural ingredients could differ depending on the geographical location and the plant species from which they were sourced.

Even in the oldest herbaria, one can encounter the use of various types of writing materials, including those produced much later than the herbarium itself. This is usually related to the intensive use of herbaria as scientific tools, which were updated by the addition of annotations and comments by subsequent researchers. It is common to find manuscripts by several authors within a single sheet, mainly due to the verification of identifications by later users (Fig. 2.17).

Some herbaria take the form of field documentation and, in addition to specimens, include illustrations, and extensive descriptions on species names, vegetation, and usage (Fig. 2.18 and Figs. 2.19 and 2.20).

Such herbaria may serve as records of systematic ethnobotanical research, containing a catalogue of names used by the local community and descriptions of the ways in which particular plants are utilised (Figs. 2.21 and 2.22).

In such cases, the handwritten component may occupy more space than the specimens themselves, which usually also means, in regard to techniques and technology, a greater diversity of materials used for descriptions (inks, Indian ink, coloured pencils, graphite pencils, ballpoint pens, felt-tip pens). In addition, personal or institutional stamps of the herbarium's creators are often present.

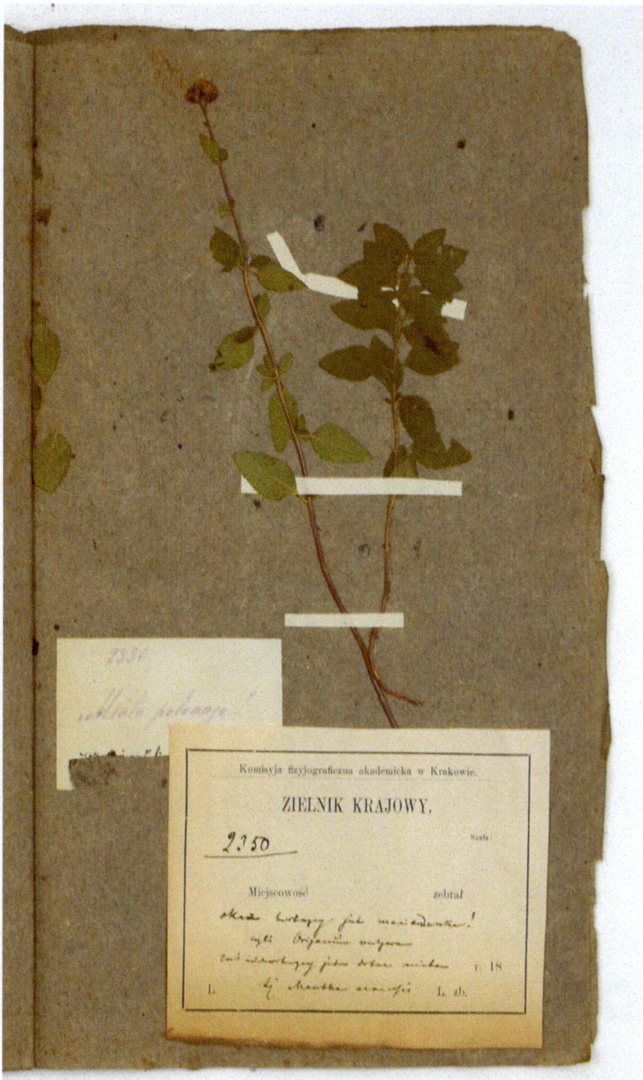

Fig. 2.23 Printed, handwritten, and mixed labels in herbaria. Herbarium of Michał Fedorowski [Fedorowski M., (*Folk Names of Plants*), Warsaw, Herbarium of the Faculty of Biology, University of Warsaw (WA), ref. WA-KH-5.1.–5.10, ca. 1880]. (Photo: M. Grenda-Kurmanow)

The descriptive layer may also appear on the label in printed form, which was a common method of marking specimens in herbaria in the nineteenth century, although handwritten descriptions continued to be used as well. Institutional printed labels are often completed with handwritten specimen data and bear the signature of the collection's author (Figs. 2.23, 2.24 and 2.25).

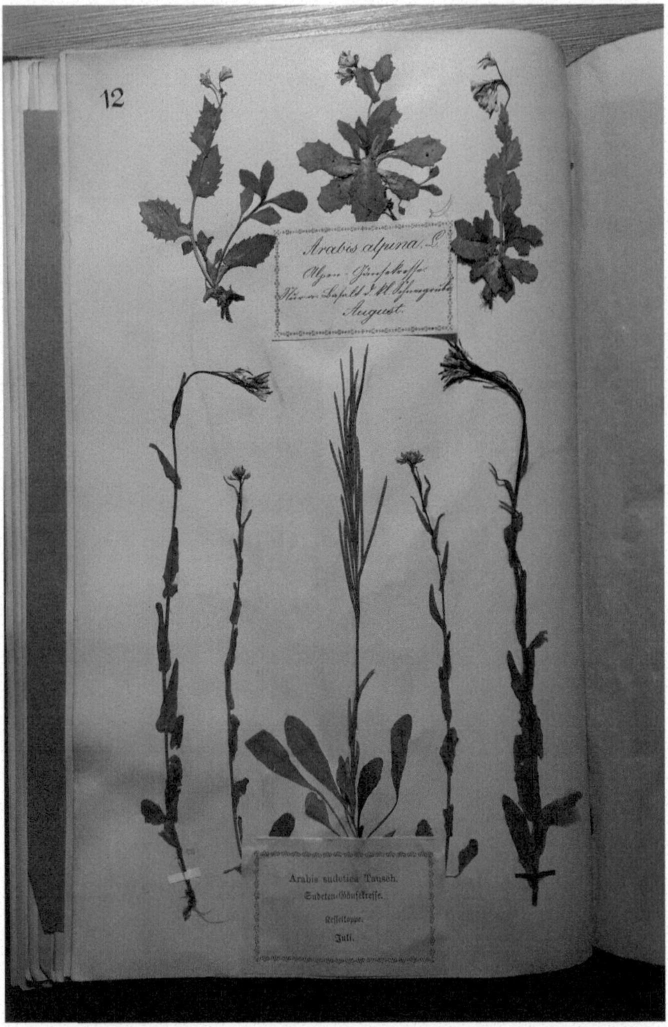

Fig. 2.24 Printed, handwritten, and mixed labels in W. Winkler's herbarium. Winkler W., untitled, Wrocław, Herbarium of the Museum of Natural History in Wrocław (WRSL), without ref. no., 1831. (Photo: M. Grenda-Kurmanow)

In the case of historical sheets, a single specimen may be accompanied by multiple labels, reflecting the addtion of scientific information while respecting the original material prepared by the author and previous users of the herbarium (Fig. 2.25).

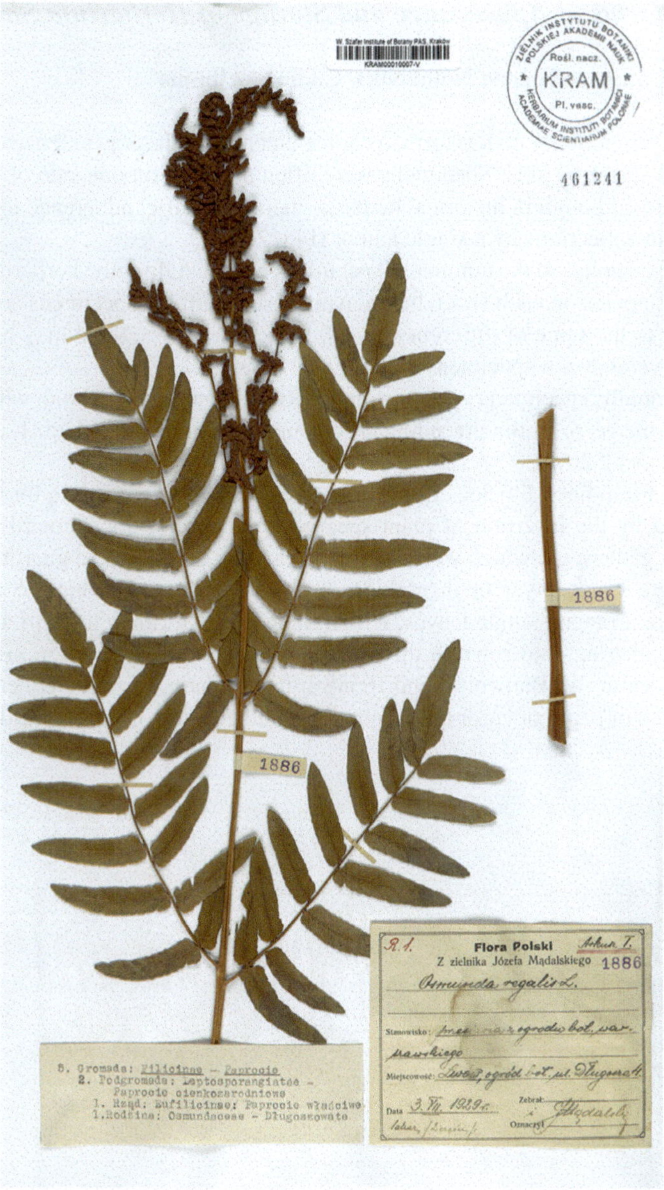

Fig. 2.25 Printed, handwritten, and mixed labels on a herbarium sheet of Józef Mądalski; Mądalski J., untitled, Kraków, Herbarium of the Institute of Botany, Polish Academy of Sciences in Kraków (KRAM), ref. 461241, barcode: KRAM00010007-V, twentieth century, with specimens from the nineteenth century, new mounting sheet with preserved older labels. (Photo: Władysław Szafer Institute of Botany, Polish Academy of Sciences)

2.1.6 Forms of Appearance and Storage of Herbarium Sheets

2.1.6.1 Compact Forms: Notebooks, Codices, Albums

Herbaria were initially codex-form, a choice dictated by the convenience of storage and use as scientific aids. Specimens were often mounted on one side of the sheet, on the *recto*, although in historical herbaria, there is no strict adherence to this rule, even within collections by a single author (Fig. 2.26).

This also applies to the number of specimens per sheet. In some herbaria, a single specimen appears on each sheet, but in many cases, multiple specimens are present, belonging to the same or different species. In extreme cases, there may be a dozen or even several dozen specimens on one sheet (Fig. 2.27).

Occasionally, specimens were accompanied by illustrative material, which could appear on the *verso* of the preceding sheet (Figs. 1.5 and 1.6 in Chap. 1, as well as Figs. 2.19 and 2.20).

In herbarium book blocks, efforts were often made to compensate for the swelling caused by the insertion of plant specimens by placing loose guards between individual gatherings, which were then sewn into the block. These guards could be present in a single layer or in multiple layers at the same location. Sometimes, sheets were arranged single leaves, with a folded edge forming a guard alternately within a gathering, and sewn in this manner. An exceptional solution, used in the sixteenth century in Rauwolf's and Reinwardt's herbaria, involved adhering additional layers of paper or cardboard along the trimmed edge of the herbarium sheets,

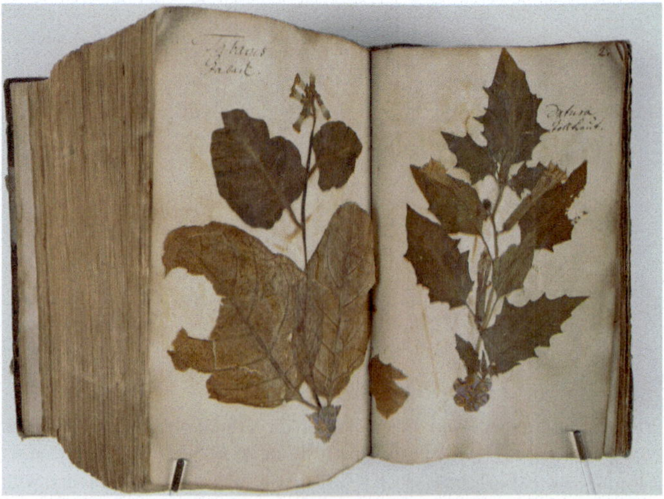

Fig. 2.26 The herbarium of Johann Friedrich Zeidler (Zeidler J.F., *Hortus Perennis*..., Lublin, Main Library of the University of Life Sciences, Volume III, ref. Zb. Specj. Starodruki XVIII.14; D. 104.57.646, 1751). In some folios, specimens are attached to both the *recto* and *verso* sides. (Photo: K. Stasiuk)

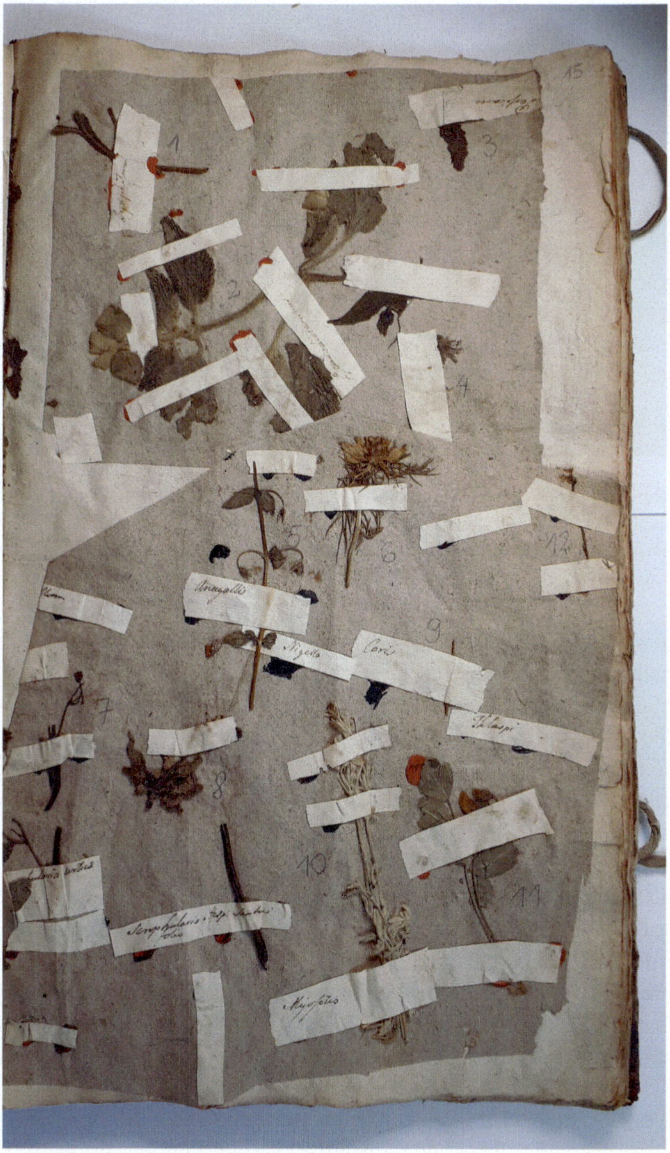

Fig. 2.27 Herbarium of Antoni Camelin or Jan Szaster: Camelin A. or Szaster J., *Herbarium, probably…*, Kraków, Herbarium of the Institute of Botany, Jagiellonian University (KRA), without ref. no., first half of the eighteenth century. Each sheet typically contains a dozen or so specimens. (Photo: M. Grenda-Kurmanow)

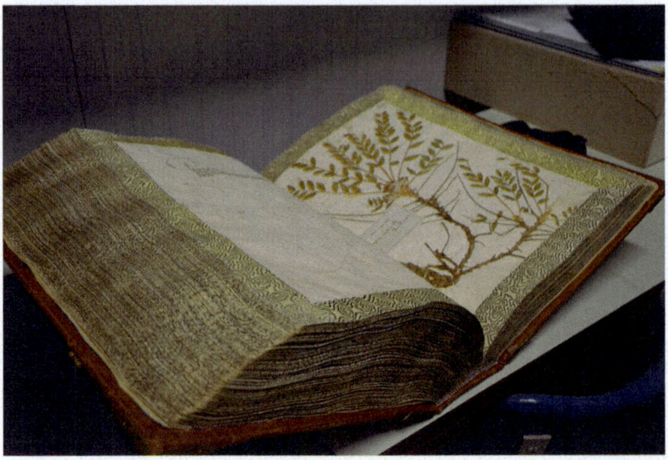

Fig. 2.28 Rauwolf's herbarium [Rauwolf L., (*Kreütterbuech*), Leiden, Naturalis Biodiversity Center (L), vol. IV, ref. *Codex Vossianus Germanicus in Folio*, L.2077656, 1573–1575]. Raised edges the margins of the sheets protect the specimens from mechanical damage and insect access. (Photo: M. Grenda-Kurmanow)

which also served to offset the swelling and, additionally, created protective edges for the specimens.[47] This not only prevented the specimens from falling out of the block, but also protected them from insect attack, as the tightly closed block was inaccessible to pests (Figs. 2.28 and 2.29).[48] The gatherings were sewn onto supports made of parchment, leather, or cord.

The bindings of historical herbaria are highly diverse. The simplest in construction are herbaria in the form of notebooks, where the protective function for the single-section block is provided by covers and additional paper gatherings, either sewn to the block or attached to it (Figs. 2.30 and 2.31).

Among the oldest herbaria, parchment bindings are encountered, where parchment is typically stretched over cardboard covers (Figs. 2.32, 2.23 and 2.34). These bindings are most often undecorated. An exception is the herbarium of Jerzy Andrzej Helwing from the National Library in Warsaw, Poland, which is a codex bound in parchment in an incredibly decorative manner, with covers painted in botanical and mythological motifs (Fig. 2.33).

The most common types of herbarium bindings are cardboard covers in full cloth, half-leather, and full leather, with half-cloth bindings less frequent (Figs. 2.35, 2.36 and 2.37). In the nineteenth century, when herbaria were still produced in codex form, they typically featured full cloth bindings.[49] Bindings may have single

[47] See also Dillenius herbarium in Thiers 2020.

[48] Saint-Lager 1885, p. 72; Thijsse 2016

[49] An example of such a codex is the herbarium of Eliza Orzeszkowa [Orzeszkowa E., (*Herbarium of Eliza Orzeszkowa*), Poznań, Poznań Society for the Advancement of Arts and Sciences, ref. Rkp. 880, 1887–1898]; (see also photographs of the interior of the block in Figs. 3.7 and 3.8 in Chap. 3).

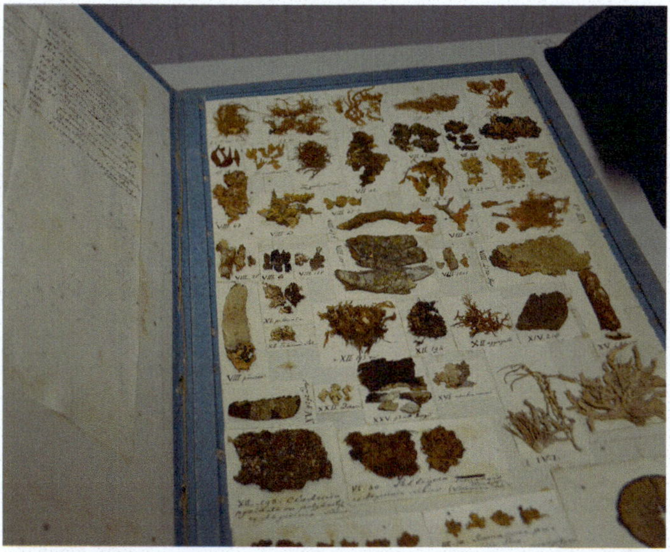

Fig. 2.29 Herbarium of Caspar Georg Carl Reinwardt, Reinwardt C. G. C., untitled, Leiden, Naturalis Biodiversity Center (L), ref. L.2077648-L.2077650, 1773–1854. Similar to Rauwolf's herbarium, raised edges the margins of the sheets protect the specimens from mechanical damage and insect access. (Photo: M. Grenda-Kurmanow)

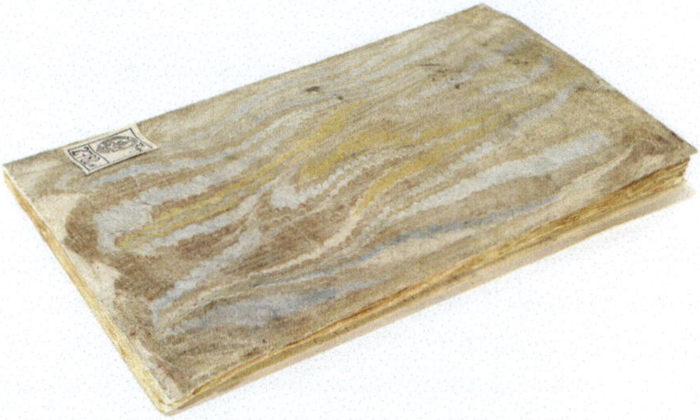

Fig. 2.30 N.n., *Herbarium Vivum…*, [Izabela Czartoryska Herbarium], Kraków, National Museum in Kraków, Czartoryski Princes Library, ref. Rkps. 2782, 1746. The herbarium has a simple cover enclosing the text block, attached to the spine. (Photo: T. Rizov-Ciechański)

or double ties, although even quadruple ties can be found, as in the *En Tibi* herbarium (Fig. 2.37), most often made of cloth tapes and less commonly of leather.

The construction of the bindings generally reflects the time and place of the herbarium's origin, but they are also frequently the result of later bookbinding practices. Herbarium bindings were often replaced, probably because of the condition of the original binding and the tendency of the text block to deform from overfilling with plant specimens or to adjust the binding to the existing collection. For this reason, in many cases the binding is not contemporary with the contents of the

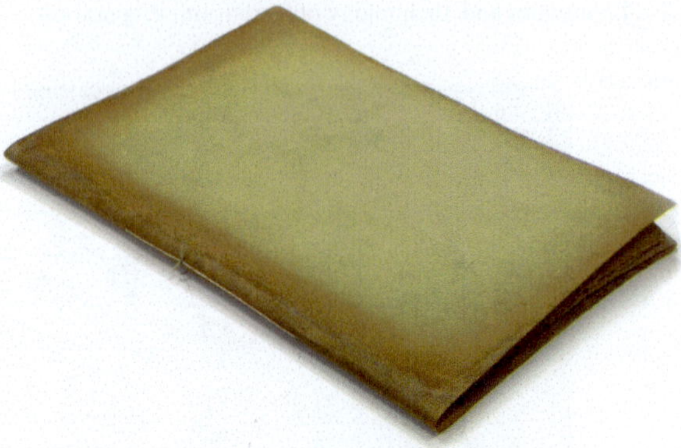

Fig. 2.31 Michał Fedorowski's herbarium [Fedorowski M., *Zielnik Litewski*, Warsaw, Herbarium of the Faculty of Biology, University of Warsaw (WA), ref. WA-KH-3, ca. 1880]. The herbarium is in the form of a notebook, with a simple cover enclosing the block, sewn to its spine. (Photo: M. Grenda-Kurmanow)

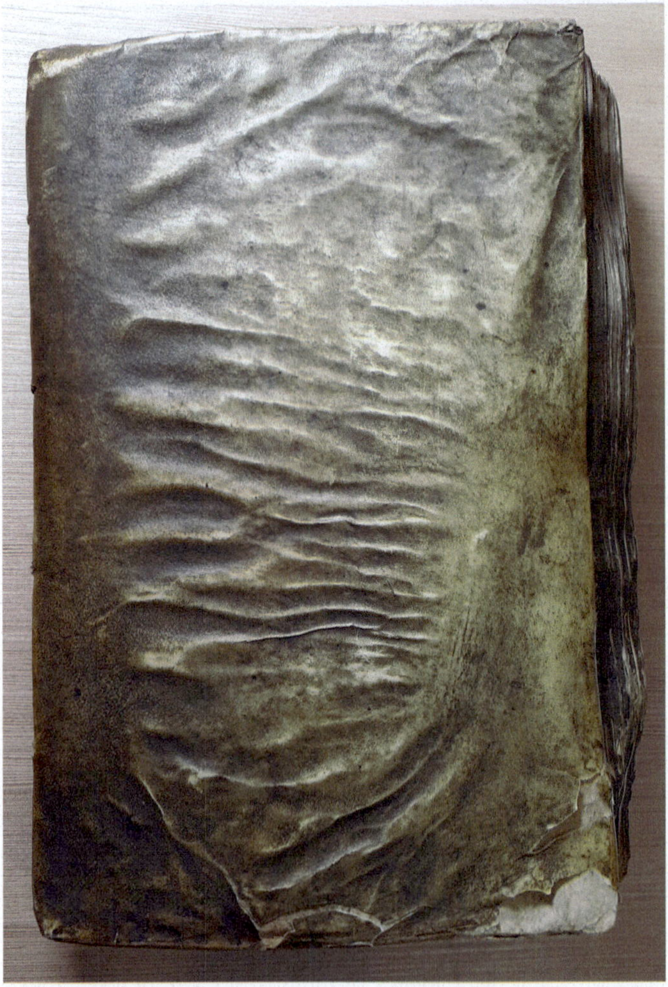

Fig. 2.32 Parchment binding on cardboard covers of Paolo Silvio Boccone's herbarium: Boccone P.S., [*Herbarium of Paolo Silvio Boccone*], Wrocław, Herbarium of the Museum of Natural History in Wrocław (WRSL), without ref. no., 1674–1695. (Photo: M. Grenda-Kurmanow)

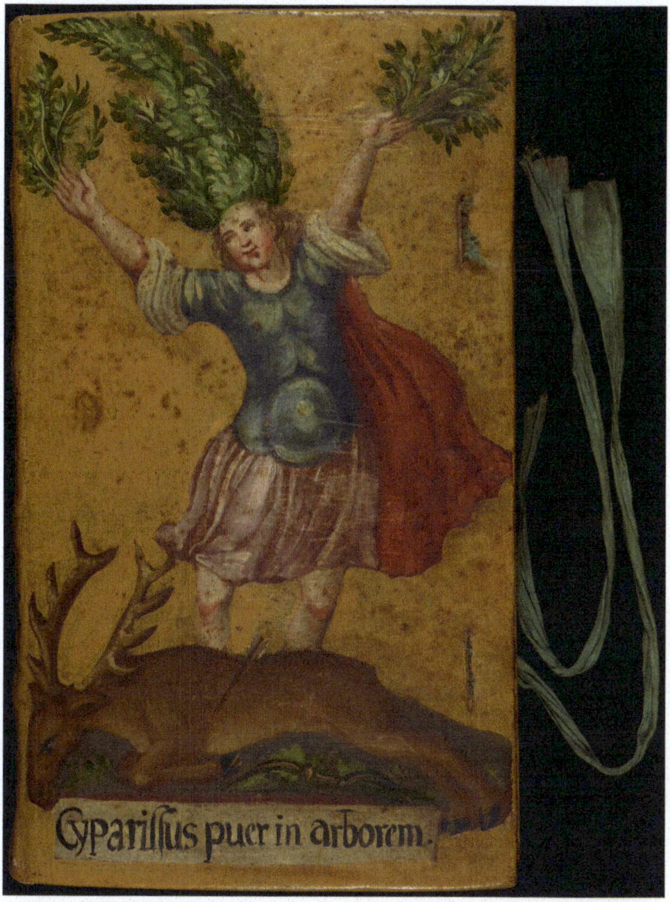

Fig. 2.33 Cover of Volume II of Georg Andreas Helwing's herbarium, Helwing, J. A., *Florae Napeisque*..., Warsaw, National Library, ref. Rps akc. 200/2, c. 1695–1705, (Polona)

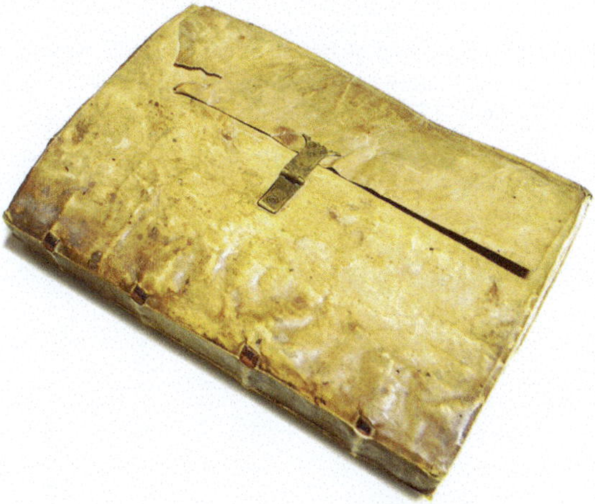

Fig. 2.34 Parchment binding of Petrus Cadé's herbarium [Cadé P., (*Cadé Herbarium*), Leiden, Naturalis Biodiversity Center (L), without ref. no., 1566]. (Photo: M. Grenda-Kurmanow)

Fig. 2.35 Paper cover of Johann Friedrich Zeidler's herbarium (Zeidler J. F., *Hortus Perennis*..., Lublin, Main Library of the University of Life Sciences, Volume I, ref. Zb. Specj. I Starodruki 14, D. 104.57.646, 1732). (Photo: T. Rizov-Ciechański)

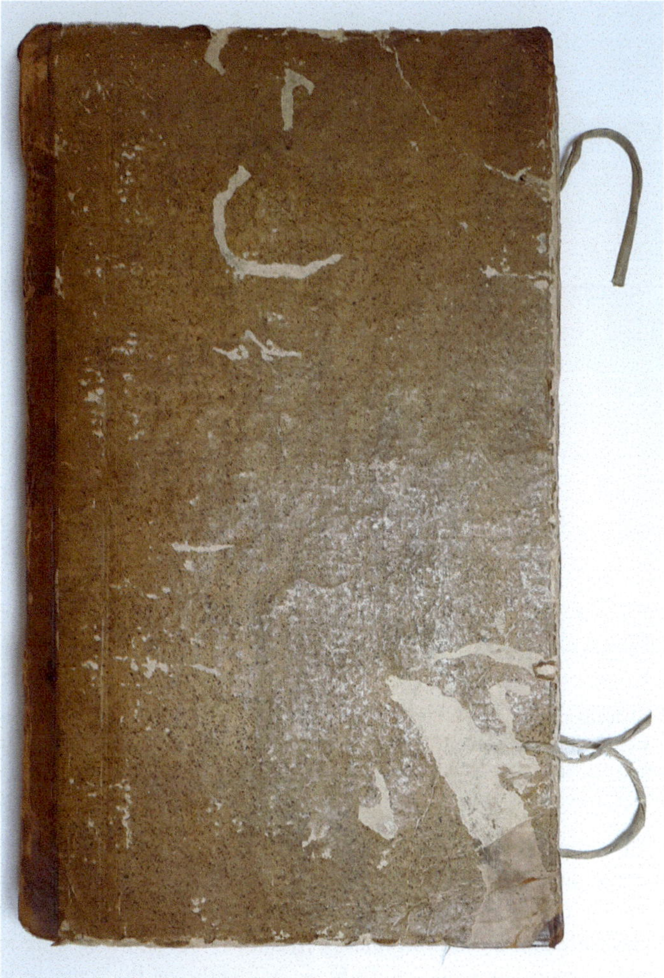

Fig. 2.36 Half-leather binding of the herbarium of Antoni Camelin or Jan Szaster [Herbarium of Antoni Camelin or Jan Szaster; Camelin A. or Szaster J., *Herbarium, probably…*, Kraków, Herbarium of the Institute of Botany, Jagiellonian University in Kraków (KRA), without ref. no., first half of the eighteenth century]. (Photo: M. Grenda-Kurmanow)

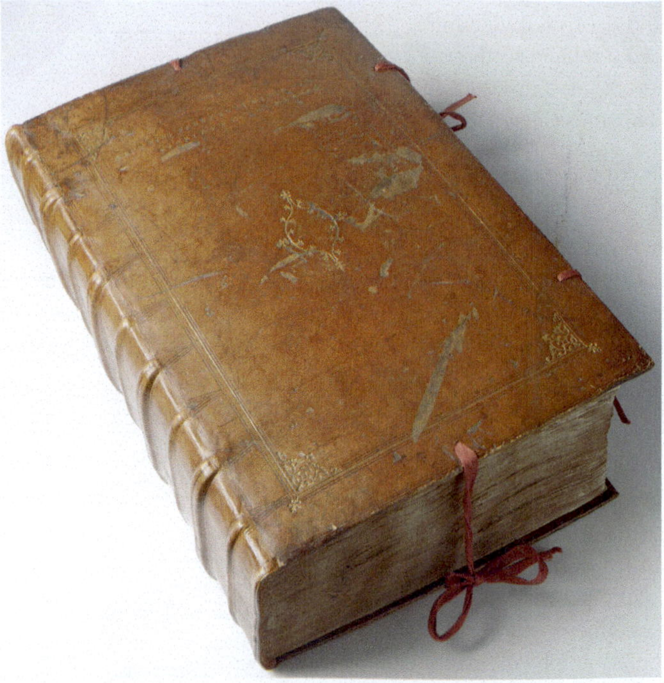

Fig. 2.37 Full leather binding of the *En Tibi* herbarium [N.n., *En Tibi*…, Leiden, Naturalis Biodiversity Center (L), ref. Codex Vossianus Germanicus in Folio No. 1 Vol. 1 Part 2, 1558]. (Photo: Naturalis Biodiversity Center)

herbarium.[50] Examples of secondary bindings include the half-leather covers of the Camelin/Szaster and Badurski herbaria from the Herbarium of the Institute of Botany of the Jagiellonian University in Kraków (KRA). Both collections, dating from the eighteenth century but originating from different sources, were rebound in the nineteenth century in identical fashion, evidently in the same bookbinding workshop (Köhler 1999).

[50] It is often difficult to determine whether the binding is original or a later replacement. In several herbaria preserved in Poland from the seventeenth and eighteenth centuries, the sewing supports are threaded over the joints of the binding through incisions made at the edges of the joints, suggesting that the binding was replaced. It should be noted that none of the bindings under consideration is a so-called limp binding. The ends of the sewing supports (made of parchment or leather) were glued to the inside of the covers, sometimes between the cover board and the spine board. While in the case of parchment bindings, the passage of sewing supports over the joints is a regular feature, the use of such a construction in paper bindings remains unclear. However, the construction itself may indicate the development of a binding scheme that enabled easy replacement if the text block became overfilled.

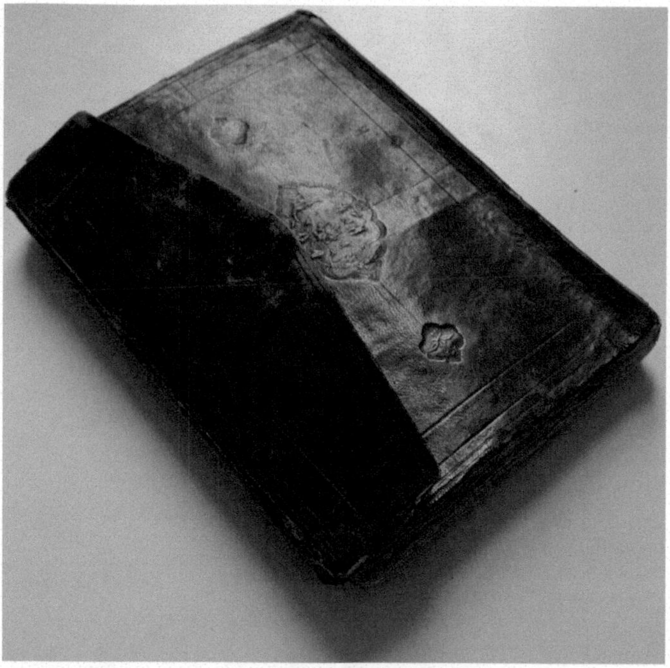

Fig. 2.38 Binding in the Turkish style, herbarium of Jean de Thévenot; Thévenot, de J., untitled, Paris, Muséum national d'Histoire naturelle (P), without ref. no., 1664–1666. (Photo: M. Grenda-Kurmanow)

The binding styles of herbaria found in scientific collections are not limited to the European cultural sphere. Among the less typical bindings, one can find, for example, Eastern (most likely Turkish) bindings of Jean de Thévenot's herbaria (Fig. 2.38) as well as Japanese bindings of Philipp Franz von Siebold's herbaria (Fig. 2.39).

2.1.6.2 Single Sheets

Linnaeus is credited with popularising the practice of mounting specimens on individual, physically unbound sheets. This method had certainly been used earlier, at least occasionally, given the intensive contacts among botanists and the numerous exchanges and shipments of plant specimens associated with them. Nevertheless, Linnaeus was the most renowned and influential botanist to adopt this type of specimen storage systematically, officially recommending the method in his seminal *Philosophia Botanica* (1751) (Linnaeus 1751, p. 7). From the mid-eighteenth century onwards, the standard practice became keeping herbarium specimens as single sheets or folders (Figs. 2.40 and 2.41, as well as Fig. 2.21 and 2.22 and Fig. 2.25).

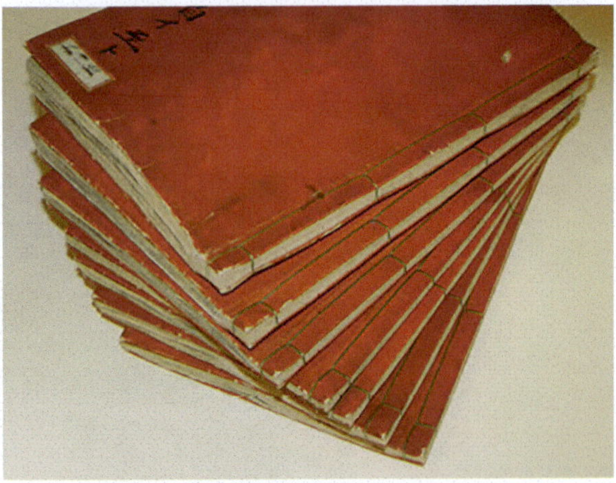

Fig. 2.39 Japanese herbarium bindings of Philipp Franz von Siebold; Siebold, von F., Leiden, Naturalis Biodiversity Center (L), ref. nos. L. 2077627–207730, 2078204–207812, 211011, 1823–1830 [Jacobi, Luu 2012]

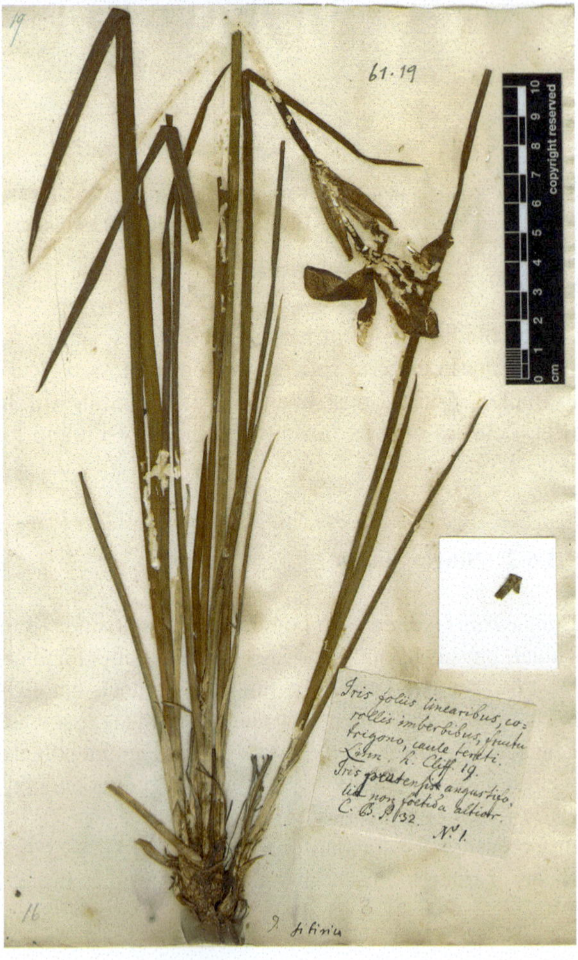

Fig. 2.40 A sheet from Linnaeus's herbarium, featuring a specimen of *Iris sibirica*; Linnaeus C., (*Linnaeus Herbarium*), London, Linnean Society, ref. LINN 61.19, before 1741 [Linnean Society of London (LINN)]

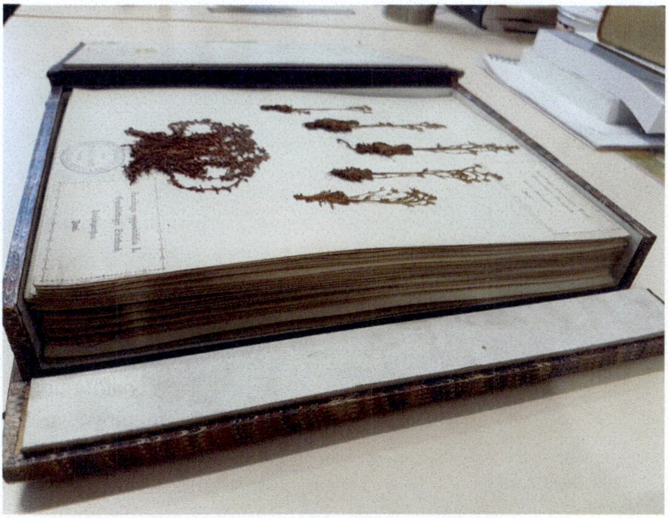

Fig. 2.41 Ornamental box for Winkler's herbarium sheets (Winkler, untitled, Warsaw, Herbarium of the Faculty of Biology, University of Warsaw (WA), nineteenth century. (Photo: Rewars)

This method was convenient and helpful to maintain systematic order, taking into account the development of botany and the discovery of new species. However, it required a different storage system, similar to techniques developed during field collection. As a result, folders, envelopes, and boxes—already previously used for storing and transporting specimens intended to be ultimately placed in the herbarium in codex form—became a permanent feature of herbarium collections. Boxes were sometimes decorative, serving as an intermediate form between the codex and the wrapped herbarium fascicle (Fig. 2.41). In individual collections, there are often consistently uniform series of boxes, which serve as a distinctive feature of a given collection (Figs. 2.42; Figs. 2.44 and 2.45).

As collective packaging, boxes and folders were the elements most likely to be replaced. The commonly used fascicles, in which specimens mounted on sheets were grouped into stacks, covered on both sides with cardboard and tied with string or cloth tapes, did not provide as much protection as additional protective packaging (Fig. 2.43).[51]

[51] See the section *Physical degradation of plant material* in Chap. 3.

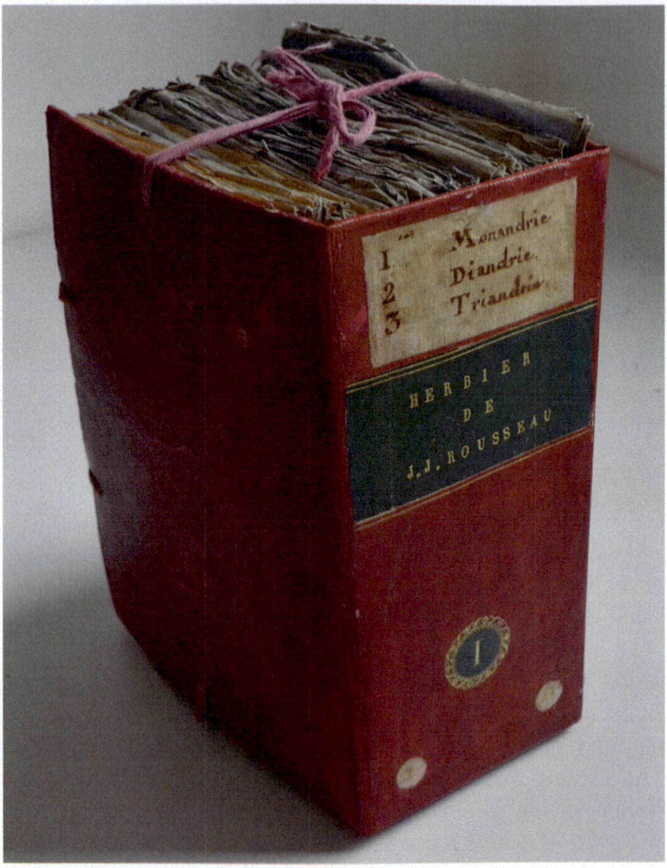

Fig. 2.42 Herbarium belonging to Jean-Jacques Rousseau [Aublet, J.B.F., (*Herbier Rousseau*), Paris, Muséum national d'Histoire naturelle, Paris (P), without ref. no., c. 1760. (Photo: M. Grenda-Kurmanow)

2.1.6.3 Unconventional Technological Solutions Found in Artistic Herbaria

The artistic and symbolic herbaria mentioned in the previous chapter[52] often diverged from the traditional form of herbaria in terms of technology. The velvet-bound herbaria of Eliza Orzeszkowa were frequently modelled on nineteenth-century photographic albums. The pages in these albums are joined with stubs, and fragments of specimens are arranged in compositions on pages reminiscent of photographic mounts, sometimes covered with coloured satin and fitted with a

[52] See the section *Special Examples of Herbaria: Artistic and Symbolic Herbaria* in Chap. 1.

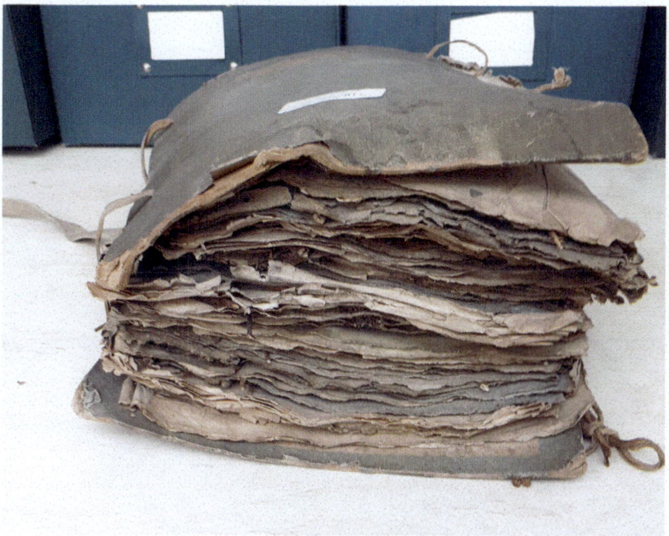

Fig. 2.43 The so-called Treviranus herbarium—a fascicle from the collections of the Herbarium of the Museum of Natural History in Wrocław (WRSL) [N.n., (*Treviranus Herbarium*), Wrocław, Herbarium of the Museum of Natural History in Wrocław (WRSL), without ref. no., undated]. It is not known whether it actually belonged to Ludolf Christian Treviranus (1779–1864), as indicated by the modern label. (Photo: M. Grenda-Kurmanow)

passe-partout with a gilded edge.[53] Albums prepared for the mounting of plant compositions were made for Orzeszkowa by Antoni Kramkowski in Grodno (Popławska 2014a, pp. 24–33).

Another example of an artistic herbarium is the work of Janina Jenko-Sokołowska from around 1900 (Figs. 2.46 and 2.47).

It features a rich form and complex symbolism, placing it in the category of artistic craft objects. Like Orzeszkowa, Sokołowska mounted plants onto cardboard sheets, to which passe-partout with gilded edges were attached. Some of her compositions represent an even further transformation of the herbarium concept, creating intricate landscapes in which it is difficult to distinguish individual plant fragments. The herbarium's substantial binding (17 × 64.5 × 43 cm), executed in the

[53] Herbaria created by Orzeszkowa, constructed in the style of photographic albums, can be found in the collections of the National Museum in Kraków, the Ossolineum, the Adam Mickiewicz Museum of Literature in Warsaw, the Rev. Jarzębowski Museum in Licheń Stary, and the Historical and Archaeological Museum in Grodno (Popławska 2014a, pp. 24–33). The writer also produced an ethnobotanical herbarium, now held in the Library of the Poznań Society for the Advancement of Arts and Sciences [Orzeszkowa E., (*Herbarium of Eliza Orzeszkowa*), Poznań, Poznań Society for the Advancement of Arts and Sciences, ref. Rkp. 880, 1887–1898]. This herbarium is constructed differently. It is bound in full cloth, with double ties made of satin ribbons. The specimens are arranged in the classical manner of scientific collections, with several specimens mounted on a single sheet. Only the title page forms a decorative composition (Fig. 3.7 in Chap. 3).

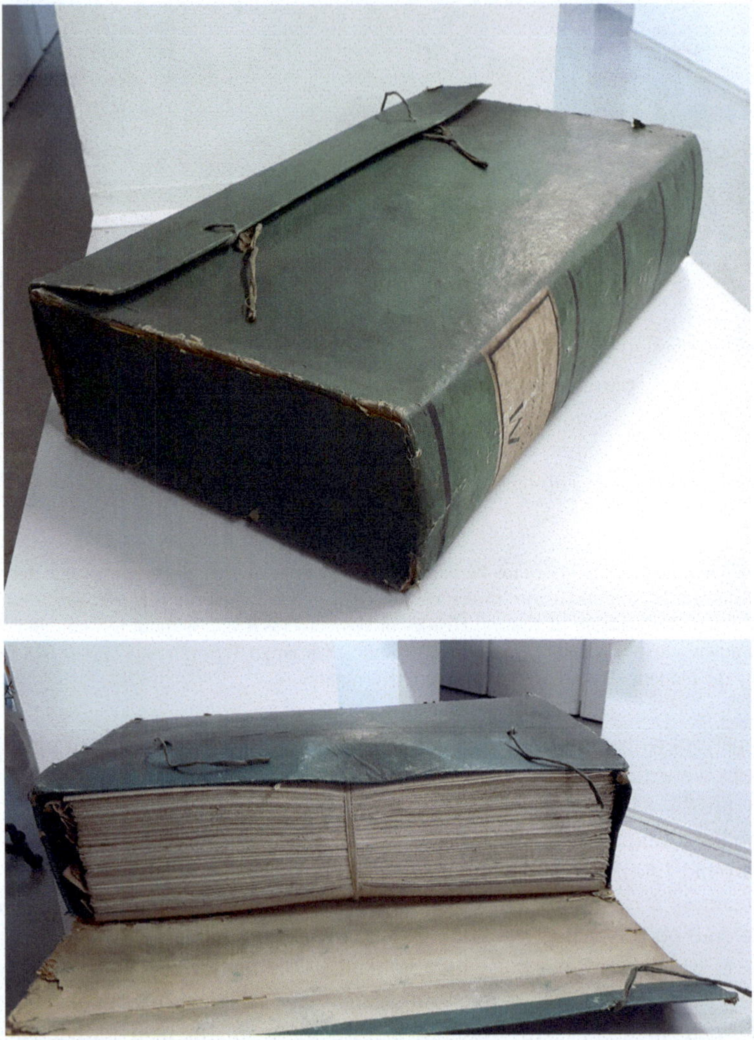

Figs. 2.44 and 2.45 Boxes for fascicles from the collections of Józef Jundziłł; Jundziłł J., (*Herbarium of Józef Jundziłł*), Kraków, Herbarium of the Institute of Botany, Polish Academy of Sciences in Kraków (KRAM), without ref. no., 1820s, containing specimens dated from the eighteenth century to 1876. In Fig. 62, a fascicle filling the box is visible. (Photo: M. Grenda-Kurmanow)

batik technique on wood, was produced at the Lviv bookbinding workshop of Ludwik Wierzbicki. The herbarium was exhibited at the industrial products exhibition in Przemyśl in 1904.[54]

[54]As Monika Paś writes, industrial exhibitions during the period of the partitions enabled the presentation of national artistic and cultural achievements. This is confirmed by the award given to Eliza Orzeszkowa at the exhibition in Lviv in 1894 (Paś 2017), see also (Kiljańska 2005).

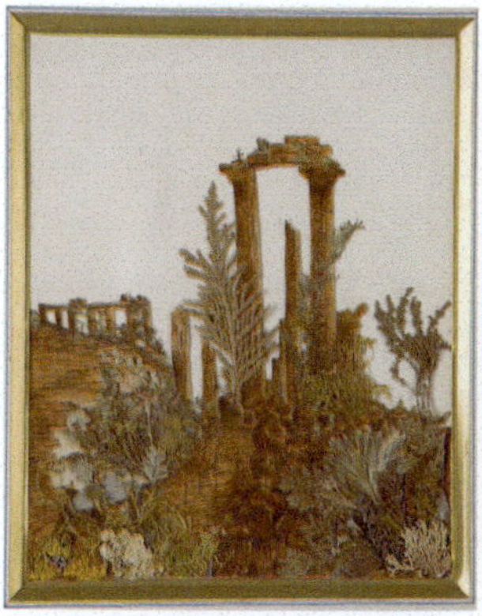
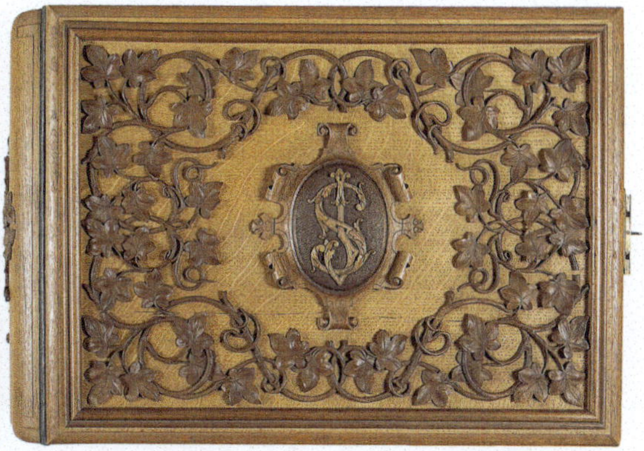

Figs. 2.46 and 2.47 Janina Jenko-Sokołowska's herbarium (Sokołowska J., bookbinding workshop: Wierzbicki, untitled [*Album ("herbarium")*], Kraków, National Museum in Kraków, ref. MNK IV-MO-1046/2, c. 1900). Fig. 2.46 shows one of the pages with an artistic composition and the binding (NMK), while Fig. 2.47 presents the binding made by Wierzbicki (Photographic Archive of the National Museum in Kraków)

In the French herbarium of Louise Gailleton, created between 1914 and 1918, additional technological elements are visible, such as fabric scraps, paint layers, and others (Fig. 2.48).

2.2 Physicochemical Characteristics of the Basic Components of Herbarium Structure

2.2.1 Chemical Compounds in the Cell Wall of Plant Specimens and in the Paper Substrate

In the context of plant specimen structure and degradation, understanding the composition of the cell wall is of key importance. The cell wall serves as a protective layer for the plant, and its disruption initiates further degradation processes in the specimen. Paper, as a plant-derived material, shares certain structural features with herbarium specimens. For both paper and plant cell walls, the main structural components are cellulose and hemicelluloses. Lignin is also present in both. These are chemical compounds that determine the physical and chemical properties of plant-based materials and their susceptibility to degradation. The proportions of these components in the plant cell wall are characteristic of the species.

The papermaking process aims to remove most substances other than cellulose, which is present in sheets in a highly processed form. In addition to cellulose, hemicelluloses, and lignin, paper may also contain residual components of plant fibres, generally referred to as extractives—organic compounds soluble in organic solvents that are not constituents of the cell wall, such as fatty acids, resins, and natural

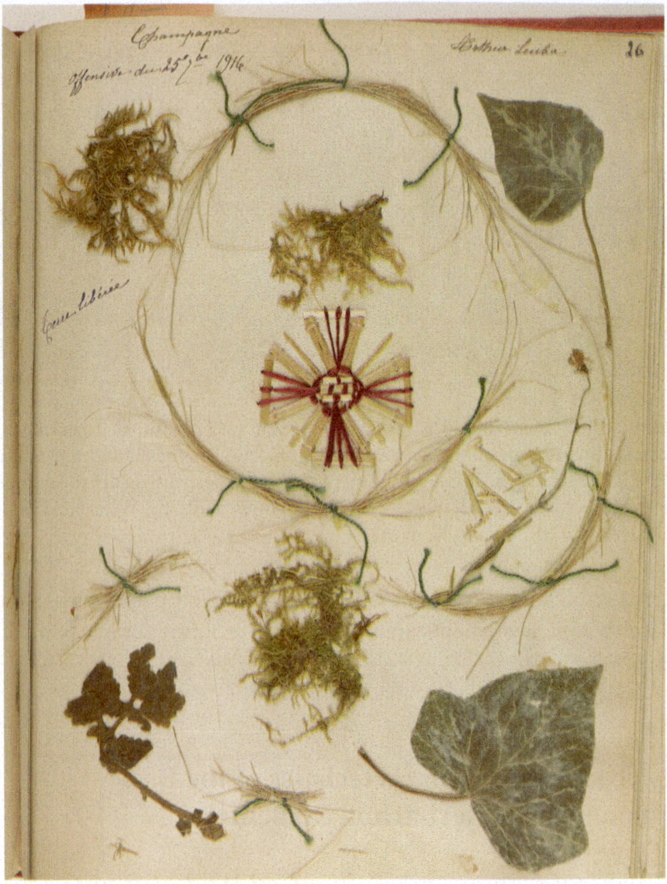

Fig. 2.48 A page from Louise Gailleton's "trench herbarium" [Gailleton L., (*Herbier des tranchées*), Paris, Muséum national d'Histoire naturelle (P), without ref. no., 1914–1918.] © MNHN—E. Lerat

fungicides. During the production of cellulose pulps, efforts are made to eliminate these substances, as they can cause complications in the manufacturing process (Sobucki 2013, p. 23; Brückle 2012a, p. 123).[55] Furthermore, paper may also contain so-called bulk additives, such as: sizing agents—carbohydrate-based (starches, dextrins, gums), resins [rosin, alkyl ketene dimer (AKD), alkenyl succinic

[55] Brückle draws attention to the potential effect of fibre self-adhesion. Sobucki, on the other hand, highlights the challenges associated with the use of resins, which are present in greater quantities in coniferous wood species. "(…) Their harmfulness does not lie in bonding the fibres, but rather in contaminating the components of the papermaking machine, including clogging the screen. For this reason, for example, pine wood is processed only by alkaline methods, in which resin acids are saponified and removed (…)" [personal communication, 7.04.2021].

anhydride (ASA)], proteinaceous substances (gelatine and other animal glues), cellulose derivatives (methylcellulose, carboxymethylcellulose), polyvinyl alcohols, styrene-acrylic copolymers (SAC); various types of alum (aluminium-potassium alum, aluminium sulphate); mineral substances serving as fillers (kaolin, chalk, talc, titanium and barium whites); colourants (dyes and pigments); and auxiliary substances (starches, animal glues) (Sobucki 2013, pp. 32–36; Banik et al. 2012).[56]

In the plant cell wall, in addition to cellulose, hemicelluloses and lignin, pectins, proteins, suberin and cutin are also present. The proportions of substances forming the structures of plant cell walls and paper are shown in Table 2.3. Figure 2.49 illustrates the distribution of cellulose, hemicelluloses, lignin and extractives content for selected plant species.

While many publications provide the percentage content of cellulose, hemicelluloses, and lignin for individual plant species, information regarding their proportions in paper is generally not reported. In the production of papers intended for archival purposes, the goal is to achieve "100% cellulose"; however, it must be assumed that even in such paper, at least trace amounts of other components are present. The cellulose content in paper determines its quality; therefore, isolating cellulose in as intact form as possible and without loss is the aim of pulp production, from which paper is manufactured (Sobucki 2013, p. 16). The most important step in this process is removing as much lignin as possible, as lignin reduces paper quality. However, it is not possible to remove it completely, since the prolonged aggressive treatment required for such removal would also destroy the cellulose itself. For comparison, if paper were made solely from mechanical pulp, it would have the same chemical composition as the wood used as raw material; thus, the lignin content would be relatively high and the cellulose content low (Sobucki 2013, p. 31). Pulp obtained from wood in the high-yield pulp process may contain over 20% lignin, whereas in the low-yield pulp process, the lignin content may not exceed 3% (Fig. 2.50) (Brückle 2012b). In a paper with such a low lignin content, the cellulose content may reach over 95%. During the pulping process, up to 75% of hemicelluloses may be dissolved (Brückle 2012b).

2.2.2 *Mineral Compounds in the Structure of Botanical Specimens and in the Structure of Paper*

In both in paper and plant specimens, ions of various mineral elements, including metal ions, may be present. In plants, it relates to the uptake of nutrients essential for the construction of their own tissues, as well as the acquisition of energy and

[56] The substances listed were used in paper production during very different periods; chronological order has not been maintained in this paragraph. Aware of the complex issues surrounding the history of papermaking, the range of materials found in paper is presented here in a summarised form. The history of the use of papermaking additives is discussed in greater detail in publications on the history of papermaking (e.g. Hunter 1978; Dąbrowski and Siniarska-Czaplicka 1991, pp. 30–227; Sobucki and Jeżewska 2015, pp. 129–139).

Table 2.3 Distribution of structural components in the cell wall and in cellulose pulp

Structural component	Cell wall		Cellulose mass
	Primary	Secondary	
Polysaccharides, including:	90%	65–95%	Up to approx. 97%
Cellulose	30%	40–90%	40–95+%
Hemicelluloses	30%	2–30%	Approx. 2%–25%
Pectins	30%	–	–
Proteins	10%	–	–
Lignin	–	15–35%	3–20%
Extractive substances	0.4–10	?	≤8%
Carbohydrate-based sizing agents: Starches, dextrin, gums; resins [e.g. rosin, alkyl ketene dimer (AKD)], alkenyl succinic anhydride (ASA); protein-based: Gelatine, other animal-derived adhesives; cellulose derivatives: Methylcellulose, carboxymethylcellulose, polyvinyl alcohols, styrene-acrylic copolymers (SAC)	–	–	≤1%
Fillers: Kaolin, chalk, talc, titanium white, baryte white	–	–	2–30%
Additives: Dyes (natural, plant extract-based, or synthetic organic dyes); pigments	–	–	<1%?
Excipients	–	–	<1%?

Based on Kopcewicz and Lewak (2012)

Modified after: Klemm et al. (2002), Banik et al. (2012), Brückle and Banik (2012), Brückle (2012b) and Sobucki (2013)

A question mark is used for values where unambiguous data are lacking

[a]Lignin is formed in the cell protoplast, but its concentration in the cell wall occurs during wall modification. Depending on the species, after lignin synthesis, its highest concentration may be found either in the primary wall and the adjacent first layer of the secondary wall, or within the secondary wall itself (Beck 2010, p. 65; Florian 1990, p. 22; Nick and Optarny 2014, p. 372; Simon et al. 2018; Wagner et al. 2012)

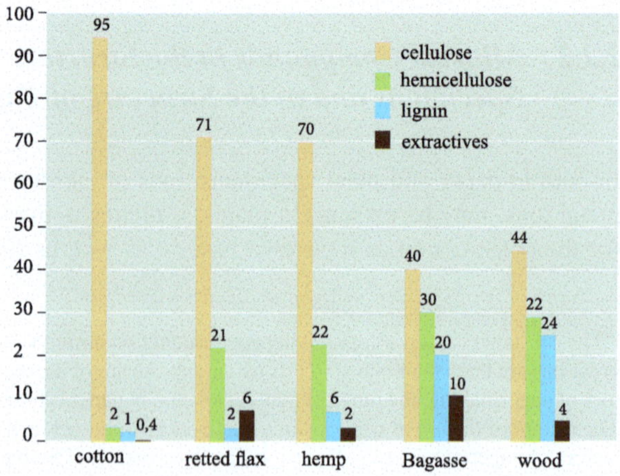

Fig. 2.49 Average content of cellulose (light beige), hemicelluloses (green), lignin (brown), and extractives (burgundy) in selected species (from left to right): cotton, retted flax, hemp, bagasse (sugarcane stems), and wood (mean values) (Based on: Brückle 2012b)

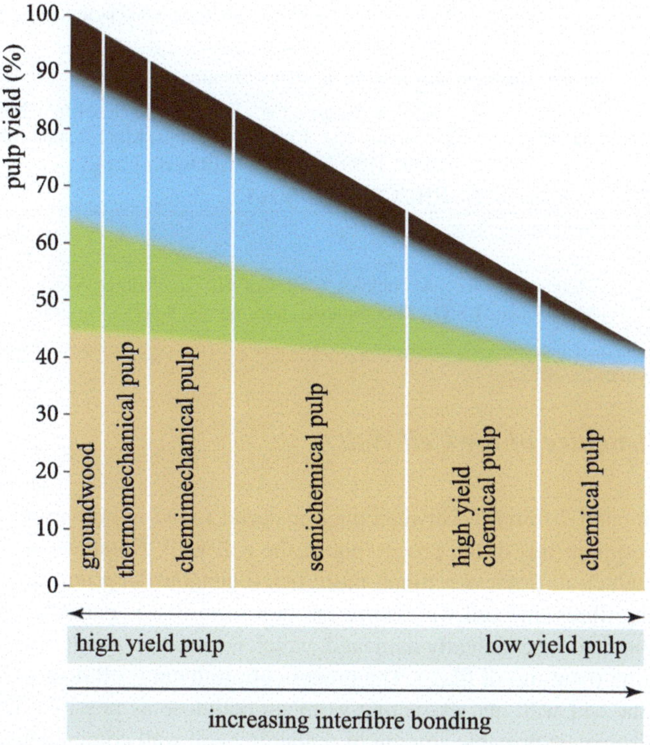

Fig. 2.50 Distribution of components in cellulose pulps obtained by various methods (from left to right): groundwood, thermomechanical, chemomechanical, semichemical, high-yield chemical, chemical. Light beige indicates cellulose content, green—hemicelluloses, brown—lignin, burgundy—extractives (Based on Brückle 2012b)

substances required for fundamental life processes such as respiration and photosynthesis. Leaves and storage organs contain the highest concentrations of mineral components. The nutrient content depends on the nutritional requirements and uptake capacity, which are genetically determined, as well as on the developmental stage, the availability of specific nutrients in the soil, and climatic conditions.

In the case of paper, the presence of mineral elements primarily results from production processes and is associated with water quality, the tools and machines used in manufacturing, and the chemicals applied in fibre processing. The lists of elements that may be present in plant specimens and in paper are shown in Tables 2.4 and 2.5. The tables do not consider contaminants arising from the use of biocidal agents.[57]

[57] See the section *Damage Caused by the Use of Biocidal Agents* in Chap. 3. For more on environmental pollution and its impact on collection storage, refer to the section *Environmental Pollution in Collection Storage Areas* in Chap. 3.

Table 2.4 Summary of macro- and microelements as well as so-called beneficial elements in plant nutrition

Source	Ions and compounds present in plant structures
Soil	Metals: K^+, Mg^{2+}, Ca^{2+}, a chelates, Fe^{2+}, Fe^{3+}, Fe chelates, Mn^{2+}, Mn^+, Mn chelates, Zn^{2+}, Zn chelates, Cu^+, Cu^{2+}, Cu chelates, MoO_4^{2-}, non-metals: NH_4^+, NO_3^-, S, SO_4^{2-}, H_2PO_3, HPO_4^{2-}, BO_3^{3-}, H_3BO_3, $B_4O_7^{2-}$, Cl^-
Air	Non-metals: N_2, NH_3, $CO(NH_2)_2$, SO_2, Cl
Industrial pollutants	Metals: Ni^{2+}
Soil and fertiliser additives	Metals: Na^+, Al^{3+}, Al chelates, Co^{2+}, $CoOH^+$, Co chelates, VO_4^{2-} Metalloids: H_2SiO_4, Si complexes, non-metals: Se (IV), Se (VI)

Based on Szymańska 2012

2.2.3 *Structure of the Cell Wall*

The fundamental difference between plant material found in herbarium specimens and cellulose pulp lies in the processing of the cell wall. Botanical specimens, as biological material, possess a much more heterogeneous structure than paper. In papermaking fibres, the cell wall is present in a form that is partially delaminated from the fibre and mechanically damaged, which is a normal result of the mechanical processing (beating) of fibres. The process of producing cellulose pulp involves loosening the cell wall and extracting as much cellulose as possible. During processing, the greatest possible amount of remaining cell wall components, primarily lignin, is removed, and the structure of fibril segments is reconfigured (Brückle 2012b).

The cell wall is an integral component of the plant cell and, with few exceptions, is present in almost all plant cells, located outside the cell membrane, which together with the rest of the metabolically active part of the cell is referred to as the protoplast. Most of the precursor elements for the substances that constitute the wall are synthesised within the cell and subsequently secreted outside the protoplast. There, they undergo polymerisation and organisation. Alongside cellular plastids, the wall is one of the main determinants of plant cell function. As it is semipermeable, it does not act as a barrier to chemical compounds; this role is fulfilled by the cell membrane, which is selectively semipermeable.[58] The passage of chemical compounds and ions through the membrane occurs either actively or passively. The cell wall contains pits through which cytoplasmic extensions, known as plasmodesmata, pass, connecting the protoplasts of adjacent cells. The system of neighbouring cell walls and intercellular spaces, known as the apoplast, forms a channel through which water, along with dissolved ions and chemical compounds, is transported.

In a young, metabolically active cell, only the primary wall is present, composed of cellulose, hemicelluloses, pectic substances, and structural and enzymatic proteins (see Table 2.3). On the inner or outer surface of the primary cell wall,

[58] An exception is made for walls covered with suberin or cutin.

Table 2.5 Summary of mineral compounds present in paper

Source	Components	Ions and compounds present in the paper structure
Soil	Clay, limestone	metals: Al^{3+}, Ca^{2+}, Mg^{2+}, Zn^{2+}, Fe^{2+}
Igneous rocks	Pyroxene, biotite	metals: Si^{4+}, Na^{+}, K^{+}, Mg^{2+}, Fe^{2+}, Fe^{3+}, Al^{3+}, Ca^{2+}
Sedimentary rocks, sandstone, limestone	Feldspar, quartz, calcite (calcium carbonate), magnesium carbonate, gypsum (calcium sulphate, $CaSO_4 \cdot 2H_2O$)	metals: Ca^{2+}, Al^{3+}, K^{+}, Mg^{2+}, Na^{+}, Si^{4+}
Metamorphic rocks	Granite, schist, marble, feldspar, mica, hornblende, quartz (SiO_2), calcite ($CaCO_3$), kaolin, haematite (FeO_3), magnetite (Fe_3O_4)	metals: Ca^{2+}, Al^{3+}, K^{+}, Si^{4+}, Mg^{2+}, Fe^{2+}, Fe^{3+}, Na^{+}
Runoff from agricultural and contaminated areas	Animal manure, fertilisers, mining waste, floodwaters	metals: Cu^{2+}, Zn^{2+}, As^{3+}, Ca^{2+}, Al^{3+}, K^{+}, Si^{4+}, Mg^{2+}, Fe^{2+}, Fe^{3+}, Se^{4+}, U^{6+}, Ni^{2+}, Pb^{2+}, Cd^{2+}, Sr^{2+}
Air	Manufacturing industry, fuel combustion products, photochemical smog, atmospherically oxidised NO	Non-metals: N_2, NH_3, SO_2, SO_3, NO_2, NO
Wood	Various ground woods	metals: Al^{3+}, Ca^{2+}, Mg^{2+}, Zn^{2+}, Fe^{2+}, Mn^{2+}, Cu^{2+}, Co^{3+}, Ba^{2+}
Lignin removal, bleaching of fibrous pulp	Sodium hypochlorite (NaOCl), calcium hypochlorite ($CaClO_2$), chlorine dioxide (ClO_2), sodium sulphide and other Sulphur compounds, lignosulphonic acid, carboxylic acid salts	metals: Na^{+}, Ca^{2+}, Mg^{2+} Non-metals: ClO_2^-, ClO_3^-, SO_2
Sizing, processing of sizing agents	Rosin, aluminium-potassium sulphate [$KAl(SO_4)_2 \cdot 12H_2O$]; aluminium sulphate [$Al_3(SO_4)_2 \cdot 18H_2O$]	metals: Al^{3+}, non--metals: SO_3
Fillers	Kaolin, calcined kaolin $Al_2Si_2O_5(OH)_4$, barium sulphate, titanium dioxide, ultra-finely ground fillers	metals: Al^{3+}, Ca^{2+}, Mg^{2+}, Zn^{2+}, Fe^{2+}, Cu^{2+}, Co^{3+}, Ba^{2+}, Ti^{2+}, K^{+}, Na^{+}, Si^{4+}
Coating	Calcium carbonate, magnesium carbonate, kaolin, titanium dioxide, talc (magnesium silicate hydroxide)	metals: Ti^{2+}, Mg^{2+}, Pb^{2+}, Ca^{2+}, Al^{3+}, Si^{4+}, Fe^{2+}
Coating pigments	*Blanc fixe* (precipitated barium sulphate), satin white (aluminium-calcium sulphate)	metals: Ba^{2+}, Ca^{2+}, Al^{3+}
Pigments	Chrome yellow ($PbCrO_4$), lead white [$PbCO_3 \cdot Pb(OH)_2$], red lead (Pb_3O_4), vermilion (HgS), orpiment (As_2S_3), lemon yellow ($BaCrO_4$); Venetian, Hamburg, and Dutch whites ($BaSO_4$)	metals: Pb^{2+}, Hg^{2+}, As^{3+}, Ba^{2+}
Deacidification, fibre loosening	Zinc oxide, magnesium carbonate, magnesium bicarbonate, calcium hydroxide, calcium bicarbonate, potassium hydroxide	metals: Zn^{2+}, Mg^{2+}, Ca^{2+}, K^{+}

Based on Purewal (2012), Brückle (2012b) and Banik et al. (2012)

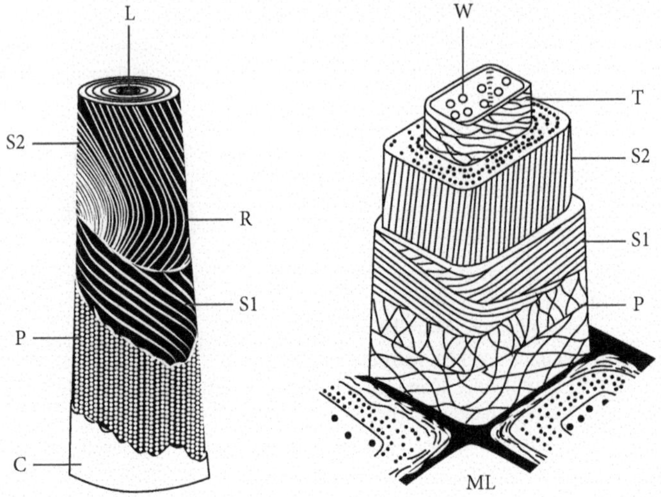

Fig. 2.51 Diagram of plant cell wall layers illustrated using a fibre: (**a**) cotton and (**b**) spruce purified from lignin. Legend: C—cuticle (rich in pectins and waxes), P—primary cell wall, R—fibril twist reversal, S1—secondary cell wall layer 1, S2—secondary cell wall layer 2 (main source of cellulose), T—tertiary wall layer, L—lumen, ML—middle lamella (in conifers—mainly lignin), W—warty layer (Based on Klemm et al. 2002)

adcrustation may occur, that is, the deposition of organic compounds such as suberin, cutin, waxes, mucilages, and gums on the wall surface. In mature cells, after elongation growth is complete, synthesis of the secondary cell wall begins on the inner side of the primary wall, adjacent to the protoplast. The secondary wall may undergo incrustation. Incrustation involves the impregnation of the cell wall framework with lignin (in a process known as lignification) as well as with mineral and organic compounds, including silica, calcium carbonate, tannins, resins, essential oils, and proteins. The microfibrillar structures of the primary and secondary walls differ. Classical descriptions of the cell wall present it as a rather ordered structure, with a hierarchical arrangement of cellulose molecules (microfibrils, fibrils, macrofibrils), between which a matrix composed of hemicelluloses locally bound to cellulose, as well as pectins and proteins—especially expansins (in the primary wall)—and also lignin, suberin, cutin, simple sugars, and water, is found (Gunning and Steer 1996, p. 14; Beck 2010, p. 61). In the primary wall, the arrangement of microfibrils is relatively irregular, whereas in the secondary wall, it is organised. The secondary wall usually consists of three layers, with the number of layers varying by species. In each layer, the fibrils are oriented at specific angles, which affects their mechanical strength and swelling capacity. The layered structure of cell walls influences their reactivity with water and other solvents (Brückle 2012a). A schematic of the layered structure of cell walls, using cotton and spruce as examples, is shown in Fig. 2.51.

In recent years, partly due to the growing interest in the use of biomass as an energy source, the structure of the plant cell wall, particularly the primary wall, has

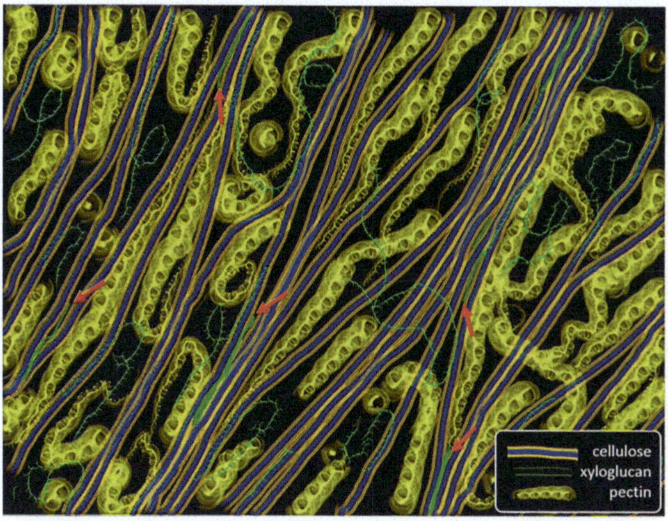

Fig. 2.52 Conceptual diagram of the structural features of the primary cell wall. Cellulose microfibrils are depicted as thick fibres with hydrophobic regions (marked in blue) and hydrophilic regions (marked in yellow). Xyloglucan (the predominant hemicellulose, marked in green) occurs in formations associated with the hydrophobic regions of cellulose, in the form of areas surrounded by it and stretched across its structure. It is also visible as trapped between the fibrils. Pectins (yellow) are present as coiled formations that fill the space between the microfibrils and bind the hydrophilic surfaces. The microfibrils are cross-linked at sites where cellulose interlaces with xyloglucan. Red arrows indicate cellulose–xyloglucan–cellulose linkages, which are regions of cell wall loosening. The diagram emphasises direct connections between cellulose microfibrils, in contrast to earlier representations in which microfibrils are shown as isolated and surrounded by matrix, connected only at discrete points (Cosgrove 2018)

been the subject of numerous analyses (e.g. Cosgrove 2001, 2014, 2018; Zheng et al. 2017). The latest concepts suggest that its individual components are more fragmented than previously assumed, and their mutual arrangement is more complex, with the general premise that cellulose microfibrils are interwoven with the inter-fibrillar capillaries of the matrix (Fig. 2.52) (Beck 2010, pp. 61–64). The proportional composition of the matrix depends on the function performed by the cell and on the living conditions of the plant.[59]

In the paper, the complex network of interactions between cellulose, hemicelluloses, and lignin is lost. Structurally, paper consists mainly of cross-linked cellulose chains, locally covered with residual hemicelluloses. Lignin residues accumulate on the surface of the fibres, which results from the mechanisms of pulping and bleaching of papermaking fibres. Pectins and waxes are removed during the earlier beating and softening of the fibres (Brückle 2012b).

[59] For example, cells provide structural support to the plant will contain more lignin, while cells involved in water regulation may contain higher amounts of cutin, which is impermeable to water.

2.2.4 *Characteristics of Compounds Present in the Cell Wall and in the Paper Substrate*

2.2.4.1 Cellulose

Cellulose is a natural polymer—a polysaccharide composed of β-D-glucose residues linked by β-1,4-glycosidic bonds between the first carbon atom of one glucose molecule and the fourth carbon atom of the next. Glucose has a ring structure containing five carbon atoms and one oxygen atom, known as a pyranose ring (in the case of glucose, this is glucopyranose). The ring does not form a flat structure but adopts a chair conformation (Fig. 2.53), which enables the molecules to join into long, ordered chains, as the functional groups are positioned in specific planes of the ring (Brückle 2012a). In the cellulose chain, glucopyranose residues are also referred to as anhydroglucose, since the formation of the polymer involves the loss of a water molecule. The smallest structural unit of the cellulose polymer is the dimer cellobiose, which consists of two β-D-glucose residues rotated 180° relative to each other (Fig. 2.53).

This polymer has a linear structure, and its molecules are polar, exhibiting strong intermolecular interactions and associating with other chains via hydrogen bonds. As a result, cellulose molecules arrange themselves in a ladder-like structure (Fig. 2.54). Hydrogen bonds also occur within a single cellulose chain, forming connections between neighbouring anhydroglucose units (Brückle 2012a).

Cellulose can exhibit varying degrees of structural order. As the degree of order and the tightness of molecular packing increase, the level of crystallinity also rises. Where hydrogen bonds are less numerous, and the polymer chains are less densely arranged, the structure of cellulose gradually transitions into an amorphous, non-crystalline region. The proportions of crystalline and amorphous domains determine the polymer's flexibility and permeability. The degree of crystallinity is an individual characteristic. The average crystallinity for plant-derived raw material is approximately 70%, and for cellulose pulps about 65% (Sobucki and Jeżewska 2015, pp. 98–99). A higher degree of crystallinity results in greater dimensional stability and tensile strength, as well as reduced swelling tendency and lower flexibility. Amorphous regions provide flexibility and allow cellulose to be penetrated by other chemical substances.

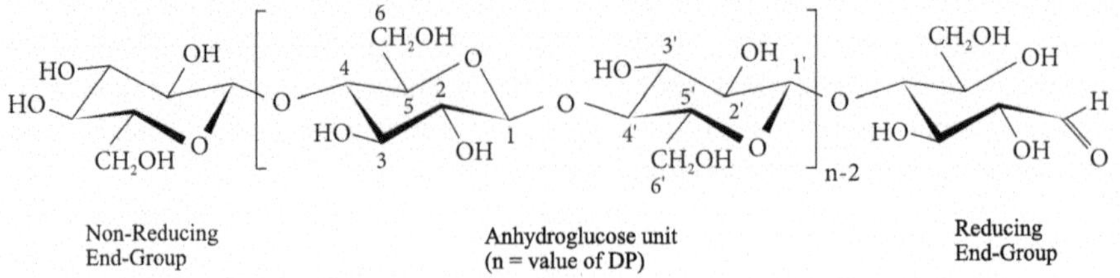

Fig. 2.53 Structure of a cellulose molecule. On the left, the non-reducing end of the cellulose chain; in the centre, an anhydroglucose unit; on the right, the reducing end of the cellulose chain

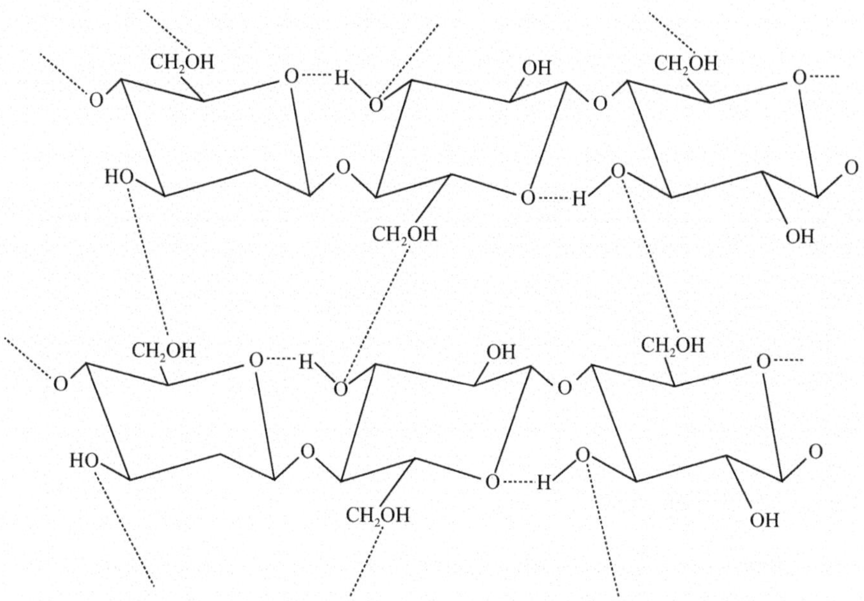

Fig. 2.54 Arrangement of cellulose molecules connected by hydrogen bonds, resembling a ladder (Based on Kronkright 1990)

The length of the cellulose chain determines the degree of polymerisation (DP), that is, the number of D-glucose residues. This parameter influences the material's resistance to degradation factors. In plant raw material, the degree of polymerisation of cellulose chains ranges from 2000 to 10,000. After processing into cellulose pulp, the polymer length decreases to approximately 700–2000. When DP falls below 1000, differences in paper mechanical strength become apparent. At DP below 100, the cellulose polymer exhibits no strength or cohesion and can be ground into a powder (Sobucki 2013, p. 16). Cellulose chains form fibrous structures of varying complexity: molecules, microfibrils, macrofibrils, and fibres. In the plant cell wall, cellulose microfibrils are interwoven with hemicelluloses, pectin, and sometimes lignin in both the primary and secondary walls.[60]

Cellulose is hygroscopic and therefore has the ability to attract and absorb water molecules. Water acts as a plasticiser, causing the swelling of amorphous regions. During the drying process, the proportion of hydrogen bonds increases, leading to recrystallisation and greater brittleness of the molecule (Brückle 2012a). The crystalline regions then undergo changes in crystalline organisation (Florian 1990). The history of water content in cellulose affects its capacity for further absorption.[61]

[60] See the section *Structure of the cell wall* in this chapter.

[61] This phenomenon is known as hysteresis, and, for cellulosic materials that have at some point been overdried, it means that under given climatic conditions, they are able to absorb less water than materials whose previous water content was comparatively higher. During continuous changes in water content associated with absorption and desorption from the environment, ongoing structural changes occur in cellulose, which are never fully reversible (Brückle 2012a).

The presence of water within the paper structure causes the spaces between cellulose chains to expand and weakens the bonds between fibres. In cases of severe swelling, the porosity of the paper changes, and the crystalline structure may also be destroyed. The manner and rate of the drying process irreversibly affect the arrangement of pores in the paper. During drying, the water content in paper is reduced from 50–70% (wet paper) to 5–10% (dry paper) at its maximum extent (Brückle and Banik 2012). Paper is considered dry when it has reached equilibrium moisture content with its environment. Drying by sublimation (lyophilisation) causes the fibre network to expand during the initial freezing, while the final sublimation stage increases the porosity of the fibres (Brückle and Banik 2012).

In plant specimen tissues, a slight water content is also retained, depending on current climatic conditions; however, this is not defined in the literature (Drobnik 2009, p. 65).

2.2.4.2 Hemicelluloses

Hemicelluloses are primarily amorphous carbohydrate polymers, with small crystalline or semicrystalline regions where they intertwine with cellulose molecules. They can also form bonds with lignin molecules (Brückle 2012b). Hemicelluloses consist of short chains, typically arranged in branched structures, without forming microfibrils. Their composition and structure are species-specific. This is a heterogeneous group of compounds with complex, not fully understood structures, which is why their classification has changed over time. Hemicelluloses include xyloglucans, found predominantly in the primary cell wall, as well as xylans, mannans, glucomannans, and β(1 → 3, 1 → 4) glucans (Scheller and Ulvskov 2010). Their structure is composed of monosaccharides such as D-xylose, D-glucose, D-galactose, D-mannose, L-arabinose, L-rhamnose, and L-fucose, as well as D-glucuronic acid. Galactans, arabinans, and arabinogalactans were once classified within this group, but these polysaccharides are now considered components of pectins (Scheller and Ulvskov 2010).

The individual units of hemicellulose chains are linked by 1–4, 1–2, 1–3, or 1–6 β- and α-glycosidic bonds. Hemicellulose molecules contain hydroxyl groups capable of forming hydrogen bonds both within and between molecules. Its degree of polymerisation is relatively low, ranging from 30 to 300 (Sobucki and Jeżewska 2015, pp. 99–100). In the cell wall, hemicelluloses intertwine with cellulose fibrils in their amorphous regions, as well as with lignin in the secondary wall and in the middle lamella. Hemicelluloses form a protective gel for cellulose in the form of a hydrated matrix, inhibiting its excessive crystallisation and aggregation, thereby ensuring the proper flexibility of cellulose structures (Florian 1990).[62]

Hemicelluloses are highly hygroscopic and readily swell. They act as regulators of cellulose flexibility, including in finished paper. During the production of

[62] See the section *Structure of the Cell Wall* in this chapter.

cellulose pulps, up to 75% of hemicelluloses can be dissolved, but complete removal is not pursued, as paper containing hemicelluloses exhibits greater tensile strength and a higher tendency to swell, which promotes the formation of bonds between fibres (Brückle 2012b).

Hemicelluloses undergo hydrolysis in alkaline and acidic aqueous solutions, as well as through the enzymatic activity of microorganisms (Kopcewicz and Lewak 2012, p. 46; Florian 1990). Low-molecular-weight hemicelluloses may dissolve in water [Florian 1990]. In the process of producing fibrous pulps, the most stable hemicelluloses are xylan and glucomannan, and these compounds most commonly constitute the hemicellulose residues found in paper (Brückle 2012b).

2.2.4.3 Lignin

Lignin is an amorphous natural polymer of phenylpropanoids with an irregular, highly cross-linked structure. It may contain residues of coniferyl, sinapyl, or p-coumaryl alcohols (Kopcewicz and Lewak 2012, pp. 50 and 378). The composition of lignin is characteristic of a given species and may also vary within a single species depending on the function and location of lignin in the plant organism. The structure of lignin is not yet fully understood. Structurally, it consists of a dense network of ring compounds and contains numerous functional groups, including hydroxyl, methoxyl, and carbonyl groups, which are highly reactive. It is covalently bonded to hemicelluloses, which intertwine with cellulose microfibrils.

Lignin is found primarily in the cell walls of vascular plants, mainly perennials, although in recent years it has also been identified in red algae (Martone et al. 2009). Depending on the plant species, it may be located in various layers of the cell wall, penetrating all its layers as well as the middle lamella (the intercellular layer) (Beck 2010, p. 65; Florian 1990; Nick and Optarny 2014, p. 372; Simon et al. 2018). Lignin provides chemical reinforcement and increases the cell wall's chemical resistance. Its function is to stiffen the wall, thereby enabling the plant to grow vertically. It also protects plants against microbial attack and prevents the penetration of water and other substances into the cell interior. Excessive lignin content makes the cell wall brittle. Lignin is insoluble in water and reduces the ability of fibres to swell and form inter-fibre bonds. It is partially soluble in ethanol and methanol and swells in the presence of certain solvents. It is thermoplastic and sensitive to alkalis. As previously mentioned, in the production of cellulose pulps, the aim is to remove lignin as much as possible, since its hydrophobic nature limits the formation of hydrogen bonds between cellulose fibres. This is achieved through of pulping, using chemical methods and during bleaching by chlorination, followed by dissolution in alkaline solutions (Sobucki and Jeżewska 2015, pp. 106–111; Brückle 2012b). As a protective substance for cellulose, lignin can be considered an antioxidant. However, lignin itself undergoes oxidation, forming acid derivatives and coloured degradation products, which have a destructive effect on cellulose (Brückle 2012b).

Lignin is a highly durable component of plant structure and, in an altered form, can be identified in archaeological wood (Florian 1990).

2.2.4.4 Pectins

Pectins are poly- and oligosaccharides of diverse composition. As they primarily consist of D-galacturonic acid residues linked by α-1,4-glycosidic bonds, they are classified as polyuronides. In addition, their structure includes sugars such as D-galactose, L-arabinose, and L-rhamnose (Noreen et al. 2017). Pectins possess linear anionic backbones with regions lacking side chains, as well as segments containing non-ionic side chains. Based on the structure of the backbone, three structural classes of pectins are distinguished: the most common homogalacturonan, and rhamnogalacturonan I and II (Noreen et al. 2017). The precursor substances of this group of compounds are protopectins, which are water-insoluble, probably due to their ability to form complexes with calcium ions. Pectins may be covalently attached to these complexes. They can also form bonds between two pectin molecules or directly with the cell wall, or become mechanically interwoven with other polymers present in the cell wall (Florian 1990).

Pectins are the main component of the middle lamella and are also present in the amorphous matrix between cellulose microfibrils in the primary cell wall, where they play a role in stiffening and act as an adhesive between the amorphous cuticle and the surface of epidermal cells. They provide structural integrity to the cell wall and regulate its permeability to ionic substances (Florian 1990). A recently discovered function of pectins is their protective effect on genetic material, observed in desert plants. Pectins form a protective mucilaginous envelope around seed embryos, supporting the repair processes of DNA damage resulting from desiccation (Zhenying et al. 2008).

Pectins are water-soluble and hydrophilic; in the presence of water, they form a gel whose rigidity increases with polymer length. They undergo hydrolysis in acids and by enzymes. Pectins can serve as a nutrient source for bacteria and fungi (Florian 1990).

2.2.4.5 Protein Present in the Plant Cell Wall

The most extensively studied group of plant cell wall proteins are extensins—structural proteins from the glycoprotein family, rich in hydroxyproline (hydroxyproline-rich glycoproteins, HRGPs) (Florian 1990). This group also includes lectins, present in species from the nightshade family (*Solanaceae*), which serve a defensive role against insects and pathogens, as well as arabinogalactan proteins (Srivastava 2002). Other cell wall proteins include the group of proline-rich glycoproteins (PRPs) and glycine-rich glycoproteins (GRPs) (Srivastava 2002).

Since hydroxyproline is a major component of collagen, extensins are sometimes referred to as "plant collagen". In addition to hydroxyproline, extensins contain amino acids such as lysine, serine, tyrosine, valine, and histidine (Srivastava 2002). Extensins are located in the primary cell wall, accounting for approximately 1–5% of the dry mass. The role of extensins is not fully understood. They have been attributed with influencing the plasticity of the cell wall during growth (hence the name extensins) and with limiting the ability of the wall to swell by cross-linking with cellulose molecules (Florian 1990). Currently, it is believed that these proteins provide reinforcement and stabilisation for cells that have completed elongation (Srivastava 2002). Loss of this protein weakens the cell wall (Florian 1990).

Additionally, enzymes are present in the cell wall. The full complement and precise localisation of all enzymatic proteins within the cell wall are not yet precisely known. However, several groups of enzymes have been confirmed, including various synthases, transferases, hydrolases, peroxidases, invertases, as well as chitinase and (1 → 3) β-glucanase, which serve a defensive role against pathogens (Srivastava 2002).

2.2.4.6 Cutin, Suberin, Waxes

Cutin and suberin are hydrophobic, amorphous polymers composed of high-molecular-weight esters of hydroxylated fatty acids. They provide a protective surface layer for the cell wall.

Suberin, like lignin, is a phenylpropanoid polymer found in the primary cell wall within the endodermal layer, impregnating the secondary protective tissue (cork).

The cutin is located on the outer surface of epidermal cells and forms a protective surface layer known as the cuticle, whose components include low-molecular-weight waxes and fatty acids.

Both suberin and cutin may contain waxes, which are soluble in organic solvents, as well as tannins that are water-soluble. At room temperature, in an alkaline environment, suberin can undergo saponification. Waxes serve to protect against ultraviolet radiation and regulate the permeability of plant tissues. They maintain the proper hydration level of tissues, preventing both desiccation and excessive swelling (Florian 1990).

References

Allen DE (1965) Some further light on the history of the vasculum. Proc Bot Soc Br Isles 6:105–109

Archer W (1950) New plastic aid in mounting herbarium specimens. Rhodora 52(624):298–299

Archer WA (1952) Aerosol for controlling herbarium pests. Science 116:233–234

Baer NS, Indictor N, Phelan WH (1978) An evaluation of poly(vinyl acetate) adhesives for use in paper conservation. Restaurator 2(2):121–138. https://doi.org/10.1515/rest.1978.2.2.121

Banik G, Brückle I, Lacher R, Wegele G (2012) Effect of sizing on paper–water interaction. In: Banik G, Brückle I (eds) Paper and water. Routledge, New York, pp 145–171

Beck CB (2010) An introduction to plant structure and development plant anatomy for the twenty-first century. Cambridge University Press, Cambridge

Bedford DJ (1999) Vascular plants. In: Carter D, Walker A (eds) Care and conservation of natural history collections. Butterworth Heinemann, Oxford, pp 61–80

Berli J, Belhadj O (2020) Consolidating herbarium specimens using two-sided hydroxylpropyl-cellulose pre-coated paper. J Pap Conserv 21(1):31–34. https://doi.org/10.1080/18680860.2020.1835112

Bridson D, Forman L (1999) The herbarium handbook. Royal Botanic Gardens, Kew
Briggs M, Damas K (2023a) Methods for drying plant specimens. In: Davies NMJ, Drinkell C, Utteridge TMA (eds) The herbarium handbook. Kew Publishing, pp 46–49
Briggs M, Damas K (2023b) The alcohol/"Schweinfurth" method for preserving plant specimens. In: Davies NMJ, Drinkell C, Utteridge TMA (eds) The herbarium handbook. Kew Publishing, Kew, pp. 50–51
Briggs D, Sell PD, Block M, I'ons RD (1983) Mercury vapour: a health hazard in herbaria. New Phytol 94:453–457
British Museum (2014–2018) Oddy test results: exhibition adhesives and tapes. https://www.conservationwiki.com/wiki/Oddy_Test_Results:_Exhibition_Adhesives_and_Tapes. Accessed 21.01.2026
Brückle I (2012a) Structure and properties of dry and wet paper. In: Banik G, Brückle I (eds) Paper and water. Routledge, New York, pp 81–120
Brückle I (2012b) Effect of pulp processing on paper–water interactions. In: Banik G, Brückle I (eds) Paper and water. Routledge, New York, pp 121–144
Brückle I, Banik G (2012) Drying paper in conservation practice. In: Banik G, Brückle I (eds) Paper and water. Routledge, New York, pp 389–418
Clarck S (1986) Preservation of herbarium specimens: an archive conservator's approach. Taxon 35(4):675–682. https://doi.org/10.2307/1221610
Collins M (2000) Medieval herbals: the illustrative traditions. British Museum and University of Toronto Press
Coradin L, Giannasi DE (1980) The effects of chemical preservations on plant collections to be used in chemotaxonomic surveys. Taxon 29(1):33–40. https://doi.org/10.2307/1219594
Cosgrove DJ (2001) Wall structure and wall loosening. A look backwards and forwards. Plant Physiol 125:131–134. https://doi.org/10.1104/pp.125.1.131
Cosgrove DJ (2014) Re-constructing our models of cellulose and primary cell wall assembly. Curr Opin Plant Biol 22:122–131. https://doi.org/10.1016/j.pbi.2014.11.001
Cosgrove DJ (2018) Diffuse growth of plant cell walls. Plant Physiol 176:16–27. https://doi.org/10.1104/pp.17.01541
Croat TB (1978) Survey of herbarium problems. Taxon 27(2/3):203–218. https://doi.org/10.2307/1220243
Dąbrowski J, Siniarska-Czaplicka J (1991) Rękodzieło papiernicze. Dzieje polskiego papiernictwa 1491–1991. Wydawnictwo Czasopism i książek technicznych Sigma Not, Warszawa
Dauwalder L (2012) Das Herbarium des Felix Platter. Die Erhaltung eines historischen Buch-Herbariums. Dissertation. Fachochshule Bern
Dauwalder L (2013) Felix platter's herbarium: the preservation of a historical 'bound herbarium'. J Pap Conserv 14(3):26–32
Davies NMJ, Drinkell C, Utteridge TMA (eds) (2023) The herbarium handbook. Kew Publishing, Kew
DeWolf G (1968) Notes on making an herbarium. Arnoldia 28(8/9):69–111
Down J (1999) Adhesive research at the Canadian conservation institute as it relates to herbarium collections. In: Metsger DA, Byers SC (eds) Managing the modern herbarium—an interdisciplinary approach. SPNHC, Ontario, pp 205–223
Down JL (2014) The evaluation of selected poly(vinyl acetate) and acrylic adhesives: a final research update. Stud Conserv 60(1):33–54. https://doi.org/10.1179/2047058414Y.0000000129
Down J (2015) Adhesive compendium for conservation. Canadian Conservation Institute, Ottawa
Down JL (2016) The effect of modifiers on the stability of a vinyl acetate/ethylene copolymer dispersion. Stud Conserv 61(1):26–45. https://doi.org/10.1179/2047058414Y.0000000130
Down JL, MacDonald MA, Tétreault J, Williams RS (1996) Adhesive testing at the Canadian Conservation Institute: an evaluation of selected poly(vinyl acetate) and acrylic adhesives. Stud Conserv 41(1):19–44. https://doi.org/10.1179/sic.1996.41.1.19
Down JL, Guild S, Hill G, St.-Jacques D, Westbury K, O'Loughlin E, Kaminska E, Williams RS, Iraci J, Tse S (2011) Update on the CCI adhesive tape and heat-set tissues Project, [in:]

Symposium 2011: Adhesives and consolidants for conservation; Research and applications; Proceedings = Symposium 2011: Adhésifs et consolidants pour la conservation; Recherche et applications; les Actes. Ottawa: Canadian Conservation Institute: 57–84.

Drobnik J (2009) Zielnik i zielnikoznawstwo. Wydawnictwo Naukowe PWN, Warszawa

Dupont AL i Tétreault J (2000) Cellulose degradation in an acetic acid environment. Stud Conserv 45 (3): 201–210. doi:https://doi.org/10.2307/1506766

Eusebio MA, Stern WL (1964) Preservation of herbarium specimens in the humid tropics. Philipp Agric 48:16–20

Fallon D, Peters M, Hunt M, Koehler K (2016) Cleaning protocol for mercuric chloride–contaminated herbarium cabinets at the Smithsonian Museum Support Center. Collect Forum 30(1–2):51–62

Fassett N (1952) Uses of cellulose acetate in the herbarium. Rhodora 54(647):286–288

Feller RL, Wilt M (1990) Evaluation of cellulose ethers for conservation. Getty Conservation Institute, Marina del Rey

Florian MLE (1990) Plant anatomy: an illustrated aid to identification. In: Florian MLE, Kronkright DP, Norton R (eds) The conservation of artifacts made from plant materials. The J. Paul Getty Trust, pp 1–27

Fuchs R (2008) Glues in paper restoration—new insights for preparation and application. In: Fellows-Jensen G, Springborg P (eds) Care and conservation of manuscripts 10, proceedings of the tenth international seminar held at the University of Copenhagen, 19th–20th October 2006. Museum Tusculanum Press, University of Copenhagen, pp 235–248

Gates KS (2009) An overview of chemical processes that damage cellular DNA: spontaneous hydrolysis, alkylation, and reactions with radicals. Chem Res Toxicol 22(11):1747–1760. https://doi.org/10.1021/tx900242k

Geiger T, Michel F (2005) Studies on the polysaccharide JunFunori used to consolidate matt paint. Stud Conserv 50(3):193–204. https://doi.org/10.1179/sic.2005.50.3.193

Gersten T, Michineau M, Paternotre A, Thys N (2017) Herbarii Bruxellenses, le projet de conservation des herbiers de la Bibliothèque Royale de Belgique. In Monte Artium 10:83–101. https://doi.org/10.1484/J.IMA.5.114683

Green D, Thickett LR (1995) Testing materials for use in the storage and display of antiquities—a revised methodology. Stud Conserv 40(3):145–152. https://doi.org/10.1179/sic.1995.40.3.145

Grenda M (2013) Ethical considerations concerning the restoration of a herbarium from the 19th century. In: ICOM-CC Graphic Documents Working Group Interim Meeting | Vienna 17–19 April 2013. ICOM-CC, Vienna, pp 93–96

Grenda M (2015a) Remedial conservation of a severely deteriorated 19th century bound herbarium. J Nat Sci Collect 2:54–59

Grenda M (2015b) Konserwacja zielników Michała Fedorowskiego ze zbiorów Zielnika Wydziału Biologii Uniwersytetu Warszawskiego, Opis popularyzatorski, dostępny pod adresem: http://www.zielnik.biol.uw.edu.pl/wp-content/uploads/2015/01/Fedorowski-opis-popularyzatorski.-compressed.pdf. dostęp 21.01.2026

Grenda-Kurmanow M (2017) Conservation versus genetics. Challenges of conservation planning for historic herbaria. In: Bridgeland J (ed) ICOM-CC 18th triennial conference preprints, Copenhagen, 4–8 September 2017. International Council of Museums, Paris, p Art 1103

Grenda-Kurmanow M (2021) Adhesives used in herbaria: current practice with regard to what we know from written sources on mounting herbarium specimens and conservation. Taxon 70:1–15. https://doi.org/10.1002/tax.12413

Gunn A (1994) Past and current practice: the botanist view. In: Child RE (ed) Conservation and the herbarium. The Institute of Paper Conservation, Leigh, pp 11–14

Gunning BES, Steer MW (1996) Plant cell biology. Structure and function. Jones and Bartlett Publishers Inc., London

Hall AV (1988) Pest control in herbaria. Taxon 37(4):885–907

Havermans J, Dekker R, Sportel R (2015) The effect of mercuric chloride treatment as biocide for herbaria on the indoor air quality. Herit Sci 3:39. https://doi.org/10.1186/s40494-015-0068-8

Hawks C, Makos K, Bell D, Wambach PF, Burrows GE (2004) An inexpensive method to test for mercury vapor in herbarium cabinets. Taxon 53:783–787

Hill SR (1983) Microwave and the herbarium specimen: potential dangers. Taxon 32:614–615. https://doi.org/10.2307/1221732

Horie V (2010) Materials for conservation: organic consolidants, adhesives, and coatings, 2nd edn. Elsevier, London

Hunter D (1978) Papermaking: The History and Technique of an Ancient Craft. New York: Dover Publications

Kaczkowski RA, Makos KA, Hawks C, Hunt M (2017) Investigation of residual contamination inside storage cabinets: collection care benefits from an industrial hygiene study. J Am Inst Conserv 56(2):142–160. https://doi.org/10.1080/01971360.2017.1326242

Karmann W, Kummer AB (2000) Tapes, adhesive. In: Ullmann's encyclopedia of industrial chemistry, vol 35. Wiley-VCH Verlag GmbH & Co. KGaA, Weinheim, pp 611–631. https://doi.org/10.1002/14356007.a26_085

Kataeva M, Panichev N, van Wyk AE (2008) Monitoring mercury in two South African herbaria. Sci Total Environ 407(3):1211–1217

Keijzers V (2013) Historische herbaria: inzicht in de conservatie problematiek en een aanzet tot een leidraad voor de conservering en restauratie van gedroogd plantenmateriaal, Dissertation. Artesis Hogeschool Antwerpen

Kiljańska A (2005) Album—zielnik w kasecie. In: Leszczyńska-Cyganik B (ed) Fin de siècle w Krakowie. Grafika użytkowa, tkaniny, rzemiosło artystyczne ze zbiorów Muzeum Narodowego w Krakowie, exhibition catalogue. Muzeum Narodowe w Krakowie, Kraków, reg. 181, pp 108–110

King C (2023) Floral dissection. In: Davies NMJ, Drinkell C, Utteridge TMA (eds) The herbarium handbook. Kew Publishing, Kew, pp 94–95

Kite M, Thomson R (2006) Conservation of leather and related materials. Butterworth-Heinemann, Oxford. https://doi.org/10.4324/9780080454665

Klemm D, Schmauder HP, Heinze T (2002) Cellulose. Biopolymers 6:275–319

Köhler P (1999) Historia Zielnika Instytutu Botaniki Uniwersytetu Jagiellońskiego (KRA) w latach 1780–1910. Kwart Hist Nauki Tech 44(2):7–60

Kopcewicz J, Lewak S (eds) (2012) Fizjologia roślin. Wydawnictwo Naukowe PWN, Warszawa

Kronkright DP (1990) Deterioration of artifacts made from plant materials. In: Florian MLE, Kronkright DP, Norton R (eds) The conservation of artifacts made from plant materials. The J Paul Getty Trust, pp 139–193

Kumar SS, Nasidze I, Walimbe SR, Stoneking M (2000) Brief communication: discouraging prospects for ancient DNA from India. Am J Phys Anthropol 113(1):129–133. https://doi.org/10.1002/1096-8644(200009)113:1<129::aid-ajpa12>3.0.co;2-2

Lellinger DB (1972) Dichlorvos and Lindane as herbarium insecticides. Taxon 21(1):91–95. https://doi.org/10.2307/1219227

Lindahl T, Nyberg B (1972) Rate of depurination of native deoxyribonucleic acid. Biochemistry 11:3610–3618. https://doi.org/10.1021/bi00769a018

Linnaeus C (1751) Philosophia Botanica in qua explicantur fundamenta botanica cum definitionibus partium, exemplis terminorum, observationibus rariorum adjectis figuris aeneis. Godofr. Kiesewetter, Stockholm

Lundell CL, Kirkham R (1966) A method for applying mystox (lauryl pentachlorophenate) to protect mounted herbarium specimens. Wrightia 3:177–180

Mądalski J (1951) Zbieranie i konserwowanie rośliny do celów naukowych (z opisem nowej metody suszenia). PWN Wrocław

Mądalski J (1955) Jak należy zbierać i konserwować rośliny do celów naukowych. PWN, Warszawa

Mądalski J (1958) A new Method of Plants' Drying for Herbarium. Fragmenta Florstica et Geobotanica 3(2):69–76

Margez M (2004) L'herbier Haller du Muséum national d'Histoire naturelle: un objet d'intérêt historique et scientifique, Dissertation. Institut national du patrimoine, Departement des restaurateurs, Paris

Marota I, Basile C, Ubaldi M, Rollo F (2002) DNA decay rate in papyri and human remains from Egyptian archaeological sites. Am J Phys Anthropol 117(4):310–318. https://doi.org/10.1002/ajpa.10045. PMID: 11920366
Martone PT, Estevez JM, Lu F, Ruel K, Denny MW, Somerville C, Ralph J (2009) Discovery of lignin in seaweed reveals convergent evolution of cell-wall architecture. Curr Biol 19(2):169–175. https://doi.org/10.1016/j.cub.2008.12.031
Massey JR (1974) Chapter 31: The herbarium. In: Radford AE, Dickinson WC, Bell CR (eds) Vascular plant systematics. Harper & Row, New York, pp 751–774
Menei E (2005) Conservation et restauration d'herbiers: un cas exemplaire à la Bibliothèque de l'Institut de France. In: Actes du colloque Voyages en botanique, Besançon 16–17 juin 2005. ACCOLAD, Agence régionale de cooperation de Franche-Comte, Besançon. https://papyrusetpapierconservation.com/wp-content/uploads/2020/08/2005-Actes-Colloque--Voyages-en-botanique-Menei.pdf. dostęp 21.01.2026
Merrill E (1926) An efficient and economical herbarium paste. Torreya 26(4):63–65
Merrill E (1948) On the control of destructive insects in the herbarium. J Arnold Arbor 29(1):103–110
Merrill E, Wyman D (1939) Index Kewensis in improved loose leafledger form. Bull Pop Inf 7(8):37–40
Michel F (2011) Funori and JunFunori: Two related consolidants with surprising properties, [w:] Symposium 2011: Adhesives and consolidants for conservation; Research and applications; Proceedings = Symposium 2011: Adhésifs et consolidants pour la conservation; Recherche et applications; les Actes. Ottawa: Canadian Conservation Institute 285–298
Nasatto PL, Pignon F, Silveira JLM, Duarte MER, Noseda MD, Rinaudo M (2015) Methylcellulose, a cellulose derivative with original physical properties and extended applications. Polymers 7:777–803. https://doi.org/10.3390/polym7050777
Nepi C (2008) L'erbario Coltellini della Sezione Botanica del Museo di Storia Naturale. In: Nepi C, Gusmeroli E (eds) Gli erbari aretini da Andrea Cesalpino ai giorni nostri, Firenze University Press, Firenze, pp 23–28
Nick P, Optarny Z (eds) (2014) Applied plant cell biology: cellular tools and approaches for plant biotechnology. Springer
Noreen A, Nazli Z-H, Akram J, Rasul I, Mansha A, Yaqoob N, Iqbal R, Tabasum S, Zuber M, Zia KM (2017) Pectins functionalized biomaterials; a new viable approach for biomedical applications: a review. Int J Biol Macromol 101:254–272. https://doi.org/10.1016/j.ijbiomac.2017.03.029
Nowak-Kemp M (2018) William Burchell in Southern Africa, 1811–1815. In: MacGregor A (ed) Naturalists in the field. Collecting, recording and preserving the natural world from the fifteenth to the twenty-first century. Brill, Leiden/Boston, pp 500–549
Ogilvie BW (2006) The science of describing. Natural history in renaissance Europe. The University of Chicago Press, Chicago/London
Oyarzun R, Higueras P, Esbrí JM, Pizarro J (2007) Mercury in air and plant specimens in herbaria: a pilot study at the MAF herbarium in Madrid (Spain). Sci Total Environ 387:346–352
Paś M (2017) Album–zielnik w kasecie. In: #dziedzictwo, exhibition catalogue. Muzeum Narodowe w Krakowie, Kraków: reg 210, pp 554–555
Phelan H, Baer NS, Indictor N (1971) An evaluation of adhesives for use in paper conservation. J Am Inst Conserv 11(2):58–75. https://doi.org/10.1179/019713671806030017
Piekiełko A (1981) Dwa osiemnastowieczne zielniki ze zbiorów Instytutu Botaniki Uniwersytetu Jagiellońskiego. Ossolineum, Wrocław
Poncy O, Aupic C, Flament G (2012) La rénovation de l'herbier du muséum national d'Histoire Naturelle. Coré 27:1–10
Popławska S (2014a) Gdy suszone rośliny stają się zabytkiem. Historia, technologia, problem konserwacji i przechowywania zielników, Dissertation, Akademia Sztuk Pięknych w Warszawie
Popławska S (2014b) Problematyka Konserwacji Artystycznego Zielnika i papeterii autorstwa Elizy Orzeszkowej podarowanych Leopoldowi Méyetowi, przechowywanych w Muzeum Narodowym w Warszawie, Dissertation. Akademia Sztuk Pięknych w Warszawie

Purewal V (1999) The identification of hazardous pesticide and fungicide residues on herbarium material. Scott Soc Conserv Restor (SSCR) J 10(4):5–9
Purewal V (2001) The identification of four persistent and hazardous residues present on historic plant collections housed within the National Museum and Gallery of Wales. Collect Forum 16(1–2):77–86
Purewal V (2012) Novel detection and removal of hazardous biocide residues historically applied to herbaria. PhD dissertation, University of Lincoln
Purewal V, Colston B, Röhrs (2008) Developing a simple screening method for the identification of historic biocide residues on herbarium material in museum collections. X-Ray Spectrum 37:137–141. https://doi.org/10.1002/xrs.1036
Reissland B, Gaibor P, Ligterink F, Neevel JG (2017) Exploring the late 19th-century landscape of ink manufacturing via a collection of 90 bottles. In: Bridgland J (ed) ICOM-CC 18th triennial conference preprints, Copenhagen, 4–8 September 2017. International Council of Museums, Paris. Art 0105
Robinson B (1903) Inseciticides used at the Gray Herbarium. Rhodora 5(58):237–247
Rollins R (1955) The Archer method for mounting herbarium specimens. Rhodora 57(682):294–299
Rytz W (1933) Das Herbarium Felix Platters. Ein Beitrag zur Geschichte der Botanik des XVI. Jahrhunderts. Separatabdruck aus den Verhandlungen der Naturforschenden Gesselschaft in Basel. Band XLIV, 1, Teil. BuchdruckereiEmil Birkhäuser & Cie, Basel
Saint-Lager J (1885) Histoire des herbiers. J.-B, Baillère et fils, Paris
Salick J, Solomon J (2014) Herbarium curation of biocultural plant collections and vouchers. In: Salick J, Konchar K, Nesbitt M (eds) Curating biocultural collections: a handbook. Royal Botanic Gardens, Kew, pp 43–54
Scheller HV, Ulvskov P (2010) Hemicelluloses. Annu Rev Plant Biol 61(1):263–289. https://doi.org/10.1146/annurev-arplant-042809-112315
Schellmann NC (2007) Animal glues: a review of their key properties relevant to conservation. Stud Conserv 52(suppl):55–66. https://doi.org/10.1179/sic.2007.52.Supplement-1.55
Scheper K (2005) Een onderzoek naar Evacon-R. Gedrag en toepassingen van een witte lijm. CR: Interdisciplinair Vakblad voor Conservering en Restauratie 6(1):32–34
Schofield EK, Crisafulli S (1980) A safer insecticide for herbarium use. Brittonia 32(1):58–62. https://doi.org/10.2307/2806221
Sharp AJ (1964) A new method for mounting evergreen conifer twigs with deciduous leaves. Rhodora 66(765):216
Shchepanek M (2001) In defence of using adhesives and low-temperature pest control for botanical specimens. Taxon 50(1):169–173. https://doi.org/10.2307/1224517
Simon C, Spriet C, Hawkins S, Lion C (2018) Visualizing lignification dynamics in plants with click chemistry: dual labeling is BLISS! J Vis Exp 131:e56947. https://doi.org/10.3791/56947
Smith A (2010) Herbaria and entomology preservation course. 18th–21st October 2010. Institut National du Patrimoine, Paris. NatSca News 21:17–23
Sobucki W (2013) Konserwacja papieru. Zagadnienia chemiczne. Ministerstwo Kultury i Dziedzictwa Narodowego, Biblioteka Narodowa, Warszawa
Sobucki W, Jeżewska E (2015) Wiedza o papierze dla konserwatorów zbiorów. Biblioteka Narodowa, Warszawa
Srivastava LM (2002) Cell Wall, cell division, and cell growth. In: Plant growth and development. Hormones and environment. Academic, Amsterdam/Boston, pp 23–74. https://doi.org/10.1016/b978-012660570-9/50142-8
Staats M, Cuenca A, Richardson JE, Ginkel RV, Petersen G, Sebery O, Bakker FT (2011) DNA damage in plant herbarium tissue. PLoS One 6:e28448. https://doi.org/10.1371/journal.pone.0028448
Stern WL, Hagen, Gillenwater B, Eason G, Garcia-Quintana A, Cail RS (1968) Lindane and Dichlorvos for protection of herbarium specimens against insects. Taxon 17(6):629–632. https://doi.org/10.2307/1218003
Stevens R, Garside P, Russell E (2011) A review of current and recent practice in the use of adhesives by the conservation department at the British library. In: Symposium 2011: adhesives and consolidants for conservation; research and applications; proceedings=symposium 2011:

Adhésifs et consolidants pour la conservation; Recherche et applications; les Actes. Canadian Conservation Institute, Ottawa, pp 28–40
Szymańska M (2012) Odżywianie mineralne roślin. In: Kopcewicz J, Lewak S (eds) Fizjologia roślin. Wydawnictwo Naukowe PWN, Waszawa, pp 234–273
Thiers B (2020) Herbarium: the quest to preserve & classify the world's plants. Timber Press
Thijsse G (2016) Tusschen pampier geleyt, ontstaan, verspreiding en gebruik van de vroegste herbaria. In: IJapelaar I, Chavannes-Mazel LCA (eds) De gorene middeleeuwen. Duizend jaar gebruik van planten (600–1600). Lecturis B.V., Eindhoven, pp 64–93
Tillet SS (1979) Technical aids for systematic botany II: new adhesives. Taxon 28(4):383–384. https://doi.org/10.2307/1219751
Tillet SS (1989) Technical aids for systematic botany III. More Ideas on Methyl-Cellulose Adhesives. Taxon 38(4):597–601. https://doi.org/10.2307/1222635
Tournefort de JP (1694) Élémens de botanique: ou Méthode pour connoître les plantes, vol 1. Imprimerie Royale, Paris
Valmont de Bomare JC (1775) Dictionnaire raisonné universel d'histoire naturelle, contenant l'histoire des animaux, des végétaux et des minéraux, et celle des corps célestes, des météores et autres principaux phénomènes de la nature T. IV. Brunet, Paris
van den Spiegel A (1606) Isagoges in rem herbariam libri duo: Paulus Meiettus, Padua (Patavsia)
Wagner A, Donaldson L, Ralph J (2012) Lignification and lignin manipulations in conifers. In: Jouanin L, Lapierre C (eds) Advances in botanical research, vol 61. Academic, Amsterdam/Boston, pp 37–76. https://doi.org/10.1016/b978-0-12-416023-1.00002-1
Walker N, Hughes D (1994) Conservation and the herbarium: the Royle herbarium—a conservation approach. In: Child RE (ed) Conservation and the Herbarium. Institute of Paper Conservation, Leigh
Webber WB, Ernest LJ, Vangapandu S (2011) Mercury exposures in university herbarium collections. J Chem Health Saf 18:9–12
Whitmore TC, Fosberg FR (1965) Lauryl Pentachlorphenate protecting herbarium specimens. Taxon 14(5):164. https://doi.org/10.2307/1217552
Wilbraham J (2023) The collection of special plant groups. Algae and bryophytes. In: Davies NMJ, Drinkell C, Utteridge TMA (eds) The herbarium handbook. Kew Publishing, Kew, pp 24–31
Yesilyurt J (2009) Botanical related adhesives. NatSCA News 16:30–31
Yesilyurt JC, Dominguez-Santana F, Carine MA (2025) Herbarium specimens: is there a best approach to mount dried plant specimens? J Nat Sci Collect 13:52–63
Yoo YJ. Um IC (2013) Examination of thermo-gelation behavior of HPMC and HEMC aqueous solutions using rheology. Korea-Austral Rheol J 25(2):67–75. https://doi.org/10.1007/s13367-013-0007-8
Zemanek A (1996) Odnalezienie prawdopodobnych śladów pierwszego polskiego zielnika królewny Anny Wazówny. Kwart Hist Nauki Tech 41(3–4):197–205
Zheng Y, Wang X, Chen Y, Wagner E, Cosgrove DJ (2017) Xyloglucan in the primary cell wall: assessment by FESEM, selective enzyme digestions and nanogold affinity tags. Plant J Cell Mol Biol 93(2):211–226. https://doi.org/10.1111/tpj.13778
Zhenying H, Boubriak I, Osborne DJ, Dong M, Gutterman Y (2008) Possible role of pectin-containing mucilage and dew in repairing embryo DNA of seeds adapted to desert conditions. Ann Bot 101(2):277–283. https://doi.org/10.1093/aob/mcm089

Chapter 3
Degradation Processes of Structural Elements of Herbarium Specimens and Paper Substrate

Abstract This chapter describes degradation processes occurring at the macroscale of herbarium structures and at the molecular level. Subsequent chapters are devoted to acid hydrolysis, alkaline degradation, oxidation, contamination, biodeterioration, and the destructive effects of biocidal agents. A separate section discusses known processes of genetic material degradation, citing numerous publications that demonstrate that methods of preparation, storage, and preservation significantly influence the state of preservation of collections.

Keywords Herbarium • Degradation • Paper degradation • DNA degradation • Biocides • Pests

The degradation of heritage objects encompasses a range of diverse processes that never occur in isolation. Phenomena of various natures take place simultaneously, and it is their mutual interaction that determines the overall effect of material degradation. For clarity and to facilitate understanding of what is happening to a heritage object, these processes can be described individually, classified, utilised in simulations, and subjected to laboratory analyses. In the case of historical herbaria, it is essential to consider degradation phenomena and conservation methods comprehensively, taking into account the similarities and differences in the properties of paper and plant material, as well as the methods of preservation and conservation for each component. This is because both types of materials interact with each other from the moment they are combined in a herbarium sheet. Materials used in the conservation of plant specimens will penetrate the hygroscopic paper substrate and will also affect the plant specimens themselves. Substances present in the paper may likewise influence the condition of the dried plants. This interdependence is particularly evident in the migration of biocidal agents into the paper substrate or in the overall chemical environment of the object. The processes and degradation products resulting from these interactions will, in turn, affect the condition of the genetic material of the plants contained within the herbarium.

This section describes the mechanisms of degradation affecting herbarium specimens at both the macroscopic structural level and the molecular scale. The discussion begins with mechanisms specific to the cell wall and the paper substrate. The

M. Grenda-Kurmanow, *Herbaria*, https://doi.org/10.1007/978-3-032-21904-6_3

catalogue of degradation types opens with an overview of the principal destructive processes: acid hydrolysis, alkaline hydrolysis, and oxidation. As oxidation reactions are triggered by a variety of factors, the mechanisms associated with photodegradation, thermal degradation, and oxidation resulting from atmospheric pollutants—which also contribute to the acidification of cellulosic materials—are discussed separately. Subsequently, physical and biological damage is described. The final part addresses DNA degradation processes.

3.1 Acid Hydrolysis

In cellulose and hemicellulose molecules, acid hydrolysis leads to the cleavage of glycosidic bonds within the polymer chains, resulting in a reduction of their degree of polymerisation. In the case of hemicelluloses, degradation can proceed to the level of simple sugars that constitute the given hemicellulose molecule.

The hydrolysis process primarily occurs in amorphous regions, where polymer chains are not tightly packed and there is sufficient space for the penetration of new water molecules and molecular movement. It proceeds in the presence of unbound water molecules, which cleave the polymer by incorporating themselves at the site of the broken bond. Acid-catalysed hydrolysis is initiated by the reaction of the hydronium ion (H_3O^+) with the oxygen atom forming the linkage between polymer units, resulting in fragmentation of the polymer chain, which continues until it breaks down into individual units—D-glucose in the case of cellulose—and the formation of aldehyde groups at the new chain ends (Whitmore 2012). During hydrolysis, water acts as a reagent, a plasticiser for cellulose molecules, and a carrier of protons and hydronium ions (Whitmore 2012). The hydrolysis process is influenced by the water content within the polymer structure, and thus also by the storage conditions of the object, particularly the level of relative humidity (RH). The duration of the reaction and temperature are also significant factors (the higher the temperature, the faster the diffusion of catalytic substances). One of the consequences of hydrolysis is the shortening of polymer chains, and the shorter the polymer chains, the more rapidly further hydrolysis proceeds. As the material of plant origin breaks down into simple sugars, the proportion of water-soluble substances increases, which affects its reactivity and reduces structural integrity. For the plant cell wall, this results in a loss of structural homogeneity (Kronkright 1990).

The factors catalysing acid hydrolysis include the presence of hydronium ions derived from carboxylic acids and aldehydes, which are products of degradation processes and are also associated with oxidation. Acidic substances may also originate from acidic and acid-forming contaminants, which are typically found in amorphous regions as products of the oxidation of hydroxyl groups to carboxyl groups.

They may be residues from the manufacturing process, result from exposure to light, or arise from atmospheric pollutants (Kronkright 1990; Whitmore 2012).[1]

Acidic and acid-generating substances may also be introduced into the structure of the object in the form of sizing agents, transition metal ions (e.g. iron, copper), or salts of certain metals, such as components of alum (aluminium potassium sulphate), papermaker's alum (aluminium sulphate), or the common constituent of iron gall inks, namely iron(II) sulphate. These act as catalysts for hydrolytic reactions. The lower the pH accompanying the reaction, the faster it proceeds. In the case of cellulose, the initial stage of hydrolysis is the most detrimental to its mechanical properties, as it results in the greatest decrease in the degree of polymerisation. Further progression of hydrolytic processes gradually, but much more slowly, reduces the strength of cellulose. This is related to the sequence of subsequent stages, in which the most significant weakening of the polymer is caused by the breakdown of its longest chains (Whitmore 2012). As a result, structural continuity is disrupted and mechanical damage occurs (Fig. 3.1).

The migration of acidic substances can lead to the formation of yellow and brown discolourations both in paper and in specimens. Drobnik notes that the presence of

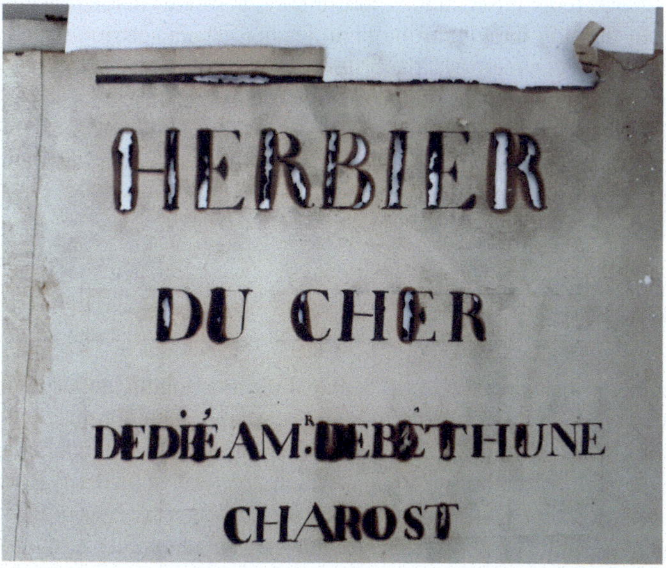

Fig. 3.1 Damage resulting from the presence of ink corrosion. Transition metal ions (in this case, most likely iron) catalyse the oxidation and acid hydrolysis of cellulose, leading to cellulose fragmentation and substrate disintegration. The photograph shows various stages of ink corrosion, from horizontal migration (the "halo" effect and the "spreading" of ink), through the formation of cracks within the letters, to the complete loss of substrate sections. N.n, *Hebier du Cher*, Wrocław, Herbarium of the Museum of Natural History in Wrocław (WRSL), without ref. no., nineteenth century. Photo: M. Grenda-Kurmanow

[1] Descriptions of degradation related to oxidation, photodegradation, and contamination are provided in the following sections.

acidic substances in paper may cause the bleaching of lichen thalli (Drobnik 2009, p. 194). The presence of acids found in certain botanical specimens—oxalic, formic, and tannic acids—also contributes to acid hydrolysis and cellulose degradation (Collins 2014).

3.2 Alkaline Degradation

Alkaline degradation of cellulose occurs in the amorphous regions that connect crystalline areas within molecules that have previously undergone oxidation. Strong alkalis have a destructive effect on cellulose, causing it to swell, break down, and dissolve. Although undegraded cellulose is sensitive to alkaline environments at $pH > 12$—which rarely occur under conservation and museum conditions—molecules that have previously undergone oxidation may prove susceptible to lower levels of alkalinity.[2] The so-called alkaline elimination reaction proceeds with the removal of a hydrogen atom from the α-carbon atom bonded to a carbonyl or carboxyl group, resulting in the acquisition of a negative charge. The internal structure of the polymer is reorganised, and as a result, the negative charge transferred to the oxygen atom forming the glycosidic bond leads to chain scission. Degradation of the amorphous regions increases the brittleness of the polymer (Whitmore 2012).

Hemicelluloses, being more amorphous and more readily susceptible to oxidation reactions than cellulose, are also more sensitive to alkalis, more easily breaking down into simple sugars and dissolving. Lignin dissolves in an alkaline environment, and its sensitivity to alkalis increases over time (Florian 1990, p. 23).

3.3 Oxidation

Oxidation, alongside acid hydrolysis, is one of the most significant degradation processes occurring in plant-derived materials. Here, the oxidation reaction is understood as the transformation of hydrocarbons into structures containing oxygen atoms, in the form of carbonyl groups, which are further oxidised to carboxylic acids (Whitmore 2012). Oxidation reactions may be triggered by a range of factors, but their general course and outcome are similar. These processes involve the formation of radical groups, which are highly reactive. In the case of cellulose, the onset of oxidation is marked by the removal of a hydrogen atom from a carbon atom in the chain. Subsequent reactions lead to the formation of carbonyl and carboxyl groups. The final stage of oxidation may involve the bonding of radicals, known as termination. For cellulose, approximately one third of oxidation reactions result in

[2] There is no universally established safe pH level. Reactions with alkalis can occur at any pH, but each one-point increase results in a tenfold acceleration of the reaction (Whitmore 2012).

chain scission and the formation of aldehyde groups at the ends of the newly formed shorter chains, while the remaining reactions involve the formation of carbonyl and carboxyl groups along the existing chains. The presence of water facilitates the course of the reaction by acting as a transport medium for oxidising agents and their reaction products, as well as a plasticiser for cellulose chains, thereby increasing their reactivity (Whitmore 2012).

The factors catalysing oxidation include: exposure to light, particularly ultraviolet radiation; the presence of contaminants resulting from transition metals such as iron and copper, including when these are components of inks and pigments (Fig. 3.1); exposure to atmospheric pollutants, also originating from the emission of volatile organic compounds (VOCs) from ageing historic materials or packaging;[3] the action of strong oxidising agents, used for example in conservation processes, such as the once commonly used chlorine-containing bleaching agents.[4]

Contaminants may also originate from biocidal agents used to protect objects against pests.[5] Certain plant species are more susceptible to oxidation processes. The effects of corrosion are visible as rust-coloured discolourations or blackened spots, for example among representatives of the family *Scrophulariaceae* Juss. (Collins 2014).

In addition to structural disintegration, oxidation promote acid hydrolysis reactions, through the presence of carboxylic acids acting as catalysts, as well as to alkaline degradation.

3.4 Photodegradation

The phenomenon of photodegradation is related to the energy of light waves. Light of a specific wavelength has a defined energy, which can break bonds between atoms. Ultraviolet radiation with a wavelength of 275 nm can break the bond between an oxygen atom and a hydrogen atom (O–H); 280 nm—the bond between a carbon atom and an oxygen atom (C–O); 305 nm—the bond between a carbon atom and a hydrogen atom (C–H); 345 nm—the bond between carbon atoms (C–C) (Kronkright 1990). For a photochemical reaction to occur, the first law of photochemistry (the Grotthuss-Draper law) must be fulfilled: light must be absorbed by the so-called reaction system. Without absorption, the reaction will not be initiated. In plants and plant-derived products, the reaction system consists of chromophore groups that can change colour, which selectively absorb light. The effect of photodegradation is therefore primarily observed as a change in colour resulting from the oxidation of polymers and reactions involving free radicals, including carbonyl groups, which are one of the sources of chromophoric substances. Photodegradation

[3] See the Sect. 3.6 in this chapter.

[4] *Ibidem*

[5] See the Sect. 3.9 in this chapter.

processes proceed more rapidly under elevated temperatures. Photodegradation occurs primarily in amorphous regions (Kronkright 1990).

Cellulose absorbs light up to 300 nm. Under ultraviolet radiation, the C–H bonds present in cellulose, particularly those located near oxygen atoms, undergo homolytic cleavage, and the resulting carbon radicals react with molecular oxygen to form peroxyl radicals. Peroxyl radicals, which tend to undergo auto-oxidation, generate carbonyl, carboxyl, and hydroxyl groups. The decomposition of peroxyl radicals also leads to the cleavage of C–C bonds, resulting in fragmentation of the cellulose chain. In the presence of oxygen, cellulose produces peroxides that strongly absorb ultraviolet radiation. Upon decomposition, these peroxides generate free radicals that cause chain fragmentation, reduce the thermal oxidative resistance of cellulose, and initiate oxidation processes that result in the formation of carbonyl and carboxyl groups. In complexes with iron, copper, and lead ions, cellulose also absorbs longer wavelengths of light, closer to the boundary between ultraviolet and visible radiation (365–370 nm); thus, the presence of these metals significantly increases the photodegradation potential of cellulose (Kronkright 1990).

The photodegradation of hemicelluloses is, to some extent, analogous to the processes occurring in cellulose, and its main consequence is the oxidation of the polymer, associated with the presence of the aforementioned carbonyl groups, which, due to their chromophoric nature, lead to yellowing. In the case of hemicelluloses, degradation results in their breakdown into soluble simple sugars. The loss of hemicelluloses, which are responsible for the elasticity of plant material, leads to increased structural stresses and mechanical damage (Kronkright 1990).

Lignin absorbs a significant range of ultraviolet radiation (Kronkright 1990). Phenolic groups can form phenoxyl (o-semiquinone) radicals, which upon further oxidation generate quinonoid structures and methyl groups. Quinonoids are coloured compounds that further increase light absorbance within the visible spectrum. The double bonds present in the lignin structure, after absorbing light, undergo oxidation and, during decomposition, form carbonyl groups which, as previously mentioned in the context of cellulose and hemicelluloses, can act as chromophores. Many of these are sensitive to visible light. In addition to the formation of chromophores, oxidation reactions also produce free radicals, which exert an oxidative effect on cellulose chains. The result of photo-oxidation in this case is lignin with a completely altered structure and properties. Degraded lignin becomes water-soluble and more sensitive to visible light. This also contributes to the degradation of hemicelluloses, which thereby lose their protective layer.

3.5 Thermal Degradation

Thermal degradation of plant-derived materials involves the absorption of heat energy. Similar to light energy, changes can occur at all structural levels and affect all components of plant structure. As a result, oxidation processes—thermo-oxidation—take place. Thermo-oxidative changes lead to the formation of peroxides, hydroperoxides, carbonyl, and carboxyl groups (Kronkright 1990). These changes influence permeability, colour, gloss, resistance to mechanical damage, solubility of resins, reduction in viscosity, swelling, and water absorption capacity. The outcome may be desiccation and shrinkage of the plant material, resulting in reduced mechanical strength. Elevated temperature also accelerates the progression of other degradation mechanisms.

Furthermore, thermoplastic components of plant structure, such as lignin, suberin, waxes, resins, and gums, become more fluid at elevated temperatures and can migrate within the tissue structure. This leads to an uneven distribution of compounds that protect the plant from light and the ingress of harmful substances, rendering elements of the internal structure more susceptible to other degradation processes. Lignin is the most sensitive to temperature-induced changes, followed by hemicelluloses, while cellulose is the least affected (Kronkright 1990).

3.6 Environmental Pollution in Collection Storage Areas

Environmental pollutants affecting the preservation state of objects made from plant-derived materials take various forms. Firstly, they may originate from atmospheric pollution present in a given geographical area, primarily caused by emissions in urban and industrial centres, and mainly resulting from the combustion of fossil fuels by vehicles, factories, and power plants. Harmful substances in gaseous form penetrate buildings, especially through windows and doors. These include ozone, nitrogen oxides, sulphides, sulphur oxides and hydroxides, and carboxylic acids (Kronkright 1990; Havermans 1995; Bégin et al. 1999; ASHRAE 2019). These compounds exhibit oxidising properties and long-term acidifying effects, initiating the process of acid hydrolysis of cellulose (ASHRAE 2019).

Contaminants may also be of internal origin, arising from activities conducted within the institution or from the construction and storage methods of the object. Such emissions may be associated with the natural ageing processes of materials used in the object's manufacture, conservation methods employed by the institution (particularly those related to disinfection), or materials introduced during conservation treatments (for example, the off-gasing of VOCs from ageing synthetic adhesives). In the case of herbaria, a specific example of contamination is the emission of volatile organic compounds (VOCs) resulting from the use of biocides, as well as those naturally released from the plant specimens themselves, which is a species-specific characteristic (Collins 2014). Some essential oils present in plant specimens may occur within the collection both as products emitted by the specimens and as naturally derived biocides (Collins 2014).

Among the pollutants emitted by the objects and packaging themselves are aldehydes, carboxylic acids, and sulphur. A summary of the types of pollutants, excluding the impact of biocidal agents,[6] is presented in Table 3.1.

[6] See the Sect. 3.9 in this chapter.

Table 3.1 Summary of indoor and outdoor air pollutants, excluding pollutants resulting from the use of biocidal agents

Type of contamination	Source of contamination	Examples of degradation processes caused by contamination
Aldehydes	**Formaldehyde**: formaldehyde-based resins in wood-based materials, solid wood, paints and adhesives, "wet" natural history specimens. **Acetaldehyde**: paints, adhesives, solid wood. Low molecular weight aldehydes can be converted into their corresponding carboxylic acids in the presence of strong oxidising agents, such as peroxides released by oil paints or any paint coatings formed through oxidative polymerization.	Formaldehyde: lead corrosion at high relative humidity (>75%)
Amines	**Ammonia (NH_3)**: alkaline silicone sealants, concrete, adhesives and emulsion paints, cleaning agents, presence of visitors, animal excrement, fertilisers, inorganic processing industry, bacterial activity. In combination with sulphate or nitrate compounds, it can form ammonium salts. Cyclohexylamine (CHA), diethylaminoethanol (DEAE), and octadecylamine (ODA): corrosion inhibitors in humidification systems, some vapour-phase corrosion inhibitors.	Ammonia: damage to ebonite and efflorescence on cellulose nitrate. Other amines: considered responsible for blemishes on paintings and corrosion of bronze, copper, and silver.
Carboxylic acids	**Acetic acid (CH_3COOH)**: acidic silicone sealants (acetoxy curing), degradation of organic materials and objects such as cellulose acetate-based items and wooden materials, most paints, floor adhesives, human metabolism, linoleum, microbiological contamination of air conditioning filters, oil paints, photographic developers, some eco-friendly cleaning solutions **Formic acid (HCOOH)**: degradation of organic materials, oil paints, wooden materials **Fatty acids (RCOOH)**: candle burning, cooking, floor adhesives, human metabolism, linoleum, lubricant in HVAC systems, microbiological activity in air conditioning or on objects, items made from animal parts (including leather, fur, insect collections), oil paints, papers, paper and wooden objects, vehicle exhaust fumes	Acetic and formic acids: yellowing of paper and photographic documents. Additionally, corrosion of copper, cadmium, lead, magnesium, and zinc alloys; efflorescence on calcareous materials (e.g. shells, corals, limestones, calcium-based fossils); fading of certain dyes; efflorescence on soda-lime glass objects; reduction in the degree of cellulose polymerisation Fatty acids: discolouration of paint layers; corrosion of bronze, cadmium, and lead; discolouration on glass

(continued)

Table 3.1 (continued)

Type of contamination	Source of contamination	Examples of degradation processes caused by contamination
Nitrogen oxides (NO_x)	**Nitric oxide (NO)**: agricultural fertilisers, fuel combustion from vehicle exhaust and thermal energy plants, gas heaters, photochemical smog **Nitrogen dioxide (NO_2)**: decomposition of cellulose nitrate, sources similar to those of NO, but primarily formed through atmospheric oxidation of NO **Nitric acid (HNO_3)** and **nitrous acid (HNO_2)**: oxidation of NO_2 in the atmosphere or on material surfaces, decomposition of cellulose nitrate	Paper degradation, fading of dyes, exacerbates degradation caused by the presence of SO_2 on leather and metals
Oxidised sulphur gases (SO_2 and SO_3)	**Sulphur dioxide (SO_2)**: decomposition of materials and objects containing sulphur, such as protein fibres, pure pyrite or mineral samples containing pyritic sulphur pigments, sulphur-vulcanised rubbers, oil refineries, pulp and paper industry, combustion of fossil fuels containing sulphur **Sulphurous acid (H_2SO_3)**: oxidation of SO_2 in the atmosphere or on the surface of materials	Paper acidification, copper corrosion, fading of dyes, structural weakening of leather
Ozone (O_3)	Electric arcing, electronic air purifiers, electrostatic filtration systems, electric insect traps, laser printers, photocopiers, UV light sources, photochemical smog	Fading of dyes and pigments; oxidation of organic materials with conjugated double bonds, such as rubber; oxidation of volatile compounds to aldehydes and carboxylic acids
Reduced sulphur gases (S^-)	**Carbon disulphide (CS_2)**: polysulphide-based sealants; fungal growth; decaying organic matter in oceans, soils, and marshes **Carbonyl sulphide (OCS)**: wool degradation, coal combustion, proximity to the ocean, soils and wetlands, oxidation of carbon disulphide. **Hydrogen sulphide (H_2S)**: thermal processing by arc welding, mineral samples containing pyrite, sulphate-reducing bacteria in impregnated objects recovered from waterlogged sites, polysulphide sealants, vulcanised rubbers, presence of visitors, combustion of fuels and coal, marshes, ocean, petroleum and pulp industries (kraft process), vehicle exhaust, proximity to volcanoes	Corrosion of bronze, copper, and silver; discolouration of gelatin-silver photographic prints; darkening of lead-based pigments

(continued)

Table 3.1 (continued)

Type of contamination	Source of contamination	Examples of degradation processes caused by contamination
Particulate contaminants	**General**: aerosol humidifiers; candle burning; concrete; cooking; laser printers; aerosol cans; contaminants deposited from clothing, carpets, packaging crates, etc. (due to abrasion, vibration, or wear); industrial activity; nearby construction work; soil **Ammonium salts**: reaction of ammonia with SO_2 or NO_2 in indoor or outdoor environments or on surfaces **Biological and organic compounds**: microorganisms, degradation of objects, human and animal dander, construction activity **Chlorides**: sea salt aerosol, combustion of fossil fuels **Soot (organic carbon)**: candle burning, fires, coal combustion, combustion of vehicle exhaust	General: mechanical degradation of object surfaces; discolouration of objects; may initiate or intensify corrosion processes due to their hygroscopic nature Ammonium salts: reduction in the degree of cellulose polymerisation, corrosion of copper, nickel, silver, and zinc; blemishes on varnished paints and furniture with natural resins, as well as on ebonite; white deposits on object surfaces Chlorine compounds: acceleration of metal corrosion Soot: discolouration of porous surfaces, increased rate of metal corrosion. Carbon and metals such as iron may reduce the degree of cellulose polymerisation by increasing the risk of oxidation reactions

Source: ASHRAE (2019)

3.7 Physical Degradation of Plant Material

3.7.1 Reduction of Mechanical Strength Properties

Physical degradation refers to changes in botanical material caused by natural ageing processes, manufacturing techniques, conservation treatments, storage conditions, handling, and exposure to chemical agents. Damage results from structural weakening, often as a consequence of chemical changes described in other sections of Chap. 3.

The strength and flexibility of plant materials are associated with the uniform distribution of cellulose, including its amorphous and crystalline regions. The cell wall is evenly covered with microcapillaries, which undergo changes, aggregation, or destruction as a result of temperature and humidity fluctuations. Each part of the plant—leaves, stems, flowers, roots—exhibits different permeability. Structural changes in plant-derived materials are associated with changes of hydrogen bond stability. Each breakage of a hydrogen bond results in a certain weakening of the material's structure in response to applied stress. This allows for compression or a change in structural configuration, involving the relative displacement of molecules (Kronkright 1990). Reorganisation occurs as a result of swelling. Repeated cycles of swelling and shrinking cause further irreversible changes in the structure of the secondary wall, allowing for the absorption of progressively smaller amounts of water from the environment, in accordance with the phenomenon of hysteresis. Subsequent shrinkage in the structurally altered wall, along with processes associated with mechano-sorptive creep, result in drastic changes in the size and arrangement of microcapillaries, which form part of the amorphous region of the wall. The loss of the hydrated hemicellulose matrix leads to the formation of empty spaces or air in its place, visible as cracks. The greater the number of altered sites in the cell wall—which itself has limited elasticity and bending strength—the greater the load borne by the unaltered portion of the tissue, and uneven loading leads to cracks and tears (Fig. 3.2) (Kronkright 1990). Furthermore, degradation processes of cellulose and hemicelluloses, such as hydrolysis and oxidation, result in their fragmentation and increased crystallinity.

A reduction in mechanical strength may also result from freezing, which is used preventively as a protection against insect infestation.[7] If specimens subjected to freezing have an excessively high moisture content (caused, for example, by an excessively high RH level), this treatment may also lead to the destruction of the cell wall structure due increased water volume resulting from freezing. Damage may also arise from the activity of microorganisms.[8]

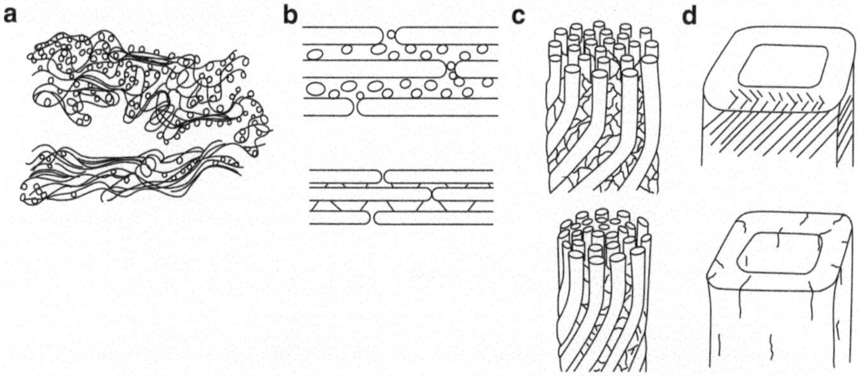

Fig. 3.2 Effects of desorption and subsequent mechano-sorptive creep on amorphous regions: (**a**) between crystalline micelles; (**b**) between cellulose aggregates within microfibrils; (**c**) between microfibrils within fibres; and (**d**) between fibres in the cell wall. (Based on Kronkright (1990))

[7] See the Sect. 4.1.1 in Chap. 4.

[8] See the Sect. 3.8 in this chapter.

3.7.2 *Mechanical Damage, Deformations, Damage Resulting from Conservation Treatments*

Mechanical damage to plant-derived materials includes cracks, tears, and losses, which disrupt of tissue continuity and impair the ability to receive and transmit stresses to adjacent structural elements. Mechanical damage may result from factors leading to structural disintegration, as previously described, including hydrolytic and oxidative processes. It can also be caused by the action of materials used during conservation, as well as by accretions that penetrate the tissue structure and reduce its strength. Damage may result from the techniques used in herbarium specimen preparation, poor storage conditions, handling, exhibition, and the use of biocides as a method of collection preservation.

A common phenomenon observed in bound herbaria is the deformation and mechanical damage of specimens resulting from overfilling of the block or, in the case of herbaria on separate sheets, storage in a distorted fascicle (Figs. 3.3 and 3.4).[9]

A block that was unsuitable or insufficiently adapted for herbarium purposes, meaning it was too tight, could undergo characteristic deformation, with the most pronounced bulging typically observed at the midpoint of the block's width, where the greatest accumulation of specimen thickness occurred. Deformation of herbarium object blocks also promoted further mechanical damage due to difficulties in handling (such as tears or creases caused by users), and facilitated access for insects and rodents. Additionally, these deformations enabled the accumulation of dust, further increasing the risk of microbial infection (Fig. 3.5).

In the case of herbaria, the most common types of damage are caused by insect activity, particularly larvae, which, as they feed, leave so-called larval galleries—structural losses in both the botanical specimens and the paper substrate.[10]

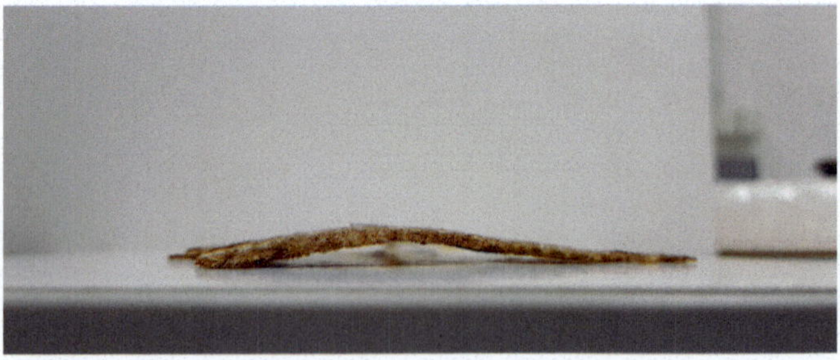

Fig. 3.3 Specimen removed from herbarium volume. Deformation caused by prolonged storage in a deformed block. Helwing A.J. or Boretius M., untitled, Warsaw, Herbarium of the Faculty of Biology, University of Warsaw (WA), ref. WA-KH-13.2.2, 1724–1745. (Photo: M. Grenda-Kurmanow)

[9] See also Sect. 5.3 in Chap. 5.

[10] See the Sect. 3.8.2 in this chapter.

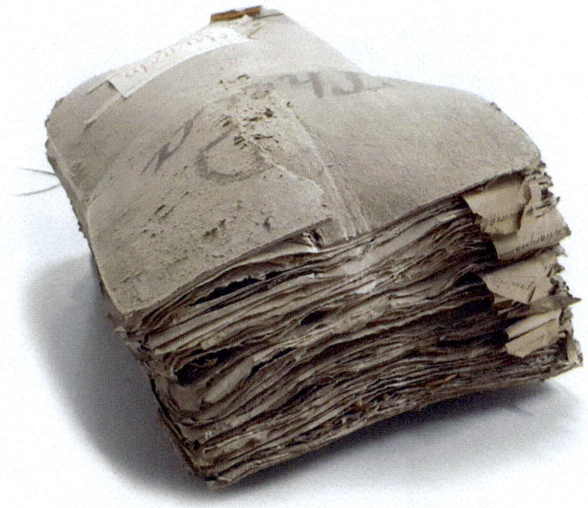

Fig. 3.4 Deformed fascicle. Jundziłł J., (*Józef Jundziłł Herbarium*), Kraków, Herbarium of the Institute of Botany, Polish Academy of Sciences in Kraków (KRAM), without ref. no., 1820s, with specimens dated from the eighteenth century to 1876. (Photo: M. Grenda-Kurmanow)

Specimens and substrate may also become deformed as a result of improper drying methods and unsuitable storage conditions, particularly due to sudden fluctuations in relative humidity and temperature (Fig. 3.6).

Attaching specimens either across the entire surface or at specific points can generate a range of mechanical stresses and strains, leading to cracking, detachment, and potential loss of plant material (Collins 2014). This is due to the differing physicochemical properties of dried plants and adhesive bonds (Figs. 3.7 and 3.8).

At the same time, residual traces of adhesive should not be routinely removed, as they may serve as identifying evidence relating to a detached or no longer existing specimen (Fig. 3.9).

Additional stresses are caused by changes in climatic conditions, which affect the moisture content of the technological components of the object, initiating expansion and contraction processes that occur differently in each element. When hygroscopic adhesives and adhesive tapes are used to mount specimens, an increase in relative humidity may activate the adhesive layer, leading adjacent sheets and specimens to stick together, which in turn can result in mechanical damage. Furthermore, cellulose or synthetic tapes degrade and may decompose under the influence of certain fumigants (Bridson and Forman 1999, p. 41).

Another type of damage, often irreversible, is the embedding of parts of the specimen's leaf in a layer of adhesive used for mounting. Attaching the specimen to the substrate with its entire surface remains a common practice in institutions.[11] This method assumes that the specimen will be studied exclusively from the side not covered with adhesive. Unlike mounting with strips or thread, gluing the entire specimen prevents its removal from the substrate. Adhesive residues may also occur on the *recto* of the specimen if the mounting is performed imprecisely. Covering the

[11] See the Sect. 2.1.4 in Chap. 2.

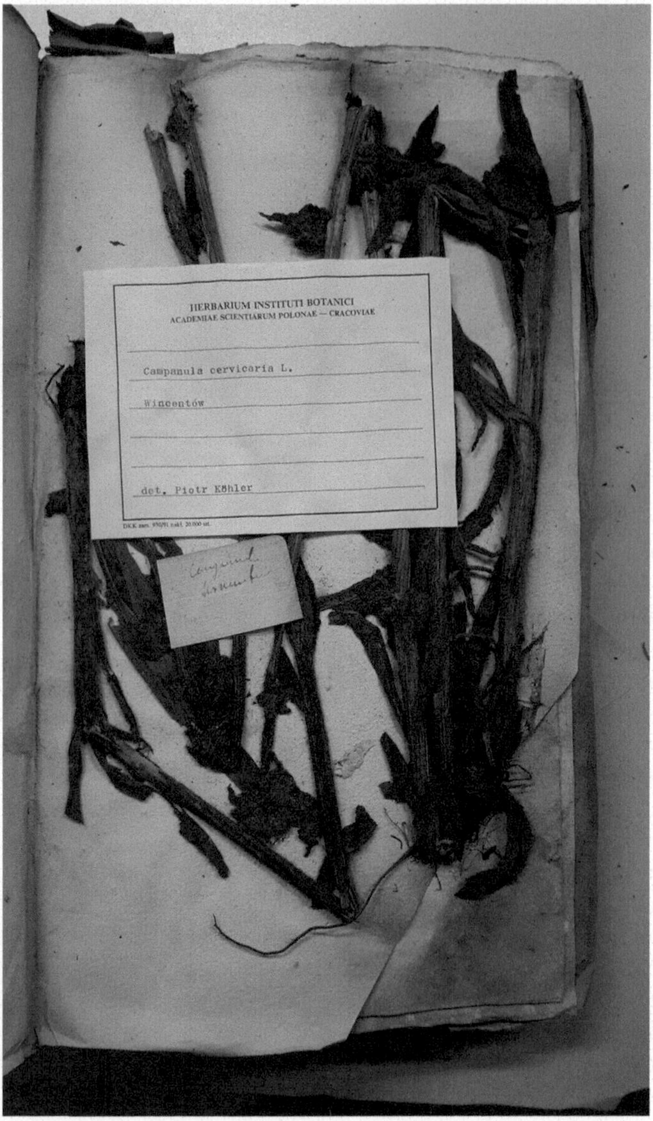

Fig. 3.5 Dust accumulation in sheet deformations. Jundziłł J., (*Józef Jundziłł Herbarium*), Kraków, Herbarium of the Institute of Botany, Polish Academy of Sciences in Kraków (KRAM), without ref. no., 1820s, with specimens dated from the eighteenth century to 1876. (Photo: M. Grenda-Kurmanow)

specimen's surface with adhesive disrupts its taxonomic features. This is particularly evident in the case of emulsion adhesives, such as popular PVA glues (Figs. 3.10 and 3.11), as well as acrylic and some other adhesives at higher concentrations. Adhesives may form various types of coatings on specimens (Figs. 3.12 and 3.13).

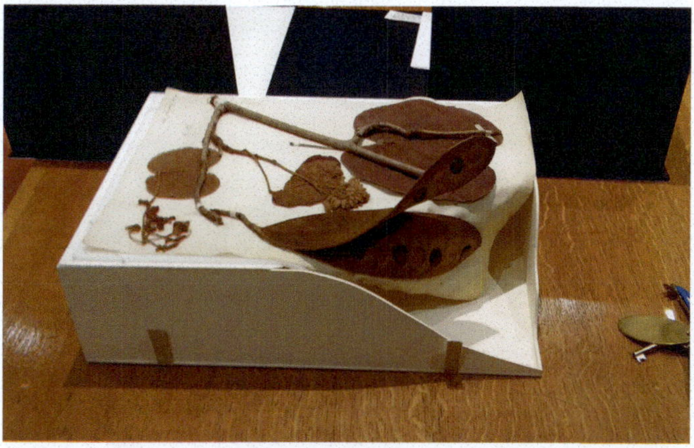

Fig. 3.6 Severe deformation of the specimen adhered to the sheet caused distortion of the substrate, making it impossible to store the object flat. Consequently, a special protective box was made to accommodate the deformation, allowing for the safe storage of the specimen. Linnaeus Collection at the Linnaean Society of London (LINN), 2015. (Photo: M. Grenda-Kurmanow)

Solvents and alkalis used during conservation can have a destructive effect on the protective cuticle layer and penetrate deep into the specimen, initiating the disintegration of plant material and accelerating processes of physical degradation. They may also cause swelling of the specimen and alter the organisation of the cell wall, which, after such interference with its structure, does not return to its previous arrangement. During drying, shrinkage occurs within the new arrangement of fibrils and microfibrils, and with each change in relative humidity, the internal structure of the cell wall becomes tighter.[12] Components of the cell wall sensitive to alkaline environments include hemicelluloses, which in their low-molecular-weight form are also water-soluble, as well as suberin and lignin (Florian 1990). Lignin is also partially soluble in alcohols: ethanol, methanol, butanol, and benzyl alcohol. It also swells under the influence of other solvents (Florian 1990). The solubility of lignin increases over time with its degree of degradation. In hot water, pectins and tannins may dissolve, while in volatile organic solvents, waxes and other extractive substances may be removed (Kronkright 1990).

The manner in which herbarium specimens are handled is of paramount importance. As previously mentioned, specimens in herbaria could be either loosely placed between sheets or attached to pages within a block, making them highly susceptible to damage and loss of botanical material. The mechanical damage described by Saint-Lager is associated with frequent relocations of collections, theft of specimens, and careless application of biocidal agents (Saint-Lager 1885, p. 43).[13]

---

[12] This is the process of mechano-sorptive creep.

[13] See also Sect. 1.3.6 in Chap. 1.

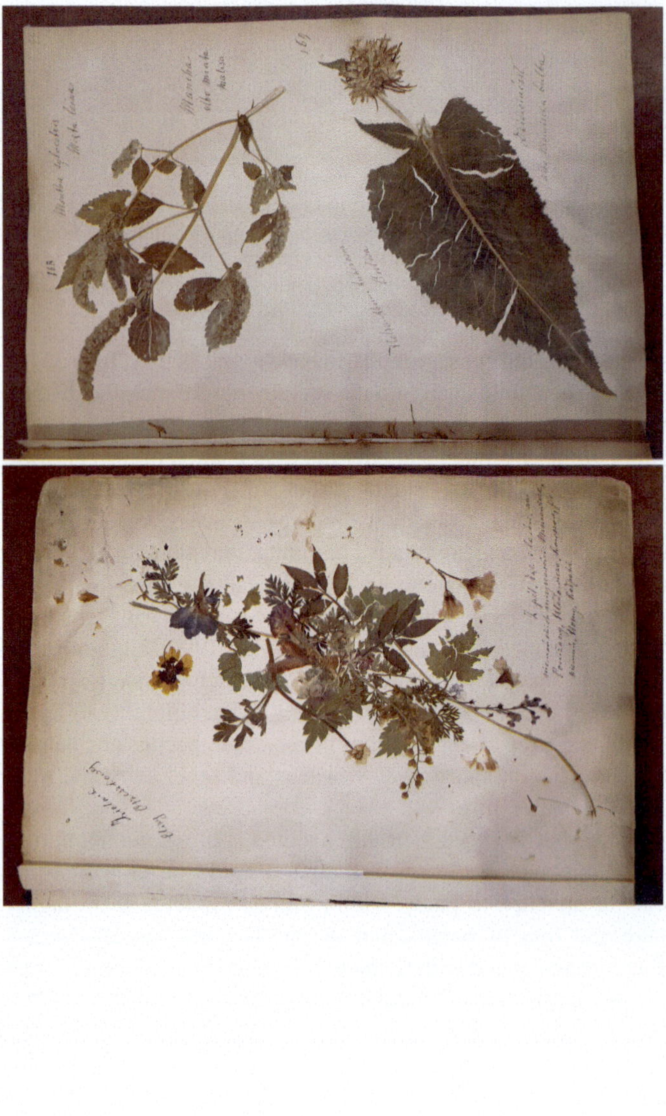

Figs. 3.7 and 3.8 Title page (Fig. 3.7) and no. 44 (Fig. 3.8) from Eliza Orzeszkowa's herbarium, [Orzeszkowa E., (*Herbarium of Eliza Orzeszkowa*), Poznań, Poznań Society for the Advancement of Arts and Sciences, ref. Rkp. 880, 1887–1898]. Numerous cracks and losses of specimens are visible, caused by the mounting technique in which specimens were glued to the substrate over their entire surface. (Photo: M. Grenda-Kurmanow)

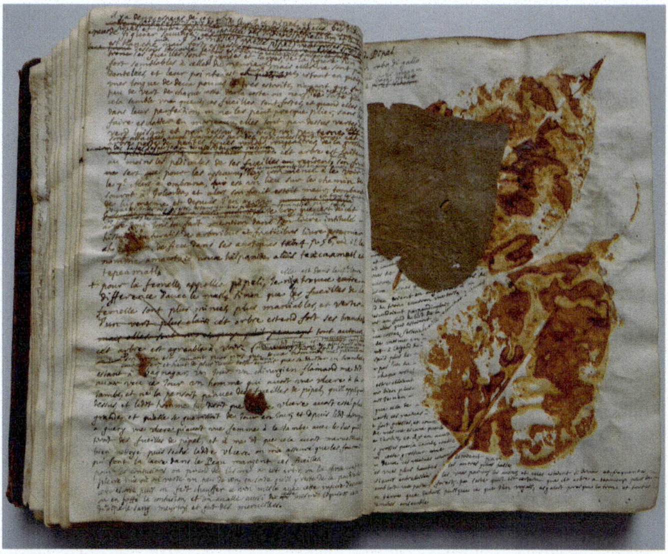

Fig. 3.9 Traces of adhesive replicating the shape of the specimen, thus serving as a guide for identifying and restoring the specimen's remains to their original position. Thévenot, de J., untitled, Paris, Muséum national d'Histoire naturelle (P), without ref. no., 1664–1666. (Photo: M. Grenda-Kurmanow)

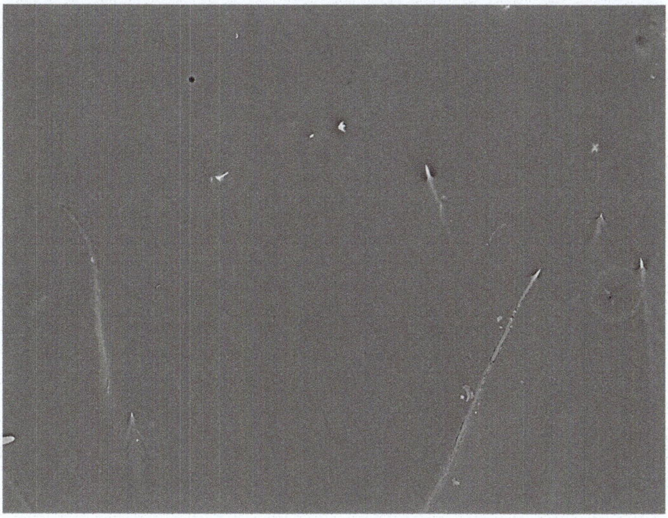

Fig. 3.10 Surface of a *Fragaria vesca* leaf with Hewit M218 adhesive applied. (Photo: J. Kotowski)

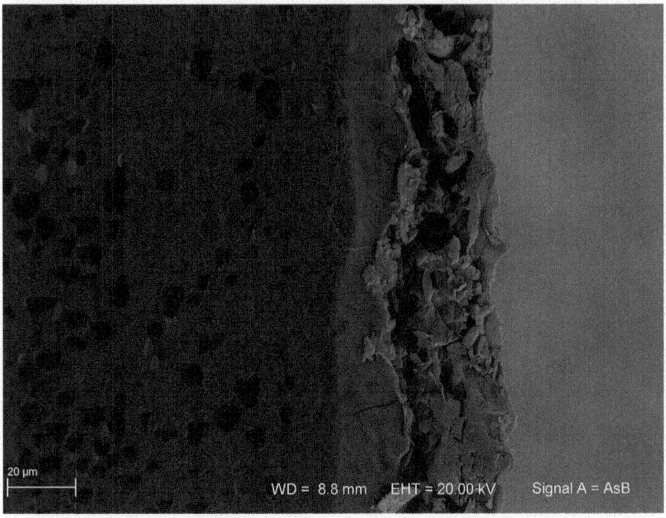

Fig. 3.11 Cross-section of a *Fragaria vesca* leaf with Jade 403 adhesive applied. (Photo: J. Kotowski)

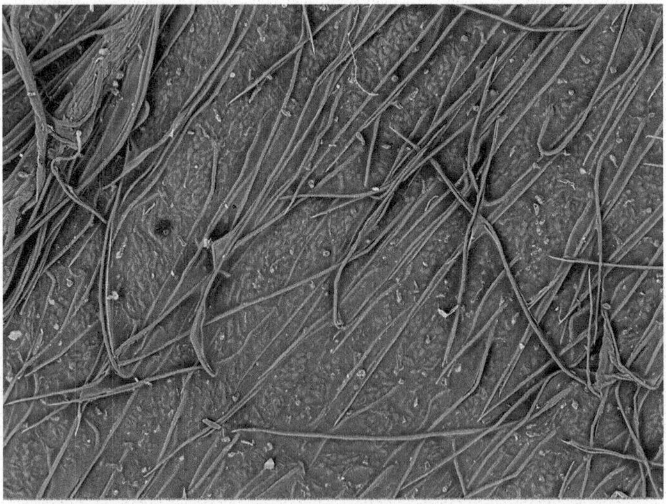

Fig. 3.12 Surface of a *Fragaria vesca* leaf with Aquazol 500 adhesive applied at a concentration of 10%. (Photo: J. Kotowski)

3.7.3 Colour Change

Another form of physical degradation, naturally occurring in botanical specimens, is discolouration. Yellowing is a characteristic process observed in specimens after pressing and drying. This is related to natural ageing processes and the darkening of

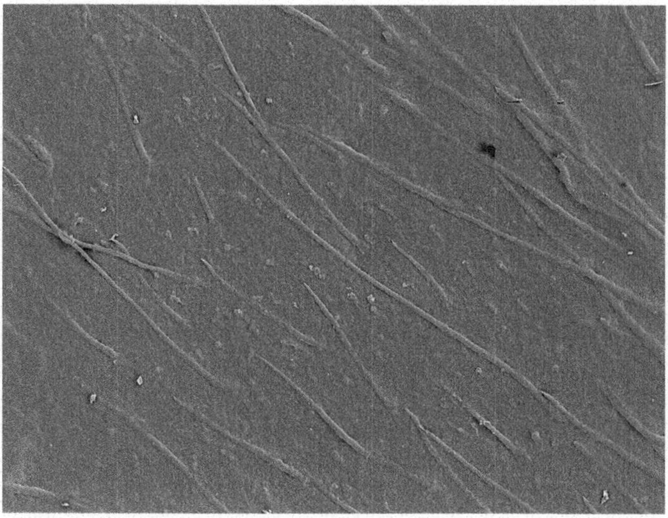

Fig. 3.13 Surface of a *Fragaria vesca* leaf coated with a 10% solution of purified wheat starch paste. (Photo: J. Kotowski)

plant glands (Collins 2014). Yellowing is typical for bulbous and tuberous plants from the following genera: *Lilium* L., *Galanthus* L., *Leucojum* L., *Ornithogalum* L., *Muscari* Mill., *Gagea* Salisb., *Scilla* L., *Allium* L., *Hemerocallis* L. (Drobnik 2009, p. 86). These plants should be dried after dissection, separating the bulbs or tubers from the leaves and flowering stem, because as long as the plant is not divided into its individual parts, the bulb or tuber continues to nourish the plant, but without access to light. In the absence of light, the specimen becomes yellowed (Drobnik 2009, p. 86).

Among the plants that naturally blacken or brown during drying, Drobnik lists: *Galium odoratum*, *Galium uliginosum*, *Galium palustre*, *Salix myrsinifolia*, *Lembotropis nigricans*, the genus *Melampyrum*, as well as the thick leaves of certain poplars, pears, and apples, the leaves of *Sambucus racemosa* and *Sambucus nigra*, and *Orchidaceae* (Drobnik 2009, pp. 86–88). In addition, the leaf blades of species rich in latex, such as some spurges (*Euphorbiaceae*), opium poppy (*Papaver somniferum*), or greater celandine (*Chelidonium majus*), also tend to blacken. In the case of other species, blackening can be considered a result of improper drying, either due to excessively slow water removal from the specimen or excessive heating (Drobnik 2009).

The white colour of flowers typically turns yellow, and in some cases may become brown or grey. Certain species temporarily, for several years, change colour during drying to turquoise, for example, the leaves and stems of *Mercurialis perennis*, the stem of *Dipsacus sylvestris*, or *Melampyrum arvense* (Drobnik 2009). Some blue and violet flowers fade, such as those of *Campanula*, *Centaurea cyanus*, and *Cichorium intybus*. Others darken, acquiring shades of violet: for instance, pink-flowering species of the family *Onagraceae*, and the purple flowers of *Vicia*,

Lathyrus, and *Boraginaceae*. Colour changes also occur in *Lathyrus sylvestris*, which turns grey; *Medicago x varia*, (*Trifolia*), and *Pulmonaria* (Drobnik 2009). In general, yellow is the most durable colour in herbarium specimens (Drobnik 2009).

Throughout the history of herbarium preparation, numerous attempts have been made to preserve the natural colours of living plants using various chemical substances.[14] For many years, there has been consensus that the most effective method is to dry the specimen as quickly and carefully as possible, thereby allowing rapid reduction of its water content to a level in equilibrium with the ambient moisture content (Norton 1990; Drobnik 2009, pp. 88–86). Colour may also change due to improper storage conditions and exposure. An example of this is the previously mentioned risk of lichen thalli discolouration when specimens are stored in an environment with excessively high pH (Drobnik 2009, p. 194). Additionally, colour changes may occur as a result of photodegradation, particularly in the presence of highly photoreactive cell wall components such as lignin or other pre-degraded cell wall elements, whose photoreactivity increases with the degree of degradation caused by other factors.[15]

3.8 Biological Degradation (Biodeterioration)

Biological damage is caused by the activity of fungi, moulds, bacteria, insects and other invertebrates, as well as rodents.

Certain species of herbarium specimens are more susceptible to insect and mould attack than others, particularly if they contain nutritional substances (for example, flowers rich in protein-containing pollen from *Brassicaceae*, *Ranunculaceae*, or *Asteraceae*). Among monocotyledons, the most vulnerable families include: *Amaryllidaceae* J. St.-Hryc., *Cyperaceae* Juss., *Iridaceae* Juss., *Liliaceae* Juss., and *Orchidaceae* Juss.; among dicotyledons, the most sensitive families are: *Aizoaceae* F. Rudolphi, *Apiaceae* Lindl., *Apocynaceae* Juss., *Araliaceae* Juss., *Asteraceae*, *Bignoniaceae* Juss., *Brassicaceae* Burnett, *Capparaceae* Juss., *Celastraceae* R. Br., *Euphorbiaceae* Juss., *Fabaceae* Lindl., *Gentianaceae* Juss., *Lamiaceae* Juss., *Malvaceae* Juss., *Nymphaeaceae* Salisb., *Ranunculaceae* Juss., and *Scrophulariaceae* Juss. (Hall 1988; Moore and Woodgyer 2023). In addition, certain species of fungi and pteridophytes are also susceptible to insect attack. Bryophytes and lichens, on the other hand, are generally more resistant to insect infestation (Hall 1988).

[14] See Sect. 2.1.3 in Chap. 2.

[15] See Sect. 3.4 in this chapter.

3.8.1 Damage Caused by Microorganism Activity

Microbiological deterioration occurs in the presence of water, which is essential for the development of microorganisms. The activity of cellulolytic and hemicellulolytic bacteria and fungi leads to enzymatic degradation. In structures where cellulose and hemicelluloses have been partially dissolved by enzymes, bacterial pits and fungal hyphal overgrowths are observed penetrating the cell wall, and aligning along the cellulose macrofibrils. This results in physical weakening of the cell wall structure, and structural weakening of the paper substrate (Fig. 3.14).

Incompletely dried specimens may pose a risk of microbiological infection. Fleshy succulent specimens are difficult to dry thoroughly and may be prone to mould growth. A similar issue arises with the drying of mosses and lichens (Collins 2014). Numerous moulds also occur naturally in the environment, making their complete elimination impossible (Purewal 2012, p. 17). The activation of dormant mould spores occurs with unexpected changes in the microclimate, associated with an increase in relative humidity (RH) to around 75%. This may be related to both seasonal microclimatic fluctuations and the effects of random events (malfunctions, flooding, or the presence of water due to improper thawing of herbarium collections). Lack of ventilation and poor air exchange also contribute to mould development. However, a high RH level (≥75%) alone does not unconditionally indicate the presence of active moulds, as the key factors are the type of collection microclimate and its stability. This is evidenced by the good preservation state of herbarium collections in tropical countries, where relative humidity consistently remains above 70% (Townsend 1999).

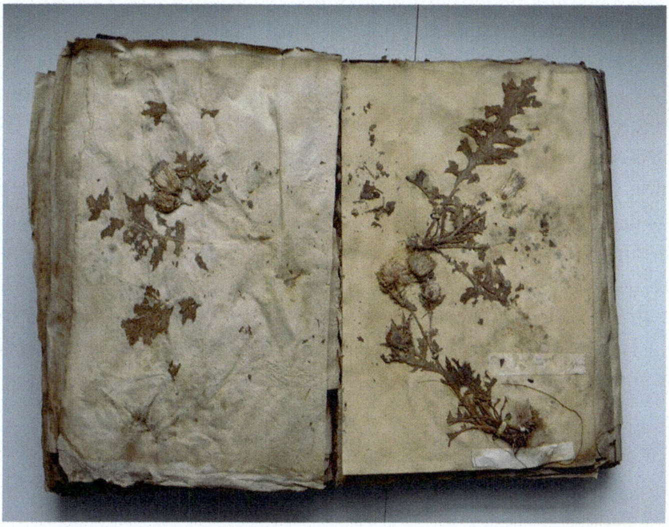

Fig. 3.14 Herbarium specimen affected by microbial infection. N.n, untitled, Paris, Muséum national d'Histoire naturelle (P), without ref. no., undated. (Photo: M. Grenda-Kurmanow)

3.8.2 Damage Caused by Insect Activity

As previously mentioned, one of the major issues and topics addressed in the context of herbarium collection preservation is insect activity. Although adhesives used to mount specimens are particularly attractive to insects, herbaria in which plants were not glued to the substrate but instead kept loosely between sheets were not immune to the threat posed by these organisms. When stored alongside other collections, they too fell victim to pests. Furthermore, as already noted, certain species are more susceptible to insect attack than others.

In the case of insects undergoing complete metamorphosis (metamorphosis with a pupal stage, such as beetles and butterflies), damage is most often caused by larvae, which, while feeding, bore larval tunnels, thereby creating losses in herbarium specimens and paper substrates (Figs. 3.15 and 3.16).

These tunnels typically take the form of round or oval holes, visible on many adjacent sheets. The tunnels may also have a more complex structure, forming winding, curved galleries. They can occur in all structural elements of herbaria, including the binding, the block, and the botanical specimens themselves. For species that develop through incomplete metamorphosis (such as silverfish and booklice), it is generally assumed that both nymphs and adults are equally damaging, leaving losses in the form of holes of various sizes. In addition to boring holes and tunnels, insects leave faeces, larval exuviae, and remnants of cocoons at feeding sites, which, like the bodies of dead adults, attract additional pests and increase the potential for mechanical and structural damage to herbaria. Insect bodies remaining within the collection, which contain water, may also contribute to microbiological attack inside the objects.

The species feeding on herbarium specimens include the biscuit/drugstore beetle (*Stegobium paniceum*), cigarette/tobacco beetle (*Lasioderma serricorne*), and Indian meal moth (*Plodia interpunctella*) (Pinniger 2015). Other reported species are the Berlin/Stockholm beetle (*Trogoderma angustum*), khapra/cabinet beetle (*Trogoderma granarium*), and varied carpet beetle (*Anthrenus verbasci*) (Hall 1988; Drobnik 2009, pp. 159–162; Querner 2015; Moore and Woodgyer 2023). Additionally, collections may contain other insect species that feed on paper and other plant-derived materials: silverfish (*Lepisma saccharina*), common furniture beetle (*Anobium punctatum*), spider beetles: *Ptinus fur*, *Ptinus tectus*, and *Niptus hololeucus*, as well as booklice, Psocids (*Liposcelis*, with *Liposcelis bostrychophilus* being the most frequently cited example) (Pinniger 2015; Querner 2015; Karbowska-Berent 2016). Table 3.2. presents a summary of the insect species most commonly found in herbaria.

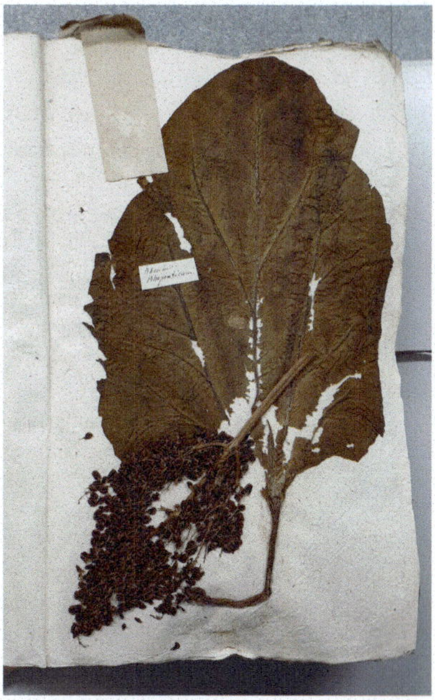

Fig. 3.15 Traces of insect feeding, with damage mainly apparent in the botanical specimen. Jundziłł J., (*Józef Jundziłł Herbarium*), Kraków, Herbarium of the Institute of Botany, Polish Academy of Sciences in Kraków (KRAM), without ref. no, 1820s, with specimens dated from the eighteenth century to 1876. (Photo: M. Grenda-Kurmanow)

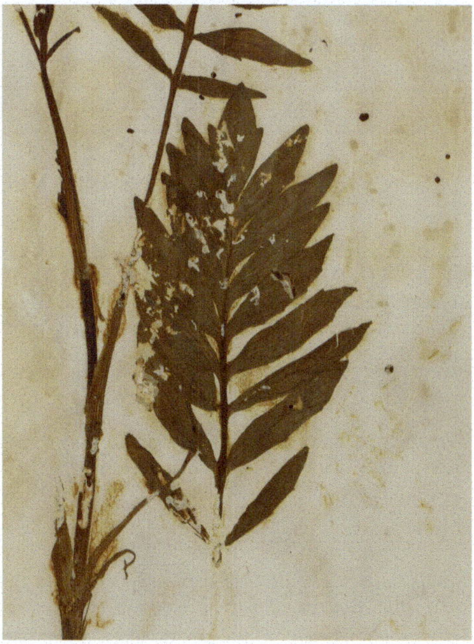

Fig. 3.16 Traces of insect feeding, losses apparent in the botanical specimen, in the adhesive layer, and in the paper substrate. N.n., *Herbarium Vivum…*, [*Izabela Czartoryska's Herbarium*], Kraków, National Museum in Kraków, Czartoryski Princes Library, ref. Rkps 2782, 1746. (Photo: T. Rizov-Ciechański)

Table 3.2 List of insects posing the greatest threat to herbarium collections

Insect species	Feeding behaviour	Size of the harmful insect stage	Time and conditions of hatching and occurrence
Biscuit/drugstore beetle (*Stegobium paniceum*)	Herbarium specimens, dried vegetables, nuts, cereal products, products with high starch content. Damage is caused mainly by larvae.	Larvae: up to 5 mm; adults: 2–3 mm	Dependent on food availability and temperature; at 30 °C with access to food, the life cycle is 5–6 weeks, under less favourable conditions up to a year. High reproductive capacity. Thermophilic and photophilic.
Cigarette/tobacco beetle (*Lasioderma serricorne*)	Larvae: herbarium specimens, animal proteins, hides. Adults do not feed	Larvae: approx. 4 mm	Thermophilic and photophilic. Hatching time depends on temperature. They die within a few days at temperatures below 4 °C
Indian meal moth (*Plodia interpunctella*)	Larvae: cereal products, seeds, nuts, dried fruit. Adults do not feed	Larvae: up to 12–14 mm	Preferred temperature: 20–25 °C
Berlin/Stockholm beetle (*Trogoderma angustum*), khapra/cabinet beetle (*Trogoderma granarium*)	Plant and animal specimens	Adults: 2–4 mm	n/a
Varied carpet beetle (*Anthrenus verbasci*)	Adults: pollen and floral nectar. Larvae: entomological collections, animal material, chitin, keratin	Larvae: 4–6 mm; adults: up to 3.5 mm	Thermophilic and photophilic. Produce 1–2 generations per year
Silverfish (*Lepisma saccharina*), firebrat (*Thermobia domestic*)	Starch, animal glues, microfungi on cellulosic materials	Adults: 10–15 mm	Requires high local relative humidity (75–80%). Avoids light. Preferred temperature for silverfish: approx. 20 °C. Firebrat prefers higher temperatures
Common furniture beetle (*Anobium punctatum*)	Larvae: wood, cellulosic materials	Larva: up to 6 mm	Prefers RH around 55%, but can survive in cold, yet humid conditions. Optimal development temperature: approx. 23 °C
Spider beetles: (*Ptinus fur*), (*Ptinus tectus*), (*Niptus hololeucus*)	Herbarium specimens of vascular plants, fungal and moss specimens, entomological collections, animal skins, paper, textiles	Ptinus fur: larva: up to 5 mm, adult: 2–4.5 mm; Ptinus tectus: larva: up to 3.5 mm; adult: 3.5–5 mm	Capable of reproducing at temperatures below 10 °C. At higher temperatures, two generations may develop per year. Ptinus fur: RH above 70%

(continued)

Table 3.2 (continued)

Insect species	Feeding behaviour	Size of the harmful insect stage	Time and conditions of hatching and occurrence
Booklice, Psocids (*Liposcelis*, e.g. *Liposcelis bostrychophilus*)	Mould on paper and cereal products, entomological collections	Adults: less than 1 mm	Reproduce very rapidly at temperatures above 25 °C. Can develop at RH above 60%

Based on Pinniger (2015); Karbowska-Berent (2016); Moore and Woodgyer (2023)

3.9 Damage Caused by the Use of Biocidal Agents[16]

Since the earliest days of herbarium development, the persistent problem of pest attacks (insects, rodents, microorganisms) has been addressed through the use of various biocidal agents or repellents. Natural substances were often employed, although their effectiveness was not always satisfactory. Spiegel mentions clove powder and the addition of aloe, which he incorporated into the adhesive used for mounting specimens (van den Spiegel 1606, p. 81),[17] de Tournefort provides a critical note on plant-derived agents, among which he lists an aloe decoction ("*aloe hepatica*"), as well as decoctions of wormwood ("absinthe", *Artemisia absinthium* L.) and santonica (*Artemisia cina* O. Berg.) (de Tournefort 1694, pp. 547–548), which caused discolouration of specimens. Many other natural substances were also in use.[18] Many of these were eventually synthesised, which facilitated their production and standardised their composition and efficacy. Some, such as pyrethrins, are still used today, both in their natural and synthetic forms.

[16] Based on the author's work (Grenda-Kurmanow 2019).

[17] The translation of the original text can be found in Sect. 1.3.2 in Chap. 1.

[18] For example, camphor—a component of camphor tree oil [*Cinnamomum camphora* (L.) J. Presl.]; cassia oil from Chinese cinnamon [*Cinnamomum cassia* (L.) J. Presl.]; thymol and carvacrol—constituents of thyme oil (*Thymus vulgaris*), wild thyme (*Thymus serpyllum* L.), and ajwain (*Trachyspermum ammi* L. or *Carum copticum* L.); neem (*Azadirachta indica* A. Juss.); pyrethrin contained in Dalmatian pyrethrum [*Tanacetum cinerariifolium* (Trevir.) Sch. Bip., formerly known as Dalmatian chrysanthemum, *Chrysanthemum cinerariifolium* (Trevir.) Sch. Bip.]; linalool, a component of true lavender oil (*Lavandula angustifolia* Mill., formerly *Lavandula officinalis* Chaix); turpentine from the distillation of Scots pine resin (*Pinus sylvestris* L.); leafy shoots of wild rosemary (*Rhododendron tomentosum* Harmaja, syn. *Ledum palustre* L.), now under species protection [Drobnik 2009, p. 165]; sweet flag (*Acorus calamus* L.); plai ginger (*Zingiber cassumunar* Roxb.); tobacco (from cultivated tobacco, *Nicotiana tabacum* L.); strychnine, present in the seeds of the strychnine tree (*Strychnos nux-vomica* L.); Javanese long pepper (*Piper retrofractum* Vahl); seeds of ginkgo (*Ginkgo biloba* L.); citronella oil (*Cymbopogon nardus* (L.) Rendle or *Cymbopogon winterianus* Jowitt); rotenone found in the roots of many species in the legume family (*Fabaceae*) (Drobnik 2009, pp. 164–165; Prance and Nesbitt 2005; Purewal 2012); as well as menthol, cedar oil, and bitter almond oil (Hawks 2001).

The most well-known and, until recently, most commonly used biocide in herbaria was mercuric chloride.[19] This is an example of a biocidal agent that creates persistent contamination in the collection and poses a health risk to humans, even long after its application.[20]

The classification of biocides may be based on their mode of action or their form of application. According to the first criterion, the types of biocidal agents include stomach poisons (which must be ingested by pests); contact agents; residual agents; desiccants, which cause dehydration and subsequent death of insects; insect growth regulators; and fumigants. Biocides may be formulated in mixtures with solvents or inert substances; as oil or emulsion concentrates, finely ground powders, water-dispersible dusts, baits, capsules releasing a toxic substance, or plastic strips impregnated with biocide (Dawson and Strang 1992).

The list of biocides used in herbarium collections is presented in Table 3.3, together with references.[21] For each compound, the CAS (Chemical Abstracts Service) registry number[22] is provided. For biocides that occur as a group of compounds (e.g. pyrethrins or carbamates), the CAS number of a representative substance is given. The third column of the table contains information on the negative impact on the genetic material of objects found in museum collections. The information regarding genetic effects has been generalised and applies to a broader range of natural history collections, not only herbaria.[23] The final columns provide infor-

[19] The first mention can be found in Tournefort, who used it in the form of monovalent mercury compound (*mercure doux*) and divalent mercury compound (sublimate, Fr. *sublimé corrosif*), as additives to animal glue with which he mounted specimens (de Tournefort 1694, pp. 547–548).

[20] In institutions with a long history of using mercuric chloride, mercury vapours can be expected in the air, particularly in storage cabinets and their immediate surroundings. As recently as the 1980s, mercuric chloride was used in the Netherlands and at the Royal Botanic Gardens, Kew. In 1988, mercuric chloride was still in use in African herbaria, and continued to be used in France until the end of the twentieth century (Grenda-Kurmanow 2019).

[21] The table is based on Grenda-Kurmanow (2019). The literature referenced in the compilation pertains to the use of biocides in herbarium collections. Information on the biocides themselves can also be found in numerous other publications concerning museum collections in general (Dawson and Strang 1992; Hawks 2001; Sirois 2001; Odegaard and Sadongei 2005; Odegaard and Zimmt 2008; Pfister 2008), as well as other types of collections in which biocidal agents have been commonly used, e.g. ethnographic, wet collections (i.e. *fluid collections*, meaning specimens preserved in conservation solutions), entomological, taxidermy, or economic botany specimens. These sources also mention other toxic substances (e.g. glyphosate, borax, or methoxychlor) that have not yet been identified in herbaria (Glastrup 1987; Hawks 2001; Odegaard and Zimmt 2008). However, this does not mean that they are not present there.

[22] Chemical Abstract Service. https://commonchemistry.cas.org/. Accessed 13 Jan 2026.

[23] Due to the limited number of studies in this area, the data presented here have been compiled from publications concerning the effects of biocides and preservatives on the genetic material of various biological specimens forming part of museum collections (Brown 1999; Whitten et al. 1999; Kigawa et al. 2003, 2011; Kigawa and Strang 2011; Strang 1999, Carter 2003; Eklund 2007; Espeland et al. 2010; Purewal 2012). In certain cases, the research findings are inconclusive. In such instances, the table presents the assessment that is critical of the given substance, on the assumption that if a particular agent has demonstrated destructive effects in any study, it should be considered a potential threat to heritage objects.

Table 3.3 List of biocides used in herbarium collections

Name of biocide, CAS number	Literature—use of biocides in herbaria	Form/method of application	Negative impact on DNA of natural history collection specimens	Carcinogenicity (according to EPA and IARC)	Characteristics
Inorganic compounds					
Mercury(II) chloride, CAS: 7487-94-7; mercury(I) chloride, CAS: 10112-91-1	de Tournefort (1694); Robinson (1903); Merrill (1948); Croat (1978); Briggs et al. (1983); Clarck (1986); Hall (1988); Bridson and Forman (1999); Hawks and Bell (1999); Purewal (1999, 2001, 2012); Rader and Ison (1999); Townsend (1999); Hawks (2001); Sirois (2001); Hawks et al. (2004); Oyarzun et al. (2007); Kataeva et al. (2008); Purewal et al. (2008); Pfister (2008); Drobnik (2009); Fellowes et al. (2011); Webber et al. (2011); Dauwalder (2012); Havermans et al. (2015); Fallon et al. (2016); Grenda-Kurmanow (2016, 2017); Popławska and Zając (2018)	Crystalline, powder/used in solutions, added to adhesive	Yes	Possible human carcinogen (EPA) Not classifiable as to its carcinogenicity to humans (IARC)	Occurs as calomel (mercury in oxidation state I, Hg_2Cl_2), or, more commonly, as a sublimate (mercury in oxidation state II, $HgCl_2$). The earliest references are found in de Tournefort (1694, pp. 547–548). Calomel, when exposed to UV radiation, can decompose into pure mercury and mercury (II) chloride, i.e. sublimate. Sublimate is volatile at room temperature. It was used in alcoholic solutions, in various proportions, sometimes with the addition of phenol, or mixed with arsenic or lauryl pentachlorophenate (LPCP) (Briggs et al. 1983). Purewal cites older, historical recipes in which sublimate is also mixed with alcohol and phenol or its derivative, cresol (Purewal 2012, p. 20). Whole botanical specimens were immersed in the solution or the mixture was applied with a brush. After removal from the solution, specimens could become brittle. May leave white deposits in the form of hair-like crystals, which can be mistaken for taxonomic features of the specimen. To prevent recrystallisation, paraffin was added to the alcoholic sublimate solution. Mercury (II) chloride sublimes slowly from the area to which it has been applied, and therefore the treatment was usually repeated several times. It was long believed that mercuric chloride loses its biocidal properties over time. In fact, the opposite is true, as mercuric chloride is permanently deposited within the structure of objects. The mercury present in mercuric chloride reacts with sulphur, which is found both as an air pollutant, a component of paper substrates, and in animal glues, forming black mercury sulphide (metacinnabar, HgS) and leaving a mark on paper in the form of concentrated or diffuse stains with black edges (Figs. 3.17, 3.18 and 3.19). Over the years, it is reduced to pure mercury, which is related to its tendency to disproportionate, i.e. to undergo simultaneous oxidation and reduction. The reduction of mercury accelerates the acid hydrolysis of cellulose. It has a destructive effect on plant tissues and paper substrates, causing brittleness and structural changes (Clarck 1986). It may cause the cuticle to disintegrate. It is a potent poison and neurotoxin.

(continued)

Table 3.3 (continued)

Name of biocide, CAS number	Literature—use of biocides in herbaria	Form/method of application	Negative impact on DNA of natural history collection specimens	Carcinogenicity (according to EPA and IARC)	Characteristics
Arsenic (arsenic trioxide), CAS: 1327-53-3, lead arsenate, CAS: 7784-40-9, and other arsenic compounds	Robinson (1903); Merrill (1948); Purewal (1999, 2001, 2012); Townsend (1999); Sirois (2001); Pfister (2008); Purewal et al. (2008); Drobnik (2009); Dauwalder (2012); Grenda-Kurmanow (2016, 2017); Popławska and Zając (2018)	White powder/ dusting, addition to adhesives	Yes	Carcinogenic to humans (EPA, IARC)	Known since antiquity, in museum collections used since the early eighteenth century, mainly in taxidermy specimens (arsenic and sodium arsenate). Herbarium collections were dusted with arsenic, lead arsenate ($PbHAsO_4$), or potassium arsenate (*sel de Macquer*, KH_2AsO_4) (Purewal 2012, p. 20; Péquignot et al. 2006). Also applied in solution with mercuric chloride and phenols. It is permanently deposited in the structure of objects and is sometimes visible as a white residue. Highly toxic not only if ingested, but also if inhaled or absorbed through the skin; carcinogenic. Phased out since the 1960s, but used in some institutions until the 1990s.
Hydrogen cyanide, CAS: 74-90-8	Merrill (1948); Purewal (2001, 2012); Drobnik (2009); Grenda-Kurmanow (2016)	Gas/fumigation	–	Inadequate information to assess carcinogenic potential (EPA)	Other names: prussic acid Used as a biocidal agent since the nineteenth century. It was also an ingredient in Zyklon B, patented in 1922 in Germany. Later used by the Nazis in extermination camps during the Second World War. In the post-war period, it was used in disinfection chambers and for fumigating entire rooms. It is readily absorbed by porous materials (such as paper) and is desorbed slowly, posing a continuous health hazard. In reaction with water molecules, it forms formic acid and ammonia, making it particularly harmful under conditions of elevated humidity, causing damage to certain pigments (copper-based pigments) and plant dyes, yellowing of paper, embrittlement of animal glues, and corrosion of base metals (Unger et al. 2001, pp. 279–280, 315; Hahn 1999).

Phosphine, CAS: 7803-51-2	Hall (1988); Purewal (1999, 2001, 2012); Drobnik (2009); Grenda-Kurmanow (2016)	Solid, crystalline, colour ranging from yellow to grey/fumigation	–	Not classifiable as to human carcinogenicity (EPA)	Other names: Phostoxin; Celphos; Delicia Gastoxin. Biocide intended for use in agriculture, but also used in herbarium collections. Until a few years ago, it was used in Poland as a disinfectant in herbarium collections (Grenda-Kurmanow 2019). Effective in controlling insect eggs (Unger et al. 2001, p. 280). Occurs in the form of aluminium phosphide and magnesium phosphide compounds, as a powder. In the presence of atmospheric moisture, these substances release phosphine gas. A strong reducing agent, extremely flammable and highly toxic. It is also available in combination with ammonium carbamate, which decomposes into ammonia and carbon dioxide. In the presence of water, it oxidises to form phosphoric acids. Under conditions of elevated temperature and humidity, it may cause corrosion of copper and its alloys, silver, gold, aluminium, nickel, as well as sulphur compounds. Consequently, it is destructive to pigments such as ultramarine and copper greens, while gilding fades when exposed to phosphine. Exposure to phosphine causes many adverse health effects, but no carcinogenic effect has been established.
Sodium fluorosilicate, CAS: 16893-85-9	Bridson and Forman (1999); Purewal (2012)	Colourless, added to the adhesive used to coat wooden furniture	Not excluded	No data	Used interchangeably with barium fluorosilicate, mainly as an agent against silverfish. The sodium salt may damage herbarium specimen seeds.
Barium fluorosilicate, CAS: 17125-80-3	Hall (1988); Bridson and Forman (1999); Purewal (1999, 2001, 2012); Purewal et al. (2008); Grenda-Kurmanow (2016)	Colourless, added to the adhesive used to coat wooden furniture	–	No data	Patented as a pesticide in 1827. Used interchangeably with sodium fluorosilicate, primarily as an agent against silverfish. Barium fluorosilicate was more effective. Both were used in bait form, as a paste made by mixing with sugar, flour, and gum arabic in water. The paste was applied to wooden storage furniture (Hall 1988).

(continued)

Table 3.3 (continued)

Name of biocide, CAS number	Literature—use of biocides in herbaria	Form/method of application	Negative impact on DNA of natural history collection specimens	Carcinogenicity (according to EPA and IARC)	Characteristics
Sulphuryl fluoride, CAS: 2699-79-8	Whitten et al. (1999); Purewal (2012)	Gas/fumigation	Not excluded	No data	Other names: Vikane; sulphuric oxyfluoride Used as an alternative to methyl bromide and phosphine fumigation. Fumigation with sulphuryl fluoride caused yellowing and acidification of papers, especially those containing lignin (Burgess and Binnie 1990a, b). According to Whitten (Whitten et al. 1999), it does not destroy genetic material in herbarium specimens; however, Kigawa and Strang (2011)—studying typically proteinaceous samples, such as chicken muscle—identified changes in protein structure. Condensation of the gas during fumigation resulted in damage to wallpapers and bronze handles. Unvarnished azurite and malachite, cobalt, and Prussian blue in linseed oil binder, as well as protein-based binders, were also damaged. Changes were also observed in textile dyes, polyvinyl acetate layers, and epoxy resins (Unger et al. 2001, p. 316).
Sulphuryl chloride, CAS: 7791-25-5	Drobnik (2009)	Colourless liquid/ fumigation	–	No data	Action similar to sulphuryl fluoride; used in a similar manner.
Silica gel, CAS: 112926-00-8	Schofield and Crisafulli (1980); Hall (1988); Dawson and Strang (1992); Bridson and Forman (1999)	Powder, aerosol	–	No data	The most popular desiccant, widely used in the museum environment. It is available as a finely ground powder and is often mixed with pyrethrins and pyrethroids, which act as repellents. Such mixtures are also sold in aerosol form. The use of the agent as an aerosol provides protection in less accessible areas (such as shelf joints and the backs of shelving units) and reduces the accumulation of silica gel layers. Contact with finely ground silica gel may cause dryness and irritation of the skin as well as respiratory tract irritation. Although spraying is not carried out directly on specimens, excess silica gel powder residues may enter the interior of objects and cause micro-damage, acting as an abrasive layer. The agent is used against many insect species, including: the varied carpet beetle (*Anthrenus verbasci* L.), the silverfish (*Lepisma saccharina* L.), and booklice (psocids, belonging to the order *Psocoptera*). The action of silica gel powder is based on the destruction of the outer layer of the insect cuticle, leading to fatal dehydration. Some silica gel packets use cobalt chloride as a moisture indicator (turning from blue to pink). This compound is carcinogenic.

Organic compounds					
Aromatic hydrocarbons					
Naphthalene, CAS: 91-20-3	Robinson (1903); Merrill (1948); Croat (1978); Hall (1988); Dawson and Strang (1992); Bridson and Forman (1999); Fenn (1999); Purewal (1999, 2001, 2012); Strang (1999); Pfister (2008); Purewal et al. (2008); Drobnik (2009); Dauwalder (2012); Grenda-Kurmanow (2016)	Solid, white/ passive fumigation	No	Possibly carcinogenic to humans (EPA, IARC)	First synthesised in 1821, used in collections since 1887. It is a polycyclic aromatic hydrocarbon. Occurs as a white powder or pellets, and was used in storage cabinets and added to packaging as a passive fumigant. It can be mistaken for paradichlorobenzene, which appears in a similar form and is used in a similar manner. Under storage conditions, naphthalene preparations slowly release an odour that repels insects. It can recrystallise on the surface of specimens, potentially being confused with taxonomic features. It penetrates deeply into the structure of paper, making it difficult to remove from objects. Contact with naphthalene may cause numerous adverse health effects. In 2008, the use of naphthalene was banned in the European Union.
Chloroorganic compounds					
DDT (dichlorodiphenyltrichloroethane), CAS: 50-29-3	Merrill (1948); Bridson and Forman (1999); Purewal (1999, 2001, 2012); Pfister (2008); Dauwalder (2012); Grenda-Kurmanow (2016); Popławska and Zając (2018)	White powder/ dusting, spray	–	Probable human carcinogen—based on sufficient evidence of carcinogenicity in animals (EPA) Probably carcinogenic (IARC)	Other names: Chlorophenothane, Dicophane Its use in the treatment of malaria and typhus during the Second World War, as well as its post-war popularity in agriculture, made this agent widely available and extensively used (Grenda-Kurmanow 2019). It was used in agricultural production from the 1940s until at least the 1970s, when it was banned in the USA due to significant environmental contamination. It was applied directly as a powder, as well as in solution for spraying, sometimes mixed with Lindane or mineral oils. It may have a destructive effect on botanical specimens (Bridson and Forman 1999, p. 22). DDT breakdown products, mainly DDE (dichlorodiphenyldichloroethylene), are also harmful to health. Until 2008, it was produced in China and is still manufactured in India (van den Berg et al. 2017). Almost completely phased out thanks to the Stockholm Convention, it is classified as a group B toxic compound. Permitted for use in malaria control in certain regions of the world.

(continued)

Table 3.3 (continued)

Name of biocide, CAS number	Literature—use of biocides in herbaria	Form/method of application	Negative impact on DNA of natural history collection specimens	Carcinogenicity (according to EPA and IARC)	Characteristics
Lindane (gamma-hexachloro-cyclohex-ane), CAS: 58-89-9	Lellinger (1972); Hall (1988); Purewal (1999, 2001, 2012); Pfister (2008); Drobnik (2009); Dauwalder (2012)	Crystalline/ fumigation, dusting	Not excluded	Carcinogenic to humans (IARC)	Other names: Gamma-BHC, gamma-HCH, Gammexane, Forlin, Gamophex. Synthesised in 1825, its insecticidal properties were discovered in 1942. Soluble in many organic solvents. During fumigation, the gas decomposes to phosgene ($COCl_2$) and hydrochloric (muriatic) acid (HCl), which is a strong catalyst for the acid hydrolysis of cellulose. For this reason, it is particularly unsuitable for use on objects composed of cellulose, such as paper or herbarium specimens. Classified as Group A under the Stockholm Convention.
LPCP/ PCPL—lau-ryl pentachloro-phenolate, CAS: 3772-94-9	Whitmore and Fosberg (1965); Clarck (1986); Hall (1988); Bridson and Forman (1999); Purewal (2001, 2012); Drobnik (2009); Grenda-Kurmanow (2016)	Liquid/fluid for lubricating and soaking specimens, spray, fumigation	–	No data	Other names: Mystox. First used in 1962 at the Natural History Museum in London (Bridson and Forman 1999, p. 21). Employed both for fumigation and for individual application, including preventive soaking, lubrication, and spraying of specimens being added to collections. Used at a concentration of 5%, in solution with paraffin or mineral turpentine. When using the solution, it was recommended to first conduct resistance tests on labels. It was also necessary to remove coated papers and specimens of grasses and ferns from the collection. The treatment of specimens with LPCP was usually not a single procedure. The solution left stains on paper, which were expected to fade after several years. The substance was used in herbaria both in temperate and tropical climates. Withdrawn in 1984.
Pentachloro-phenol (PCP), CAS: 87-86-5	Coradin and Giannasi (1980); Dauwalder (2012); Purewal (2012)	Solid, colourless crystals/ dusting, soaking, spray	Cannot be excluded	Likely to be carcinogenic to humans (EPA) Carcinogenic to humans (IARC)	Other names: Santophen, Pentachlorol, Chlorophen, Chlon, Dowicide 7, Pentacon, Penwar, Sinituho. First synthesised in the 1930s, it was mainly used in liquid form for soaking and spraying specimens. Pentachlorophenol, its salts and esters were included in Annex A of the Stockholm Convention in 2015.
Sodium pentachloro-phenolate, CAS: 131-52-2	Bridson and Forman (1999)		Not excluded	No data	Sodium salt of PCP.

Carbon tetrachloride, CAS: 56-23-5	Croat (1978); Purewal (1999, 2001, 2012); Drobnik (2009); Grenda-Kurmanow (2016)	Colourless liquid/ fumigation, spray	Not excluded	Likely to be carcinogenic to humans (EPA) Possibly carcinogenic to humans (IARC)	Other names: Tetrachloromethane, Benziform, Benzinoform, Carbon chloride, Carbon tet, Freon-10, Refrigerant-10, Halon-104, Methane tetrachloride, Methyl tetrachloride, Perchloromethane, Tetraform, Tetrasol. Colourless liquid with a sweetish odour. Formerly used as a solvent, fire extinguishing agent, and refrigerant. First synthesised in 1839, it was used on an industrial scale from the 1950s to the 1980s. In the 1980s, it was withdrawn from widespread use due to its toxicity to humans and its destructive effect on the ozone layer.
Paradichlorobenzene (1,4-dichlorobenzene), CAS: 106-46-7	Merrill (1948); Croat (1978); Schofield and Crisafulli (1980); Hall (1988); Bridson and Forman (1999); Fenn (1999); Purewal (1999, 2001, 2012); Pfister (2008); Purewal et al. (2008); Drobnik (2009); Dauwalder (2012); Grenda-Kurmanow (2016)	White crystals/ passive fumigation	Not excluded	Possibly carcinogenic to humans (IARC)	Other names: P-dichlorobenzene; 1,4-dichlorobenzene, p-DCB; 1,4-DCB; PDB; PDCB. Used since 1913 in collections for passive fumigation as well as a repellent, fungicide, and rodent control agent. Typically applied in a similar manner to naphthalene, inside cabinets, but also in solution form. More volatile than naphthalene. It is difficult to maintain an even concentration in storage cabinets. It is five times heavier than air, and therefore should be placed on upper shelves, never in direct contact with specimens. A toxic substance causing numerous adverse health effects upon exposure. Reacts with certain pigments and dyes, altering their colour: zinc white, lithopone, scarlet pigments, ultramarine, acetylcellulose-based dyes. Also causes yellowing of paper, fading of inks, and increased shrinkage of some resins and plastics. Upon dissociation, it may have a bleaching effect on specimens and archival materials, even when tightly packaged. In the event of paradichlorobenzene vapour leakage from unsealed storage areas, vapour clouds may form in the air near the source, posing a health risk. Still used in some institutions today.
Para-chloro-meta-cresol (4-chloro-3-methyl-phenol, PCMC), CAS: 59-50-7	Grenda-Kurmanow (2016)	Fumigation	–	No data	Other names: 4-chloro-3-methylphenol, p-chlorocresol, PCMC, rachit, Preventol CMK Chlorinated phenol, used for passive fumigation as well as by swabbing with a 0.3% solution, either directly or by soaking interleaving sheets in a 10% PCMC solution in 70% ethanol (Sobucki 2013, pp. 128–129; Zerek 2017)

(continued)

Table 3.3 (continued)

Name of biocide, CAS number	Literature—use of biocides in herbaria	Form/method of application	Negative impact on DNA of natural history collection specimens	Carcinogenicity (according to EPA and IARC)	Characteristics
Ethylene dichloride (EDC, 1,2-dichloroethane) in a 3:1 mixture with carbon tetrachloride, CAS: 107-06-2	Croat (1978); Drobnik (2009); Purewal (2012), Grenda-Kurmanow (2016)	Gas/fumigation, passive fumigation	Not excluded	Probable human carcinogen—based on sufficient evidence of carcinogenicity in animals (EPA) Possibly carcinogenic to humans (IARC)	Chlorinated hydrocarbon. Used in a 7:3 mixture with carbon tetrachloride—applied for fumigation (Dawson and Strang 1992; Drobnik 2009, p. 166). Deregistered for use in 1984.
Aldrin, CAS: 309-00-2	Dauwalder (2012)	Solid, white/dusting	–	Probable human carcinogen—based on sufficient evidence of carcinogenicity in animals (EPA)	Other names: HHDN, Octalene Compound invented in the mid-twentieth century. Used until approximately the 1990s, with gradual bans introduced in successive countries from the 1970s onwards. Belongs to the group of most persistent biocides, highly toxic, potential carcinogen. Oxidised within the bodies of insects to dieldrin. Classified as Group A under the Stockholm Convention.
Dieldrin, CAS: 60-57-1	Dauwalder (2012)	Solid, white in colour/dusting, spray	–	Probable human carcinogen—based on sufficient evidence of carcinogenicity in animals (EPA) Probably carcinogenic to humans (IARC)	Other names: HEOD A compound invented in the mid-twentieth century. Used until approximately the 1990s, with gradual bans introduced in successive countries since the 1970s. Belongs to the group of most persistent biocides, highly toxic, potential carcinogen. Classified as group A under the Stockholm Convention.

Endrin, CAS: 72-20-8	Dauwalder (2012)	White crystals/ dusting, spray	–	Not classifiable as to its carcinogenicity to humans (EPA, IARC)	Other names: Mendrin, Endrex Compound discovered in the mid-twentieth century. Used until approximately the 1990s, with gradual bans introduced in successive countries from the 1970s onwards. Belongs to the group of the most persistent biocides, highly toxic. It is a stereoisomer of dieldrin. Classified as Group A under the Stockholm Convention.
Chlordane, CAS: 57-74-9 (or 12789-03-6)	Croat (1978)	Powder/passive fumigation	–	Probable human carcinogen—based on sufficient evidence of carcinogenicity in animals (EPA) Possibly carcinogenic to humans (IARC)	Other names: Heptachlor, Octachlor, Chlorindan, Kypchlor, Toxichlor, Belt, Ortho-Klor, Chlor Kil, Chlorotox, Dowchlor, Oktaterr, Starchlor, Topiclor, Sydane, Termex, Intox A compound from the group of diene compounds, similar to aldrin, endrin, and dieldrin. It is a mixture of chlorinated hydrocarbon isomers. Decomposes to phosgene, chlorides, hydrochloric acid, and carbon monoxide. It is a highly persistent compound, classified in group A of the Stockholm Convention.
Organophosphorus compounds					
Dichlorvos (DDVP, 2,2-dichloro-vinyl dimethyl phosphate), CAS: 62-73-7	Lellinger (1972); Croat (1978); Schofield and Crisafulli (1980); Hall (1988); Bridson and Forman (1999); Purewal (1999, 2001); Pfister (2008); Drobnik (2009); Dauwalder (2012); Fenn (1999); Grenda-Kurmanow (2016)	Liquid/dusting, spray, passive fumigation	Yes	Probable human carcinogen—based on sufficient evidence of carcinogenicity in animals (EPA) Possibly carcinogenic to humans (IARC)	Other names: DDVP, Dichlorphos, Vapona. Available as emulsions, aerosols, pesticide-impregnated strips, or oil concentrates. Soluble in many organic solvents, including chlorinated solvents and alcohols. Introduced to the market as an insecticide in the 1960s. Used for dusting, spraying, or as a passive fumigant. When used in collections, it may leave a film on object surfaces and cause colour changes in dyes, especially reds, as well as in the paper itself. Under conditions of elevated humidity, it becomes acidic and causes corrosion of silver, tin, lead, and mild steel. It is a highly toxic substance. Working in proximity to a dichlorvos source (e.g., a dispenser releasing the toxin) results in numerous adverse health effects.
Malathion, CAS: 121-75-5	Croat (1978)	Spray	–	Probably carcinogenic to humans (IARC)	Other names: Carbophos, Maldison, Mercaptothion Used in agriculture, horticulture, and healthcare, mainly for the control of mosquitoes and lice. Available in liquid, powder, emulsion, and as a powder for preparing a paste. Introduced into use in the 1950s. It is a compound from the group of phosphoric acid esters and derivatives of succinic acid.

(continued)

Table 3.3 (continued)

Name of biocide, CAS number	Literature—use of biocides in herbaria	Form/method of application	Negative impact on DNA of natural history collection specimens	Carcinogenicity (according to EPA and IARC)	Characteristics
Chlorpyrifos, CAS: 2921-88-2	Hall (1988)	Powder, spray or emulsion concentrate/spray	–	No data	Other names: Dursban; Lorsban; Dowco, Chlorpyriphos-ethyl; Brodan, Bolton, Detmol, Eradex, Empire, Hatchet, Nufos, Piridane, Scout, Stipend, Tricel, Warhawk. Introduced as a pesticide in 1965. Occurs in liquid form, prepared for spraying. Corrosive to copper and bronze. Also causes discolouration of red dyes. Highly toxic; exposure to this agent results in a range of adverse health effects, especially in children. Withdrawn since 2014, but is still occasionally detected in orchard plants.
Phenols					
Phenol, CAS: 108-95-2	Clarck (1986); Hawks and Bell (1999); Purewal (2001, 2012); Pfister (2008); Dauwalder (2012); Grenda-Kurmanow (2016)	Fumigation	–	Not classifiable as to its carcinogenicity to humans (EPA, IARC)	The antiseptic properties of phenol have been known since the nineteenth century. Phenol, like creosote, was added to a solution of mercuric chloride in alcohol, sometimes in combination with arsenic. It was also placed in liquid form in cabinets as a passive fumigant.
Thymol (2-isopropyl-5-methylphenol), CAS: 89-83-8	Hall (1988); Bridson and Forman (1999); Fenn (1999); Purewal (1999, 2012); Pfister (2008); Drobnik (2009); Dauwalder (2012); Grenda-Kurmanow (2016, 2017)	Fumigation	–	No	Thymol, previously obtained from natural sources, was first synthesised in the nineteenth century. It was used as a fungicide applied either as a solution or by passive fumigation. A 1% solution of thymol in ethanol was sprayed or applied to specimens affected by microbiological infection. Fumigation is carried out at elevated temperatures by heating solid thymol. Thymol dissolves certain inks and adhesives and may cause discolouration of paper. As a toxic substance, it may cause adverse health effects upon direct contact or ingestion.

Creosote, CAS: 8001-58-9	Pfister (2008); Drobnik (2009); Grenda-Kurmanow (2016)	Fumigation	–	Probable human carcinogen—based on limited evidence of carcinogenicity in humans (EPA) Probably carcinogenic to humans (IARC)	Similarly to phenol, creosote was added to a solution of mercuric chloride in alcohol, sometimes in combination with arsenic. It was also placed in liquid form in cabinets as a passive fumigant.
Pyrethrins and pyrethroids					
Pyrethrins and pyrethroids, example CAS numbers: CAS: 121-21-1 (pyrethrin I), CAS: 121-29-9 (pyrethrin II), CAS: 52645-53-1 (permethrin)	Schofield and Crisafulli (1980); Hall (1988); Croat (1978); Bridson and Forman (1999); Purewal (1999, 2001, 2012); Pfister (2008); Dauwalder (2012)	Liquid, powder/spray, granules, dusting	–	Not classifiable as to its carcinogenicity to humans (permethrin) (IARC)	Pyrethrins are naturally occurring substances obtained from Dalmatian pyrethrum (*Tanacetum cinerariifolium* (Trevir.) Sch. Bip, formerly known as Dalmatian chrysanthemum, *Chrysanthemum cinerariifolium* (Trevir.) Sch. Bip). The pyrethrin group comprises six natural compounds that are constituents of the crude extract from Dalmatian pyrethrum flowers. Their insecticidal properties have been known since the nineteenth century. Pyrethrins are biodegradable under the influence of oxygen and ultraviolet radiation. Since the 1970s, pyrethroid-based pesticides—synthetic analogues of pyrethrins—have been available, including permethrin ($C_{21}H_{20}Cl_2O_3$), cypermethrin ($C_{22}H_{19}Cl_2NO_3$), and deltamethrin ($C_{22}H_{19}Br_2NO_3$). Pyrethroids are more chemically stable than pyrethrins, but are also readily biodegradable. Pyrethrins and pyrethroids are contact insecticides. They are used in the form of microcapsules, powders, oil solutions, and as liquids for spraying; in the case of herbarium specimens, they are mainly mixed with silica gel. They are also combined with piperonyl butoxide, which serves to increase their stability and efficacy. They are still widely used today, both preventively and as an intervention measure.

(continued)

Table 3.3 (continued)

Name of biocide, CAS number	Literature—use of biocides in herbaria	Form/method of application	Negative impact on DNA of natural history collection specimens	Carcinogenicity (according to EPA and IARC)	Characteristics
Other					
Carbon disulphide, CAS: 75-15-0	Robinson (1903); Croat (1978); Purewal (1999, 2001, 2012); Pfister (2008); Drobnik (2009); Dauwalder (2012); Grenda-Kurmanow (2016)	Liquid, ranging from colourless to yellow/ fumigation	–	Insufficient data	Used in collections since 1887, mainly in disinfection chambers, but also as a fumigant for specific rooms. Suspected of having a destructive effect on varnishes (Unger et al. 2001, p. 296). Highly toxic—deregistered in some countries in 1984. According to Pfister (2008), some institutions still use it.
Ethylene oxide, CAS: 75-21-8	Croat (1978); Hall (1988); Purewal (1999, 2001); Drobnik (2009); Purewal (2012); Popławska and Zając (2018)	Fumigation	Yes	Carcinogenic to humans (EPA, IARC)	Other names: 1,2-epoxyethane, oxirane, Rotanox, Carboxide, ETO. Used for fumigation in specialised fumigation chambers, most commonly in libraries, applied against microorganisms and insects. However, it has also been used as a fumigant for storage rooms. It has been used in mixtures with carbon dioxide (CO_2), methyl bromide (CH_3Br), freons, and phosphine (PH_3) (Unger et al. 2001, p. 306). If a vacuum can be maintained in the chamber, ethylene oxide also kills insect eggs. It persists in objects made of leather, rubber, vinyl, and fats, being released gradually (Hall 1988; Hengemihle et al. 1995). Fumigation with ethylene oxide may cause methylation or ethylation of crystalline regions at the boundary of amorphous areas where hydrogen bonds occur (Kronkright 1990). It acts as a cross-linking agent on free hydroxyl groups in materials such as wood or paper, resulting in reduced hygroscopicity (Unger et al. 2001, p. 316). It may have a negative impact on certain pigments (lead-tin yellow) and plant dyes, as well as on egg white casein (Hall 1988; Hahn 1999). It oxidises copper and its alloys (for example, bronze). It reacts with proteins present in leather and parchment, damaging their structure—they become stiff, brittle, and less resistant to biological deterioration. It also reacts with textiles that have previously been disinfected with sodium pentachlorophenate. Polyvinyl chlorides strongly absorb ethylene oxide, simultaneously losing tensile strength (Unger et al. 2001, pp. 316–317). It is a mutagen and carcinogen.

Propylene oxide, CAS: 75-56-9	Drobnik (2009)	Fumigation	Yes	Probable human carcinogen—based on sufficient evidence of carcinogenicity in animals (EPA) Possibly carcinogenic to humans (IARC)	Other names: 1,2-epoxypropane, 2-methyloxirane, PPO Weaker than ethylene oxide and not as effective. Has been mixed with methyl bromide (CH_3Br). Used as a fumigant.
Methyl bromide—an organobromine compound, CAS: 74-83-9	Croat (1978); Coradin and Giannasi (1980); Hall (1988); Purewal (1999, 2001, 2012); Drobnik (2009); Grenda-Kurmanow (2016, 2017)	Fumigation	Yes	Not classifiable as to its carcinogenicity to humans (EPA, IARC)	Other names: bromomethane, methylbromine, Meth-O-Gas, Maltox. Its insecticidal properties were discovered in 1932 (Unger et al. 2001, p. 301). In its pure form, it is odourless. It disperses rapidly and penetrates walls and floors. It is more effective under conditions of elevated relative humidity and temperature. In reaction with water, it forms aggressive bromine water, which is corrosive. It is highly reactive, undergoing methylation and bromination reactions with various substances. It should not be used on materials containing sulphur, including specimens, leathers, coated papers, photographic papers, and parchment, as reaction with methyl bromide will alter their colour and cause them to emit a strong odour of thiols (thioalcohols), which are acidic substances. It is corrosive to zinc, tin, iron, and lead. It is therefore destructive to pigments such as lead white, Naples yellow, lead yellow, and red lead, which blacken upon reaction with methyl bromide (Unger et al. 2001, p. 316). It is a strong solvent for rubbers and other organic materials. It may cause embrittlement of animal glues and softening of natural resins and varnishes. It was often mixed with chloropicrin (CCl_3NO_2), which is phytotoxic. It is highly toxic and has carcinogenic effects. It was widely used for fumigating herbarium collections, including for passive fumigation. It was withdrawn in 2004 due to its destructive impact on the ozone layer.
Methyl iodide, CAS: 74-88-4	Kosuge et al. (2005); Drobnik (2009)	Fumigation	Yes	Not classifiable as to its carcinogenicity to humans (IARC)	Used as a substitute for methyl bromide, for room fumigation and passive fumigation inside storage cabinets.

(continued)

Table 3.3 (continued)

Name of biocide, CAS number	Literature—use of biocides in herbaria	Form/method of application	Negative impact on DNA of natural history collection specimens	Carcinogenicity (according to EPA and IARC)	Characteristics
Formaldehyde, formalin, CAS: 50-00-0 Paraformaldehyde, CAS: 30525-89-4	Robinson (1903); Coradin and Giannasi (1980); Pfister (2008); Drobnik (2009); Dauwalder (2012); Grenda-Kurmanow (2016)	Colourless gas (formaldehyde), powder, crystals (paraformaldehyde)/ fumigation	Yes	Carcinogenic to humans (formaldehyde) (EPA, IARC)	Used for fumigation. Paraformaldehyde, a derivative of formaldehyde, was used for fumigation in institutions, leaving a white residue on objects, including those not directly exposed to formaldehyde but located near fumigated items (Unger et al. 2001, p. 314). It reacts with free amino groups present in protein-based binders, causing their hardening. It also hardens parchment and leather, and accelerates the degradation of wool, furs, and hair. Formaldehyde was also used as a passive fumigant. It is a strong reducing agent.
Carbamates and thiocarbamates CAS: 63-25-2 (carbaryl), CAS: 34681-10-2 (Butocarboxim)	Pfister (2008); Dauwalder (2012); Grenda-Kurmanow (2017) (Butocarboxim)	Crystalline, liquid/spraying	–	Not classifiable as to its carcinogenicity to humans (carbaryl) (IARC)	Derivatives of carbamic acid, developed in the 1950s, used in institutions at least until the 1970s. Poorly soluble in water, more soluble in organic solvents, also used as fungicides. Products encountered under the names: Bendiocarb, carbaryl, Propoxur. These are contact insecticides or require ingestion by the insect. Available as solutions, powders, dusts for preparing pastes, in the form of granules and emulsions. They are highly toxic.
Alcohol, CAS: 64-17-5 (ethyl alcohol)	Coradin and Giannasi (1980); Bedford (1999); Bridson and Forman (1999); Purewal (2001)	Liquid/soaking	Ambiguous results		Mainly ethanol C_2H_5 OH, often used as a solvent in solutions of mercuric chloride, arsenic, thymol, PCMC, but also on its own. Specimens were usually brushed with or immersed in alcohol. Alcohol may cause discolouration of plants and make them brittle.
Petrol, CAS: 8006-61-9	Hall (1988)	Liquid/soaking	Not excluded		Used for soaking specimens. Has a destructive effect on xanthophylls (pigments from the carotenoid group).

Pyridine, CAS: 110-86-1	Drobnik (2009)	Fumigation	–	Possibly carcinogenic to humans (IARC)	First obtained in the second half of the nineteenth century. Used for the fumigation of collections, including passive fumigation. It is a starting material for various pesticides, including chlorpyrifos.
Quaternary ammonium cations, CAS: 7281-04-1	Pfister (2008); Dauwalder (2012)	Liquid/spraying	–	No data available	An example of a preparation belonging to this group is Sterinol (or Atoxyn) (a 10% aqueous solution of dimethyllaurylbenzylammonium bromide) (Karbowska-Berent 2015). This group comprises ionic, surface-active agents that were first synthesised in 1890 (Lipińska-Ojrzanowska and Walusiak-Skorupa 2014). These agents increase the permeability of the cell membrane in botanical specimens by disrupting its wall. Upon contact with the cell membrane, adsorption of ammonium cations occurs on the negatively charged cell wall, enabling the compound to penetrate into the cytoplasm. They may cause skin irritation and induce contact allergy.
Thiosemi-carbazide, CAS: 79-19-6	Grenda-Kurmanow (2017)	White or yellow powder	Not excluded	No data	Rodenticide. The presence of this biocide was detected in the Izabela Czartoryska Herbarium, 1746.
Karatan/ Dinocap (dinitrophe-nol derivative), CAS: 39300-45-3	Grenda-Kurmanow (2017)	Liquid/spraying	–	No data	Fungicide. The presence of this biocide was detected in the Izabela Czartoryska Herbarium, 1746.

Based on Grenda-Kurmanow (2019)

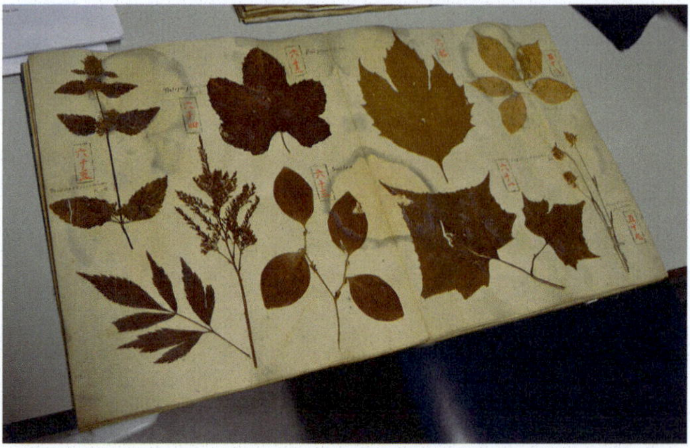

Fig. 3.17 Black discolourations caused by the use of mercury (II) chloride for specimen preservation. Siebold, von F., Ito, K., Leiden, Naturalis Biodiversity Center (L), ref. L. 2077627–207730, 2078204–207812, 211011, 1823–1830. (Photo: M. Grenda-Kurmanow)

mation on the carcinogenic effects of the listed biocides, based on the EPA (United States Environmental Protection Agency) and IARC (International Agency for Research on Cancer) databases,[24] as well as descriptions of their effects and applications, with particular emphasis on their destructive impact on elements of heritage objects (see also Figs. 3.17, 3.18 and 3.19). The descriptions of selected agents indicate whether they are listed on the Stockholm Convention list which regulates the use of persistent organic pollutants (POPs).[25]

3.10 Degradation of Genetic Material

DNA in historical objects undergoes progressive fragmentation as they age. Genetic material obtained from archaeological or museum specimens is referred to as ancient DNA (aDNA). Although herbarium specimens are often not as old as archaeological tissues dating back tens or hundreds of thousands of years—whose genetic material is classified as aDNA—they are nonetheless included in this

[24] United States Environmental Protection Agency (EPA). https://iris.epa.gov/AtoZ/?list_type=erd. Accessed 13 Jan 2026; International Agency for Research on Cancer (IARC). https://monographs.iarc.who.int/list-of-classifications/. Accessed 13 Jan 2026.

[25] Stockholm Convention. http://www.pops.int/. Accessed 13 Jan 2026. The Stockholm Convention classifies toxic substances into three groups: Group A—intentionally produced toxic agents that should be eliminated, with specific exemptions for certain uses; Group B—toxic agents whose intentional production should be strictly limited and restricted to particular purposes (e.g. DDT for malaria control); Group C—toxic agents that are by-products of the breakdown of other substances (e.g. by-products of manufacturing processes), whose presence should be minimised. The Stockholm Convention was adopted at a conference on 22 May 2001 and entered into force on 17 May 2004.

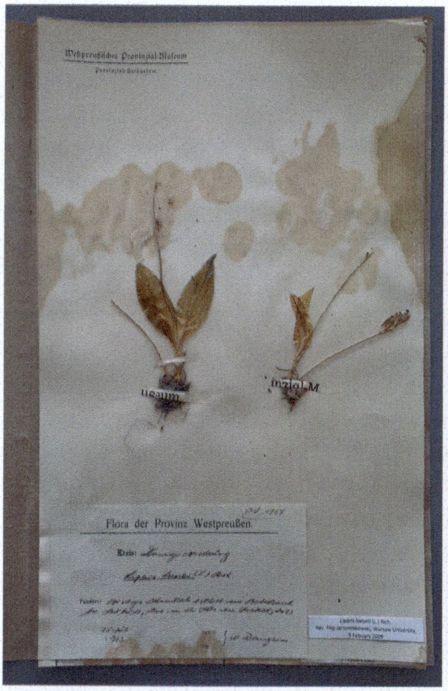

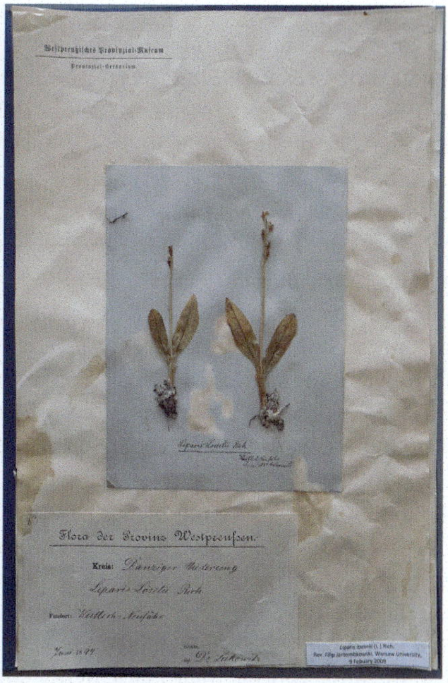

Figs. 3.18 and 3.19 Damage probably caused by DDT. Part of the herbarium in Toruń was also affected by flooding in 1945. Wangerin(?), W., *Flora der Provinz Westpreussen*, Toruń, Herbarium of the Nicolaus Copernicus University in Toruń (TRN), without ref. no., 1913; and Lakowitz?, *Flora der Provinz Westpreussen*, Toruń, Herbarium of the Nicolaus Copernicus University in Toruń (TRN), without ref. no., 1894. (Photo: M. Grenda-Kurmanow)

category due to the nature of the damage they sustain (Bakker 2018). For many years, analyses of degradation processes have been conducted alongside the development of improvements and innovations in research methodology, aimed at addressing the challenges of aDNA analysis resulting from ageing processes (e.g. Pääbo 1989; Pääbo et al. 2004; Rohland and Hofreiter 2007; Rohland et al. 2010; Kistler 2012; Sawyer et al. 2012; Rizzi et al. 2012; Burrell et al. 2015; Wales et al. 2014; Hart et al. 2016; Weiss et al. 2016; Gutaker et al. 2017; Latorre et al. 2020; Kistler et al. 2020 and many others). One of the general conclusions regarding the stability of genetic material is that DNA is better preserved under low-temperature conditions.[26] Genomes derived from historical plant DNA account for a much smaller proportion of publications than those of bacteria, fungi, and mammals (Hofreiter et al. 2014; Weiss et al. 2016), making historical herbaria particularly attractive for new scientific discoveries. These studies are also challenging because, as estimated from studies on the kinetics of DNA degradation in herbarium specimens, herbarium material degrades six times faster than aDNA from bone (Weiss et al. 2016).

[26] Based on this assumption, maps are created to estimate the likelihood of aDNA survival in different regions of the world (Hofreiter et al. 2014).

Degradation processes in genetic material occur simultaneously with the time of its formation. In a living cell, the integrity of genetic material is maintained by repair processes involving enzymes. Errors arising during replication, transcription, and translation are, to the extent possible for a given organism, continuously detected and repaired (Pääbo et al. 2004). The desiccation of a specimen in preparation for inclusion in a herbarium triggers a series of processes that lead to cell death by dehydration, often due to exposure to high temperatures. However, since these processes are not programmed by the plant, as is the case with naturally occurring abiotic (physical) stresses, the resulting changes in the genetic material of herbarium specimens are also different.[27] Furthermore, as described in previous chapters, specimens were often subjected to additional treatments and exposed to various factors that may have a destructive effect on DNA.

Due to the absence of repair mechanisms in dead cells, degradative changes accumulate, leading to DNA disintegration. The most common damage to ancient DNA (aDNA) DNA strand fragmentation, with the average length variously defined as 30–300 base pairs for herbarium specimens (e.g. Särkinen et al. 2012; Bakker 2018; Canales et al. 2022). Many authors emphasise that the condition of genetic material depends not only on the age of the sample, but also on the kinetics of degradation in a given case. The degree of degradation in historical specimens can be highly variable, even among objects of similar age. In general, aDNA strands are significantly shorter than DNA extracted from comparable fresh material (Pääbo et al. 2004). An exception is historical genetic material preserved in permafrost (Hofreiter et al. 2014). In the case of herbarium collections, the influence of specimen preparation, preservation methods, and storage conditions is particularly emphasized.[28] For this reason, the necessity of collaboration between researchers and curators in selecting appropriate specimens for genetic studies is also highlighted (Canales et al. 2022).

In the literature concerning historical DNA, the degradation of genetic material is considered primarily in the context of subsequent identification challenges.[29] The main types of damage include depurination, β-elimination, single-strand breaks, and deaminated cytosine, particularly at the ends of shortened DNA fragments (Rizzi et al. 2012; Sawyer et al. 2012; Dabney et al. 2013). When DNA is extracted from historical samples and analysed, destructive factors manifest in three distinct ways: by reducing the size of DNA fragments; by introducing modifications that block the replication of DNA molecules by polymerases used in analytical proce-

[27] According to Staats et al., in herbarium specimens, provided they have been dried sufficiently quickly, DNA fragmentation into ladder-like ("multimeric") oligonucleosomal fragments, characteristic of programmed cell death processes, does not occur (Staats et al. 2011, see also Reape and McCabe 2008).

[28] See also Sect. 3.10.7 in this chapter.

[29] This represents a somewhat different attitude towards material that may be considered historical, compared to the approach typical of conservators. While conservators tend to focus on slowing down degradation and preserving the material *per se* as a document that should remain available for future generations, scientists assess the quality of genetic material in terms of its current utility, where the significance lies in present technological capabilities and overcoming the obstacle of DNA degradation.

dures, thereby hindering various forms of analysis; and by causing changes that result in the incorporation of incorrect nucleotides during DNA replication (Dabney et al. 2013). In the case of herbarium specimens, it has been found that DNA strand breaks occur particularly before purines, and that depurination-induced DNA breaks occur continuously over time and may largely account for the progressive shortening of DNA fragments (Weiss et al. 2016).

The analysis of plant samples may also be hindered by the presence of cellular components that interfere with analysis, such as polyphenols (e.g. tannins), polysaccharides, proteins, and lipids (Kistler 2012; Särkinen et al. 2012; Staats et al. 2013; Wales et al. 2014; Bressan et al. 2014). Moreover, archaeological plant materials are often rich in humic acids, some of which originate from associated sediments that are not always removed and may also impede analysis. The processes contributing to aDNA degradation are described below.

3.10.1 Enzymatic Degradation

After the death of an organism and the breakdown of phospholipid subcellular compartments capable of sequestering nucleases, which are catabolic enzymes, the genetic material undergoes damage caused by the action of released endogenous enzymes (Hofreiter et al. 2001; Molak and Ho 2011; Dabney et al. 2013). Enzymatic changes following cell death lead to non-specific shortening of DNA chains. In addition, DNA is enzymatically degraded as a result of the activity of bacteria, fungi, and insects that feed on material already partially degraded by enzymes. Most often, ancient DNA (aDNA) is a mixture of short fragments of the original genetic material and fragments of microbial DNA (Dabney et al. 2013; Weiss et al. 2016). Damage can be slowed if the tissue is rapidly desiccated or if DNA is absorbed into a mineral matrix, as well as if it is stored at low temperatures and in the environments with high salt concentrations. Such conditions may occur especially in the case of archaeological samples (Lindahl 1993; Hofreiter et al. 2001; Pääbo et al. 2004; Willerslev and Cooper 2005). The "protective" effect results from the deactivation of nucleases, which may precede the process of these enzymes breaking down nucleic acid chains to mononucleotides (Hofreiter et al. 2001).

Nevertheless, even in a desiccated cell, DNA remains partially hydrated, and as a result, slow, continuous, and irreversible ageing processes still occur, sometimes similar to those observed in living cells (Lindahl 1993).

3.10.2 Hydrolysis

As a result of acid hydrolysis, the DNA chain may be cleaved and directly fragmented within one strand of the double helix.

Spontaneous hydrolysis of phosphodiester bonds at neutral pH occurs at a slow rate; however, it can be accelerated in the presence of specific compounds that catalyse the reaction, such as transition metal ions or formaldehyde (Srinivasan et al. 2002; Gates 2009).

N-glycosidic bonds, which link nitrogenous bases to sugars, may undergo cleavage. These bonds are susceptible to catalytic action in acidic environments. As a result, there is a loss primarily of guanine and adenine, which are purines. This process is known as depurination (Lindahl 1993; Pääbo et al. 2004). The changes occur within a single DNA strand, weakening the DNA backbone. The hydrolysis product may take the form of a closed acetal ring or an open-chain aldehyde. Abstraction of the acidic proton adjacent to the aldehyde group leads to β-elimination of the phosphate residue on the 3′ side of the abasic site. Further γ,δ-elimination of the phosphate on the 5′ side of the abasic site is slow under physiological conditions, but occurs readily under alkaline conditions, resulting in strand breakage with 3′- and 5′-phosphate termini. Additionally, the aldehyde product tends to undergo cross-linking (Gates 2009).

This results in the loss of genetic information, which is not compensated for as it would be in a living, metabolically active, fully hydrated molecule.[30] Chain shortening occurs at a rate similar to depurination, and the pace of this degradation is associated with the specimen's innate hypersensitivity to chemical agents and may vary between specimens originating from the same period (Pääbo et al. 2004). According to studies by Weiss et al., in herbarium specimens the process of depurination proceeds continuously, resulting in the accumulation of numerous short fragments in the ageing genetic material (Weiss et al. 2016). Hydrolysis may also lead to depyrimidination, that is, the loss of pyrimidines analogous to the loss of purines, although this occurs to a much lesser extent. The process leads to the formation of an AP site (apurinic/apyrimidinic site). The remaining sugar-phosphate backbone is unstable and rapidly degrades, leaving a gap if the DNA molecule is double-stranded (Brown 2018, pp. 394–398).

Furthermore, nitrogenous base residues may undergo hydrolytic deamination, a process involving the removal of an amino group ($–NH_2$) from the molecule. This reaction can proceed either via hydroxide attack on a neutral nitrogenous base or via water molecule attack on a base protonated at the third nitrogen atom (Gates 2009). This process most commonly affects cytosine and its homologue, 5-methylcytosine. As a result of deamination by a water molecule attack on a positively charged (protonated) nitrogenous base, cytosine is converted to uracil, leading to the formation of incorrect base pairs (G–U) instead of (G–C).[31] Methylcytosine may be converted to thymine. To a much lesser extent, deamination can also affect purines, resulting in the conversion of guanine to xanthine and adenine to hypoxanthine. Both forms

[30] In a metabolically active cell, the repair of genetic information lost in this way is carried out by enzymes. First, the damaged sites are excised by the appropriate nuclease (AP), sugar residues are removed by phosphodiesterases, and the resulting gaps are then filled in by DNA polymerases and ligases (Lindahl 1993).

[31] In living organisms, repair processes are ensured by the presence of DNA uracil glycosylase (UDG), which recognises and removes uracil. Subsequent enzymes restore cytosine at the damaged site. If uracil formed by deamination is not removed, this leads to transcriptional errors and mutations (Lindahl 1993; Pääbo et al. 2004).

preferentially pair with cytosine (Lindahl 1993) Alterations in base configuration cause errors during genetic material analysis. Weiss et al. observed a strong correlation between deamination-driven accumulation of cytosine-to-thymine substitutions and the passage of time (Weiss et al. 2016). Therefore, for herbarium specimens, as in the case of bone studies, the presence of such increased substitutions is evidence of the authenticity of historical DNA and allows the exclusion of contamination with modern material (Weiss et al. 2016).

3.10.3 Oxidation

Oxidative DNA damage is caused by reactive oxygen species (ROS), which include hydroxyl radicals (OH·); alkoxyl radicals (RO·), typically formed as a result of reactions involving hydroxyl radicals; alkylperoxyl radicals (ROO·); superoxide anion radicals ($O_2^{\cdot-}$); as well as singlet oxygen (O_2) and hydrogen peroxide (H_2O_2), which are not radicals but are also classified as reactive oxygen species.

The endogenous source of reactive oxygen species (ROS) is cellular metabolic processes. However, ROS may also be introduced by external factors. Hydroxyl radicals (HO·) can be generated by ionising radiation; the Fenton reaction, which involves iron (II) ions or other transition metals [e.g. copper (I)] with hydrogen peroxide; or by the photolytic degradation of alkyl hydroperoxides (Burrows and Muller 1998). Among the precursor substances for the formation of free radicals are chloric acid and hypochlorous acid (HOCl), and mercuric chloride (a biocidal agent) for the superoxide anion radical, hydrogen peroxide for the hydroperoxyl radical, singlet oxygen for the alkoxyl radical, and ozone (O_3) for the peroxyl radical (Costa et al. 1991). Hofreiter et al. and Pääbo et al. also cite residual radiation as one of the sources (Hofreiter et al. 2001; Pääbo et al. 2004).[32] DNA strand fragmentation associated with oxidation may result in cross-linking and modification of nitrogenous bases.[33]

DNA degradation associated with oxidation occurs primarily at the sites of double bonds in pyrimidine and purine rings, leading to the cleavage of ring structures. The bonds in the deoxyribose molecule are also susceptible to oxidation and may be broken, leading to the disintegration of the sugar rings (Pääbo et al. 2004). Fragmentation is not always a direct effect, but may represent a subsequent stage following hydrolysis of the glycosidic bond or nucleophilic substitution.[34] Moreover,

---

[32] Residual (relic) radiation—microwave background radiation, a remnant of the Universe's evolutionary processes, the relic noise from the Big Bang.

[33] In a living cell, an imbalance resulting from oxidation of genetic material that cannot be compensated by repair processes is referred to as oxidative stress.

[34] Electron-rich purines and pyrimidines readily react with so-called electrophiles, i.e. molecules that are electron-deficient and, under appropriate conditions, can act as electron acceptors. Substitution reactions between electrophiles and nucleophiles (molecules with an excess of electrons) are known as nucleophilic substitution reactions. Electrophiles include, among others, halides, oxidising agents, and alkylating agents (Burrows and Muller 1998).

the harmful nature of hydrogen peroxide and the superoxide anion radical arises from their reaction with transition metal ions (iron, copper) in the course of the Fenton reaction, the product of which is the hydroxyl radical. Oxidative processes generate alkali-labile sites, which are sensitive to elevated temperatures (Burrows and Muller 1998).

The most significant damage is caused by the action of the hydroxyl radical, which is one of the most aggressive oxidising agents. It can induce direct degradation by abstracting a hydrogen atom from the sugar-phosphate backbone (Gates 2009). It also causes indirect degradation by attaching to bases, forming so-called adducts, which are subsequently reduced or oxidised (depending on the nature of the adduct), resulting in various products, including different forms of formamidopyrimidines and glycols (Cooke et al. 2003). These transformations can affect all bases, although not all are equally susceptible.[35] The best-characterised degradation process involves the transformation of guanine, the base most sensitive to oxidation, into 8-oxoguanine. 8-oxoguanine forms stable pairs with adenine (instead of cytosine, as guanine does), creating a risk of errors during the identification of genetic material (Lindahl 1993; Burrows and Muller 1998; Cooke et al. 2003). Radicals formed after base attachment may, under the influence of subsequent radicals, cross-link or generate so-called tandem lesions, i.e., complexes of adjacent damaged sites (Gates 2009). They may also react with aromatic amino acids of proteins or amino acid radicals, leading to DNA–protein cross-linking (Cooke et al. 2003).

Oxidation may also be associated with UV radiation, which can cause damage either directly or indirectly through the generation of free radicals. The changes depend on the wavelength. UVB radiation (280–320 nm) can act directly on DNA when photons are absorbed by the nucleotide chain. In this way, it induces various pathological alterations in DNA bases, rendering their unstable in an alkaline environment (Burrows and Muller 1998). One such alteration is the formation of a covalent bond between two adjacent pyrimidine bases in DNA, leading to the production of cyclobutane pyrimidine dimers, primarily thymine dimers. If these changes are not corrected during DNA replication, they result in the deletion of one or more base pairs or the substitution of base pairs within the DNA strand. UVA (320–400 nm) does not induce changes directly, but generates free radicals through reactions with molecular oxygen in its basic, triplet state, resulting in the formation of the superoxide anion radical, which can subsequently be converted into hydrogen peroxide and the hydroxyl radical (Sinha and Häder 2002). Further reactions are typical radical reactions as described above.

Ionising radiation also exerts a detrimental effect on DNA, and its nature likewise depends on the type and intensity of the radiation. Similar to ultraviolet radiation, it can generate free radicals, particularly the hydroxyl radical, through the radiolysis of water molecules, including intracellular water. Certain types of ionising radiation act directly on DNA by removing a hydrogen atom, resulting in strand breaks or, with repeated dose deposition, cleavage of the entire chain. Ionising

[35] Cooke et al. distinguish more than 20 types of pathologies associated with reactions involving reactive oxygen species (Cooke et al. 2003).

radiation may also act indirectly by stimulating the formation of reactive molecules such as peroxides. External sources of radiation include devices emitting X-rays, γ-rays, or neutrons (Ward 1988; Brown 2018, pp. 394–398).

3.10.4 Alkylation

Alkylation is a process involving the attachment of alkyl groups (particularly methyl groups) to DNA nucleotides. Sources of alkyl groups include, among others, methyl halides, used as biocidal agents (Brown 2018, pp. 394–398).[36] These include methyl bromide and methyl iodide, which participate in DNA methylation, a specific type of alkylation reaction. Other biocidal agents that directly alkylate DNA are ethylene oxide and propylene oxide, under the influence of which a hydroxyethyl radical is incorporated into the nucleophilic regions of DNA in place of a hydrogen atom (Kigawa et al. 2003; Kigawa and Strang 2011; Kigawa et al. 2011).[37]

The effect of alkylation depends on the position at which the nucleotide is modified and on the type of alkyl group added. Certain methylations alter the base-pairing properties of the modified nucleotide and lead to point mutations. The changes may involve deglycosylation (removal of sugar residues from the glycoside) and opening of ring structures (Gates 2009). Alkylation at the third nitrogen position of cytosine significantly accelerates its deamination. There are also alkylations that cause cross-linking between the two strands of the DNA molecule (Brown 2018, pp. 394–398).

The most frequently targeted site by alkyl groups is the nitrogen at position 7 of the guanine residue, due to its nucleophilic reactivity and exposure within the DNA structure (this applies to the majority of mutations induced by ethylene and propylene oxides as well as methyl halides) (Gates 2009; La et al. 2010). Alkylation of DNA phosphodiester residues leads to the formation of phosphotriesters, which are significantly more susceptible to hydrolysis.

3.10.5 High Temperature and Humidity

Elevated temperature accelerates the degradation of DNA, particularly through hydrolysis (Lindahl and Nyberg 1972; Staats et al. 2011). Heat stimulates water-induced cleavage of the β-N-glycosidic bond, which links the base to the sugar

[36] The characteristics of methyl bromide and methyl iodide are described in Sect. 3.9 in this chapter.

[37] The characteristics of ethylene oxide and propylene oxide are described in Sect. 3.9 in this chapter. Among methylating biocidal agents, dichlorvos can also be mentioned, although the mechanism of its degradative action may be considered ambiguous. Dichlorvos is an alkylating agent for DNA *in vitro*, but *in vivo* its effect is marginal (Wooder and Wright 1981). Espeland et al. observed a detrimental effect of dichlorvos on the genetic material of entomological specimens, but no explanation for the DNA degradation mechanism was proposed (Espeland et al. 2010).

component of the nucleotide in double-stranded DNA, resulting in the formation of an apurinic/apyrimidinic site in the polynucleotide, which is unstable. Combined with the spontaneous breakdown of the phosphodiester backbone via β-elimination, this leads to strand breaks in the DNA.

Temperature plays a crucial role in preserving the integrity of genetic material *post mortem*. Numerous studies have demonstrated that the best-preserved material is that which has survived at reduced (relative to so-called room temperature) or very low temperatures.[38] In contrast, genetic material from archaeological specimens that have persisted in hot and extremely arid or tropical climates—characterised by high temperatures and high humidity—has undergone complete or near-complete degradation (Kumar et al. 2000; Marota et al. 2002).

In studies on the impact of relative humidity on specimens of eastern red cedar (*Juniperus virginiana*), Adams determined a safe RH range of 23.1–55.4%. However, the storage temperature of the samples was not specified (see Adams 2011).[39] In research conducted by Kigawa and Strang, protein samples (from muscle tissue) and fungal samples, conditioned at 100% RH and in water, and subsequently exposed to 60 °C, underwent complete or significant degradation (Kigawa and Strang 2011).[40]

3.10.6 Cross-Linking

DNA cross-linking occurs as a consequence of hydrolytic and oxidative processes, as well as alkylation and other reactions associated with the action of biocidal agents. As a result, mutations may arise within the DNA strand, DNA–DNA complexes, Maillard reaction products—which are formed during the condensation of sugars and primary amine groups in proteins and nucleic acids—and DNA–protein complexes, due to the action of aldehydes (Pääbo 1989; Srinivasan et al. 2002; Pääbo et al. 2004; Molak and Ho 2011).

A summary of DNA degradation processes following organismal death, along with their impact on DNA analysis, is presented in Table 3.4.

---

[38] As with the aforementioned permafrost (Hofreiter et al. 2001, 2014; Pääbo et al. 2004). Molak and Ho propose a "thermal age" model, which, starting from a temperature of 10 °C assumed to correspond to the actual age of the sample, allows estimation of the level of genetic material degradation under different thermal storage conditions (Molak and Ho 2011).

[39] Furthermore, the samples were not ventilated but sealed in a plastic container. Above 75% RH, fungal growth was observed on the specimens. In the range of approximately 69–75% RH, after 2 months the DNA in the samples was clearly degraded, and after 12 months genetic material was detected only in samples stored at RH between 23.1% and 54.4%. However, the author concluded that a safe RH level is approximately 55%.

[40] The authors also tested conditioning at RH = 33%, 53%, and 84%. Samples conditioned under these conditions allowed for effective extraction of genetic material.

Table 3.4 Degradation processes of aDNA and their impact on identification potential

Type of damage incurred	Type of destruction	Impact on DNA molecule analysis
Nucleotide chain breakage	Enzymatic degradation caused by microbial activity	Small amounts of DNA, reduction in DNA molecule size Degradation of the phosphodiester backbone and sugar backbone via β-elimination, formation of single-stranded fragments
	Degradation caused by nucleases in the cell *post mortem*	
	Depurination and depyrimidination during hydrolysis, formation of abasic sites	
	Direct hydrolytic degradation	
	Desiccation, high temperature	
Formation of erroneous code fragments as a result of hydrolysis	Loss of amino groups; this leads to the generation of erroneous damage codes, e.g. deamination of cytosine to uracil; 5-methylcytosine to thymine; adenine to hypoxanthine or guanine to xanthine	Results in the incorporation of incorrect nitrogenous bases during amplification and alteration of the code: A to G, C to T, G to A
Formation of erroneous code fragments and fragments blocking the polymerase enzyme as a result of oxidation	Modifications of nitrogenous bases: 5-Hydroxy-5-methylhydantoin; 5-Hydroxyhydantoin—blocking; 8-Oxoguanosine—alters coding from G to T	No amplification, enhancement of chimeric sequences through "jumping PCR"
		Incorporation of an incorrect nitrogenous base
Cross-linking	DNA–DNA cross-linking via alkylation	May prevent amplification of the original DNA
	DNA cross-linking with proteins following the Maillard reaction	Increases the risk of contamination

Based on Pääbo et al. (2004); Fulton (2012); Rizzi et al. (2012)

3.10.7 The Impact of Storage Conditions and Historical Preservation Methods on DNA

Authors of studies concerning historic genetic material consistently emphasise that storage conditions are of key importance for the preservation of DNA (Lindahl 1993; Savolainen et al. 1995; Pääbo 1989; Kumar et al. 2000; Marota et al. 2002; Pääbo et al. 2004; Kigawa and Strang 2011; Kigawa et al. 2011; Molak and Ho 2011; Staats et al. 2011; Dabney et al. 2013; Choi et al. 2015; Weiss et al. 2016). Acidic environments, high temperatures, and increased or decreased relative humidity are detrimental. However, conditions that are unequivocally safe for DNA have not been clearly defined.[41] Low pH resulting from the use of preservation agents such as formaldehyde, phenols, or alcohol can significantly accelerate the hydrolytic degradation of genetic material (Carter 2003, pp. 88–105). The climatic conditions maintained in collections as part of Integrated Pest Management generally define the concept of "safe conditions" for collections in broad terms.[42]

In addition, studies have found that many biocides and preservatives used in the past have a harmful effect on the preservation of genetic material.[43] These include, among others, the aforementioned alkylating agents: methyl bromide, methyl iodide, ethylene oxide, and propylene oxide. Destructive effects have also been observed in the case of mercuric chloride, which directly induces single-strand breaks in DNA and leads to degradation associated with the action of reactive oxygen species (Costa et al. 1991). Arsenic is also classified as a harmful biocidal substance, as it enables but weakens DNA extraction from biological specimens (Töpfer et al. 2011). Studies on the destructive impact of formaldehyde on DNA have also enabled the identification of numerous mechanisms contributing to the degradation of genetic material. Formaldehyde initiates DNA denaturation (disruption of interchain hydrogen bonds and base unpairing) in adenine-thymine-rich regions of double-stranded DNA, creating sites for chemical interactions (Srinivasan et al. 2002). In addition, it contributes, among other things, to hydrolytic processes and DNA cross-linking both within the double helix and between DNA and proteins. The degree of formaldehyde interaction is influenced by temperature, concentration, and the pH of the reaction environment. The higher the temperature and the lower the pH, the greater the degree of DNA degradation in the preserved specimen (Srinivasan et al. 2002). Dichlorvos, a compound with DNA-methylating activity *in vitro*, has also been classified as destructive to the DNA of preserved biological specimens (Espeland et al. 2010). Other agents classified as carcinogenic and harmful to the genetic material in biocultural collections include lindane, pentachlorophenol, carbon tetrachloride, paradichlorobenzene, and ethylene dichloride.[44]

The harmfulness of alcohol as a preservative for specimens has been ambiguously determined. Most authors consider alcohol to have a destructive effect on DNA, indicating the destruction or significant reduction of genetic material stored in alcohol (Pyle and Adams 1989; Bridson and Forman 1999, pp. 292–293; Staats et al. 2011; Särkinen et al. 2012; Salick and Solomon 2014). However, studies have reported that DNA extraction from herbarium specimens stored in 96% alcohol as comparable to that from leaves of various plant species preserved in either alcohol or liquid nitrogen (Bressan et al. 2014).[45] In a study concerning entomological collections, Carter emphasised that high-concentration alcohol and denatured alcohol (90–100%) allow for the preservation of long DNA fragments in large quantities, especially when specimens are stored at low temperatures (e.g. in a refrigerator)

[41] See comments on Adams's research (Adams 2011) in Sects. 4.1.5 and 4.3 in Chap. 4.

[42] See Chap. 4.

[43] See the Sect. 3.10.4 in this chapter.

[44] See the Sect. 3.9 in this chapter.

[45] See also Bakker (2018) and Eklund (2007), who, after *in vitro* tests, defined the use of denatured alcohol as safe.

(Carter 2003). However, the widespread use of lower-concentration alcohols and denatured alcohol (below 80%) and the storage of specimens at room temperature, often for economic reasons, leads to significant degradation, and in the study conducted, made it impossible to extract genetic material after just 15 years. In Eklund's research, which used high-concentration alcohols (99% ethanol and 100% denatured alcohol), ethanol was assessed as ambiguously safe, while denatured alcohol was considered safe for DNA under the conditions applied in the study.

Among non-biocidal preservation methods, microwaves have been assessed as harmful to DNA (Pyle and Adams 1989; Bridson and Forman 1999, p. 23).[46] Studies from 2013 confirmed that microwaves have a destructive effect on high-molecular-weight DNA present in plant specimens (Lander et al. 2013).

References

Adams RP (2011) DNA from herbarium specimens: II. Correlation of DNA degradation with humidity. Phytologia 93:351–359

American Society of Heating, Refrigerating and Air-Conditioning Engineers (ASHRAE) (2019) Museums, libraries and archives. In: ASHRAE handbook: heating, ventilating and air-conditioning: applications. ASHRAE, Atlanta, pp 24.1–24.43

Bakker FT (2018) Herbarium genomics: plant archival DNA explored. In: Lindqvist C, Rajora OP (eds) Paleogenomics, population genomics. Springer. https://doi.org/10.1007/13836_2018_40

Bedford DJ (1999) Vascular plants. In: Carter D, Walker A (eds) Care and conservation of natural history collections. Butterworth Heinemann, Oxford, pp 61–80

Bégin P, Deschâtelets S, Grattan D, Gurnagul N, Iraci J, Kaminska E, Woods D, Zou X (1999) The effect of air pollutants on paper stability. Restaurator 20(1):1–21. https://doi.org/10.1515/rest.1999.20.1.1

Bressan EA, Rossi ML, Gerald LT, Figueira A (2014) Extraction of high-quality DNA from ethanol-preserved tropical plant tissues. BMC Res Notes 7(1):268. https://doi.org/10.1186/1756-0500-7-268

Bridson D, Forman L (1999) The herbarium handbook. Royal Botanic Gardens, Kew

Briggs D, Sell PD, Block M, I'ons RD (1983) Mercury vapour: a health hazard in herbaria. New Phytol 94:453–457

Brown TA (1999) Chapter 6: genetic material. In: Carter D, Walker A (eds) Care and conservation of natural history collections. Butterworth Heinemann, Oxford, pp 133–138

Brown TA (2018) Genomes 4. Garland Science, New York/London

Burgess HD, Binnie NE (1990a) The effect of Vikane™ on the stability of cellulosic and ligneous materials – measurement of deterioration by chemical and physical methods. MRS Proc 185:791–798. https://doi.org/10.1557/proc-185-791

Burgess HD, Binnie NE (1990b) The development of a research approach to the scientific study of cellulosic and ligneous materials. J Am Inst Conserv 29(2):133–152

Burrell AS, Disotell TR, Bergey CM (2015) The use of museum specimens with high-throughput DNA sequencers. J Hum Evol 79:35–44. https://doi.org/10.1016/j.jhevol.2014.10.015

Burrows CJ, Muller JG (1998) Oxidative nucleobase modifications leading to strand scission. Chem Rev 98(3):1109–1152. https://doi.org/10.1021/cr960421s

[46] Microwaves as an element of Integrated Pest Management (IPM) policy are described in Sect. 4.1.3 in Chap. 4.

Canales NA, Clarke AC, Nesbitt M, Gutaker R (2022) Chapter 2. DNA from museum collections. In: de Boer H, Rydmark MO, Verstraete B, Gravendeel B (eds) Molecular identification of plants: from sequence to species. Advanced Books. https://doi.org/10.3897/ab.e68634

Carter JD (2003) The effects of preservation and conservation treatments on the DNA of museum invertebrate fluids preserved collections. Dissertation, University of Wales

Chemical Abstract Service. https://commonchemistry.cas.org/. Accessed 13 Jan 2026

Choi J, Lee H, Shipunov A (2015) All that is gold does not glitter? Age, taxonomy, and ancient plant DNA quality. PeerJ 3:e1087. https://doi.org/10.7717/peerj.1087

Clarck S (1986) Preservation of herbarium specimens: an archive conservator's approach. Taxon 35(4):675–682. https://doi.org/10.2307/1221610

Collins C (2014) Standards in the care of botanical materials. http://conservation.myspecies.info/node/35. Accessed 21 Jan 2026

Cooke MS, Evans MD, Dizdaroglu M, Lunec J (2003) Oxidative DNA damage: mechanisms, mutation, and disease. FASEB J 17:1195–1214

Coradin L, Giannasi DE (1980) The effects of chemical preservations on plant collections to be used in chemotaxonomic surveys. Taxon 29(1):33–40. https://doi.org/10.2307/1219594

Costa M, Christie NT, Cantoni O, Zelikoff JT, Wang XW, Rossman TG (1991) DNA damage by mercury compounds: an overview. In: Suzuki T, Imura N, Clarkson TW (eds) Advances in mercury toxicology. Rochester series on environmental toxicity. Springer, Boston. https://doi.org/10.1007/978-1-4757-9071-9_16

Croat TB (1978) Survey of herbarium problems. Taxon 27(2/3):203–218. https://doi.org/10.2307/1220243

Dabney J, Meyer M, Pääbo S (2013) Ancient DNA damage. Cold Spring Harb Perspect Biol 5(7):a012567. https://doi.org/10.1101/cshperspect.a012567

Dauwalder L (2012) Das Herbarium des Felix Platter. Die Erhaltung eines historischen Buch-Herbariums. Dissertation, Fachochshule Bern

Dawson JE, Strang TJK (1992) Solving museum insect problems: chemical control, Technical bulletin no. 15. Canadian Conservation Institute, Ottawa

de Tournefort JP (1694) Élémens de botanique: ou Méthode pour connoître les plantes, vol 1. Imprimerie Royale, Paris

Down JL, Guild S, Hill G, St.-Jacques D, Westbury K, O'Loughlin E, Kaminska E, Williams RS, Iraci J, Tse S (2011) Update on the CCI adhesive tape and heat-set tissues Project. In: Symposium 2011: adhesives and consolidants for conservation; research and applications; proceedings=symposium 2011: Adhésifs et consolidants pour la conservation; Recherche et applications; les Actes. Canadian Conservation Institute, Ottawa, pp 57–84

Drobnik J (2009) Zielnik i zielnikoznawstwo. Wydawnictwo Naukowe PWN, Warszawa

Espeland M, Irestedt M, Johanson KA, Akerlund M, Bergh JE, llersj M (2010) Dichlorvos exposure impedes extraction and amplification of DNA from insects in museum collections. Front Zool 7:2. https://doi.org/10.1186/1742-9994-7-2

Fallon D, Peters M, Hunt M, Koehler K (2016) Cleaning protocol for mercuric chloride–contaminated herbarium cabinets at the Smithsonian Museum Support Center. Collect Forum 30(1–2):51–62

Fellowes J, Pattrick RAD, Green DI, Dent A, Lloyd JR, Pearce CI (2011) Use of biogenic and abiotic elemental selenium nanospheres to sequester elemental mercury released from mercury contaminated museum specimens. J Hazard Mater 189:660–669. https://doi.org/10.1016/j.jhazmat.2011.01.079

Fenn J (1999) Plastic materials used in the herbarium. In: Metsger DA, Byers SC (eds) Managing the modern herbarium – an interdisciplinary approach. SPNHC, Ontario, pp 235–259

Florian MLE (1990) Plant anatomy: an illustrated aid to identification. In: Florian MLE, Kronkright DP, Norton R (eds) The conservation of artifacts made from plant materials. The J. Paul Getty Trust, pp 1–27

Fulton TL (2012) Setting up an ancient DNA laboratory. In: Hofreiter M, Shapiro B (eds) Ancient DNA, Materials and protocols. Springer, pp 1–11

Gates KS (2009) An overview of chemical processes that damage cellular DNA: spontaneous hydrolysis, alkylation, and reactions with radicals. Chem Res Toxicol 22(11):1747–1760. https://doi.org/10.1021/tx900242k

Glastrup J (1987) Insecticide analysis by gas chromatography in the stores of the Danish National Museum's Ethnographic Collection. Stud Conserv 32(2):59–64. https://doi.org/10.1179/sic.1987.32.2.59

Grenda-Kurmanow M (2016) Challenges of conservation treatment of historic herbaria. In: Green museum – how to practice what we preach: 31th annual meeting of the society for the preservation of natural history collections. Botanic Garden and Botanical Museum Berlin, Freie Universitat, Berlin, pp 117–119. https://doi.org/10.3372/SPNHC2016

Grenda-Kurmanow M (2017) Conservation versus genetics. Challenges of conservation planning for historic herbaria. In: Bridgeland J (ed) ICOM-CC 18th triennial conference preprints, Copenhagen, 4–8 September 2017, Art. 1103. International Council of Museums, Paris

Grenda-Kurmanow M (2019) Review of biocides used as prevention and intervention measures for historic artefacts, with special regard to herbaria collections. Notes Konserwatorski 21:121–161. https://doi.org/10.36155/NK.21.00004

Gutaker R, Reiter E, Furtwängler A, Schuenemann VJ, Burbano HA (2017) Extraction of ultrashort DNA molecules from herbarium specimens. BioTechniques 62:76–79. https://doi.org/10.2144/000114517

Hahn O (1999) Chemische Schädlingsbekämpfung. Risike für Pigmente und Farbstoffe. Restauro 4:275–279

Hall AV (1988) Pest control in herbaria. Taxon 37(4):885–907

Hart ML, Forrest LL, Nicholls JA, Kidner CA (2016) Retrieval of hundreds of nuclear loci from herbarium specimens. Taxon 65(5):1081–1092. https://doi.org/10.12705/655.9

Havermans J (1995) Enviromental influences on the deterioration of paper. PhD dissertation, Technische Universiteit Delft

Havermans J, Dekker R, Sportel R (2015) The effect of mercuric chloride treatment as biocide for herbaria on the indoor air quality. Herit Sci 3:39. https://doi.org/10.1186/s40494-015-0068-8

Hawks C (2001) Historical survey of the sources of contamination of ethnographic materials in museum collections. Collect Forum 16(1–2):2–11

Hawks C, Bell D (1999) Removal of stains caused by mercuric chloride treatments from herbarium sheet labels. In: Bridgeland J (ed) BidICOM Committee for Conservation preprints, Vol. II, 12th triennial meeting, Lyon, 29 August–3 September. James and James, London, pp 723–727

Hawks C, Makos K, Bell D, Wambach PF, Burrows GE (2004) An inexpensive method to test for mercury vapor in herbarium cabinets. Taxon 53:783–787

Hengemihle FH, Weberg N, Shahani C (1995) Desorption of residual ethylene oxide from fumigated library materials, preservation research and testing series No. 9502. Washington, Library of Congress

Hofreiter M, Jaenicke V, Serre D, von Haeseler A, Pääbo S (2001) DNA sequences from multiple amplifications reveal artifacts induced by cytosine deamination in ancient DNA. Nucleic Acids Res 29(23):4793–4799. https://doi.org/10.1093/nar/29.23.4793

Hofreiter M, Paijmans JLA, Goodchild H, Speller CF, Barlow A, Fortes GG, Thomas JA, Ludwig A, Collins MJ (2014) The future of ancient DNA: technical advances and conceptual shifts. BioEssays 37(3):284–293. https://doi.org/10.1002/bies.201400160

Karbowska-Berent J (2015) Nowe tendencje w dezynfekcji i dezynsekcji zabytków na podłożu papierowym. Toruńskie Studia Bibliologiczne 2(15):189. https://doi.org/10.12775/TSB.2015.024

Karbowska-Berent J (2016) Zabytki na podłożu papierowym jako środowisko życia owadów. Przegląd Papierniczy 1(2):72–76. https://doi.org/10.15199/54.2016.2.2

Kataeva M, Panichev N, van Wyk AE (2008) Monitoring mercury in two South African herbaria. Sci Total Environ 407(3):1211–1217

Kigawa R, Strang T (2011) Effects of various fumigants and non-chemical treatments on DNA molecules on proteins: case studies on natural history specimens and proteinaceous components of museum objects. In: Winsor P, Pinniger D, Bacon L, Child B, Harris K, Lauder D, Phippard J, Xavier-Rowe A (eds) Integrated pest management for collections. Proceedings of 2011: a pest odyssey, 10 years later. English Heritage, London, pp 115–122

Kigawa R, Nochide H, Kimura H, Miura S (2003) Effects of various fumigants, thermal methods and carbon dioxide treatment on DNA extraction and amplification: a case study on freeze-dried mushroom and freeze-dried muscle specimens. Collect Forum 18(1–2):74–89

Kigawa R, Strang T, Hayakawa N, Kimura H, Young G (2011) Investigation of effects of fumigants on proteinaceous components of museum objects (muscle, animal glue and silk) in comparison with other non-chemical pest eradicating measures. Stud Conserv 56:196–215. https://doi.org/10.1179/204705811X13110713013272

Kistler L (2012) Ancient DNA extraction from plants. In: Hofreiter M, Shapiro B (eds) Ancient DNA, Materials and protocols. Springer, pp 71–79

Kistler L, Bieker VC, Martin MD, Pedersen MW, Madrigal JR, Wales N (2020) Ancient plant genomics in archaeology, herbaria, and the environment. Annu Rev Plant Biol 71(1):605–629. https://doi.org/10.1146/annurev-arplant-081519-035837

Kosuge K, Akiyama H, Taugchi N (2005) Optical conditions of chemical fumigation with methyle-iodide for biological collections. BUNRUI 5(1):21–32. https://doi.org/10.18942/bunrui.KJ00004649629

Kronkright DP (1990) Deterioration of artifacts made from plant materials. In: Florian MLE, Kronkright DP, Norton R (eds) The conservation of artifacts made from plant materials. The J. Paul Getty Trust, pp 139–193

Kumar SS, Nasidze I, Walimbe SR, Stoneking M (2000) Brief communication: discouraging prospects for ancient DNA from India. Am J Phys Anthropol 113(1):129–133. https://doi.org/10.1002/1096-8644(200009)113:1<129::aid-ajpa12>3.0.co;2-2

La DK, Upton PB, Swenberg JA (2010) Carcinogenic alkylating agents. In: McQueen CA (ed) Comprehensive toxicology. Elsevier Science, pp 63–83. https://doi.org/10.1016/b978-0-08-046884-6.01405-6

Lander TA, Dadonaite B, Monro AK (2013) Microwave drying of plant material for herbarium specimens and genetic analysis. Taxon 62(4):790–797

Latorre SM, Lang PLM, Burbano HA, Gutaker RM (2020) Isolation, library preparation, and bioinformatic analysis of historical and ancient plant DNA. Curr Protoc Plant Biol 5:e20121. https://doi.org/10.1002/cppb.20121

Lellinger DB (1972) Dichlorvos and lindane as herbarium insecticides. Taxon 21(1):91–95. https://doi.org/10.2307/1219227

Lindahl T (1993) Instability and decay of the primary structure of DNA. Nature 362:709–715

Lindahl T, Nyberg B (1972) Rate of depurination of native deoxyribonucleic acid. Biochemistry 11:3610–3618. https://doi.org/10.1021/bi00769a018

Lipińska-Ojrzanowska A, Walusiak-Skorupa J (2014) Czwartorzędowe związki amoniowe – nowe zagrożenie w środowisku pracy. Med Pr 65(5):675–682. https://doi.org/10.13075/mp.5893.00056

Marota I, Basile C, Ubaldi M, Rollo F (2002) DNA decay rate in papyri and human remains from Egyptian archaeological sites. Am J Phys Anthropol 117(4):310–318. https://doi.org/10.1002/ajpa.10045. PMID: 11920366

Merrill E (1948) On the control of destructive insects in the herbarium. J Arnold Arbor 29(1):103–110

Molak M, Ho SYW (2011) Evaluating the impact of post-mortem damage in ancient DNA: a theoretical approach. J Mol Evol 73(3–4):244–255. https://doi.org/10.1007/s00239-011-9474-z

Moore A, Woodgyer E (2023) Pest management. In: Davies NMJ, Drinkell C, Utteridge TMA (eds) The herbarium handbook. Kew Publishing, Kew, pp 194–209

Norton RE (1990) Technology of plant materials used in artifacts. In: Florian MLE, Kronkright DP, Norton R (eds) The conservation of artifacts made from plant materials. The J. Paul Getty Trust, pp 83–138

Odegaard N, Sadongei A (2005) Old poisons, new problems: a museum resource for managing contaminated cultural materials. Altamira Press, Walnut

Odegaard N, Zimmt WS (2008) Pesticide removal studies for cultural objects. In: Dignard C, Helwig K, Mason J, Nanowin K, Stone T (eds) Preserving aboriginal heritage: technical and traditional approaches. Canadian Conservation Institute, Ottawa

Oyarzun R, Higueras P, Esbrí JM, Pizarro J (2007) Mercury in air and plant specimens in herbaria: a pilot study at the MAF herbarium in Madrid (Spain). Sci Total Environ 387:346–352

Pääbo S (1989) Ancient DNA: extraction, characterization, molecular cloning, and enzymatic amplification. Proc Natl Acad Sci 86(6):1939–1943. https://doi.org/10.1073/pnas.86.6.1939

Pääbo S, Poinar H, Serre D, Jaenicke-Després V, Hebler J, Rohland N, Kuch M, Krause J, Vigilant L, Hofreiter M (2004) Genetic analyses from ancient DNA. Annu Rev Genet 38:645–679. https://doi.org/10.1146/annurev.genet.37.110801.143214

Péquignot A, Marte F, von Endt D (2006) L'arsenic dans les collections d'Histoire naturelle. La Lettre de l'OCIM 105:4–10

Pfister A-L (2008) L'influence des biocides sur la conservations de Naturalia, HEAA Arc, Filière Conservation-restauration, Orientation objets archéologiques et ethnographiques. Dissertation, Hautes écoles spécialisées de Suisse Occidentale

Pinniger DB (2015) Pest management in museums, archives and historic houses. Archetype Publications, London

Popławska S, Zając I (2018) Artystyczne i naukowe zielniki z zasuszonymi roślinami. Problematyka konserwacji zielników w formie kodeksu. Toruńskie Studia Bibliologiczne 1(20):67–87. https://doi.org/10.12775/TSB.2018.004

Prance G, Nesbitt M (eds) (2005) The cultural history of plants. Routledge, New York

Purewal V (1999) The identification of hazardous pesticide and fungicide residues on herbarium material. Scott Soc Conserv Restor J 10(4):5–9

Purewal V (2001) The identification of four persistent and hazardous residues present on historic plant collections housed within the National Museum and Gallery of Wales. Collect Forum 16(1–2):77–86

Purewal V (2012) Novel detection and removal of hazardous biocide residues historically applied to herbaria. PhD dissertation, University of Lincoln

Purewal V, Colston B, Röhrs (2008) Developing a simple screening method for the identification of historic biocide residues on herbarium material in museum collections. X-Ray Spectrum 37:137–141. https://doi.org/10.1002/xrs.1036

Pyle M, Adams R (1989) In situ preservation of DNA in plant specimens. Taxon 38(4):576–581. https://doi.org/10.2307/1222632

Querner P (2015) Insect pests and integrated pest management in museums, libraries and historic buildings. Insects 6(2):595–607. https://doi.org/10.3390/insects6020595

Rader L, Ison C (1999) Legacy of mercuric chloride. In: Metsger DA, Byers SC (eds) Managing the modern herbarium – an interdisciplinary approach. SPNHC, Ontario, pp 353–354

Reape TJ, McCabe PF (2008) Apoptotic-like programmed cell death in plants. New Phytol 180(1):13–26. https://doi.org/10.1111/j.1469-8137.2008.02549.x. PMID: 18631291

Rizzi E, Lari M, Gigli E, De Bellis G, Caramelli D (2012) Ancient DNA studies: new perspectives on old samples. Genet Sel Evol 44:21. https://doi.org/10.1186/1297-9686-44-21

Robinson B (1903) Insecticides used at the gray herbarium. Rhodora 5(58):237–247

Rohland N, Hofreiter M (2007) Comparison and optimization of ancient DNA extraction. BioTechniques 42(3):343–352

Rohland N, Siedel H, Hofreiter M (2010) A rapid column-based ancient DNA extraction method for increased sample throughput. Mol Ecol Resour 10(4):677–683. https://doi.org/10.1111/j.1755-0998.2009.02824.x

Saint-Lager J (1885) Histoire des herbiers. J.-B. Baillère et fils, Paris

Salick J, Solomon J (2014) Herbarium curation of biocultural plant collections and vouchers. In: Salick J, Konchar K, Nesbitt M (eds) Curating biocultural collections: a handbook. Royal Botanic Gardens, Kew, pp 43–54

Särkinen T, Staats M, Richardson JE, Cowan RS, Bakker FT (2012) How to open the treasure chest? Optimising DNA extraction from herbarium specimens. PLoS One 7(8):e43808. https://doi.org/10.1371/journal.pone.0043808

Savolainen V, Cuénoud P, Spichiger R, Martinez MD, Crèvecoeur M, Manen JF (1995) The use of herbarium specimens in DNA phylogenetics: evaluation and improvement. Plant Syst Evol 197:87–98. https://doi.org/10.1007/BF00984634

Sawyer S, Krause J, Guschanski K, Savolainen V, Paabo S (2012) Temporal patterns of nucleotide misincorporations and DNA fragmentation in ancient DNA. PLoS One 7(3):e34131. https://doi.org/10.1371/journal.pone.0034131

Schofield EK, Crisafulli S (1980) A safer insecticide for herbarium use. Brittonia 32(1):58–62. https://doi.org/10.2307/2806221

Sinha RP, Häder DP (2002) UV-induced DNA damage and repair: a review. Photochem Photobiol Sci 1(4):225–236. https://doi.org/10.1039/b201230h
Sirois J (2001) The analysis of museum objects for the presence of arsenic and mercury: non-destructive analysis and sample analysis. Collect Forum 16(1–2):65–75
Sobucki W (2013) Konserwacja papieru. Zagadnienia chemiczne. Ministerstwo Kultury i Dziedzictwa Narodowego, Biblioteka Narodowa, Warszawa
Srinivasan M, Sedmak D, Jewell S (2002) Effect of fixatives and tissue processing on the content and integrity of nucleic acids. Am J Pathol 161(6):1961–1971. https://doi.org/10.1016/s0002-9440(10)64472-0
Staats M, Cuenca A, Richardson JE, Ginkel RV, Petersen G, Sebery O, Bakker FT (2011) DNA damage in plant herbarium tissue. PLoS One 6:e28448. https://doi.org/10.1371/journal.pone.0028448
Staats M, Erkens RHJ, van de Vossenberg B, Wieringa JJ, Kraaijeveld K, Stielow B (2013) Genomic treasure troves: complete genome sequencing of herbarium and insect museum specimens. PLoS One 8(7):e69189. https://doi.org/10.1371/journal.pone.0069189
Strang TJK (1999) A healthy dose of the past: a future direction in herbarium pest control? In: Metsger DA, Byers SC (eds) Managing the modern herbarium – an interdisciplinary approach. SPNHC, Ontario, pp 59–80
Töpfer T, Gamauf A, Haring E (2011) Utility of arsenic-treated bird skins for DNA extraction. BMC Res Notes 4:197. https://doi.org/10.1186/1756-0500-4-197
Townsend J (1999) Preventive conservation: concept and strategy for long-term preservation. In: Metsger DA, Byers SC (eds) Managing the modern herbarium – an interdisciplinary approach. SPNHC, Ontario, pp 23–35
Unger A, Schniewind AP, Unger W (2001) Conservation of wood artifacts: a handbook. Springer Verlag, New York
van den Berg H, Manuweera G, Konradsen F (2017) Global trends in the production and use of DDT for control of malaria and other vector-borne diseases. Malar J 16(1):401. https://doi.org/10.1186/s12936-017-2050-2
van den Spiegel A (1606) Isagoges in rem herbariam libri duo. Paulus Meiettus, Padua (Patavia)
Wales N, Andersen K, Cappellini E, Avila-Arcos MC, Gilbert MT (2014) Optimization of DNA recovery and amplification from non-carbonized archaeobotanical remains. PLoS One 9(1):e86827. https://doi.org/10.1371/journal.pone.0086827
Ward JF (1988) DNA damage produced by ionizing radiation in mammalian cells: identities, mechanisms of formation, and reparability. Prog Nucleic Acid Res Mol Biol 35(3):95–125. https://doi.org/10.1016/s0079-6603(08)60611-x
Webber WB, Ernest LJ, Vangapandu S (2011) Mercury exposures in university herbarium collections. J Chem Health Saf 18:9–12
Weiss CL, Schuenemann VJ, Devos J, Shirsekar G, Reiter E, Gould BA, Stinchcombe JR, Krause J, Burbano HA (2016) Temporal patterns of damage and decay kinetics of DNA retrieved from plant herbarium specimens. R Soc Open Sci 3:160239. https://doi.org/10.1098/rsos.160239
Whitmore PM (2012) Paper ageing and the influence of water. In: Banik G, Brückle I (eds) Paper and water. Routledge, New York, pp 219–254
Whitmore TC, Fosberg FR (1965) Lauryl pentachlorphenate protecting herbarium specimens. Taxon 14(5):164. https://doi.org/10.2307/1217552
Whitten WM, Williams NH, Glover KV (1999) Sulphuryl fluoride fumigation: effect on DNA extraction and amplification from herbarium specimens. Taxon 48(3):507–510
Willerslev E, Cooper A (2005) Ancient DNA. Proc Biol Sci 272(1558):3–16. https://doi.org/10.1098/rspb.2004.2813
Wooder MF, Wright AS (1981) Alkylation of DNA by organophosphorus pesticides. Acta Pharmacol Toxicol 49:51–55. https://doi.org/10.1111/j.1600-0773.1981.tb03252.x
Zerek BF (2017) The Warsaw school of paper conservation. Przegląd Biblioteczny 85:89–103

Chapter 4
Preventive and Interventional Collection Preservation of Herbarium Collections

Abstract This chapter addresses issues related to the preservation of herbarium specimens. The focus is on evaluating the strategic principles of Integrated Pest Management (IPM), describing the evolution of perspectives, and assessing the mixed evaluations of individual IPM components. The section also discusses challenges associated with decontamination and the preservation of genetic material.

Keywords Integrated Pest Management (IPM) · Freezing · Decontamination · DNA preservation · Climate control

The following sections are devoted to the strategies currently employed for the preservation of natural history collections, which constitute an integral part of collection management in many institutions housing herbaria. Numerous publications emphasise the importance of preventive measures, which are designed to ensure the overall safety of entire collections. At the same time, a range of intervention activities is outlined, which become necessary in cases of neglect or unforeseen incidents. The significance of comprehensive staff training and effective communication among employees is also highlighted as key factors enabling the successful implementation of an integrated pest management (IPM). Over the course of developing IPM, various solutions have been adopted, some of which have, over time, been found to have adverse effects on collections, particularly with regard to different disinfection methods. This section addresses the issues associated with certain practices, such as exposing objects to varying temperatures or employing alternative disinfection techniques. Discrepancies in the recommended climatic conditions for collection storage are also discussed, as these pose challenges for the preservation of genetic material. Furthermore, the section explores issues related to the study of genetic material and the resulting dilemmas concerning DNA preservation. As a point of reference, research on genetic material derived from other types of objects (including those belonging to biocultural collections) is also cited, due to the limited number of publications addressing the impact of materials used in preservation and conservation on the material contained in herbarium specimens.

M. Grenda-Kurmanow, *Herbaria*, https://doi.org/10.1007/978-3-032-21904-6_4

4.1 Integrated Pest Management (IPM) for Herbarium Collections

Integrated Pest Management (IPM) is a multifaceted strategy adopted for museum collections, primarily aimed at the preventive control of pest infestations within collections. The system was developed as an alternative to earlier collection preservation methods, which relied on the continuous application of successive biocides. Such practices, especially when used over many years, led to chronic illnesses and allergies among staff working in collection-holding institutions (Pinniger 2011, 2015; Strang 1999a). From the perspective of conservation care for historic objects, particularly important are the intervention measures characteristic of herbaria, which, in addition to the continued use of selected biocidal agents, also include freezing, heating, and exposing collections to microwaves.

The concept of IPM was adopted from the field of crop protection. In relation to museum institutions, it began to be applied in the 1980s and 1990s, with its development and widespread implementation occurring in the first decade of the twenty-first century (Querner and Simon 2011; Hall 1988). For herbarium collections, the first experiences and steps towards introducing prevention instead of toxic intervention were undertaken and published as early as 1948; however, this was a pioneering approach that did not find global continuation for a long time (Merrill 1948; Strang 1999a). A system of integrated preventive measures is of particular importance for collections stored in historic buildings, as well as for institutions housing natural history collections, including herbaria. Among museum pests targeted by IPM activities, selected insects are of primary concern, as well as rodents and birds. The system is based on comprehensive control and management of interconnected degradation factors: light, climatic conditions, the presence of microbiological infections, and insects, all of which have a decisive impact on the condition of collections (Pinniger 2015, pp. 1–7). There is now a substantial body of literature on IPM, supplemented by publications from regular meetings on IPM topics organised by the international group The MuseumPests Working Group, which also edits an online compendium of IPM knowledge.[1]

Modern IPM involves the implementation of a structured policy of prevention and the prioritisation of actions related to the preservation of collections. The prevention policy should be based on the identification of the most significant pest-related issues affecting specific collections and the establishment of key detailed objectives for the local IPM policy. The next step should be the formation of a team of appropriately trained staff from various departments (for example, a team comprising staff from administration, inventory, conservation, and subject specialists associated with the given collection), whose task will be to implement IPM

[1]The literature on IPM includes, above all, numerous publications by David Pinniger (including those already cited (Pinniger 2011 and 2015) and many others) and Thomas Strang (1996, 1999a, b, 2012), among others. One of the online resources dedicated to this subject is the website www.museumpests.net [accessed 13.01.2026], created by The MuseumPests Working Group.

procedures in accordance with the list of priorities established for the institution. The long-term responsibility of the team of experts should be to establish procedures for the continued operation of IPM within the institution, including the development of a budget and the regular evaluation and adjustment of the adopted system (Pinniger 2015, pp. 1–7, 125–132).

The priorities of IPM, which are intended to ensure the effectiveness of both preventive and intervention measures, are presented in the following order (from most important): avoiding the presence of pests; blocking their access to collections; detecting their presence and proper species identification; responding to the presence of pests with a selected method, evaluating the policy applied, and implementing necessary improvements; remedial actions (for example, conservation treatments) following the application of intervention measures.[2] In the implementation of IPM, particular emphasis is placed on educating all staff regarding appropriate procedures and the risks associated with the presence of pests.

The first two priorities are strictly preventive in nature and impose the requirement to maintain a certain sanitary regime within the institution, primarily regarding the consumption of food inside the building; outside the building, in terms of waste storage and the design of greenery in its surroundings; as well as securing the building by installing physical barriers to prevent pests from accessing the collections (for example, mesh screens in windows and ventilation grilles). Preventive measures also include the appropriate arrangement of storage areas to facilitate thorough cleaning, inspection of the plumbing system, lighting, the tightness of windows and other openings, and the climatic conditions in the building (Strang 1996, 1999a).[3]

Dirt and dust accumulating in all forgotten corners of the storage area and other rooms, as well as bird and rodent nests and droppings, other dead insects, the presence of mould, and food residues, also create favourable conditions for insect development. These must be removed in order to effectively prevent insect feeding, as their presence negates the effects of intervention measures by creating conditions for the return of pests (Hall 1988; Strang 1999a; Pinniger 2015; Moore and Woodgyer 2023).

Detection of pests presence involves regular inspections of rooms housing collections, as well as monitoring for pests using bait or adhesive traps, mechanical traps, and species-specific pheromone traps. It is also essential to raise awareness among staff and external visitors to report any observed signs of pest presence. Such signs include nests, droppings, larvae, eggs, dead pests or their body parts. Traces may also be evident as characteristic damage visible on collection items. Locations where evidence of pest activity has been observed should be marked and given particular attention. The most important aspect of this priority is the correct identification of the pest and the planning of appropriate intervention measures.

---

[2] According to Strang, the priorities are briefly named as follows: *Avoid, Block, Detect, Respond, Recover/Treat* (Strang 1996).

[3] A discussion of the climatic conditions recommended for herbarium collections can be found in the section *Stable Climatic Conditions* in this chapter.

The primary preventive and intervention measure is quarantine, which should obligatorily include objects newly acquired for the collection as well as items on loan or returning from other institutions. When quarantine is applied to items within the collection, it is essential to inspect and thoroughly clean the area where the objects were stored, removing any pest residues or by-products of their activity (Pinniger 2015, pp. 1–7; Hall 1988; Moore and Woodgyer 2023).

As mentioned earlier, treatments aimed at eradicating insects present or potentially present in collections include freezing, exposing collections to high temperatures in special chambers or using microwaves, as well as storing objects in a low-oxygen (anoxic) environment. These treatments are described below. Selected biocidal agents are also still used, depending on the institution.

According to the principles of IPM, following intervention, an evaluation of the effectiveness of the system should be conducted, and, if necessary, modifications should be introduced to improve its efficacy. The final stage after intervention should be a "return to normality", which may involve conservation procedures, primarily consisting of cleaning the objects and their surroundings, as well as the continuation of preventive measures.

4.1.1 Freezing

Freezing is the most commonly used procedure in herbarium institutions as both a preventive and intervention tool against insects. The method operates by rapidly lowering the storage temperature to kill pests, and involves keeping objects tightly sealed in impermeable materials for a certain period in a freezer at a specified, sufficiently low temperature. The literature reveals a wide range of recommended temperatures and freezing durations (Strang 1992). Typically, a temperature between −18 and − 20 °C is cited, but lower temperatures (−30, or even −50 °C) are also recommended (see Strang 1992, 1997, 2012; Bridson and Forman 1999; Pinniger 2015). The freezing period should be at least 2 days, but may last longer, up to 7 or 14 days; the lower the freezing temperature, the shorter the required duration. Some authors provide specific combinations of temperature and time, for example, Pinniger: 3 days at −30 °C, 7 days at −25 °C, 14 days at −18 °C (Pinniger 2015, pp. 72–96). He also notes that the freezer should operate efficiently enough to lower the temperature of the entire object within 24 h, due to the risk of some insects adapting to changing conditions. It should be noted that cold air penetrating the object requires time, and the temperature indicated by the cooling device may not reflect the temperature inside the object. Bridson and Forman report an average time for complete freezing of an object (achieving the target temperature throughout the structure) as 17 h (Bridson and Forman 1999, pp. 22–26). Strang points out that there is no "magic" temperature value suitable for eradicating all pests at all developmental stages, and that thermal adaptation in insects is short-term; therefore, a sufficiently long freezing period is important (Strang 1992, 1997, and 2012, pp. 151–188). A key stage is identifying the specific threat present in the collection and adjusting the freezing conditions accordingly. At the same time, Strang states that freezing at temperatures between −20 and − 40 °C for about 7 days should effectively kill all insects present in the object, although lowering the temperature below −20 °C is more energy-intensive and costly, and may also cause greater damage to the objects themselves than treatment at slightly higher temperatures (between −18 and − 20 °C) (Strang 1997 and 2012, pp. 151–188). With an appropriately selected freezing duration, there is no need to repeat the procedure (Strang 1997). After freezing, objects must remain in their packaging until they reach the target (storage) temperature to avoid moisture condensation. Transitional rooms are sometimes used to allow gradual attainment of the target temperature, but many institutions lack such spaces. The time required to reach thermal equilibrium with the environment is estimated at several hours to about 1 day (see also Bridson and Forman 1999, pp. 22–26 and Strang 1997). Bridson and Forman note that insufficiently dried botanical specimens may blacken as a result of freezing (Bridson and Forman 1999, pp. 22–26).

An unpublished survey conducted by the author in 2013 indicates that Polish herbarium institutions readily employ periodic freezing as a preventive measure, using temperatures ranging from −12 to as low as −50 °C, for varying durations of 24 h up to 30 days.[4]

4.1.2 High Temperatures

For natural history collections, including herbaria, heat treatment has also been employed, taking advantage of the fact that most insects die at temperatures above 55 °C (Pinniger 2015, pp. 72–96). This method is faster than freezing, but poses a greater risk to heritage objects. In the past, ovens were used for this purpose, which caused objects to become brittle and deformed (Pinniger 2015). Strang cites the use of 60 °C as a common solution (Strang 1995, 2001), while Bridson and Forman recommend a temperature of 45 °C for 2–3 h, but also mention temperatures as high as 80–100 °C as being used in some herbaria, emphasising that high temperatures are harmful to all components of a herbarium specimen (Bridson and Forman 1999, pp. 22–26).

In the process of developing an appropriate methodology for this treatment, the Thermo Lignum thermal chamber system was devised, in which the temperature is gradually increased over 3 h to 48–55 °C, maintained at the highest level for a further 3 h, and then reduced to the initial temperature, with RH as a controllable factor. This latter aspect distinguishes the method from traditionally used thermal treatments, where only temperature is regulated and RH is consequently kept at a very low level (according to Ackery, approximately 15%), leading to damage and

[4] Grenda (2013) Methods of preserving herbarium collections from pests, survey conducted among herbarium institutions, Warsaw; unpublished survey report

deformation of the objects' structure (Ackery et al. 2004). The Thermo Lignum method was developed with particular consideration for biological collections, and has therefore also been the subject of studies concerning its potential harmfulness to genetic material. According to Ackery's team, who conducted research on entomological collections, the process used in Thermo Lignum does not have a destructive effect on DNA. However, as previously demonstrated, high temperature has an adverse impact on genetic material.[5] The authors also excluded changes in bronze materials with visible verdigris corrosion and in elements containing fat, while simultaneously citing unpublished reports of noticeable changes in oily fish specimens following the application of the method (Ackery et al. 2004). The assessment, however, was based solely on visual impressions. Much more critical of this method are the detailed studies by Ball, Bisulca, and Odegaard, who, after conducting a series of tests on various materials, observed changes occurring in the structure of adhesive layers, especially protein-based adhesives, as well as migration of fatty components within the objects' structure (Ball et al. 2011). This poses a particular risk to herbarium specimens, which are adhered to the substrate either at specific points or over their entire surface. Furthermore, observations by botanical collection conservators indicate that the Thermo Lignum process results in the migration of biocides such as DDT, lindane, or mystox, and their concentration on the surface of the object (Collins 2014).

4.1.3 Microwaves

Another method used in combating insects was the exposure of herbarium specimens to microwaves. This approach gained popularity in the 1980s, when microwave-generating devices, in the form of microwave ovens, became widely available.[6] Although even at that time the harmful side effects of microwaves on specimens were recognised, they were recommended as a rapid means of disinfection, based on heating the water contained in the bodies of insects to the boiling point. The detrimental effects of microwaves on specimens resulted from the highly uneven distribution of temperature during heating and the consequent limited control over the process (Pinniger 2015, pp. 72–96; Strang 1999b). Microwave treatment also caused discolouration of specimens, weakening of adhesives specimens were mounted with to the substrate, disintegration of certain botanical specimens in parts containing more water (such as stems), and even explosion of some plant parts (such as nuts) (Hill 1983; Bridson and Forman 1999, pp. 22–26; Strang 1999b). In addition, small metal elements present in specimens, such as paper clips, pins, or staples, could cause ignition and local charring of the specimen (Hill 1983; Hall

[5] See the section *Degradation of Genetic Material* in Chap. 3.

[6] Strang provides an extensive review of the most important publications from the 1980s on the use of microwaves in herbarium collections (Strang 1999b).

1988; Strang 1999b; Pinniger 2015, pp. 72–96). According to a 2013 study, microwaves have a destructive effect on high-molecular-weight DNA contained in plant specimens (Lander et al. 2013). Furthermore, they have a damaging effect on the cell wall and membrane, and reduce or eliminate seed viability (Hill 1983; Hall 1988; Bridson and Forman 1999, pp. 22–26; Strang 1999b).

4.1.4 Anoxia

A non-chemical method that does not rely on temperature manipulation, is storing objects in a low-oxygen (anoxic) environment. Controlled atmospheric treatments (CATs), which exploit the oxygen requirements of insects, have been introduced as a direct replacement for fumigation with toxic gases such as methyl bromide or ethylene oxide (Pinniger 2015, pp. 72–96). Nitrogen, carbon dioxide, as well as argon and other noble gases, are used to create anoxic conditions. Special chambers or bags are required to achieve anoxia, enabling the maintenance of oxygen levels between 0.3 and 0.5% (Pinniger 2015, pp. 72–96). The duration of exposure in a nitrogen-filled chamber depends on the insect species being targeted and the temperature applied: at 25 °C, the treatment lasts approximately 2–3 weeks, but if the temperature is reduced to 20 °C, considered the minimum for anoxic procedures, the duration must be extended to 4–5 weeks to effectively control species tolerant of low-oxygen conditions. High nitrogen concentrations result in low relative humidity; therefore, Pinniger recommends humidifying the chamber along with the supplied nitrogen (Pinniger 2015, pp. 72–96). When using carbon dioxide, the temperature may be increased to 30 °C. However, carbon dioxide is not an inert gas, and its use requires special precautions. Argon and other noble gases have been tested in anoxic treatments, but not on a large scale due to high costs (Pinniger 2015, pp. 72–96). Institutions also sometimes employ more modest anoxic procedures, using oxygen absorbers in individual airtight packages containing the objects.

4.1.5 Stable Climatic Conditions

Maintaining appropriate climatic conditions a key aspect of preventive collection care. In the case of herbaria, the primary focus is on the insect activity, as insects pose the main threat to these collections, and on creating conditions within the collections that are unfavourable for their survival. Accordingly, the general recommendation for storage conditions, as with other heritage objects, is to maintain the lowest possible temperature and relative humidity (RH), and to avoid sudden fluctuations in climatic conditions. At the same time, as described above, controlled periodic temperature manipulation of individual objects is permitted in order to eradicate insects. Particular attention is also paid to proper room ventilation, also due to the emission of volatile organic compounds from objects contaminated with biocides (Hall 1988).

However, the detailed recommendations found in publications concerning herbaria are no longer consistent. Bridson and Forman cite an "ideal" temperature range of 20–23 °C and a relative humidity (RH) of around 55%, emphasising that due to the human factor, RH should be maintained between 40–60% (Bridson and Forman 1999, pp. 10, 19). Strang criticises these recommendations as failing to address the problem of insect infestation in herbarium collections (Strang 1999b). This aligns with Pinniger's observations, who notes that a temperature of 22 °C allows certain insect species to complete several developmental cycles and produce more than one generation per year (Pinniger 2015, pp. 65–72). Salick and Solomon recommend an optimal RH of 45% and advise that it should not exceed 60%, but do not specify a temperature range (Salick and Solomon 2014). Hall proposes an optimal RH of around 50%, preferably below 43% as a preventive measure against moulds, which serve as food for booklice (*Liposcelis*), and sets an upper limit at 72%. She cites critical RH values for the development and feeding of specific insect species: 45% for the firebrat (*Thermobia domestica*), 43% for the larvae of the cigarette beetle (*Lasioderma serricorne*), and 60% for booklice (*Liposcelis*). She also provides an example of a herbarium institution that successfully controlled pests by maintaining RH at 39% (Hall 1988). Hall's recommendations also lack information regarding the appropriate temperature. Adams recommends an RH of 55%, although his research indicates that a broader range, from approximately 23 to 54%, is beneficial for DNA preservation; however, the tests were conducted at an unknown temperature in sealed containers (Adams 2011).

Pinniger recommends not exceeding a temperature of 20 °C and a relative humidity (RH) of 60% in order to limit insect reproduction and prevent them from completing their life cycle (Pinniger 2015, pp. 1–7). Many insects, such as booklice feeding on moulds or the silverfish (*Lepisma saccharina*), reproduce at RH levels above 60–70%. Lower RH levels are not highly detrimental to insects; only extremely dry conditions (RH < 10%) are critical for certain species. However, such a low RH would also be very damaging to collections (Pinniger 2015, pp. 9–95). Drobnik states that RH in rooms and herbarium cabinets should not exceed 35%, but does not explain the rationale for such a low minimum relative humidity (Drobnik 2009, p. 159). Based on Pinniger's recommendations, Davies proposes a temperature range of 16–18 °C and RH between 40 and 60%, with fluctuations of up to ±5% (Davies 2023).

Insects, which generally have limited thermoregulatory abilities, possess preferred temperature ranges—varying between species—within which they are able to reproduce. Most often, a rapid increase in reproductive potential occurs at temperatures above 25 °C, while in the range of 15–20 °C reproduction slows down, and below 5–10 °C development and reproduction are inhibited (Drobnik 2009, p. 159). Maintaining temperatures below 5 °C in rooms occupied by people during the day is difficult to implement due to comfort considerations; however, such conditions are recommended, for example, in storage facilities where human presence is limited.[7] In storage areas, windows should also be covered to prevent localised temperature increases in areas exposed to sunlight. Areas around plumbing installations may also create local conditions favourable to insect development. In selected areas of a building (near the floor and along north-facing walls), climatic conditions may differ from those in the rest of the room. In buildings with artificially lowered temperatures, particular attention should be paid to the risk of increased relative humidity, which is a typical effect of air conditioning systems (Pinniger 2015, pp. 65–72).

Many publications concerning herbarium collections, and more broadly, natural history or biocultural collections, devote more attention to relative humidity than to temperature. The drive to eliminate the presence of insects leads to recommendations for the lowest possible RH values. However, maintaining a very dry climate in collections can be detrimental to the materials from which herbaria are made, primarily cellulose.[8] At the same time, it cannot be overlooked that collections have been created as scientific tools, and thus it is not possible to exclude the sharing of herbarium sheets with researchers or their use as educational materials. This necessitates at least the periodic presence of objects in conditions of human thermal comfort and the appropriate planning of object acclimatisation to room conditions in the event of access or use.

It should be emphasised that the recommended climatic conditions described above should serve as guidelines rather than as a rigid or universally applicable standard. The challenge of maintaining the "correct" climatic conditions for herbarium collections is part of the ongoing conservation discourse concerning the appropriate environment for heritage objects. Artificial regulation of temperature and humidity within narrowly defined ranges, without regard to the prevailing climatic conditions of a given region, may result in greater damage than adapting to the local climate within a range of minor, controllable fluctuations. Townsend provides the example of Indonesian herbarium institutions housed in buildings constructed using local methods, where, due to the tropical climate, relative humidity (RH) often exceeds 70% (Townsend 1999). This is generally considered an unacceptable level of relative humidity, conducive to mould growth and insect proliferation. However, the climate is stable, and because traditional architecture allowed for adequate ventilation, no microbiological contamination of the collections was observed in these institutions. In contrast, extensive mould damage was noted in the collections of other Indonesian institutions located in new, poorly ventilated, air-conditioned buildings constructed in the Western style. This was likely due to complete reliance on an inadequate ventilation system, which was further compromised by frequent power outages (Townsend 1999).

[7] In the Economic Botany collections storage at the Royal Botanic Gardens, Kew, a constant temperature of 12 °C is maintained, which does not allow for prolonged stays in the store, but effectively reduces the risk of insect infestation (information from Dr. Mark Nesbitt, curator of the EBC collections at Kew).

[8] See Chap. 3. *Degradation Processes of Structural Elements of Herbarium Specimens and Paper Substrates*.

This illustrates a typical issue related to climate control in collections, which could be summed up by the saying, “the perfect is the enemy of the good.” Since the 1970s and 1980s, recommendations to maintain strictly limited temperature and humidity conditions—around 21 °C and 50% RH, with fluctuations of 2–3 °C and up to 5% RH—have been repeated in publications and conservation reports in most institutions worldwide.[9] These recommendations are often artificially adopted standards that are either unattainable in practice or extremely costly, and maintaining them bears no real correlation to the climatic conditions characteristic of a given region, their seasonality, or the feasibility of maintaining a stable climate within a particular building (Michalski 2016 and many other publications by this author).

The 2019 recommendations of the American Society of Heating, Refrigerating and Air-Conditioning Engineers (ASHRAE) highlight the need for economical and sustainable energy use to achieve the desired climatic conditions in collections (ASHRAE 2019). In practice, this means that maintaining appropriate temperature and humidity conditions should not rely on the use of air conditioners, but rather on passive climate control methods, adequate room ventilation, and simple technologies that are easy to maintain (ASHRAE 2019). This approach is linked to energy conservation, reduction of the carbon footprint, and the protection of the global climate. The conservation of heritage objects should therefore be carried out with respect for nature and should be environmentally friendly. This represents a breakthrough compared to previous ASHRAE recommendations, which focused primarily on climate control based largely on air conditioning systems.[10] The ASHRAE (2019) publication also presents guidelines for individual climate control classes, depending on the climate zone in which the collections are located. This enables realistic decision-making regarding the target conditions for heritage objects. Climate design should also be based on at least a year-long observation of the climatic history of a given building, as well as on long-term planning of the desired climatic conditions, taking into account the seasonal fluctuations that naturally occur in a given region. The aforementioned climate control classes refer to the storage and display conditions of objects. The strictest control class (A), in which RH is maintained at 35–65% and temperature at 10–25 °C, allows for fluctuations of ±2 °C and from ±5% (variant AA) to ±10% RH (variant A2). The final class (D) means that collection caretakers focus solely on maintaining RH below 75%. A relative humidity of 75% has been identified as critical due to the risk of mould growth, various types of corrosion, and other damage to heritage objects (ASHRAE 2019). The acceptability of such conditions stems from the fact that the harmfulness of prolonged fluctuations is less than previously thought, and the greatest threat

[9] See the history of climatic recommendations and summaries in Bratasz (2013) and (Michalski 2016).

[10] Compare with the recommendations from the *ASHRAE Handbook* from 2011 or 2015. As Michalski notes, since 2003 the ASHRAE guidelines have already taken into account the “average historical climate” as an alternative to an artificially imposed climate, whereas earlier recommendations included values of 21 °C and 50% RH (Michalski 2007).

arises from failures of climate control systems and random events (Michalski 2016; ASHRAE 2019).

The authors also refer to the declaration of the International Institute for Conservation of Historic and Artistic Works/International Council of Museums—Committee for Conservation (IIC/ICOM-CC) from 2014, concerning climate conditions for objects included in international projects and exhibitions. The recommendations cited in the declaration extend the permissible temperature range (15–25 °C) and relative humidity (RH) (45–55%), with possible RH fluctuations from ±5% up to even ±10% within 24 h. The maximum safe RH range for the majority of collections is therefore from 40 to 60% (IIC/ICOM-CC 2014).[11]

As a result, most of the previously cited recommendations for herbarium collections fall within the ranges specified by ASHRAE (2019) and the IIC/ICOM-CC declaration. However, according to the comments of IPM specialists, the temperature should be maintained at the lowest possible level and should not exceed 22 °C. For storage areas with limited human presence, the temperature can be kept lower than in spaces intended for access or exhibition. Climate planning, however, should be rationally based on an analysis of the climatic conditions in the building throughout the year, as well as on the formulation of achievable goals and realistic assumptions for the given institution.

In this context, creating separate storage conditions that are safe for genetic material appears to be particularly problematic. In line with the previously discussed issues of DNA degradation, which may be accelerated by elevated temperature and humidity, it is essential to maintain the low temperature and humidity, as well as to prevent large fluctuations in climatic conditions. Additionally, it is necessary to ensure the proper environment for the storage of herbarium specimens. Potential air pollutants described earlier, compounds emitted by biocidal substances or degrading elements from which herbaria are made, as well as compounds contained within them, may contribute to the formation of an acidic environment and, in multiple ways, accelerate the degradation processes of genetic material. At the same time, the pH of the environment should not be excessively high, remaining within the range of physiological conditions, i.e. pH $\approx$ 7.4, which is fairly consistent with the recommendations for the storage of objects on paper substrates (see also Hofreiter et al. 2001; Carter 2003; Brown 2018, pp. 16–23).

---

[11] The document cites three sources of guidelines: the Bizot Group, the Australian Institute for the Conservation of Cultural Materials (AICCM), and the American Institute for Conservation (AIC). The Bizot Group allows the greatest fluctuation (±10%), with the proviso that particularly sensitive objects require stricter RH control. The AICCM gives an allowable RH fluctuation of ±5%, and for temperature ± 4 °C. The AIC allows an RH fluctuation of ±5%, noting that annual variations should remain within the range of 40–60%.

4.2 Decontamination of Collections Treated with Biocides

Decontamination of collections treated with biocides is not an element of IPM; nevertheless, it constitutes a significant issue in collection management due to the considerable risks it poses to user health and the preservation of the collections themselves.[12] The literature on decontamination usually concerns collections other than herbaria (Odegaard 2001; Odegaard and Zimmt 2008; Pfister 2008, pp. 75–83). The term decontamination itself can be misleading, as it literally denotes the complete removal and deactivation of toxic substances. Experience unfortunately shows that such success is unattainable in the case of biocidal agents used in biocultural collections. Therefore, for heritage objects, decontamination is only partial, and the effectiveness is reported as the degree of decontamination, usually expressed as a percentage. Additionally, the term decontamination has sometimes been used to refer to the preventive disinfection of herbarium specimens prior to their incorporation into collections (Bridson and Forman 1999, pp. 22–26).

Decontamination methods include, among others, processes focused on the surroundings of the objects themselves, such as ventilation, the use of various types of absorbents to capture toxic substances, and vacuuming (Pfister 2008, pp. 75–88). In many cases involving objects contaminated with toxic substances, a decision is made to replace the substrate (e.g. the paper sheet on which a botanical specimen is mounted), although this is generally undesirable due to the loss of the object's original.

In addition, methods requiring complex manipulation of objects are employed, which are typically divided into the following groups: non-aqueous mechanical methods, methods using various types of radiation, freezing, and ultrasonic waves; aqueous mechanical methods, chemical methods (including biological ones), and methods using carbon dioxide.

Non-aqueous mechanical methods include: vacuuming the object with a HEPA-filter vacuum cleaner and other vacuuming tools; covering with a material containing activated carbon, which can absorb certain contaminants; mechanical cleaning with various tools; using compressed air; under an extraction hood; washing with acetone; rinsing textile objects in tetrachloroethane; airing objects; airing at high temperatures (approx. 60 °C, at RH = 55%, effective for biocidal substances such as lindane or pentachlorophenol, a method also suggested for biocides such as naphthalene or paradichlorobenzene) (Purewal 2001; Odegaard and Zimmt 2008; Pfister 2008, pp. 75–88). For herbarium collections contaminated with naphthalene, the most effective method proved to be airing with a continuous flow of air over the material for 48 h. This method enabled the removal of approximately 79% of the

[12] The issue of decontamination is also significant for ethical reasons, especially in the context of the repatriation of colonial collections; see the chapter *Ethical and Legal Issues Related to Herbarium Collections* in Chap. 1.

biocide (Purewal 2012).[13] Attempts were also made to decontaminate using laser treatment and lyophilisation, but without satisfactory results. In addition, the effects of ultrasonic waves, high-energy microwaves, and UV radiation were tested (Pfister 2008, pp. 75–88).

Aqueous methods primarily concern textile objects and include immersion in hot water, sometimes with detergents, as well as treatment with steam (Odegaard and Zimmt 2008; Pfister 2008, pp. 75–88).

Chemical methods involve the use of chemical compounds designed to complex or hydrolyse biocidal substances. An example of such an approach is the application of the chelating agent 2,3-dimercaptosuccinic acid to neutralise mercuric chloride present in herbaria. However, this agent is itself toxic and may have a destructive effect on inks (Hall 1988; Hawks and Bell 1999). Attempts have also been made to remove mercuric chloride using an alcoholic solution of iodine, which, however, had a very low pH, as well as Lugol's solution (an aqueous solution of elemental iodine in potassium iodide), a time-consuming method that nevertheless yielded partially positive results (Pfister 2008, pp. 75–88).

The use of supercritical carbon dioxide was also tested, which in this state exhibits properties of both a liquid and a gas (Tello et al. 2005). Supercritical carbon dioxide is characterised by low viscosity and low surface tension, allowing for effective penetration of materials subjected to its action. The method demonstrated good efficacy against mercury compounds (70–90%) and DDT (up to 80%) (Odegaard and Zimmt 2008). Liquid carbon dioxide also showed high effectiveness against DDT (up to 91%) (Odegaard and Zimmt 2008).

Other experimental chemical methods considered even included the use of biological methods, namely the introduction of bacteria that induce the oxidation of substances such as lindane or DDT. However, these methods do not appear to be feasible for safe implementation as a solution for institutional biocultural collections.

4.3 Preservation of Genetic Material in Collections—Studies on the Impact of Preservation and Conservation Methods on aDNA

The analysis of genetic material obtained from historical herbarium specimens has been addressed multiple times in the literature, particularly over the past two decades.[14] These studies have focused on the techniques for analysing genetic

[13] However, the concentration of naphthalene increases approximately 48 hours after the procedure, which, according to the author, is caused by the migration of another "portion" of naphthalene from the interior of the object to the surface of the structure.

[14] E.g. Rogers and Bendich 1985; Pyle and Adams 1989; Taylor and Swann 1994; Savolainen et al. 1995; Brown 1999; Drábková et al. 2002; Ames and Spooner 2008; Erkens et al. 2008; Lister et al. 2008; Adams 2011; Lehtonen and Christenhusz 2010; Adams and Sharma 2010; Staats et al. 2011;

material, seeking to answer whether the age of a specimen affects the quality and quantity of DNA in the sample, or whether the appearance of a specimen can be used to preliminarily assess the likelihood of successful DNA extraction. They have also aimed to determine the causes of genetic material fragmentation, to improve the extraction process, and to analyse the purity and size of DNA fragments successfully extracted from herbarium specimens. Additionally, they have included studies on the kinetics of genetic material degradation in dried plants.[15] In many cases, it has been difficult to determine precisely why analyses did not yield the expected results. The development of sequencing techniques and the establishment of rigorous research protocols now make it possible to analyse even highly fragmented samples. A smaller body of literature concerns studies on the impact of preservation and conservation methods on ancient DNA (aDNA).

According to herbarium specimen researchers, the preservation of DNA in herbarium specimens is fundamentally influenced by the method of specimen preparation, the preservation techniques employed, and storage conditions (Savolainen et al. 1995; Molak and Ho 2011; Staats et al. 2011; Dabney et al. 2013; Choi et al. 2015; Weiss et al. 2016).[16] However, as they consistently emphasise, it is usually impossible to reconstruct the specimen's history, including the methods of its preparation and preservation. The main factors accelerating degradation processes are defined as acidic environments, increased humidity, and high temperatures.

The complexity of this issue is illustrated by a review of studies on the impact of climatic conditions and applied conservation methods on genetic material. Adams conducted the aforementioned tests on the effect of relative humidity on herbarium specimens, using eastern red cedar as a model species (Adams 2011). After placing dried specimens in airtight jars, he maintained a constant RH level and examined the samples at intervals of 2, 6, and 12 months. According to his results, the safe RH range was 23.1–54.4%; however, in his conclusions, he defined the safe RH level as 55%.[17] He considered an RH above 69% to be harmful (no genetic material remained after one year of storage), and above 75% he observed fungal growth on the samples. However, the method of storing the samples did not allow for air circulation, nor were the thermal conditions of the experiment specified. In studies by Kigawa and Strang, a detrimental effect of high temperature (60 °C) was found on samples conditioned under very high humidity (100%) and in water (Kigawa and Strang 2011).

Särkinen et al. 2012; Staats et al. 2013; Costa and Roberts 2014; Drábková 2014; Neubig et al. 2014; Yoshida et al. 2014; Bressan et al. 2014; Choi et al. 2015; Xu et al. 2015; Hart et al. 2016; Weiss et al. 2016; Enan et al. 2017; Gutaker et al. 2017; Kuzmina et al. 2017; Shepherd 2017; Bakker 2018; Korpelainen and Pietiläinen 2019; Lang et al. 2019; Latorre et al. 2020; Papalini et al. 2023 and many others.

[15] See the section *Degradation of Genetic Material* in Chap. 3.

[16] See also the chapter *Degradation of Genetic Material* in Chap. 3, especially section *The Impact of Storage Conditions and Historical Preservation Methods on DNA*.

[17] This conclusion did not follow directly from the results presented earlier.

Studies have also been published on the general impact of agents used in the processing and preservation of botanical specimens on their condition. Coradin and Giannasi analysed the effects of various drying methods and the use of fixatives in the field (including biocidal agents such as pentachlorophenol, methyl bromide, and formaldehyde) on the presence of flavonoids (Coradin and Giannasi 1980). The authors employed thin-layer chromatography. The results showed that storing specimens in preservatives leads to the loss or disruption of chemotaxonomic characteristics of the specimens, as well as to misleading colour changes.

A more general line of research, in terms of the material analysed, concerned the impact of various biocides and preservatives on the genetic material of biocultural collections. In these studies, the samples analysed were usually prepared from contemporary materials (Whitten et al. 1999; Williams 1999; Kigawa et al. 2003; Espeland et al. 2010; Kigawa and Strang 2011; Kigawa et al. 2011).[18] Williams's work was based on the analysis of fresh otter skin samples exposed to arsenic, mercuric chloride, sodium chloride, sodium fluorosilicate, formalin, borax, alum (ammonium aluminium sulphate), magnesium carbonate, and potassium nitrate (Williams 1999). In all cases, including the control samples, genetic material degradation was observed. The tests conducted by Whitten, Williams, and Glover were the only ones in this group that actually concerned herbarium specimens and aimed to determine whether fumigation with sulfuryl fluoride destroys DNA (Williams 1999). Analysis of four-year-old specimens after fumigation showed that comparable extraction and amplification of genetic material was possible. The authors assessed the fumigant as safe. Kigawa's studies (Kigawa et al. 2003), as well as those by Kigawa and Strang (2011) and Kigawa et al. (2011), involved analyses of samples mainly of protein origin (chicken muscle, fungi, animal glue, silk) subjected to various fumigants. These studies demonstrated the destructive effect of methyl bromide, methyl iodide, ethylene oxide, propylene oxide, and their mixtures on the DNA of the tested samples, especially muscle tissue. The study by Kigawa et al. showed that sulfuryl fluoride disrupts protein structure (Kigawa et al. 2011). In their analysis of the impact of dichlorvos, naphthalene, and paradichlorobenzene on the genetic material of housefly specimens prepared 3 weeks earlier, Espeland et al. demonstrated the destructive effect of dichlorvos, while the other two agents were considered safe, at least after the applied 20-month exposure (Espeland et al. 2010).

Research has also been conducted on the impact of specific conservation treatments on the genetic material of invertebrates, PCR product DNA, and Egyptian animal mummies (Carter 2003; Eklund 2007; Eklund and Thomas 2010). Carter carried out a study on freshly collected specimens of the common woodlouse (*Porcellio scaber*), which were subjected to various preservation fluids: ethanol; 4% formaldehyde; denatured alcohol with additives such as ethyl acetate, propylene glycol, ethoxyethanol; Steedman's solution (a mixture of formaldehyde,

[18] The origin of the term "biocultural collections", which also includes the category of ethnographic or, alternatively, ethnobiological collections, economic botany objects and others, is discussed in the section *Ethical and Legal Issues Related to Herbarium Collections* in Chap. 1.

phenoxyethanol, and propylene glycol), for periods ranging from 1 to 24 months, depending on the preservative used (Carter 2003). The study confirmed the destructive effect of ethyl acetate and ethoxyethanol on DNA. Analysis of samples preserved in formaldehyde showed that storage in this preservative did not allow for sufficient extraction of genetic material. Denatured alcohol, although it enabled extraction, yielded only a limited amount of DNA.

Eklund primarily conducted *in vitro* analyses on DNA material contained in ready-made PCR products of defined length, assuming that such a base material would transparently allow for the assessment of the tested agents' effects (Eklund 2007). This objective required testing exclusively liquid-form materials, with numerous modifications compared to the originally intended concentrations. She regarded the *in vitro* study as a screening test, since the actual impact of the materials depends, among other factors, on the type of tissue subjected to conservation (Eklund 2012). The selection of materials for testing was based on a literature review. The chosen materials mainly concerned the conservation of zoological and palaeontological specimens (bone, skin, hair), but also included substances commonly used in the conservation and preservation of other heritage objects, both historically and at present. The tested agents included, among others, biocides such as arsenic, carbon tetrachloride, and mercuric chloride, as well as other substances like hydrogen peroxide, sodium hypochlorite, acrylic adhesive, polyvinyl acetate, gum arabic, alcohol, acetone, and ethyl acetate. Following comprehensive analyses of the data obtained from the studies, the author classified the use of acetone, denatured alcohol and their mixture, amyl acetate, arsenic, chloroform, sodium chloride, toluene, trichloroethylene, and xylene as safe procedures. Furthermore, unlike Carter, she classified ethyl acetate as safe for DNA. The results also suggested that, within this group, amyl acetate, denatured alcohol, and sodium chloride may possess DNA-preserving properties. Many of the remaining procedures were assessed as ambiguous, while others were deemed unequivocally destructive (e.g. mercuric chloride and oxidising agents also used as bleaches).[19]

The author also analysed of hair from ancient Egyptian cat mummies and a modern Egyptian rabbit mummy, to determine the impact of mummification as a conservation procedure on DNA. The genetic material from the ancient mummies proved too degraded to allow for further amplification, whereas the material extracted from the five-year-old rabbit mummy was well preserved. Since, in PCR product tests, the author examined the effects of substances used in mummification—namely ethanol, sodium carbonate, sodium bicarbonate, and sodium chloride—which she assessed as safe or relatively safe for DNA, she expected to obtain genetic material from all the mummies. In her summary, she emphasised that the research failure may indicate unfavourable storage conditions or conservation treatments, about which, despite her efforts, she was unable to obtain specific information.

[19] See also the sections *The Impact of Storage Conditions and Preservation Methods on DNA* in Chap. 3.

Eklund's work also raises valid considerations about the problem of defining and distinguishing treatments performed on objects (Eklund 2007, pp. 38–46). The authors of the previously cited studies, when listing the treatments whose impact on DNA was subsequently analysed, usually referred to them as *conservation* and *preservation*, although from today's perspective these procedures have been excluded from the conservator's repertoire. These include the use of most biocidal agents or, in the case of paper conservation, strongly oxidising bleaches. The properties of various synthetic adhesives, including those from the poly(vinyl acetate) group and their impact on the condition of heritage objects, have also been discussed for years (e.g. Down et al. 1996; Down 2014, 2016).[20] Natural adhesives, on the other hand, pose a risk in the form of genetic material contamination (Bower et al. 2010; Eklund 2012). A separate issue is who carries out or has carried out these treatments. Preventive measures and simple repairs in particular were very often performed by technical staff or specialists with backgrounds other than conservation. This was frequently associated with a different perception of collection care issues and the use of materials not accepted by conservators. Terminological problems also concern the queries themselves, as researchers often encounter a lack of documentation or poor documentation, and even if they do find a list of materials used for repairs or conservation, in many cases, these are no longer available on the market, or their composition has changed. Knowledge of the object's history, storage conditions, and past conservation treatments can help estimate which objects are "promising" as sources of genetic material.

In the field of herbarium specimens, research concerning the impact of preservation and conservation methods on the integrity of genetic material has, as previously mentioned, focused on the effects of temperature and relative humidity (Adams 2011), as well as the use of biocidal agents, including alcohol and formalin (Whitten et al. 1999; Särkinen et al. 2012; Bressan et al. 2014). Many authors, in publications not entirely devoted to the study of the harmfulness of these agents, have noted the destructive impact of alcohol and formalin on the genetic material of specimens (Staats et al. 2013). This group also includes studies on the kinetics of degradation described by Weiss et al. (2016).

Accelerated ageing studies of herbarium specimens conducted by the author confirmed that exposure of specimens to elevated temperatures has a destructive effect on their genetic material (Grenda-Kurmanow 2021a, pp. 207–349). As part of research into the impact of conservation materials on the genetic material of specimens, an accelerated ageing experiment was carried out using leaf samples of *Arabidopsis thaliana* and *Fragaria vesca*. The leaves were first prepared as herbarium specimens by drying them between blotting papers. Fragments of the leaves were then placed in a climate chamber allowing for the regulation of temperature and relative humidity. Accelerated ageing was conducted under conditions of fluctuating relative humidity (25–75%) at a constant temperature. The experiment was performed in cycles at temperatures of 40 °C and 60 °C. Subsequent samples were

[20] See also the section *Adhesives Used Historically and in Contemporary Practice* in Chap. 2.

removed from the chamber after 2, 4, 8, 14, and 28 days in each cycle. The results of DNA isolation from samples aged at different temperatures showed that at 60 °C, the genetic material degraded more rapidly, yielding noticeably shorter fragments after 8 days and undergoing almost complete destruction after 28 days. In contrast, for the group exposed to the lower temperature, it was possible to isolate genetic material from samples at every stage of ageing (Grenda-Kurmanow 2021a, pp. 207–349).

This result was used as the basis for further research, in which analogous samples with applied adhesives, and in one case a deacidification agent, were subjected to ageing at 40 °C. The adhesives were selected based on a literature review and the results of an international survey conducted among conservators and curators of herbarium collections (Grenda-Kurmanow 2021b). In total, 20 different materials were tested: poly(vinyl acetates): Hewit M218, Jade 403, Evacon-R; acrylic adhesives: Lascaux 303 HV mixed with Lascaux 498 HV; cellulose ethers: Tylose MH 300 and MH 1000, hydroxypropylcelluloses: Klucel G and Klucel E; starch adhesives from wheat and rice starch; ethulose; gum arabic; protein-based adhesives: hide glue, isinglass, and gelatine; as well as Aquazol adhesive [poly(2-ethyl-2-oxazoline, PEOX)]. As in the first experiment, the samples were subjected to PCR analyses at various stages of ageing. The interpretation of the results was based on the assessment of the quantity and quality of genetic material after accelerated ageing, in relation to control samples. The study included analysis of the efficiency of genetic material isolation, contamination of samples with organic compounds and proteins, assessment of the degree of DNA degradation in plant specimens at different stages of ageing by analysing the length of isolated molecules, and analysis of the effectiveness of individual samples as templates in PCR. Additionally, the degree of degradation was analysed using a 2100 Agilent Bioanalyser.

The study identified issues with the isolation of genetic material in samples coated with PVA adhesives and reduced DNA concentrations in samples treated with Klucel E. Subtle degradative changes were also observed in most samples to which selected materials were applied, representing all groups of adhesives commonly used for specimen mounting and conservation. The research further demonstrated that the resistance of herbarium specimens to the applied accelerated ageing conditions and the effects of the applied materials may be species-dependent, which further complicates the assessment of the safety of agents used in conservation and technical repairs of herbaria with regard to entire collections.

It was not possible to unequivocally assess any of the materials studied as absolutely safe, indicating that further, more advanced research in this area is required. The results confirm that, as Jane Down stated over 20 years ago, "the perfect adhesive for herbarium collections is still elusive" (Down 1999 p. 221). One of the adhesives used in the experiment described above has since been withdrawn from the market and replaced with another "neutral" adhesive. This confirms the previously described issue regarding the availability of information on the composition and performance of materials used in conservation, as well as the fact that research does not keep pace with changes in production. An unfavourable result was also obtained for the surface-acting deacidification agent Bookkeeper, a popular product used for non-aqueous deacidification of paper-based objects (Grenda-Kurmanow 2021b, pp. 207–349). This raises the question of the safe pH range for the environments in which herbaria are stored. As mentioned earlier, the most widely accepted and intuitive solution is to maintain a neutral pH in collections[21]; however, a precise evaluation of the impact of pH on the condition of herbarium collections, with particular emphasis on historical genetic material, requires further research. The appropriate environmental pH can be maintained by using acid-free materials made from α-cellulose for packaging, labels, and inventory tags.[22] Materials used for any repairs (mounting, backing, infilling) should also be of conservation, archival or museum quality, meaning high fibre quality that ensures the long-term stability of these materials and safety of the historical objects. These materials are often marked with standards for durability and quality.[23] Such materials include papers produced by traditional methods, such as handmade papers made from long-fibre plant materials.[24]

The research results, however, enabled the preliminary development of a safe methodology for the conservation of historic herbaria.[25] As a result, adhesives from the Aquazol group[26] were selected as relatively safe materials for conservation treatments involving direct contact with specimens. Aquazols [poly(2-ethyl-2-oxazoline), PEOX] are a group of adhesives patented in 1977 by Dow Chemical; they are available in versions corresponding to different molecular weights: 50,000 (Aquazol 50), 200,000 (Aquazol 200), and 500,000 (Aquazol 500), which affects their penetration capacity (Down 2015, pp. 97–98). Aquazol, used in conservation as a consolidant, was recommended in 2011 for treatments on paper-based objects. It is soluble in a variety of solvents (including water, acetone, ethanol, and isopropanol), is thermally stable, and non-toxic (Ibidem). It forms flexible films that do not discolour over time, do not become brittle, and are not susceptible to microbiological infection. Its viscosity decreases with ageing. It is sensitive to elevated relative humidity, which weakens its adhesive strength. Rice starch paste made from purified starch was also assessed as a stable adhesive. As it is a natural adhesive, its use was accepted only for treatments that did not involve direct contact with the specimen, to avoid contamination.

The studies described, although they do not provide a definitive answer regarding the preservation and conservation of herbaria, have been cited to broaden

---

[21] See the section *Stable Climatic Conditions* in Chap. 4.

[22] See also the chapter *Physicochemical Characteristics of the Basic Components of Herbarium Structures* in Chap. 2.

[23] E.g. ISO 9706 and ISO 16245 standards. However, it should be noted that these standards allow for a high pH level in cellulosic materials (pH in the range 7.5–10).

[24] In the conservation of historic objects on paper substrates, Japanese papers produced today as well as papers made using traditional Western methods are used for this purpose.

[25] Examples of the application of this methodology are described in Chap. 5. *Herbarium Conservation in Practice—Three Visions of Ethical Conservation of Historical Herbaria*

[26] See examples of application described in Chap. 5. *Herbarium Conservation in Practice—Three Visions of Ethical Conservation of Historical Herbaria.*

knowledge of this issue among those who have a direct impact on the management of collections.

References

Ackery PR, Testa JM, Ready PD, Doyle AM, Pinniger DB (2004) Effects of high temperature pest eradication on DNA in entomological collections. Stud Conserv 49(1):35–40

Adams RP (2011) DNA from herbarium specimens: II. Correlation of DNA degradation with humidity. Phytologia 93:351–359

Adams RP, Sharma LN (2010) DNA from herbarium specimens: I. Correlation of DNA size with specimen age. Phytologia 92:346–353

American Society of Heating, Refrigerating and Air-Conditioning Engineers (ASHRAE) (2019) Museums, libraries and archives. In: ASHRAE handbook: heating, ventilating and air-conditioning: applications. ASHRAE, Atlanta, pp 24.1–24.43

Ames M, Spooner DM (2008) DNA from herbarium specimens settles a controversy about origins of the European potato. Am J Bot 95:252–257. https://doi.org/10.3732/ajb.95.2.252

Ball MD, Bisulca C, Odegaard N (2011) Assessment of the Thermo-Lignum oven pest eradication treatment on natural and synthetic polymers and resins. In: Winsor P, Pinniger D, Bacon L, Child B, Harris K, Lauder D, Phippard J, Xavier-Rowe A (eds) Integrated pest management for collections. Proceedings of 2011: a Pest Odyssey, 10 years later. English Heritage, London, pp 107–114

Bower MA, Campana MG, Checkley-Scott C, Knight B, Howe CJ (2010) The potential for extraction and exploitation of DNA from parchment: a review of the opportunities and hurdles. J Inst Conserv 33(1):1–11. https://doi.org/10.1080/19455220903509937

Bratasz Ł (2013) Allowable microclimatic variations in museums and historic buildings: reviewing the guidelines. In: Climate for collections. Standards and uncertainties. Archetype Publications, Doerner Institut, London, pp 11–19

Bressan EA, Rossi ML, Gerald LT, Figueira A (2014) Extraction of high-quality DNA from ethanol-preserved tropical plant tissues. BMC Res Notes 7(1):268. https://doi.org/10.1186/1756-0500-7-268

Bridson D, Forman L (1999) The herbarium handbook. Royal Botanic Gardens, Kew

Bakker FT (2018) Herbarium genomics: plant archival DNA explored. In: Lindqvist C, Rajora OP (eds) Paleogenomics, population genomics. Springer. https://doi.org/10.1007/13836_2018_40

Brown TA (1999) Chapter 6: genetic material. In: Carter D, Walker A (eds) Care and conservation of natural history collections. Butterworth Heinemann, Oxford, pp 133–138

Brown TA (2018) Genomes 4. Garland Science, New York/London

Carter JD (2003) The effects of preservation and conservation treatments on the DNA of museum invertebrate fluids preserved collections. Dissertation,. University of Wales

Collins C (2014) Standards in the care of botanical materials http://conservation.myspecies.info/node/35. Accessed 21 Jan 2026

Choi J, Lee H, Shipunov A (2015) All that is gold does not glitter? Age, taxonomy, and ancient plant DNA quality. PeerJ 3:e1087. https://doi.org/10.7717/peerj.1087

Coradin L, Giannasi DE (1980) The effects of chemical preservations on plant collections to be used in chemotaxonomic surveys. Taxon 29(1):33–40. https://doi.org/10.2307/1219594

Costa CM, Roberts RP (2014) Techniques for improving the quality and quantity of DNA extracted from herbarium specimens. Phyton 48:1–8

Dabney J, Meyer M, Pääbo S (2013) Ancient DNA damage. Cold Spring Harb Perspect Biol 5(7):a012567. https://doi.org/10.1101/cshperspect.a012567

Davies N (2023) Specimen storage. Environmental conditions. In: Davies NMJ, Drinkell C, Utteridge TMA (eds) The herbarium handbook. Kew Publishing, Kew, pp 182–183

Down JL, MacDonald MA, Tétreault J, Williams RS (1996) Adhesive testing at the Canadian conservation institute: an evaluation of selected poly(vinyl acetate) and acrylic adhesives. Stud Conserv 41(1):19–44. https://doi.org/10.1179/sic.1996.41.1.19

Down J (1999) Adhesive research at the Canadian conservation institute as it relates to herbarium collections. In: Metsger DA, Byers SC (eds) Managing the modern herbarium—an interdisciplinary approach. SPNHC, Ontario, pp 205–223

Down JL (2014) The evaluation of selected poly(vinyl acetate) and acrylic adhesives: a final research update. Stud Conserv 60(1):33–54. https://doi.org/10.1179/2047058414Y.0000000129

Down J (2015) Adhesive compendium for conservation. Ontario: Canadian Conservation Institute

Down JL (2016) The effect of modifiers on the stability of a vinyl acetate/ethylene copolymer dispersion. Stud Conserv 61(1):26–45. https://doi.org/10.1179/2047058414Y.0000000130

Drábková L (2014) DNA extraction from herbarium specimens. In: Besse P (ed) Molecular plant taxonomy. Springer, New York, pp 69–84

Drábková L, Kirschner J, Vlĉek Ĉ (2002) Comparison of seven DNA extraction and amplification protocols in historical herbarium specimens of Juncaceae. Plant Mol Biol Report 20:161–175. https://doi.org/10.1007/BF02799431

Drobnik J (2009) Zielnik i zielnikoznawstwo. Wydawnictwo Naukowe PWN, Warszawa

Eklund JA (2007) The effects of preparation and conservation treatments on DNA., PhD Dissertation,. University of London

Eklund JA (2012) The possible effects of preparation and conservation treatments on DNA research, using treatments for basketry as a case study. J Inst Conserv 35(1):92–102. https://doi.org/10.1080/19455224.2012.681614

Eklund JA, Thomas MG (2010) Assessing the effects of conservation treatments on short sequences of DNA in vitro. J Archaeol Sci 37(11):2831–2841. https://doi.org/10.1016/j.jas.2010.06.019

Enan MR, Palakkott AR, Ksiksi TS (2017) DNA barcoding of selected UAE medicinal plant species: a comparative assessment of herbarium and fresh samples. Physiol Molec Biol Plants 23:221–227

Erkens RH, Cross H, Maas JW, Hoenselaar K, Chatrou LW (2008) Assessment of age and greenness of herbarium specimens as predictors for successful extraction and amplification of DNA. Blumea 53:407–428. https://doi.org/10.3767/000651908X608052

Espeland M, Irestedt M, Johanson KA, Akerlund M, Bergh JE, Källersj M (2010) Dichlorvos exposure impedes extraction and amplification of DNA from insects in museum collections. Front Zool 7:2. https://doi.org/10.1186/1742-9994-7-2

Grenda M (2013) Methods of preserving herbarium collections from pests, survey conducted among herbarium institutions, Warsaw

Grenda-Kurmanow M (2021a) Adhesives used in herbaria: current practice with regard to what we know from written sources on mounting herbarium specimens and conservation. Taxon 70:1–15. https://doi.org/10.1002/tax.12413

Grenda-Kurmanow M (2021b) Konserwacja i restauracja zabytkowych zielników a zachowanie jakości materiału genetycznego roślin (Conservation and restoration of historical herbaria and preservation of plant genetic material). PhD Disseration. Akademia Sztuk Pięknych w Warszawie

Gutaker R, Reiter E, Furtwängler A, Schuenemann VJ, Burbano HA (2017) Extraction of ultrashort DNA molecules from herbarium specimens. BioTechniques 62:76–79. https://doi.org/10.2144/000114517

Hall AV (1988) Pest control in herbaria. Taxon 37(4):885–907

Hart ML, Forrest LL, Nicholls JA, Kidner CA (2016) Retrieval of hundreds of nuclear loci from herbarium specimens. Taxon 65(5):1081–1092. https://doi.org/10.12705/655.9

Hawks C, Bell D (1999) Removal of stains caused by mercuric chloride treatments from herbarium sheet labels. In: Bridgeland J (ed) BidICOM committee for conservation preprints, 12th Triennial Meeting Lyon, 29 August–3 September, vol II. James and James, London, pp 723–727

Hill SR (1983) Microwave and the herbarium specimen: potential dangers. Taxon 32:614–615. https://doi.org/10.2307/1221732

Hofreiter M, Serre D, Poinar HN, Kuch M, Pääbo S (2001) Ancient DNA. Nat Rev Genet 2:353–359

IIC/ICOM-CC (2014) Environmental guidelines—IIC and ICOM-CC declaration International Institute for Conservation of Historic and Artistic Works, and ICOM-CC. International Council of Museums Committee for Conservation., https://www.icom-cc.org/en/environmental-guidelines-icom-cc-and-iic-declaration. Accessed: 21 Jan 2026

Kigawa R, Nochide H, Kimura H, Miura S (2003) Effects of various fumigants, thermal methods and carbon dioxide treatment on DNA extraction and amplification: a case study on freeze-dried mushroom and freeze-dried muscle specimens. Collect Forum 18(1–2):74–89

Kigawa R, Strang T (2011) Effects of various fumigants and non-chemical treatments on DNA molecules on proteins: case studies on natural history specimens and proteinaceous components of museum objects. In: Winsor P, Pinniger D, Bacon L, Child B, Harris K, Lauder D, Phippard J, Xavier-Rowe A (eds) Integrated pest management for collections, Proceedings of 2011: a Pest Odyssey, 10 years later. English Heritage, London, pp 115–122

Kigawa R, Strang T, Hayakawa N, Kimura H, Young G (2011) Investigation of effects of fumigants on proteinaceous components of museum objects (muscle, animal glue and silk) in comparison with other non-chemical pest eradicating measures. Stud Conserv 56:196–215. https://doi.org/10.1179/204705811X13110713013272

Korpelainen H, Pietiläinen M (2019) The effects of sample age and taxonomic origin on the success rate of DNA barcoding when using herbarium material. Plant Syst Evol 305:319–324. https://doi.org/10.1007/s00606-019-01568-4

Kuzmina ML, Braukmann TWA, Fazekas AJ, Graham SW, Dewaard SL, Rodrigues A, Bennett BA, Dickinson TA, Saarela JM, Catling PM, Newmaster SG, Percy DM, Fenneman E, Lauron-Moreau A, Ford B, Gillespie L, Subramanyam R, Whitton J, Jennings L, Metsger D, Warne CP, Brown A, Sears E, Dewaard JR, Zakharov EV, Hebert PDN (2017) Using herbarium-derived DNAs to assemble a large-scale DNA barcode library for the vascular-plants of Canada. Appl Plant Sci 5:1700079. https://doi.org/10.3732/apps.1700079

Lander TA, Dadonaite B, Monro AK (2013) Microwave drying of plant material for herbarium specimens and genetic analysis. Taxon 62(4):790–797

Lang PLM, Willems FM, Scheepens JF, Burbano HA, Bossdorf O (2019) Using herbaria to study global environmental change. New Phytol 221(1):110–122. https://doi.org/10.1111/nph.15401

Latorre SM, Lang PLM, Burbano HA, Gutaker RM (2020) Isolation, library preparation, and bioinformatic analysis of historical and ancient plant DNA. Curr Protoc Plant Biol 5:e20121. https://doi.org/10.1002/cppb.20121

Lehtonen S, Christenhusz MJM (2010) Historical herbarium specimens in plant molecular systematics—an example from the fern genus Lindsaea (Lindsaeaceae). Biologia 65(2):204–208. https://doi.org/10.2478/s11756-010-0008-8

Lister D, Bower M, Howe C, Jones M (2008) Extraction and amplification of nuclear DNA from herbarium specimens of emmer wheat: a method for assessing DNA preservation by maximum amplicon length recover. Taxon 57(1):254–258

Merrill E (1948) On the control of destructive insects in the herbarium. J Arnold Arbor 29(1):103–110

Michalski S (2007) The ideal climate, risk management, the ASHRAE chapter, proofed fluctuations, and toward a full risk analysis model. In: Experts' roundtable on sustainable climate management strategies, Tenerife

Michalski S (2016) Climate guidelines for heritage collections: where we are in 2014 and how we got here. In: Summit on the museum preservation environment. Smithsonian Institution Scholarly Press, Washington, D.C, pp 7–32

Molak M, Ho SYW (2011) Evaluating the impact of post-mortem damage in ancient DNA: a theoretical approach. J Mol Evol 73(3–4):244–255. https://doi.org/10.1007/s00239-011-9474-z

Moore A, Woodgyer E (2023) Pest management. In: Davies NMJ, Drinkell C, Utteridge TMA (eds) The herbarium handbook. Kew Publishing, Kew, pp 194–209

MuseumPests Working Group. www.museumpests.net. Accessed 13 Jan 2026

Neubig KM, Whitten WM, Abbott JR, Elliott S, Soltis DE, Soltis PS (2014) Variables affecting DNA preservation in archival DNA specimens. In: Applequist WL, Campbell LM (eds) DNA banking in the 21st century: proceedings of the U.S. workshop on DNA banking. The William L. Brown Center at the Missouri Botanical Garde, St. Louis, pp 81–136

Odegaard N (2001) Methods to mitigate risks from use of contaminated objects, including methods to decontaminate affected objects. Collect Forum 17(1–2):117–121

Odegaard N, Zimmt WS (2008) Pesticide removal studies for cultural objects. In: Dignard C, Helwig K, Mason J, Nanowin K, Stone T (eds) Preserving aboriginal heritage: technical and traditional approaches. Canadian Conservation Institute, Ottawa

Papalini S et al (2023) Challenges and opportunities behind the use of herbaria in paleogenomics studies. Plants 12(19):3452. https://doi.org/10.3390/plants12193452

Pfister A-L (2008) L'influence des biocides sur la conservations de Naturalia, HEAA Arc, Filière conservation-restauration, orientation objets archéologiques et ethnographiques. Dissertation. Hautes écoles spécialisées de Suisse Occidentale

Pinniger DB (2011) Ten years on–from vodka beetle to risk zones. In: Winsor P, Pinniger D, Bacon L, Child B, Harris K, Lauder D, Phippard J, Xavier-Rowe A (eds) Integrated pest management for collections, Proceedings of 2011: A Pest Odyssey, 10 years later. English Heritage, London, pp 1–9

Pinniger DB (2015) Pest management in museums, archives and historic houses. Archetype Publications, London

Purewal V (2001) The identification of four persistent and hazardous residues present on historic plant collections housed within the National Museum and Gallery of Wales. Collect Forum 16(1–2):77–86

Purewal V (2012) Novel detection and removal of hazardous biocide residues historically apllied to herbaria. PhD dissertation,. University of Lincoln

Pyle M, Adams R (1989) In situ preservation of DNA in plant specimens. Taxon 38(4):576–581. https://doi.org/10.2307/1222632

Rogers SO, Bendich AJ (1985) Extraction of DNA from milligram amounts of fresh, herbarium and mummified plant tissues. Plant Mol Biol 5(2):69–76. https://doi.org/10.1007/BF00020088. PMID: 24306565

Salick J, Solomon J (2014) Herbarium curation of biocultural plant collections and vouchers. In: Salick J, Konchar K, Nesbitt M (eds) Curating biocultural collections: a handbook. Royal Botanic Gardens, Kew, pp 43–54

Savolainen V, Cuénoud P, Spichiger R, Martinez MD, Crèvecoeur M, Manen JF (1995) The use of herbarium specimens in DNA phylogenetics: evaluation and improvement. Plant Syst Evol 197:87–98. https://doi.org/10.1007/BF00984634

Särkinen T, Staats M, Richardson JE, Cowan RS, Bakker FT (2012) How to open the treasure chest? Optimising DNA extraction from herbarium specimens. PLoS One 7(8):e43808. https://doi.org/10.1371/journal.pone.0043808

Shepherd LD (2017) A non-destructive DNA sampling technique for herbarium specimens. PLoS One 12(8):e0183555. https://doi.org/10.1371/journal.pone.0183555

Staats M, Cuenca A, Richardson JE, Ginkel RV, Petersen G, Sebery O, Bakker FT (2011) DNA damage in plant herbarium tissue. PLoS One 6:e28448. https://doi.org/10.1371/journal.pone.0028448

Staats M, Erkens RHJ, van de Vossenberg B, Wieringa JJ, Kraaijeveld K, Stielow B (2013) Genomic treasure troves: complete genome sequencing of herbarium and insect museum specimens. PLoS One 8(7):e69189. https://doi.org/10.1371/journal.pone.0069189

Strang TJK (1992) A review of published temperatures for the control of pest insects in museums. Collect Forum 8(2):41–67

Strang TJK (1995) The effect of thermal methods of pest control on museum collections. In: 3rd international conference on biodeterioration of cultural property, 4–7 July 1995, Bangkok. Organizing Committee of ICBCP-3, Bangkok, pp 199–212

Strang TJK (1996) Preventing infestations: control strategies and detection methods, Canadian Conservation Institute (CCI) Notes 3/1. Canadian Conservation Institute, Ottawa

Strang TJK (1997) Controlling insect pests with low temperature. Canadian Conservation Institute (CCI) Notes 3/3. Canadian Conservation Institute, Ottawa

Strang TJK (1999a) A healthy dose of the past: a future direction in herbarium pest control? In: Metsger DA, Byers SC (eds) Managing the modern herbarium—an interdisciplinary approach. SPNHC, Ontario, pp 59–80

Strang TJK (1999b) Sensitivity of seeds in herbarium collections to storage conditions, and implications for thermal insect pest control methods. In: Metsger DA, Byers SC (eds) Managing the modern herbarium—an interdisciplinary approach. SPNHC, Ontario, pp 81–102

Strang TJK (2001) Principles of heat disinfestation. In: Kingsley H, Pinniger D, Xavier-Rowe A, Winsor P (eds) Integrated pest management for collections. Proceedings of 2001 A pest odyssey. James & James, pp 114–129

Strang TJK (2012) Studies in pest control for cultural property. PhD dissertation,. Göteborgs Universitet

Taylor JW, Swann EC (1994) DNA from herbarium specimen. In: Hermann B, Hummel S (eds) Ancient DNA. Recovery and analysis of genetic material from paleontological, archaeological, museum, medical, and forensic specimens. Springer Verlag, pp 166–181

Tello H, Jelen E, Unger A (2005) Decontamination of ethnological objects with supercritical carbon dioxide. Collect Forum 19(1–2):45–48

Townsend J (1999) Preventive conservation: concept and strategy for long-term preservation. In: Metsger DA, Byers SC (eds) Managing the modern herbarium—an interdisciplinary approach. SPNHC, Ontario, pp 23–35

Querner P, Simon S (2011) Developing and implementing an integrated pest management concept in the large collections of the National Museums in Berlin. In: Winsor P, Pinniger D, Bacon L, Child B, Harris K, Lauder D, Phippard J, Xavier-Rowe A (eds) Integrated pest management for collections, Proceedings of 2011: A Pest Odyssey, 10 years later. English Heritage, London, pp 38–45

Weiss CL, Schuenemann VJ, Devos J, Shirsekar G, Reiter E, Gould BA, Stinchcombe JR, Krause J, Burbano HA (2016) Temporal patterns of damage and decay kinetics of DNA retrieved from plant herbarium specimens. R Soc Open Sci 3:160239. https://doi.org/10.1098/rsos.160239

Whitten WM, Williams NH, Glover KV (1999) Sulphuryl fluoride fumigation: effect on DNA extraction and amplification from herbarium specimens. Taxon 48(3):507–510

Williams SL (1999) Destructive preservation: a review of the effect of standard preservation practices on the future use of natural history collections, PhD dissertation, Goteborg studies in conservation 6. Acta Universitatis Gothoburgensis, Goteborg

Xu C, Dong W, Shi S, Cheng T, Li C, Liu Y, Wu P, Wu H, Gao P, Zhou S (2015) Accelerating plant DNA barcode reference library construction using herbarium specimens: improved experimental techniques. Molec Ecol Res 15:1366–1374. https://doi.org/10.1111/1755-0998.12413

Yoshida K, Burbano HA, Krause J, Thines M, Weigel D, Kamoun S (2014) Mining herbaria for plant pathogen genomes: back to the future. PLoS Pathog 10(4):e1004028. https://doi.org/10.1371/journal.ppat.1004028

Chapter 5
Herbarium Conservation in Practice—Three Visions of Ethical Conservation of Historical Herbaria

Abstract This chapter outlines the conservation-restoration methodology for historic herbaria, developed on the basis of archival queries and technical analysis, performed on three bound eighteenth-century herbaria from Polish collections: the herbarium of Izabela Czartoryska (1746), held in the collections of the National Museum in Kraków/Princes Czartoryski Library; the herbarium of Johann Friedrich Zeidler (1732), from the Main Library of the University of Life Sciences in Lublin; and the herbarium attributed to Helwing or Boretius, from the Herbarium of the Faculty of Biology at the University of Warsaw (1724–1745). For each object, the principles of a safe conservation methodology were defined, encompassing non--invasive or micro-destructive analytical studies and technical solutions of physical intervention in the structure of the objects. The outcomes of the conservation treatments carried out are also presented.

Keywords Conservation of herbaria · Bound herbaria · Non-aqueous treatment · Deacidification · Consolidation of specimens · Specimen deformation

As demonstrated in the preceding chapters, historical herbaria are highly technologically complex objects, in which the paper substrate is combined with a variety of botanical specimens. They also contain numerous additional elements, such as materials used to mount the specimens, including various adhesives or other substances, as well as manuscript or printed elements and structural components made from different materials. Furthermore, herbaria may be contaminated with toxic biocidal substances or bear traces of additional preparatory treatments performed in the past, the presence of which is often impossible to predict, as they are rarely documented in any way. Due to this complexity, herbaria present a complicated and specific set of conservation challenges, and each object requires a highly individual approach.

This chapter presents safe conservation strategies for historic herbaria, in accordance with current knowledge. The objects described in this section illustrate various aspects of conservation issues. At the same time, they are among the oldest and most valuable of their kind in Polish collections: the herbarium owned by Izabela Czartoryska, dated 1746, from the collections of the Czartoryski Library/National

M. Grenda-Kurmanow, *Herbaria*, https://doi.org/10.1007/978-3-032-21904-6_5

Museum in Kraków; the herbarium of Johann Friedrich Zeidler from 1732, from the collections of the Main Library of the University of Life Sciences in Lublin; and the herbarium attributed to Helwing or Boretius from the years 1724–1745, from the Herbarium of the Faculty of Biology, University of Warsaw (WA). Each of these objects required slightly different solutions due to the specific nature of their construction and condition.

Prior to commencing conservation treatments, a technical analysis was carried out. All three herbaria were suspected of containing biocidal substances, which were commonly used in natural history collections. As mentioned in the section *Damage Caused by the Use of Biocidal Agents* (Chap. 3), many of these substances constitute persistent contaminants within objects, detectable even after several centuries. Consequently, it was deemed necessary to examine all three herbaria for the presence of biocides. The aim was to assess safety both when working during conservation treatment and in the future use of the collections. As already noted in the section *Decontamination of Collections Treated with Biocides* (Chap. 4), none of the decontamination methods is fully effective; therefore, if an object has previously been treated with biocidal agents, it may still pose a risk to users upon return to the owner, even with the best efforts during any attempted decontamination. The priority was to employ, as far as possible, non-invasive methods that would provide the broadest possible knowledge regarding potential contamination of the object.[1]

For the identification of metals present in objects from natural history and ethnographic collections, a variety of spectroscopic (spectrometric) methods have long been employed (Palmer 2001; Sirois 2001; Sirois and Sansoucy 2001; Purewal 2001, 2012; Pfister 2008; Salmo et al. 2017; Marcotte et al. 2014). These include atomic spectroscopy methods such as atomic absorption spectrophotometry (AAS), atomic emission spectroscopy (AES), and their derivatives. AAS is based on the absorption of radiation, the type (wavelength) of which is specific to each metal. The ability to measure the emission of such radiation for the identification of metals is utilised in AES. Variants of AAS include flame atomic absorption spectrophotometry (FAAS) and graphite furnace atomic absorption spectrophotometry (GFAAS). Variants of AES include inductively coupled plasma atomic emission spectroscopy (ICP-AES) and microwave plasma-atomic emission spectrometry (MP-AES). For the detection of biocides, inductively coupled plasma mass spectrometry (ICP-MS) is also used. All these analyses require sampling.

For the analysis of biocidal substances based on inorganic compounds, polarising microscopy, scanning electron microscopy (SEM), as well as a range of methods utilising X-ray radiation were also employed: radiography, scanning electron microscopy with X-ray emission spectrometry (SEM-XES), energy dispersive X-ray spectroscopy (EDS, EDX or EDAX), X-ray photoelectron spectroscopy

[1] In the case of biocides forming crystalline deposits, it is possible to collect a sample without damaging the object. Studies have also been conducted on dust collected from the object (Pfister 2008), as well as by taking a sample through rubbing the object's surface with cotton wool (Palmer 2001; Sirois 2001). However, in the objects under consideration, no characteristic deposits were present.

(XPS), SEM microanalysis (e.g. SEM-EDX), particle/proton induced X-ray emission (PIXE), secondary ion mass spectrometry (SIMS), X-ray diffraction (XRD), and X-ray fluorescence (XRF). The latter method enables elemental analysis of an object without the need to take a sample. The examination can be carried out using a portable device by touching the surface of the object. In the micro version (Ma-XRF), it is possible to perform the analysis without touching the surface of the object.

In addition to the techniques mentioned above, Fourier transform infrared spectroscopy (FTIR) and chromatographic methods—high-performance liquid chromatography (HPLC) and gas chromatography with mass spectrometry (GC/MS)—are also used, primarily for the analysis of organic compounds and a limited number of inorganic compounds. GC/MS in combination with solid-phase microextraction (GC/MS-SPME) enables the passive collection of volatile organic compounds (VOCs) from an object and allows for analysis without taking a physical sample. For objects containing plant material, studies using similar techniques have been conducted in conservation projects involving herbaria and in ethnographic collections (e.g. Dauwalder 2012; Ormsby et al. 2006; Palmer et al. 2003).

As mentioned above, most of the research methods listed require sampling from the object. This does not pose a problem when the poison leaves a trace in the form of crystalline deposits. A sample collected by contact, through rubbing, can also be used for testing. However, in cases where no deposits are present on the object and there is uncertainty as to which area contains visible biocide residues, non-invasive methods that enable the identification of biocidal agents may provide a solution. Therefore, for the technical analysis of herbaria in this project, it was decided to employ Ma-XRF and GC/MS-SPME techniques. These methods also offer additional advantages, described below, which were utilised in the analysis of the objects under consideration.

Ma-XRF assists in identifying the presence of inorganic compounds, particularly those containing heavy metal ions such as mercury, arsenic, and lead. The XRF scanner enables imaging of the entire area of the object, allowing for the determination of the distribution of contaminants, which cannot be analysed using point-based examination with a portable XRF device. This is of particular importance when detecting the presence of biocidal substances, which may have been applied to the specimens themselves, to the mounting substrate, or added to the adhesive used to attach the specimens. Furthermore, contamination with a biocide, even if it is known to have been applied to the specimen, migrates over time into the porous structure of the paper, making it difficult to predict in advance where it is currently located within the object (Purewal 2012, p. 25).

The Ma-XRF examination is performed by placing the object on the scanner table[2] and positioning it as flat as possible in order to achieve the highest possible mapping resolution (Figs. 5.1 and 5.2).

[2] Analysis with M6 JetStream scanner by Bruker-Nano GmbH, equipped with a rhodium (Rh) cathode and polycapillary optics, 50 kV/0.6 mA, without a filter. The analyses were conducted by Łukasz Ćwikliński from the Institute of Physics, Nicolaus Copernicus University in Toruń.

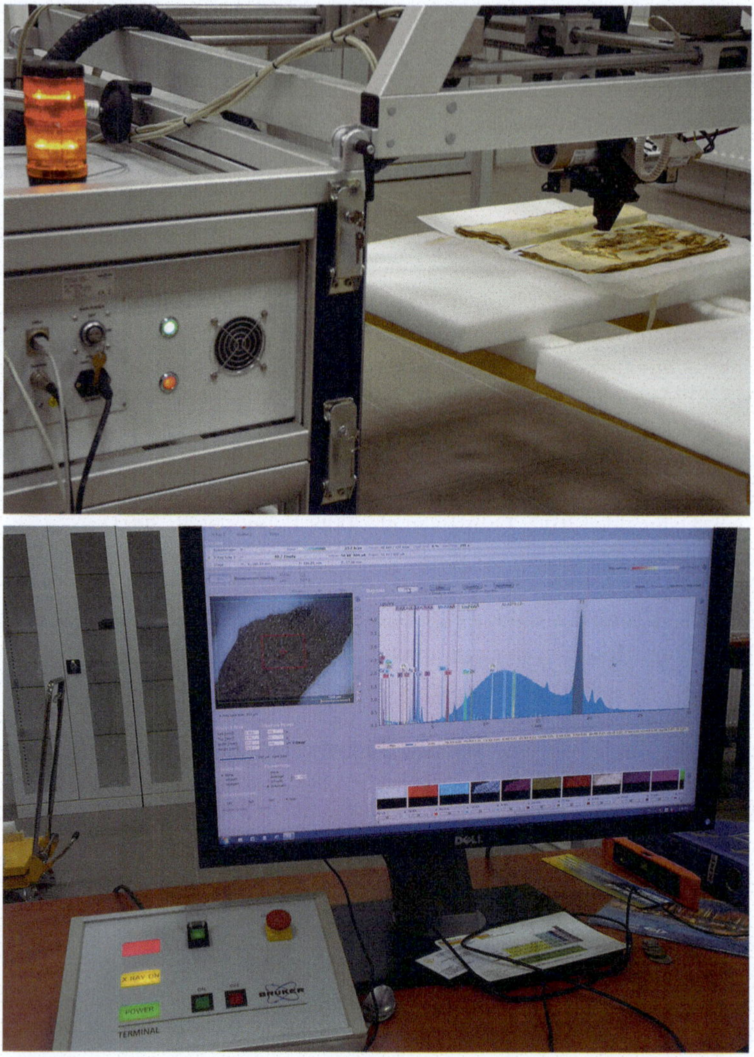

Figs. 5.1 and 5.2 Ma-XRF scanner analysis at the Centre for Modern Interdisciplinary Technologies (ICNT) in Toruń. The object (in this case, the Czartoryska herbarium) is placed in the scanner (Fig. 5.1). Figure 5.2 presents an example analysis of the scanned area. (Photo by M. Grenda-Kurmanow)

Gas chromatography with solid-phase microextraction (GC/MS SPME) enables the collection and identification of volatile organic compounds (VOCs) directly from the object in a non-destructive manner, at the storage site, followed by analysis of the collected sample in the chromatograph. Prior to sampling, the object may be wrapped in aluminium foil to concentrate the present volatile organic compounds. Sampling is performed by inserting a needle with a sorbent between the pages of the

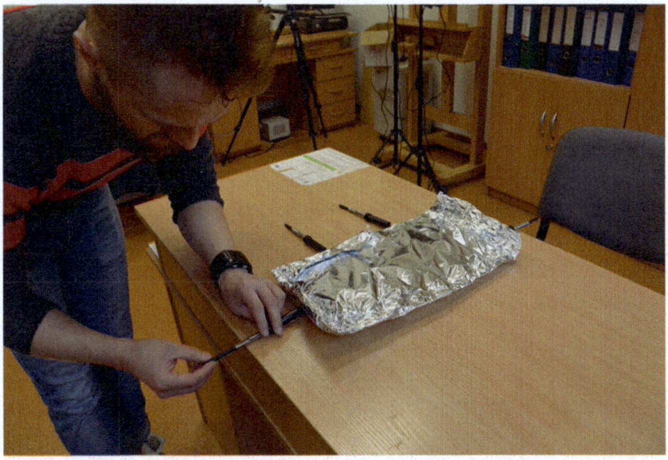

Fig. 5.3 VOCs analysis using GC/MS SPME in Czartoryska herbarium, performed by Prof. Tomasz Sawoszczuk in the National Museum in Kraków. Herbarium is wrapped in aluminum foil, and analysed with needles containing a triple sorbent (DVB/CAR/PDMS) placed between the pages of the volume. (Photo by M. Grenda-Kurmanow)

block (still wrapped in foil) for several hours (Fig. 5.3). Additionally, a reference sample is collected, i.e., VOCs from the gas phase surrounding the objects, using a separately prepared fibre. After removing the needle, securing it, and transporting it to the laboratory, the needle is unsealed and placed in the injector of the gas chromatograph, which then reads the collected sample by desorbing the fibre.[3]

Ma-XRF also enables preliminary identification of pigments and inks, while GC/MS-SPME can be used for the identification of microbiological volatile organic compounds that serve as markers of mould activity. The biological nature of the objects also precluded the use of the ethylene oxide disinfection method, which was until recently popular in Poland, as this would pose a threat to the genetic material of the plants.[4] The following chapters present the results for each object.

In planning the conservation treatments, the results of preliminary studies on the impact of conservation materials on the genetic material of herbarium specimens were also taken into account.[5] This primarily meant limiting the selection of materials used for mounting specimens and repairing mechanical damage in the paper substrate to two designated types of adhesives: adhesives from the Aquazol group and paste made from purified rice starch. For treatments requiring direct contact

[3] In this study, a sandwich fibre with triple sorbent (Divinylbenzene/Carboxen/Polydimethylsiloxane; DVB/CAR/PDMS) was used. Sampling lasted 4 h. Desorption was carried out at 250 °C for 15 minutes.

[4] See the section *The Impact of Storage Conditions and Historical Preservation Methods on DNA* in Chap. 3.

[5] Summarised in the section *Preservation of Genetic Material in Collections—Studies on the Impact of Preservation and Conservation Methods on aDNA* in Chap. 4.

between the adhesive and the specimen, it was decided to use adhesives from the Aquazol group. However, for repairing the paper substrate, an adhesive more compatible with paper was needed. Since rice starch, as a natural ingredient, may pose a risk of contamination, it was assumed that this adhesive would be used only in cases where it does not come into direct contact with the botanical specimen. Such procedures included mounting specimens using strips with adhesive applied only to the ends of the strips, as well as filling losses in the paper substrate of the sheets, when Aquazol would not provide an effective bond. The remaining conservation activities and treatment plans were determined in consultation with each owner of the objects, taking into account their individual needs and the planned policy for the use of the object.

5.1 Izabela Czartoryska Herbarium, 1746, National Museum in Kraków, Ref. Rkps 2782[6]

5.1.1 Description

The 1746 herbarium was a natural history exhibit in the extensive collection of Princess Izabela Czartoryska, née Flemming. The object is listed in the printed catalogue of the Princess's collection, published in 1828, which was displayed in the Gothic House in Puławy (Czartoryska 1828, p. 99). It is not known who compiled the herbarium or precisely how it came into Czartoryska's possession. An inscription on one of the pages suggests that the plants may have been collected in the vicinity of Lublin, although the paper used for the sheets originates from Żukowo near Kartuzy (Pomeranian Voivodeship) (Piekiełko 1977).

The herbarium is a modest, single-section booklet containing 30 sheets with specimens of 26 species attached to them. The plants have been adhered to the substrate with starch adhesive.[7] The herbarium includes a title page and two indices at the end of the block, one in Polish and one in Latin. Each specimen is accompanied by an inscription bearing both the Polish and Latin names. Throughout the block, there is handwritten pagination in ink at the centre of the upper edge of the sheets. Secondary pagination, made in pencil in the corners, has also been added to the object. This is visible in the photographs in Piekiełko's 1977 study. A loose sheet, trimmed to a smaller size than the main block, has been inserted between the last sheet and the back cover. In addition, three specimens were added secondarily, lying loose between the sheets, one of which is enclosed in a modern notebook paper

[6] N.n., *Herbarium Vivum…*, [*Izabela Czartoryska Herbarium*], Kraków, National Museum in Kraków, Czartoryski Princes' Library, ref. Rkps 2782, 1746.

[7] GC/MS analysis, performed by Dr. Bartłomiej Witkowski at the Faculty of Chemistry, University of Warsaw.

envelope. The cover of the herbarium consists of a sheet of paper decorated using the ebru technique, adhered to the spine of the section forming the block.

The object was severely damaged. Approximately 70% of the cover was preserved.[8] Many pages exhibited significant losses (Figs. 5.4 and 5.5).

Many specimens have survived only fragmentarily, in a residual form, or have become almost completely detached from the substrate. Accumulated dirt in many areas (Fig. 5.6) and the adhesive used for mounting, most likely in combination with improper storage conditions, facilitated insect infestation. Throughout the object, numerous traces of insect activity were visible as larval tunnels (Fig. 5.7).

The paper has undergone significant deformation in many areas due to stresses caused by the method of mounting the specimens (Fig. 5.8). At the same time, the starch adhesive used to secure the specimens was applied imprecisely and severely degraded. Its thick layer has formed a brown, hard crust, leading to the disintegration of the botanical specimens into numerous cracks (Figs. 5.4, 5.5, 5.7, and 5.8). The adhesive tended to crumble and detach from the paper substrate.

Throughout the object, numerous ink corrosion spots are visible, caused by the catalytic effect of Fe^{2+} ions present in the inks on cellulose degradation (Neevel and Reissland 2005). The most pronounced corrosion is observed at the sites of pagination and textual corrections—these areas contain the highest quantities of ink. Ink migration is particularly evident on folio 29, which contains the *Index Polski* (Fig. 5.9). It is possible that it was initiated by periodic increases in relative

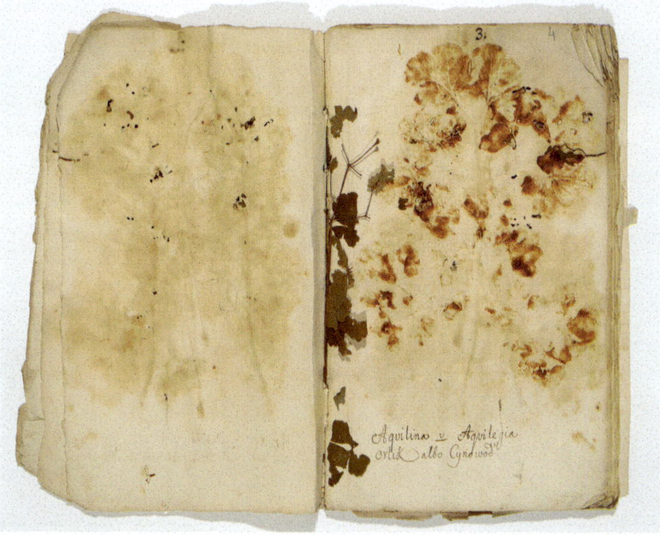

Fig. 5.4 Czartoryska Herbarium, National Museum in Kraków, Czartoryski Princes Library. Folio 3, condition before conservation. (Photo: T. Rizov-Ciechański)

[8] See the description of conservation treatment in the following section, with Fig. 5.15</InternalRef>.

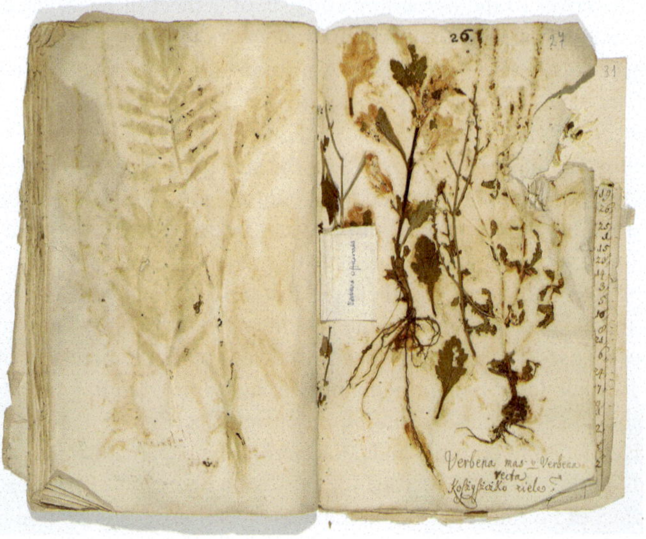

Fig. 5.5 Czartoryska Herbarium, National Museum in Kraków, Czartoryski Princes Library. Folio 26, condition before conservation. (Photo: T. Rizov-Ciechański)

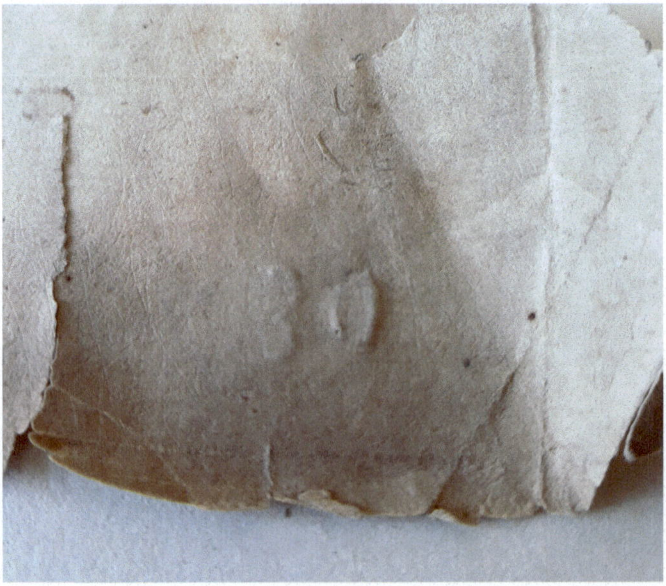

Fig. 5.6 Czartoryska Herbarium, National Museum in Kraków, Czartoryski Princes Library. Fragment of folio 4. Condition before conservation. Accumulated dirt, paper deformation caused by the addition of secondary pagination, and numerous mechanical damages. (Photo: M. Grenda-Kurmanow)

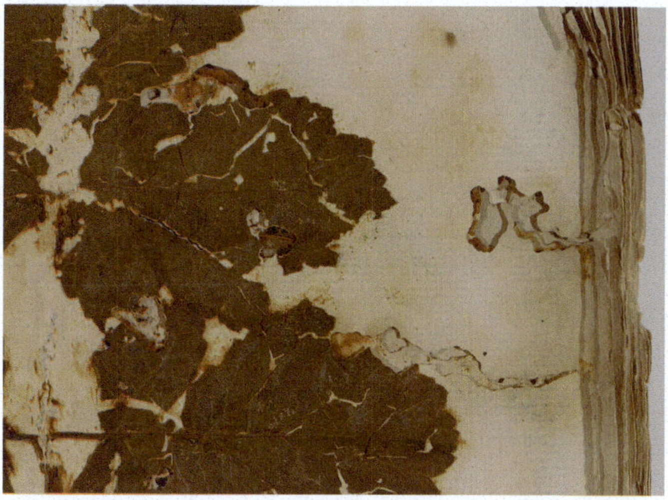

Fig. 5.7 Czartoryska Herbarium, National Museum in Kraków, Czartoryski Princes Library. Larval galleries. Condition before conservation. (Photo: M. Grenda-Kurmanow)

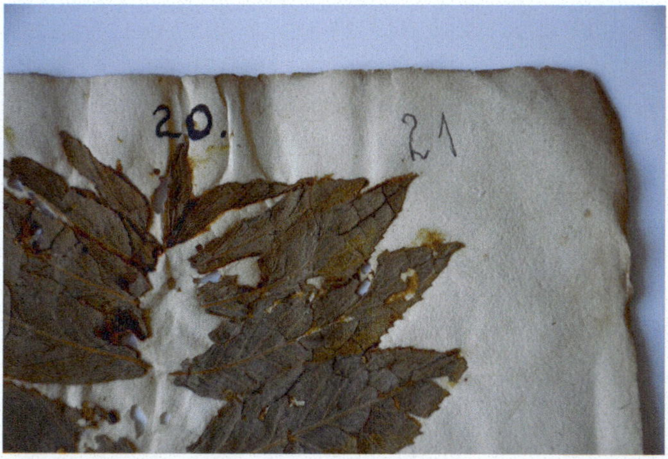

Fig. 5.8 Czartoryska Herbarium. The National Museum in Kraków, Czartoryski Princes Library. Fragment of folio 20. Condition before conservation. Substrate deformations, adhesive layers, and degradation of the botanical specimen. (Photo: M. Grenda-Kurmanow)

humidity in the object's environment and improper storage conditions. This also necessitated assessment of possible microbiological infection. An analysis for the presence of biocidal agents in the object was also conducted due to the potential health risk to users.

Fig. 5.9 Czartoryska Herbarium, National Museum in Kraków, Czartoryski Princes Library. *Verso* of the folio with the *Polish Index*. Ink migration on the *recto* side of the sheet. (Photo: T. Rizov-Ciechański)

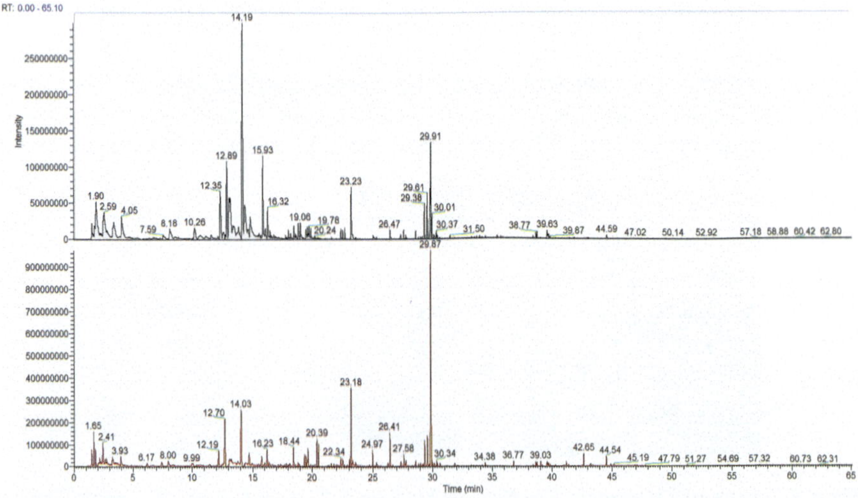

Fig. 5.10 Chromatograms showing VOCs collected inside the Czartoryska herbarium

The analysis of VOCs collected from the Czartoryska herbarium (Fig. 5.10) revealed the presence of Dinocap, a fungicide derived from dinitrophenol, as well as thiosemicarbazide and naphthalene.[9]

[9]GC/MS-SPME analysis, performed by Prof. Tomasz Sawoszczuk, Kraków University of Economics.

The results of the qualitative analysis of VOCs also showed that among the volatile compounds present inside the object, it is possible to identify, among others, furfural and acetic acid, which are products of cellulose and hemicellulose degradation; amino acids indicating the degradation of plant material contained within the objects; and essential oils derived from plants. Analysis for the presence of microbiological volatile organic compounds, which serve as markers of mould fungal activity, revealed that no active mould was present in the herbarium.

The results of the Ma-XRF analysis[10] (Fig. 5.11, see also Figs. 5.12 and 5.13) revealed the presence of arsenic in almost all scanned areas. In addition, iron and copper were detected in all scans, with a non-specific distribution.

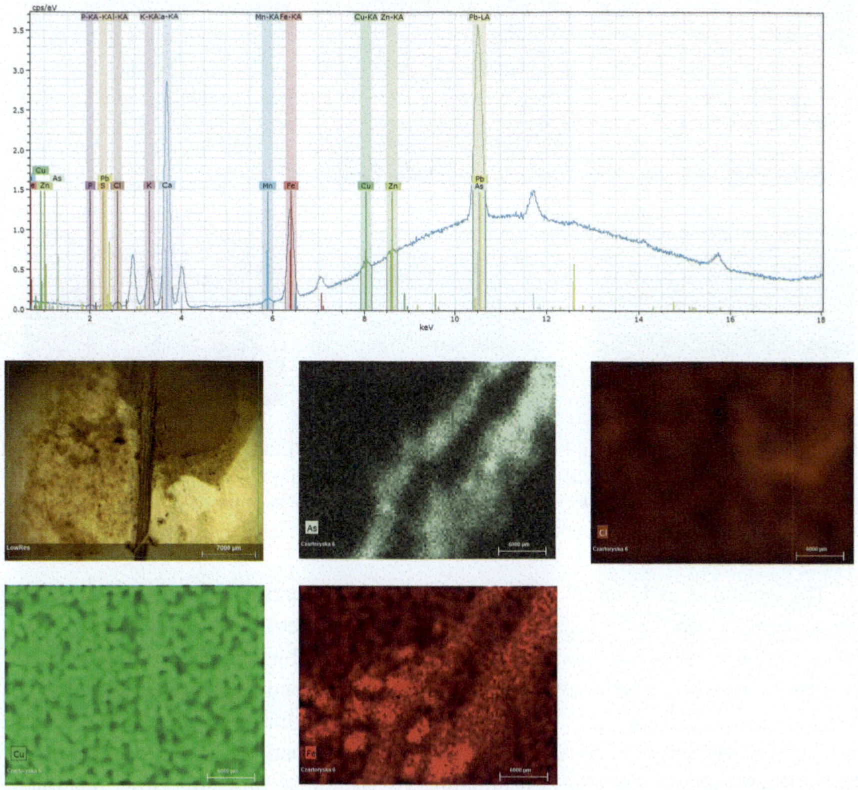

Fig. 5.11 Example Ma-XRF spectrum (**a**) and mapping for selected elements detected in Czartoryska's herbarium. VIS photograph (**b**), mapping of arsenic (**c**), chlorine (**d**), copper (**e**), and iron (**f**)

[10] Ma-XRF analysis, performed by Łukasz Ćwikliński at the Interdisciplinary Centre for Modern Interdisciplinary Technologies (ICNT) in Toruń.

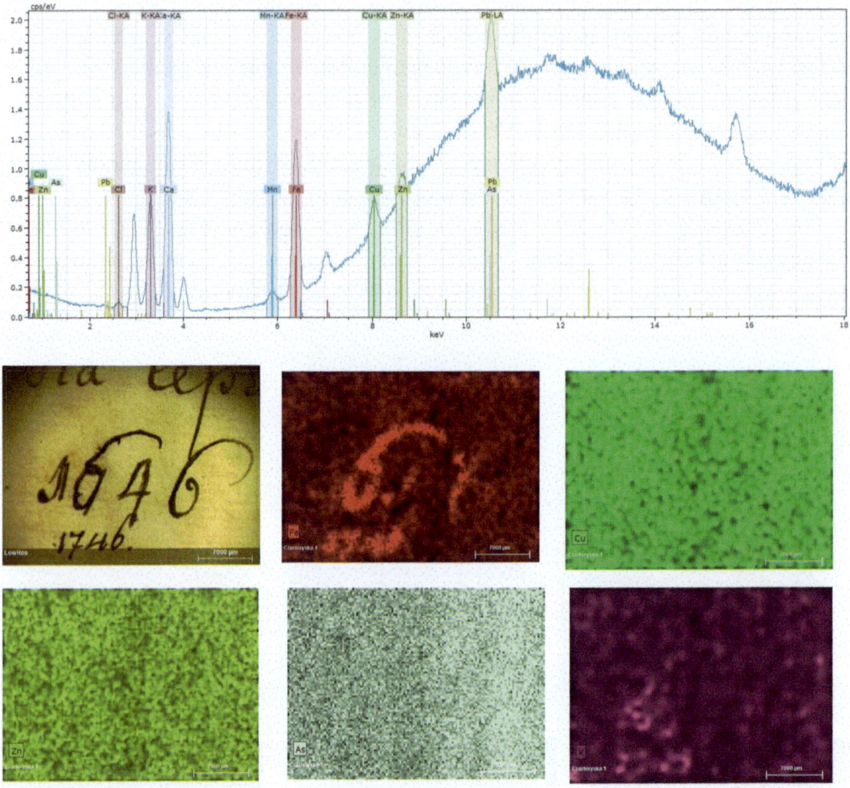

Fig. 5.12 Identification of iron-based ink, most likely iron gall ink. Ma-XRF spectrum (**a**) and mapping for selected elements detected in Czartoryska's herbarium. Manuscript fragment in VIS (**b**), mapping of iron (**c**), non-specific distribution of copper (**d**), whose presence is indicated by the spectrum, imaging for zinc (**e**), arsenic (**f**), and potassium (**g**)

The presence of biocidal substances necessitates particular caution when handling objects, especially regarding the personal protection of users. This involves strict use of synthetic gloves when manipulating the object and limiting close contact with it (e.g., by leaning over or inhaling substances emitted by the object). It has been determined that safe handling of specimens during conservation can be achieved by using tweezers and various types of flat spatulas, which are helpful for lifting and levering specimen fragments. At the same time, pressing specimens should be carried out using blunt, flexible tools, such as Teflon spatulas. The aforementioned tools allow the manipulation of specimens without direct contact. The use of gloves also minimises contamination of the specimen's genetic material by the user.

A preliminary analysis of the manuscript layers was also carried out using the Ma-XRF technique (Figs. 5.12 and 5.13).

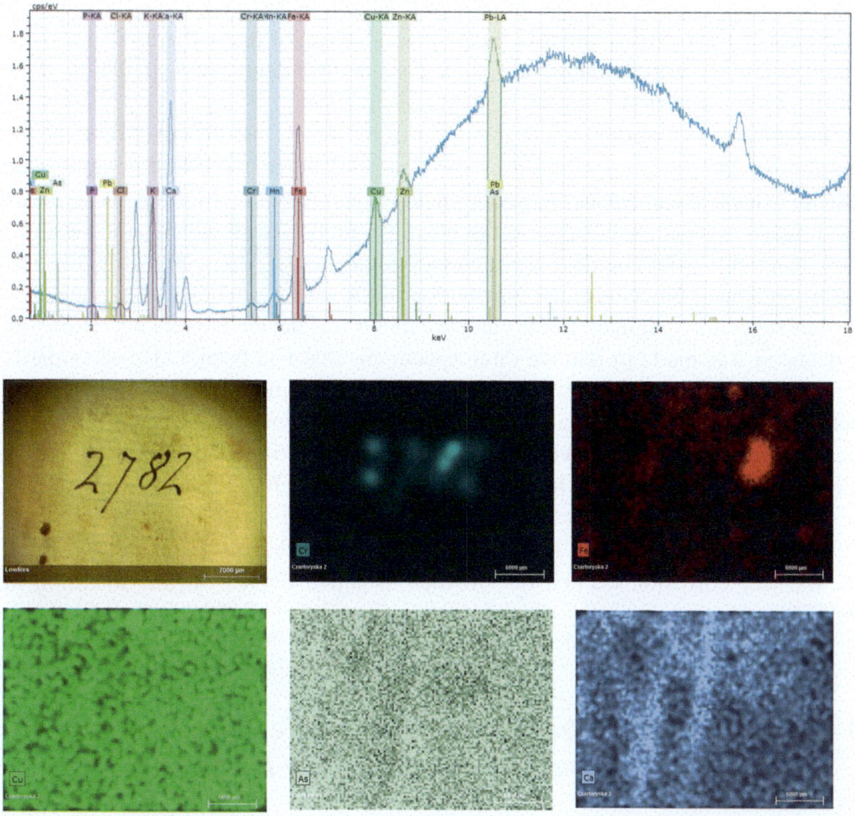

Fig. 5.13 Identification of a chromate ink, most likely logwood ink, suggesting that the inscription is a secondary signature mark (Logwood ink was introduced in 1847 as an alternative to iron-gall ink (Reissland et al. 2017)). Ma-XRF spectrum (**a**) and mapping for selected elements for selected elements detected in Czartoryska's herbarium. Manuscript fragment in VIS (**b**), mapping of chromium (**c**), iron (**d**), copper (**e**), arsenic (**f**), and calcium (**g**) in the scanned area

5.1.2 Conservation Objectives

Due to the extensive advanced deterioration of the botanical specimens and the paper substrate, the object required conservation intervention. The priority was to preserve the remaining plant fragments and to organise the numerous pieces that had fallen into the gutter. As a significant portion of the specimens had become detached (Figs. 5.4 and 5.5), it was planned to restore as many preserved fragments as possible to their original locations. It was considered that placing them in envelopes would completely compromise the legibility of the scientific document that the historic herbarium represents. In this case, the possible attachment of envelopes containing specimen fragments to the herbarium sheets was ruled out, as it would violate the integrity and authenticity of the object. It was necessary to use an adhesive for mounting the specimens that would be safe for the plants. It was assumed that attempts to analyse the genetic material of the herbarium specimens could not be excluded, although given the considerable degree of degradation of the entire object, such studies would be extremely difficult.

It was also necessary to repair the paper of the sheets and the cover by reinforcing the structure in areas affected by mechanical damage and filling in any losses. Due to extensive damage to the paper, including numerous tears along the spines of the folds, it was decided that the entire block would be disassembled, and conservation treatments would be carried out on individual sheets. After completing the necessary treatment procedures, reconstruction of the herbarium block was planned.

The secondary pagination was analysed and it was decided to retain it. However, a decision was made to remove three specimens that had been added secondarily from the block. There was no space in the object to mount them, nor would such an action be justified in any way. Leaving them loosely inserted between the sheets posed a risk both to their own safety and to the safety of the specimens originally mounted in the herbarium, which could be damaged mechanically as a result of friction between the dried plants and the added envelopes.

It also seemed necessary to limit the destructive effects of inks, particularly at sites where corrosion occurs, due to their negative impact on the condition of the object.

5.1.3 Conservation Procedures Using a Safe Conservation Methodology and Including Research Findings[11]

Conservation treatment began with securing loose fragments of botanical specimens by placing them in acid-free paper envelopes, which were carefully labelled for each sheet (Fig. 5.14).

The pages of the block were then separated by cutting the sewing threads close to the kettle stitch, in order to minimise thread loss.

Crumbled fragments in the spine folds and those located under the sewing, which become intermingled between the pages, were placed in separate envelopes. The paper of the cover was separated from the title page (Fig. 5.15), surface cleaned, and float washed, followed by structural reinforcement with Tylose MH 300 (MHEC)

[11] The following descriptions primarily cover treatments carried out directly on botanical specimens or those having a more or less direct impact on their subsequent condition. Other treatments are described in summary form. All results of technical analysis, descriptions of all treatments and specifications of the materials used are included in the conservation report [Grenda-Kurmanow M. (2019a). *Dokumentacja prac konserwatorskich i restauratorskich.* Herbarium Vivum albo Zielnik naturalnie rosnących zioł, niektorych tu wkleionych, dla lepszego ich rozeznania. Roku 1746—*zielnik Izabeli Czartoryskiej z 1746 roku ze zbiorów Muzeum Narodowego w Krakowie (dawniej w zbiorach Biblioteki Książąt Czartoryskich w Krakowie),* conservation report, Warsaw-Kraków].

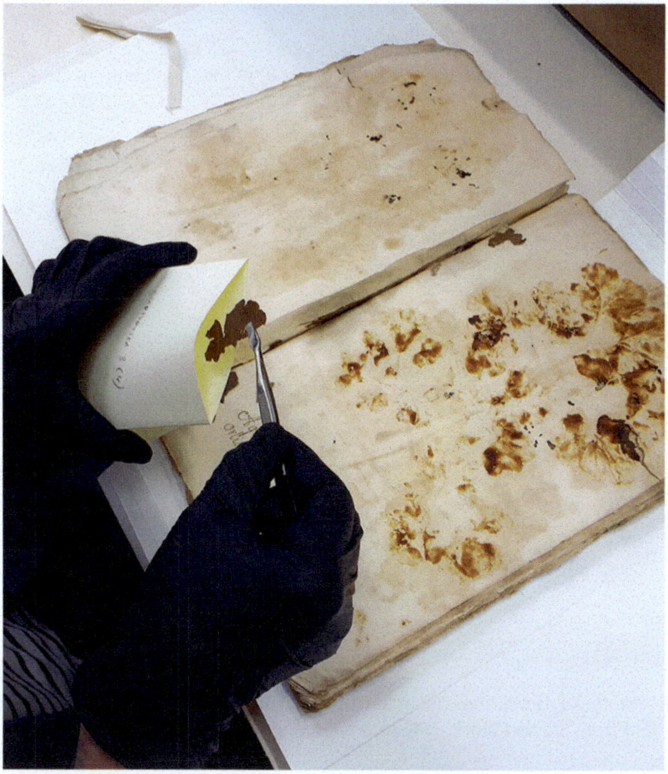

Fig. 5.14 Czartoryska Herbarium, National Museum in Kraków, Czartoryski Princes Library. Arranging detached specimen fragments. (Photo: P. Popławski)

and flattening. Losses were then filled with toned wove paper. The infilled cover paper was lined with Japanese *kozo* paper.

Folds forming the single section of the block were stored on individual supports made of rigid acid-free board and wrapped in a thin acid-free paper folder until conservation treatments could be carried out on the respective page. The pages were first surface cleaned of dust, dirt, and accretions (Fig. 5.16) with a brush, latex sponge, sulphur-free erasers, and a scalpel.

The presence of Fe^{2+} iron ions in the manuscript layer was subsequently confirmed using bathophenanthroline indicators (see Neevel and Reissland 2005; Neevel 2009). Despite the low pH (ranging from 4.6 to 5.1 for the paper of the sheets), both aqueous and non-aqueous deacidification methods were ruled out. The use of a non-aqueous method (e.g. Bookkeeper) could result in a significant surface increase in pH and also carries the risk of white deposits forming on the sheets and specimens (Boone et al. 1998; Sobucki et al. 2015). In the case of specimens, such deposits would be impossible to remove. Furthermore, due to the inconclusive effects of this product on the genetic material of botanical specimens observed in studies, the use of Bookkeeper was abandoned as a precaution. Treatments

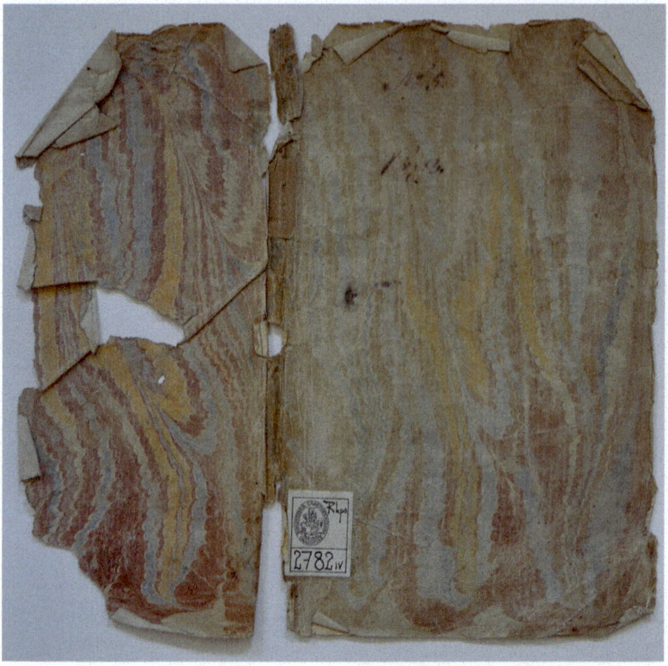

Fig. 5.15 Czartoryska Herbarium, National Museum in Kraków, Czartoryski Princes Library. Cover separated from the text block. (Photo: M. Grenda-Kurmanow)

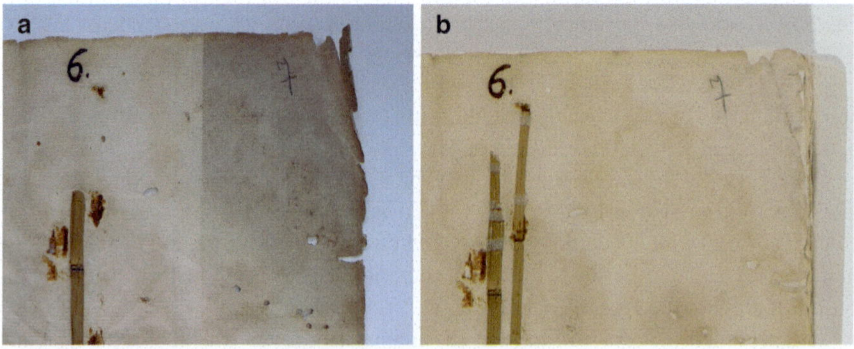

Fig. 5.16 Folio 6 of the Czartoryska herbarium (National Museum in Kraków, Czartoryski Princes Library) during surface cleaning (**a**) and after conservation (**b**). (Photo: M. Grenda-Kurmanow)

involving water, for this object, were to be limited to a minimum. Tears and pronounced, set creases present in the sheets were repaired using thin Japanese *kozo* papers, and rice starch paste from purified starch. The spines of the folds were also reinforced and repaired. The three-dimensional nature of the herbarium (delicate specimens mounted with a thick layer of adhesive on the paper substrate) made it impossible to press the sheets flat after repair. Attempts of local flattening under layers of felt proved too hard and stiff, failing to achieve satisfactory flattening and still posing a risk of damaging the specimens. Therefore, the locally moistened areas of paper during repair were shaped manually with a Teflon folder, then dried and, if needed, gently flattened using locally a heated spatula.

Local flattening of creased edges and corners was also carried out. Fragments of the sheets were moistened using demineralised water, either with an ultrasonic nebuliser producing a fine mist or, in the case of more severe creases, with a very gently moistened cotton swab. Flattening was not undertaken near specimens or in areas where deformation resulted from the presence of the dried plant. Losses were filled with Japanese papers and wove hemp paper, using the rice starch paste made from purified starch. Wove hemp paper, thicker and more rigid, provided better protection for the loss, but in cases of very large deformations it proved insufficiently flexible, and Japanese *mitsumata* paper was therefore used in such instances. It should be noted that in areas where losses affect both the botanical specimen and the paper support, the infill will always be set slightly back from the surface of the *recto* (an example is illustrated in the next case study, Fig. 5.41). Attempting to align the surface of the infill with that of the sheet would involve interference with the structure of the botanical specimen, which adheres closely to the substrate.

Paper losses present next to specimens (mainly larval galleries) were shaped during infilling, ensuring that the infills matched the shape of the deformation caused by the specimen (Fig. 5.17). In this way, the deformation was not eliminated, but botanical specimens were provided with support. Where possible, the infills were flattened in a manner similar to that used for tears. In selected cases, the infill was covered with nonwoven fabric and cotton wool to "cushion" the drying repair, and then with cardboard, onto which a small weight was placed to preserve the shape of the deformation (Fig. 5.18).

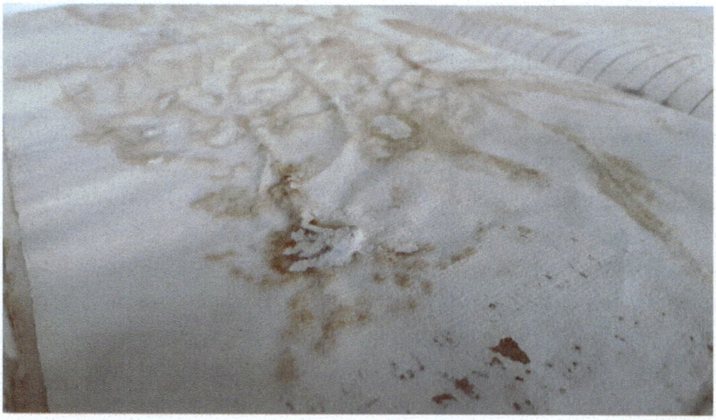

Fig. 5.17 Czartoryska Herbarium, National Museum in Kraków, Czartoryski Princes Library. Infilling fragmented loss replicating the deformation caused by the shape of the botanical specimen. (Photo: M. Grenda-Kurmanow)

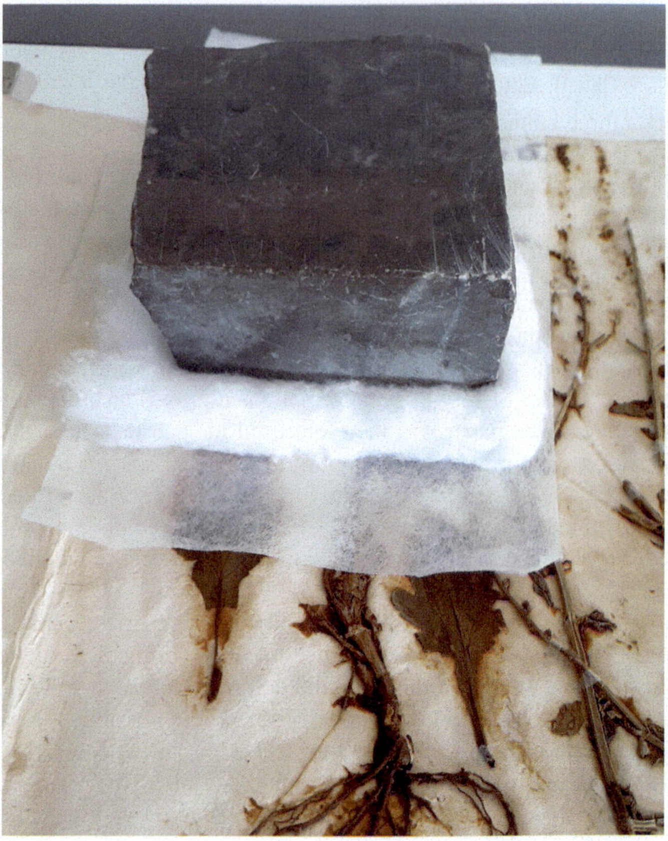

Fig. 5.18 Czartoryska Herbarium, National Museum in Kraków, Czartoryski Princes Library. Method of drying in deformed areas. (Photo: M. Grenda-Kurmanow)

Subsequently, the ink corrosion sites were secured. The procedure was carried out using an experimental method involving an ultrasonic nebuliser, to avoid the use of liquid solutions. For localised nebulisation, performed exclusively in areas containing the manuscript layer, an aqueous solution of DTPA (diethylenetriaminepentaacetic acid) with the addition of an aqueous solution of calcium hydroxide was used (Wagner and Bulska 2003, Sobucki 2013, pp. 81–84), followed by a solution of 1% gelatine.[12]

Next, detached fragments of botanical specimens and loose plant fragments were attached in their original locations. In locating these fragments, paper deformations—particularly those indicating the arrangement of stems as raised elements—proved extremely helpful, as did paper discolourations and traces of previously applied adhesive, which reveal the original shape of the botanical specimen. Where

[12] The method of DTPA and gelatine application used here was based on the assumption of avoiding liquid solutions, but its effectiveness requires further research

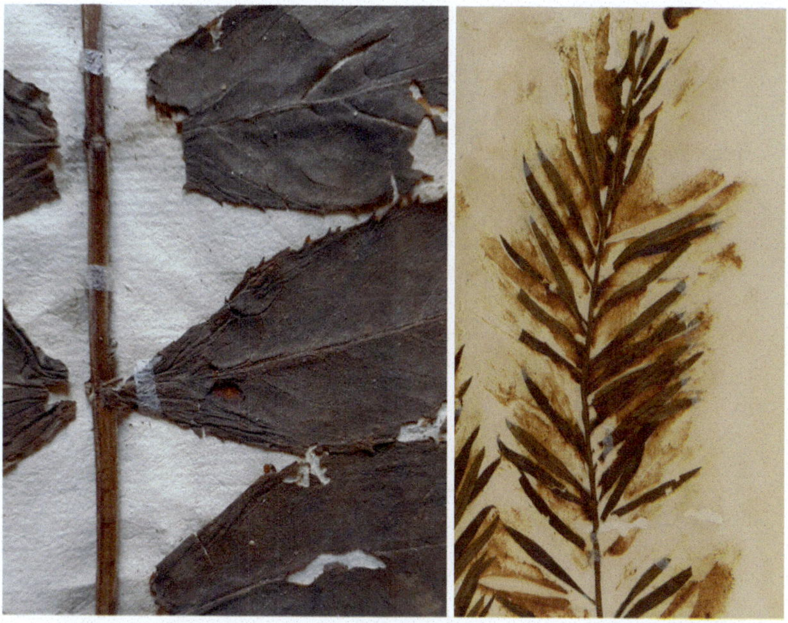

Fig. 5.19 Examples of specimen mounting in the Czartoryska Herbarium (Czartoryski Princes Library, National Museum in Kraków) using Japanese paper. (Photo: M. Grenda-Kurmanow)

it was possible to add fragments and secure them at the edges of the specimens, mounting was carried out using strips of Japanese *kozo* paper and purified rice starch paste (Fig. 5.19). The adhesive was applied only to the ends of the strip to avoid direct contact with the specimen.

In cases where fragments could not be mounted in this manner (e.g. internal leaf fragments), Aquazol 200 was used (Fig. 5.20). In addition, severely cracked and delaminating specimen fragments that could not be consolidated with brush-applied adhesive were nebulised with an aqueous solution of Aquazol 50 (Fig. 5.21).

As a result of the undertaken actions, it was possible to a large extent to restore the preserved plant fragments to their original locations (Figs. 5.22 and 5.23).

Fragments that could not be matched with certainty were left in envelopes made of thin acid-free paper and included as attachments (Figs. 5.24 and 5.25). The envelopes also contained additional loose specimens found in the block, as well as secondary envelopes made of notebook paper present in the object. Envelopes made of thin paper are particularly useful for herbarium specimens, as their slight transparency allows for preliminary identification of the contents without opening. All attachments were placed in conservation-grade polyester sleeves, which were then stored in acid-free folders.

After stabilising and securing all fragments of the specimens, the block was sewn together using the original thread according to the original sewing pattern. The cover was then attached to the spine of the single section. The herbarium is now housed in an acid-free box.

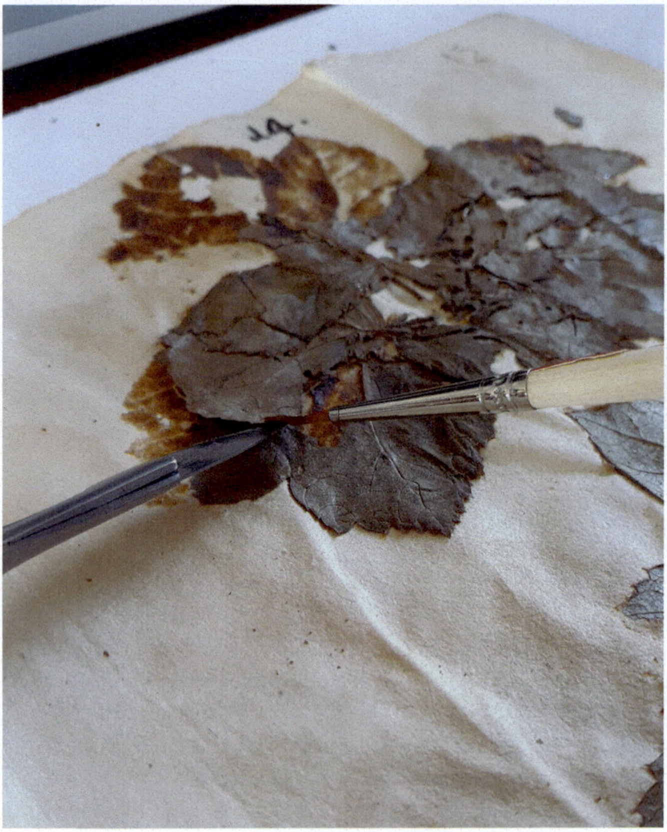

Fig. 5.20 Spot adhesion of a specimen in the Czartoryska herbarium (Czartoryski Princes Library, National Museum in Kraków) using Aquazol 200. (Photo: M. Grenda-Kurmanow)

5.2 Herbarium of Johann Friedrich Zeidler, Volume I, 1732, Main Library of the University of Life Sciences in Lublin, Ref. Zb. Specj. I Starodruki 14, 14, D. 104.57.646[13]

5.2.1 Description

The volume of Zeidler's herbarium described here is one of two surviving volumes. In addition to Volume I, Volume III from 1751 has also been preserved in the library. The second volume is currently considered lost. The herbarium has a complex and not fully understood history. Johann Friedrich Zeidler (1700–1756) was a Silesian

[13] Zeidler J.F., *Hortus Perennis*…, Lublin, Main Library of the University of Life Sciences in Lublin, Vol. I, ref. Zb. Specj. I Starodruki 14, D. 104.57.646, 1732.

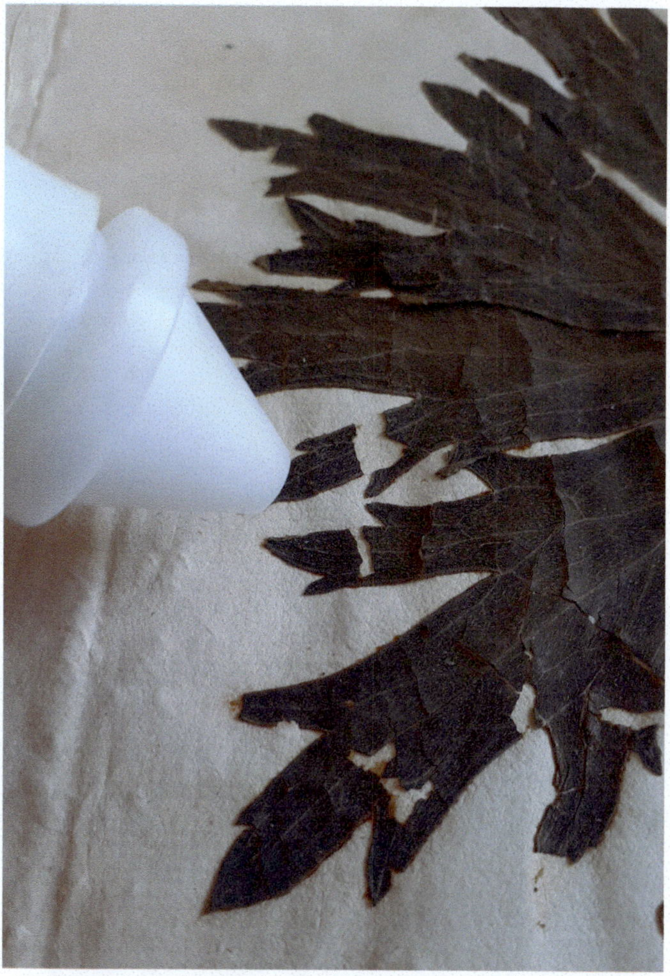

Fig. 5.21 Local consolidation of delaminating specimen edges in the Czartoryska Herbarium (National Museum in Krakow, Czartoryski Princes Library). (Photo: M. Grenda-Kurmanow)

naturalist and collector of natural specimens. Between 1732 and 1751, on commission from Count Jan Anton Schaffgotsch, he prepared a series of herbaria, which were subsequently incorporated into the Schaffgotsch family library, initially located in Sobieszów (Hermsdorf), and later in the Majorat Library in Cieplice (Majoratsbibliothek zu Warmbrunn). The object contains numerous provenance marks such as bookplates, watermarks, references to Schaffgotsch lands in the extended title of the herbarium, stamps, and inventory labels characteristic of the Cieplice library. While the herbarium remained in Warmbrunn until the Second World War, its history immediately after the war is shrouded in mystery. The Schaffgotsch collections suffered greatly after the war due to dispersal, and as a

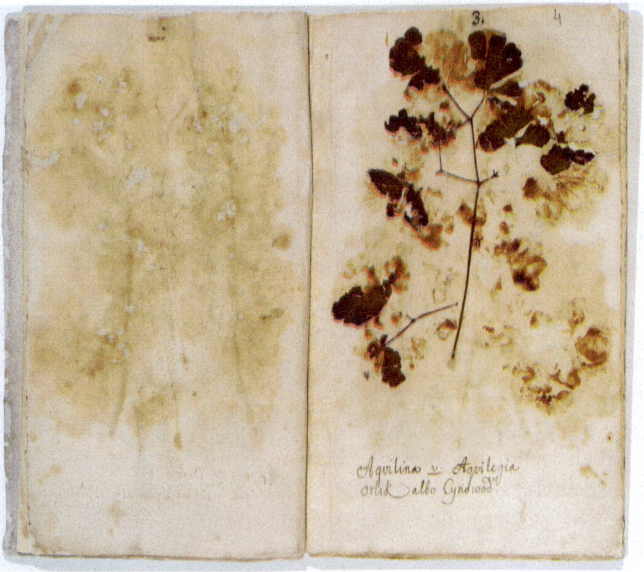

Fig. 5.22 Czartoryska Herbarium, National Museum in Kraków, Czartoryski Princes Library. Folio 3 after conservation. (Photo: T. Rizov-Ciechański)

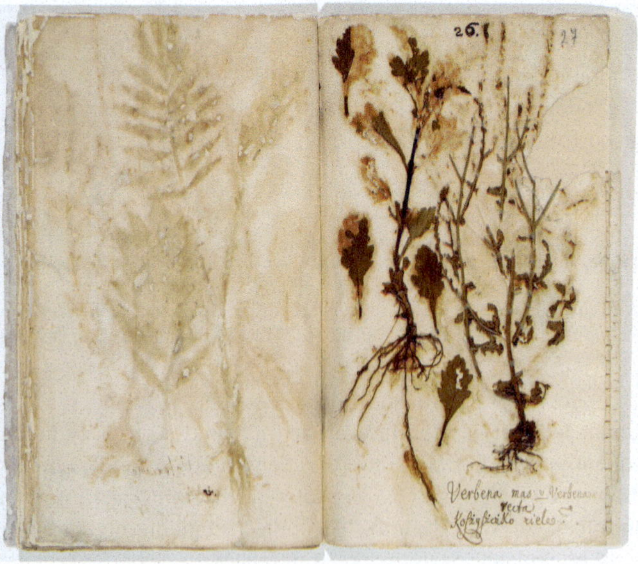

Fig. 5.23 Czartoryska Herbarium, National Museum in Krakow, Czartoryski Princes Library. Folio 26 after conservation. (Photo: T. Rizov-Ciechański)

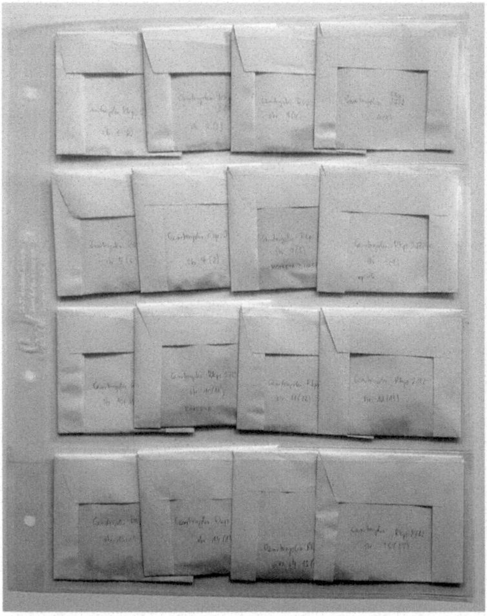

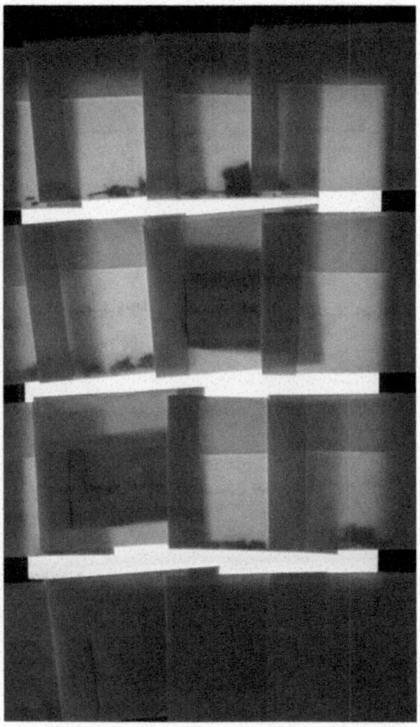

Figs. 5.24 and 5.25 Envelopes made of thin acid-free paper, allowing the contents to be pre-inspected without opening the envelope. (Photo: M. Grenda-Kurmanow)

result, surviving fragments of their collection can now be found throughout Poland (Firszt 2009, 2016).[14] It is likely that in the 1950s, two volumes (I and III) of Zeidler's herbarium found their way to the Main Library of the University of Life Sciences in Lublin. This certainly occurred after the separation of the unit from Maria Curie-Skłodowska University. The stamp of the Higher School of Agriculture in Lublin (now the Main Library of the University of Life Sciences in Lublin) suggests that the object was entered into the Library's inventory between 1955 and 1970.[15]

The Zeidler Herbarium is a very impressive volume, containing approximately 300 botanical specimens on 268 pages. The plants were attached by overall adhesion to the paper substrate. The specimens were additionally secured at the base with decorative vase-shaped labels (Fig. 5.26).

Each specimen was labelled with an inscription made in ink. The manuscript layer is also present in the form of pagination, Latin and German indexes at the end of the volume, and an ornately calligraphed title page (Figs. 5.27 and 5.28).

[14] See also the section *Herbaria as Collectible Phenomena and Components of Natural History Collections* in Chap. 1.

[15] In 1955, the university (now the University of Life Sciences), previously a branch of Maria Curie-Skłodowska University (UMCS) in Lublin, was named the Higher School of Agriculture. In 1972, it was renamed the Agricultural Academy. The institution operated under this name until 2008, when it became the University of Life Sciences.

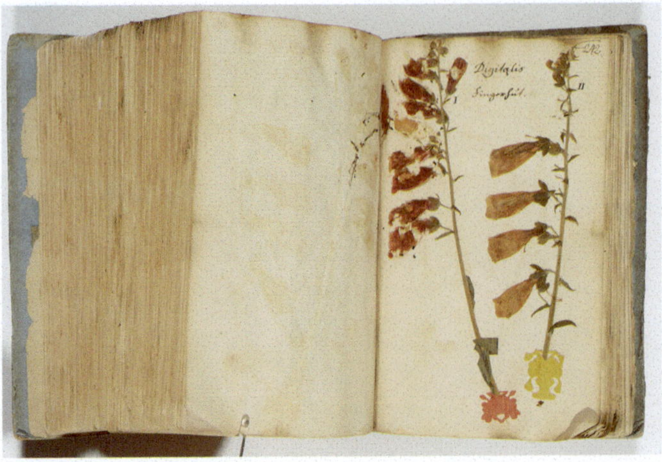

Fig. 5.26 Herbarium of Johann Friedrich Zeidler, Main Library of the University of Life Sciences in Lublin, folio 242, condition before conservation. (Photo: T. Rizov-Ciechański)

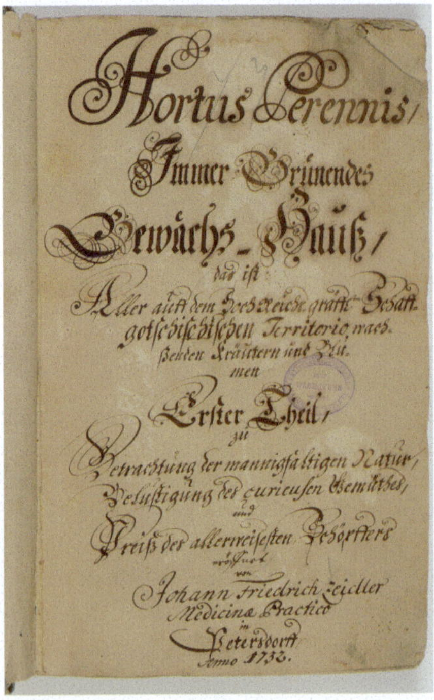

Fig. 5.27 Zeidler's Herbarium, Main Library of the University of Life Sciences in Lublin, title page, condition before conservation. (Photo: T. Rizov-Ciechański)

The Ma-XRF analysis confirmed the identification of iron gall ink. Additionally, potassium was identified in the area of the inscriptions (Fig. 5.29).[16]

[16] Ma-XRF analysis, performed by Łukasz Ćwikliński at the Interdisciplinary Centre for Modern Interdisciplinary Technologies (ICNT) in Toruń.

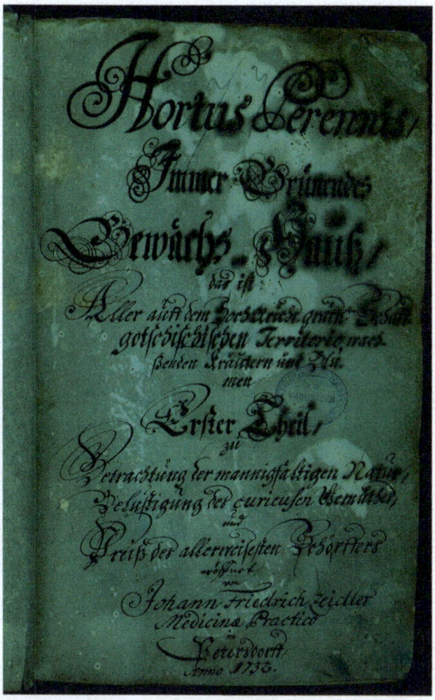

Fig. 5.28 Zeidler's herbarium, title page under UV light, before conservation. (Photo: T. Rizov-Ciechański)

The manuscript layer was preserved in varying condition. On the title page, where the concentration of ink is highest, there are pronounced ink corrosion marks, clearly visible under UV light (Figs. 5.27 and 5.28). Additionally, in over one hundred pages of the object, the presence of metal inclusions have been detected, in some cases resulting in visible corrosion of the paper substrate.

An unusual decorative technique employed in the herbarium is the application of a paint layer to selected specimens (Fig. 5.26 and 5.32, as well as Figs. 2.4, 2.5 and 2.6 in Chap. 2). It is not known whether this was done by the author of the herbarium or by a later curator of the collection. Nevertheless, paint layers are present in both surviving volumes of Zeidler's herbaria. The use of paint to decorate the specimens has contributed to their noticeable degradation and increased brittleness (Fig. 5.26 and 5.32).

Using the Ma-XRF technique, two pigments were preliminarily identified in Zeidler's herbarium: Prussian blue (Fig. 5.30) and copper green (Fig. 5.31). Microchemical analyses confirmed the identification of Prussian blue and specified the green pigment as copper green, most likely copper acetate with an addition of Prussian blue and a yellow pigment that could not be identified.[17]

[17] Microchemical analyses performed by Dr. Anna Nowicka at the Department of Specialist Research and Documentation Techniques, Faculty of Conservation and Restoration of Works of Art, Academy of Fine Arts in Warsaw.

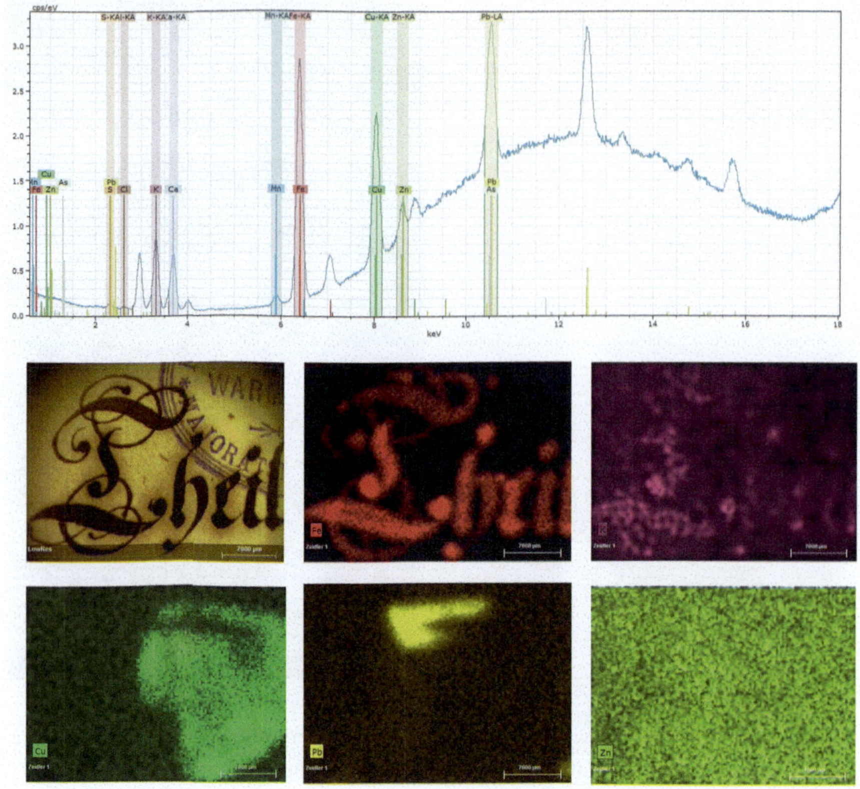

Fig. 5.29 Identification of iron-based ink, most likely iron gall ink. Ma-XRF spectrum (**a**) and mapping for selected elements detected in Zeidler's herbarium. Fragment in VIS (**b**), iron (**c**), potassium (**d**), copper (**e**), lead (**f**), and zinc (**g**)

The remaining components of the paint layer were identified by HPLC/MS analysis as cochineal and an unspecified green dye based on tannins.[18] FTIR analysis identified a binder made from stone fruit tree gum and a chalk ground onto which the green paint layer was applied. The analysis also confirmed the presence of Prussian blue.[19]

The object also exhibited numerous deformations and mechanical damage resulting from its construction. The use of animal glue[20] in the overall adhesion of the specimens caused significant stress and mechanical damage, including cracks

[18] HPLC/MS analyses performed by performed by Dr. Bartłomiej Witkowski at the Faculty of Chemistry, University of Warsaw.

[19] FTIR analyses, performed by performed by Dr. Joanna Kurkowska at the Intercollegiate Institute for Conservation and Restoration of Works of Art, Academy of Fine Arts in Warsaw.

[20] GC/MS analysis, performed by Dr. Bartłomiej Witkowski at the Faculty of Chemistry, University of Warsaw.

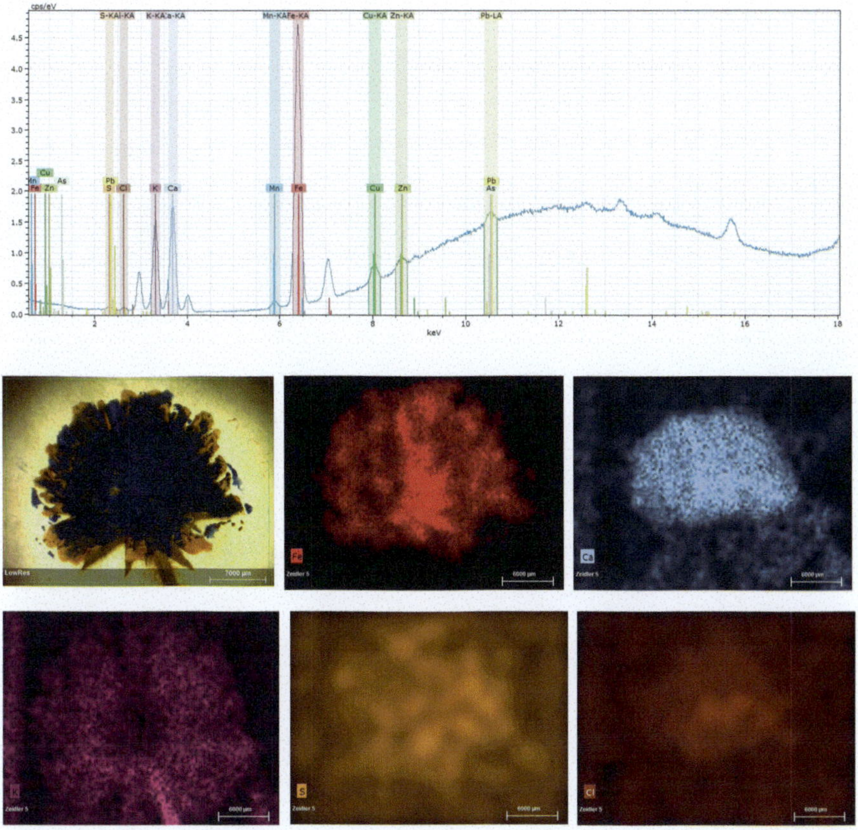

Fig. 5.30 Pigment identification, Ma-XRF spectrum (**a**) and mapping for selected elements for selected elements detected in Zeidler's herbarium. Fragment in VIS (**b**), mapping of iron (**c**), calcium (**d**), potassium (**e**), sulphur (**f**), and chlorine (**g**)

within leaves or petals and local fragmentation. The paint layer was not firmly bonded to the surface of the specimens and tended to powder, leaving traces on adjacent sheets. In the case of the green pigment applied on a ground layer, numerous losses and cracks in both the ground and the pigment are visible (Fig. 5.32). Consequently, tests for the consolidation of the paint layer were planned.

The object was previously exposed to moisture, leaving the larger stains on the title page and index pages, as well as minor stains along the trimmed edge of the entire block. Due to the visible effects of moisture, it was deemed necessary to conduct a microbiological examination of the object and to consider disinfection if microbiological contamination is confirmed. In addition, an analysis of the potential presence of biocides was considered essential.

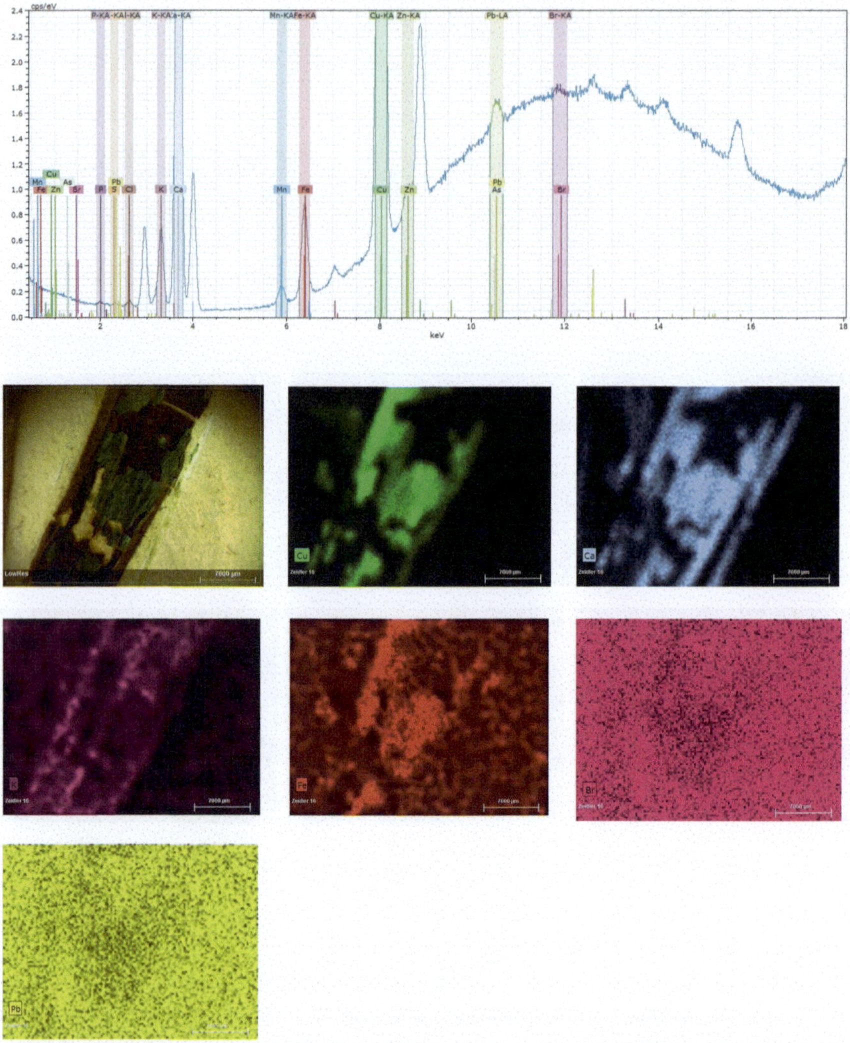

Fig. 5.31 Pigment identification, Ma-XRF spectrum (**a**) and mapping for selected elements for selected elements detected in Zeidler's herbarium. Fragment in VIS (**b**), mapping of copper (**c**), calcium (**d**), potassium (**e**), iron (**f**), bromine (**g**), lead (**h**)

VOC analysis with GC/MS-SPME (Fig. 5.33) revealed the presence of trace amounts of arsenic compounds as well as camphor and thymol.[21]

The origin of thymol and camphor may be ambiguous, as they are components of essential oils emitted by certain plants. However, in this case, thymol is released

[21] GC/MS-SPME analysis, performed by Prof. Tomasz Sawoszczuk, Kraków University of Economics

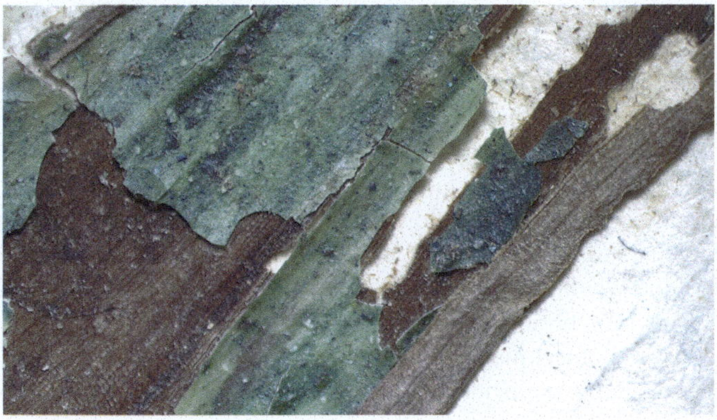

Fig. 5.32 Zeidler's Herbarium, Main Library of the University of Life Sciences in Lublin, damage to the green paint layer on the ground, photomicrograph. (Photo by M. Grenda-Kurmanow)

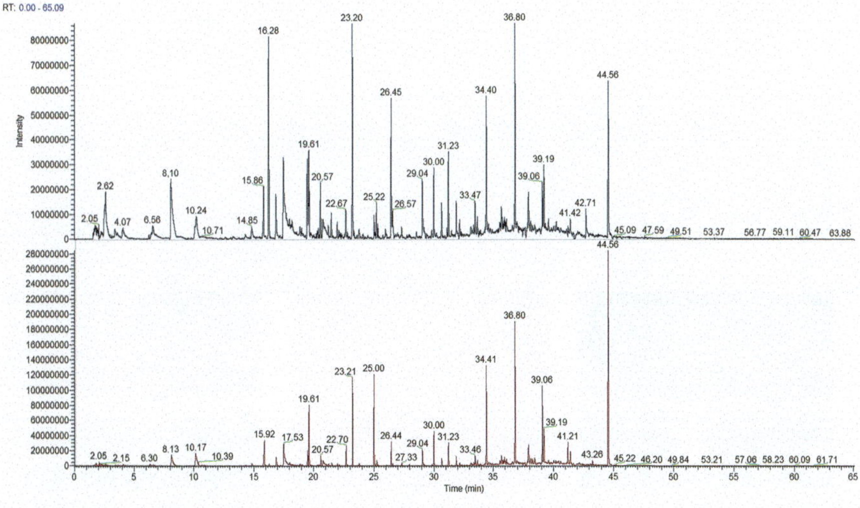

Fig. 5.33 Chromatograms showing VOCs collected inside the herbarium of Johann Friedrich Zeidler

in significant quantities, which supports the hypothesis that it was used as a preservative.[22]

Similarly to the Czartoryska herbarium, the results of qualitative analyses demonstrated that among the volatile compounds present within the objects, it is possible to identify, among others: furfural and acetic acid, which are products of cellulose and hemicellulose degradation; amino acids indicating the degradation of

---

[22] See also the remarks on natural essential oils in the section *Environmental Pollution in Collection Storage Areas* in Chap. 3.

plant material contained within the objects or animal glue used for mounting the plants; and essential oils derived from the plants themselves. Analysis for the presence of microbiological volatile organic compounds, which serve as markers of mould activity, confirmed that no active mould was present in the herbarium.

The results of Ma-XRF analysis (Fig. 5.34) indicate the presence of bromine, mercury, and lead. In addition, a large amount of iron and copper is found throughout the herbarium in a non-specific manner, usually in the form of concentrated clusters. Mercury was detected in only 1 of 16 scans, making it difficult to conclusively determine whether mercuric chloride may be present in the herbarium. In contrast, signals from bromine and lead are repeatedly observed across many scans, suggesting that the object may have been subjected in the past to fumigation with methyl bromide and to a biocide containing lead. However, analysis of the Kβ and

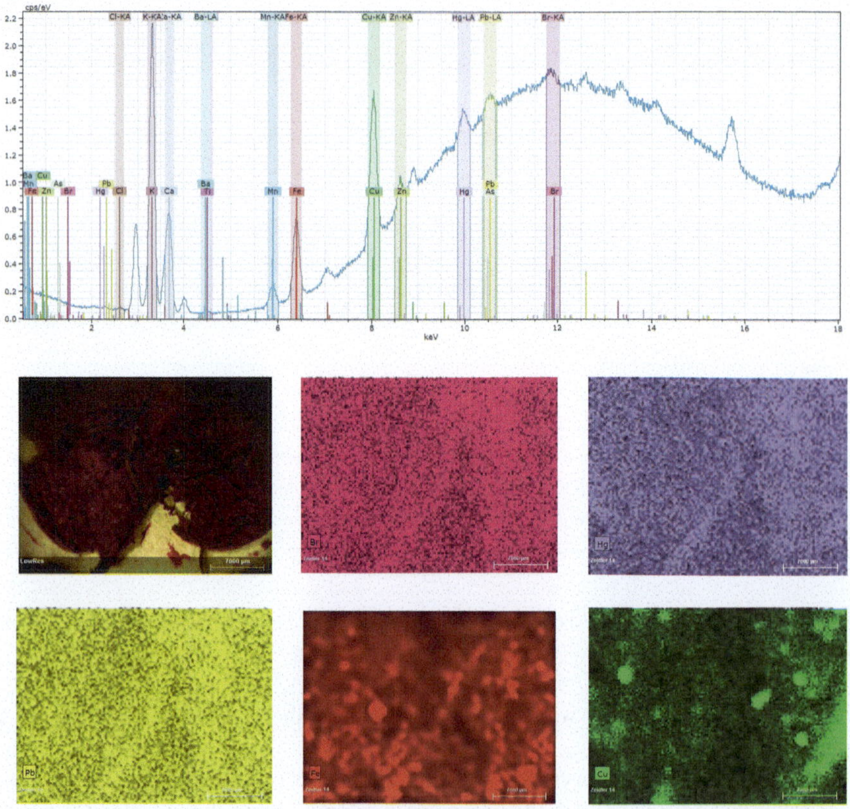

Fig. 5.34 Ma-XRF spectrum (**a**) and elemental mapping for selected elements detected in Zeidler's herbarium. Fragment in VIS (**b**), mapping for bromine (**c**), mercury (**d**), lead (**e**), iron (**f**), and copper (**g**)

$L\beta$ lines excluded the presence of arsenic, which could have indicated the use of lead arsenate.[23]

Similar to the previously described case study, the results of the biocide presence analysis for the Zeidler herbarium indicate that particular caution is required when handling the object, especially regarding the personal protection of users. This involves the strict use of synthetic gloves when manipulating the object and limiting close contact with it (such as leaning over, inhaling substances emitted by the object, etc.). The use of gloves also minimises the contamination of the specimen's genetic material by the user.

The use of adhesive for the direct mounting of specimens contributed to increased insect activity within the object, evident in the form of larval tunnels bored both in the structure of the specimens and in the substrate. Losses from this group are present in 95% of the block's sheets (Figs. 5.35 and 5.36).

Additionally, the codex construction, with a difference in flexibility between the paper substrate and the specimens, promoted detachment of specimens, mechanical damage, and the accumulation of specimen fragments towards the spine during page turning. Some fragments of broken specimens have migrated between the sheets within the block. Areas where dried plants have detached or crumbled have revealed a layer of adhesive on the paper. Mechanical damage has also been caused

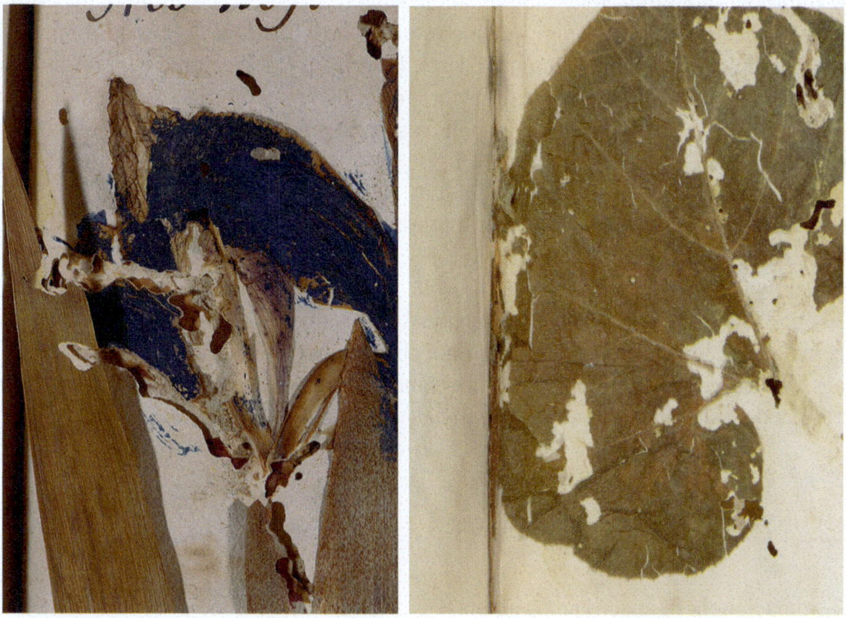

Figs. 5.35 and 5.36 Zeidler Herbarium, Main Library of the University of Life Sciences in Lublin, condition before conservation. Larval galleries in the paper substrate and botanical specimens. (Photo: T. Rizov-Ciechański)

[23] The $K\alpha$ lines of these two elements overlap, so identification should be refined based on the $K\beta$ lines.

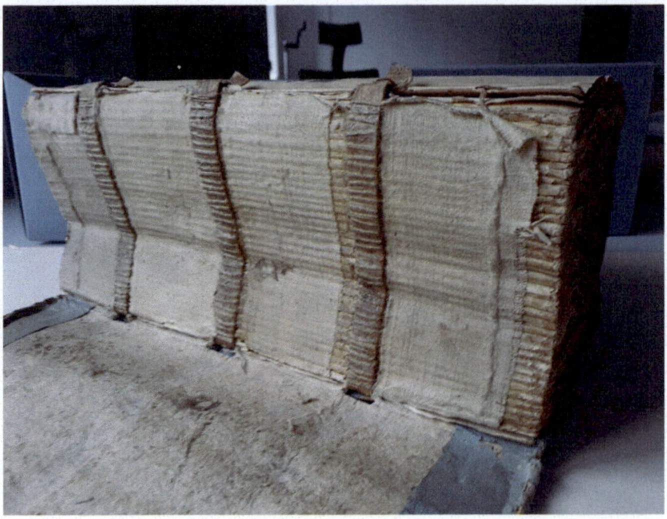

Fig. 5.37 Zeidler's herbarium, Main Library of the University of Life Sciences in Lublin, condition before conservation. Indentation of the spine. (Photo: M. Grenda-Kurmanow)

by improper mounting, for example, at the edge of the sheet, resulting in the crumbling of specimen's edge. Improper mounting or unsuitable storage conditions have also led to a few specimen fragments detaching from the sheet and adhering to the *recto* side of the preceding sheet. Furthermore, there have been instances of stem breakage, partial detachment of specimens from the sheet, and accumulation of loose specimen fragments in the gutter.

The spine of the block was deformed by an indentation (Fig. 5.37).

The construction of the binding suggests that the object was rebound several times or even specifically prepared for easy replacement of the binding, which was probably related to the incorporation of the herbarium into the library collection in Cieplice. This was confirmed by an analysis of the fibrous composition of the paper on the spine of the binding, which, unlike all the other herbarium papers made from rags, contained wood pulp.[24] This allows the time of the binding replacement to be estimated as no earlier than the second half of the nineteenth century.

5.2.2 *Conservation Objectives*

The detachment of specimen fragments, as well as the presence of broken elements of botanical specimens in the gutter, necessitated conservation intervention, especially mounting or reinforcing existing attachments of specimens. The preserved

[24] Fibre composition analysis, performed by Dr. Katarzyna Królikowska-Pataraia at the Department of Specialist Research and Documentation Techniques, Faculty of Conservation and Restoration of Works of Art, Academy of Fine Arts in Warsaw.

paint layers required consolidation. The significant presence of Prussian blue in certain areas of Zeidler's herbarium was another factor that precluded treatments aimed at alkalising the object's environment, due to the sensitivity of this pigment to alkaline conditions. Furthermore, as in the case of Czartoryska's herbarium, ink corrosion and metal inclusions present within the structure of the sheets required stabilisation.

The damage to the binding and its partial detachment from the block prior to conservation led to the decision to separate these two elements for the duration of the conservation treatment. Following the conservation of both the text block and the binding, it was planned to reunite the original components. Apart from this, only minimal intervention procedures were envisaged, focusing on securing the specimens against further degradation and minimising the loss of botanical information (specimen fragments) in the future. Consequently, all work was to be carried out within the block, without its disassembly. For mounting the specimens, it was necessary to use an adhesive that would not be destructive to plants, as the possibility of future genetic analyses involving the herbarium specimens cannot be excluded.

5.2.3 *Conservation Procedures Using a Safe Conservation Methodology and Including Research Findings*[25]

The conservation treatment began with securing loose fragments of botanical specimens and transferring them into envelopes made of acid-free paper, which were labelled with the number of the sheet where the specimens were originally found. The block was separated from the binding. The blue, original paper of the cover was surface cleaned and washed locally without disassembly. However, the brittle secondary paper made of wood pulp, which had been adhered to the spine, was removed, washed, structurally reinforced, lined, and infilled. The binding boards were repaired and locally consolidated. Losses in the blue cover paper were filled from the recto using matched, toned Japanese *kozo* papers.

The treatments on the pages, as intended, were carried out without disassembling the block. Prior to commencing the surface cleaning of the block pages, the paint layer present on certain specimens was gently consolidated by local nebulization with a 2% solution of Aquazol 50.

Subsequently, the pages were surface cleaned using a soft synthetic brush, and, outside the specimen areas, also with a latex sponge, sulphur-free erasers, and a

[25] As with the previously described herbarium, the following descriptions primarily cover treatments carried out directly on botanical specimens or those having a more or less direct impact on their subsequent condition. Other treatments are described in summary form. Descriptions of all treatments and the materials used, together with detailed specifications, are included in the conservation report [Grenda-Kurmanow M. (2019b) *Dokumentacja prac konserwatorskich i restauratorskich.zielnik Johanna Friedricha Zeidlera z 1732 roku, ze zbiorów Biblioteki Głównej Uniwersytetu Przyrodniczego w Lublinie*, conservation report, Warsaw].

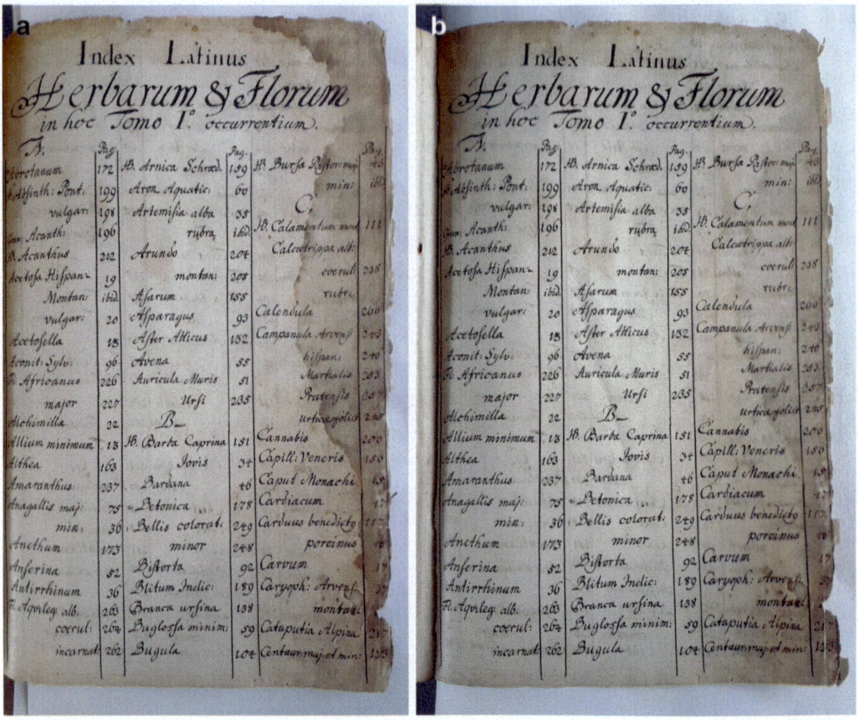

Fig. 5.38 Zeidler's herbarium, Main Library of the University of Life Sciences in Lublin, first page of the Latin index before (a) and after stain removal (b). (Photo: M. Grenda-Kurmanow)

scalpel, which was primarily used to remove traces of insects and occasional deposits. Stains present on some pages were then washed locally. During swabbing, care was taken to avoid contact between the botanical specimens and water. The most pronounced stains were found on the pages listing plant species at the end of the block, and these were locally washed repeatedly (Fig. 5.38). After local washing, the pages were flattened under weights.

After surface cleaning and local washing of the sheets, repairs were carried out on mechanical damages to the paper substrate. Tears and severe, persistent creases present in the paper substrate were reinforced with thin Japanese *kozo* papers, using rice starch paste from purified starch. As with the Czartoryska herbarium, due to the three-dimensional nature of the herbarium, it was not possible to press the sheets flat after the repairs. Therefore, the areas moistened during reinforcement were dried and straightened locally using a heated spatula. Local flattening of creased edges and corners was also performed by moistening and flattening them with the heated spatula, yielding satisfying effects. Flattening was applied only locally at the sheet edges. No such interventions were undertaken near the specimens or in areas where deformation resulted from the mounting of the dried plant (Fig. 5.39).

The losses were filled according to the same principles as in the Czartoryska herbarium, using two types of paper: a stiffer wove paper and a soft, easily

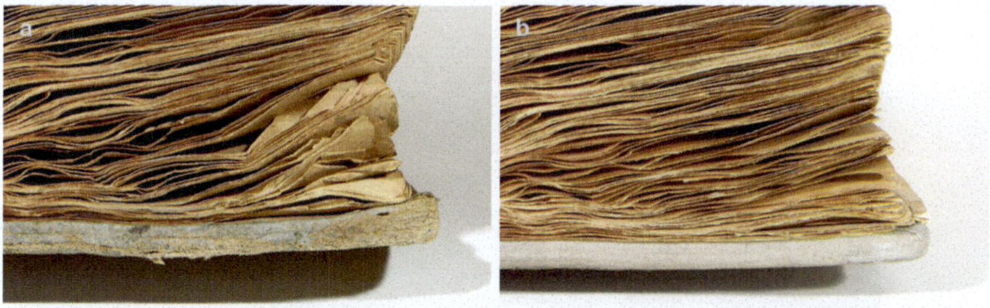

Fig. 5.39 Zeidler herbarium, Main Library of the University of Life Sciences in Lublin, section of the block edge before (**a**) and after conservation (**b**), showing the effect of local flattening of the sheets. (Photo: T. Rizov-Ciechański)

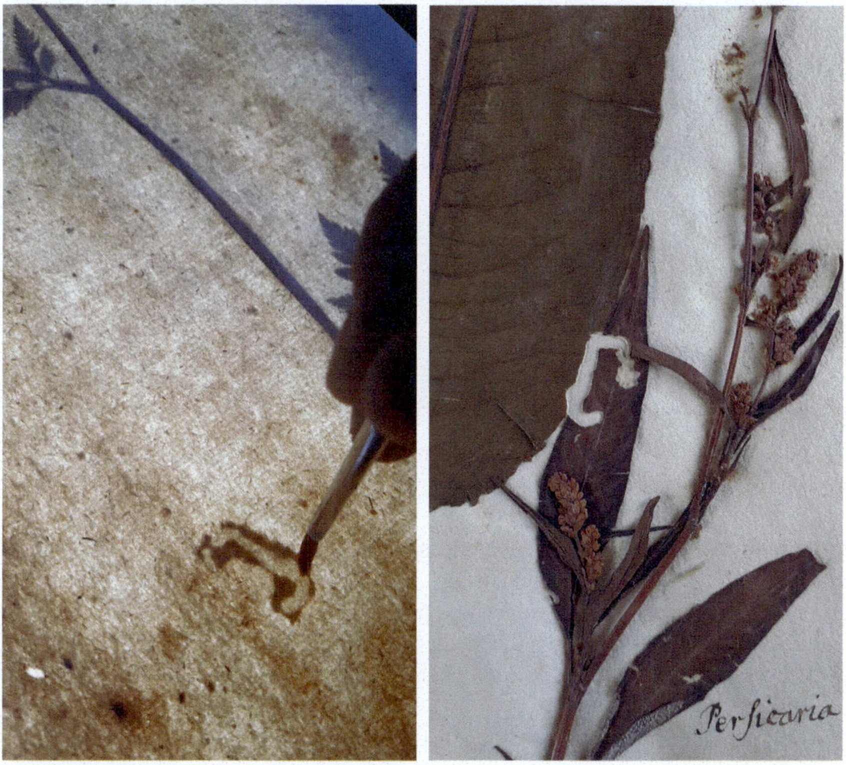

Figs. 5.40 and 5.41 Zeidler herbarium, Main Library of the University of Life Sciences in Lublin, shaping the infill (Fig. 5.40), example of infill (Fig. 5.41). (Photo: M. Grenda-Kurmanow)

mouldable Japanese *mitsumata*, depending on the nature of the loss (Figs. 5.40 and 5.41).

When attaching deformed fragments, the shape of the infill was adapted to the deformation. The infills were flattened using a heated spatula, provided the condition of the object in that area allowed it. Where it was not possible to apply pressure

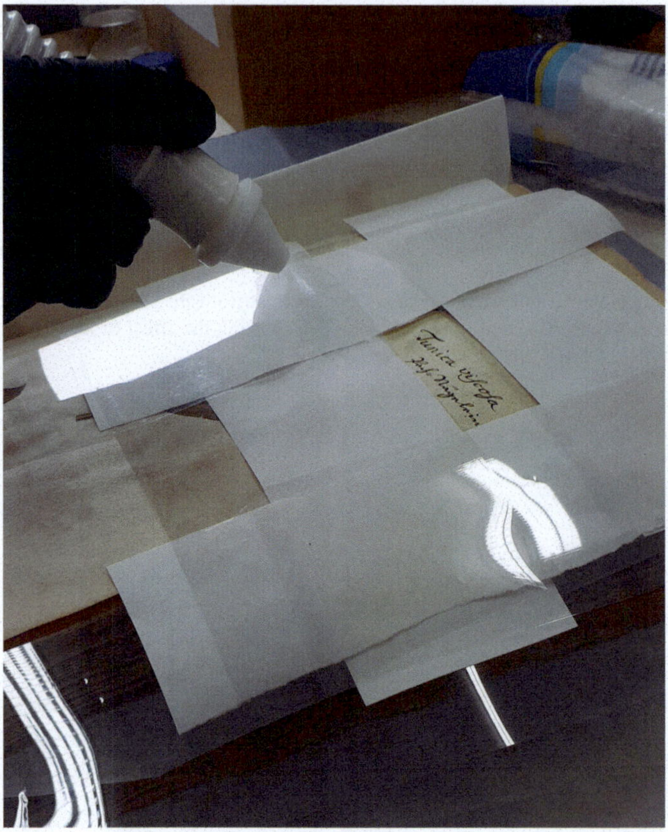

Fig. 5.42 Zeidler's herbarium sheet prepared for nebulisation, with areas covered by blotting paper and Melinex. (Photo: M. Grenda-Kurmanow)

with a hard tool, the repair was covered, as in the case of the Czartoryska herbarium, with a nonwoven fabric and "encasing" cotton wool over the infill, followed by cardboard, on which a small weight was placed.

Ink corrosion areas were nebulised in a manner similar to that used for the Czartoryska herbarium, employing a chelating DTPA solution followed by gelatin application (Fig. 5.42).

The detached fragments of botanical specimens and many loose plant fragments were attached in their original locations. The identification of the correct placement was aided by paper deformations and traces of previously applied adhesive, which reflected the original shape of the botanical specimen. Where it was possible to match fragments and attach them at the edges, assembly was carried out using strips of Japanese *kozo* paper and purified rice starch paste. The adhesive was applied only to the ends of the strip to avoid contact with the specimen itself (Fig. 5.43).

In cases where fragments could not be mounted in this manner (e.g. internal leaf fragments), the fragments were spot-adhered using Aquazol 200 (Figs. 5.44, 5.45 and 5.46 and 5.48 and 5.49).

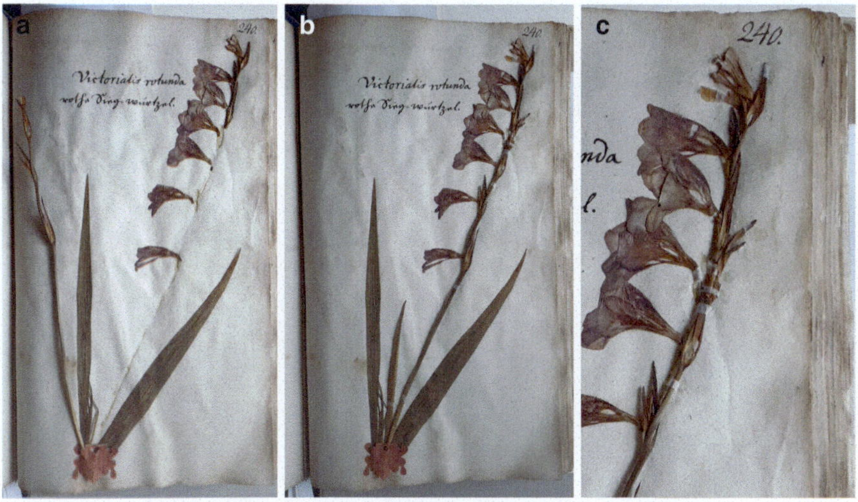

Fig. 5.43 Zeidler's herbarium, Main Library of the University of Life Sciences in Lublin, folio 240 before securing the specimen's stem in the correct position (**a**); after attaching the stem with strips of Japanese paper (**b**); detail—attachment with strips of Japanese paper (**c**). (Photo: M. Grenda-Kurmanow)

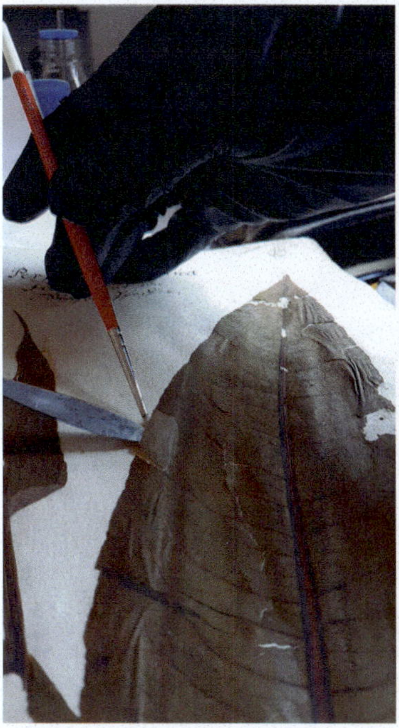

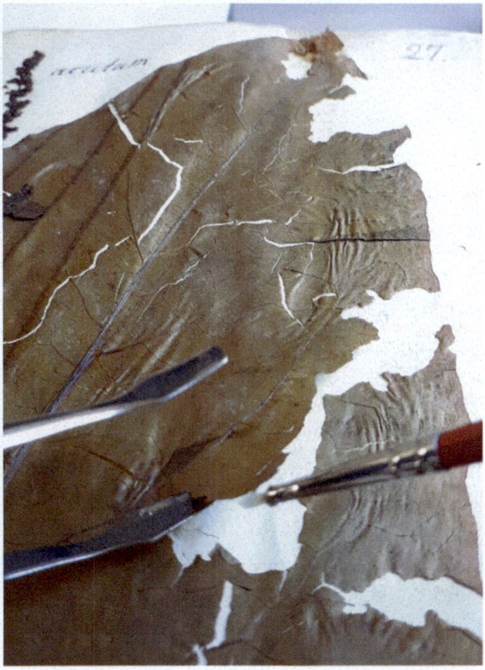

Figs. 5.44 and 5.45 Reattaching specimens in the Zeidler herbarium (Main Library of the University of Life Sciences in Lublin). (Photo: M. Grenda-Kurmanow)

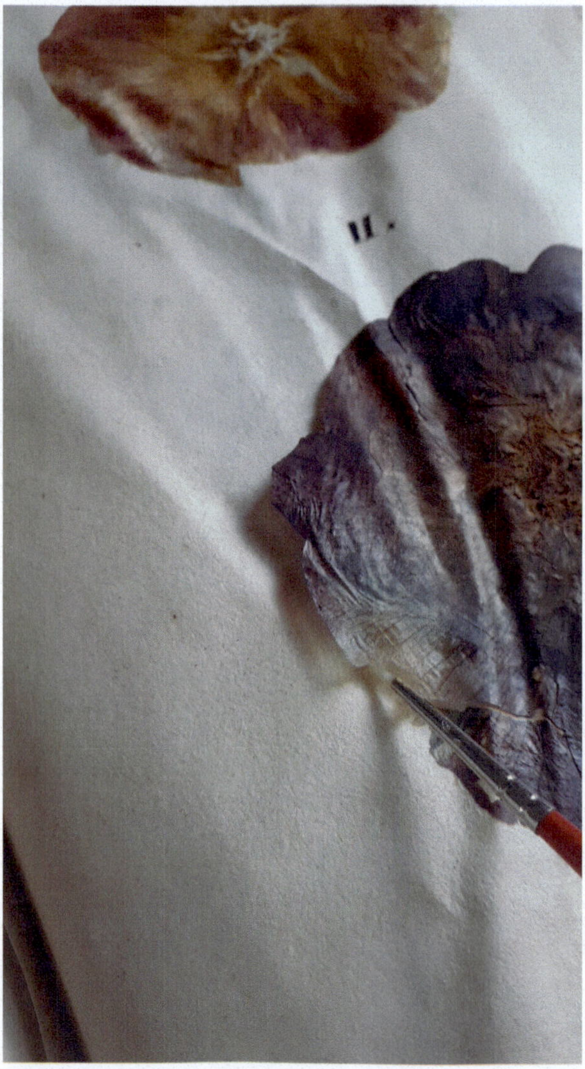

Fig. 5.46 Spot adhesion mounting of a specimen in the Zeidler herbarium (Main Library of the University of Life Sciences in Lublin). (Photo: M. Grenda-Kurmanow)

Subsequently, the consolidation procedure was repeated for specimens where the paint layer was present in significant amounts (Fig. 5.47). As a result of treatment, it was possible to a large extent to restore the plant specimens to their original locations and stabilise them (Figs. 5.48, 5.49 and 5.50).

Fragments that could not be matched with certainty were, as in the case of the Czartoryska herbarium, left in envelopes made of thin acid-free paper, which serve

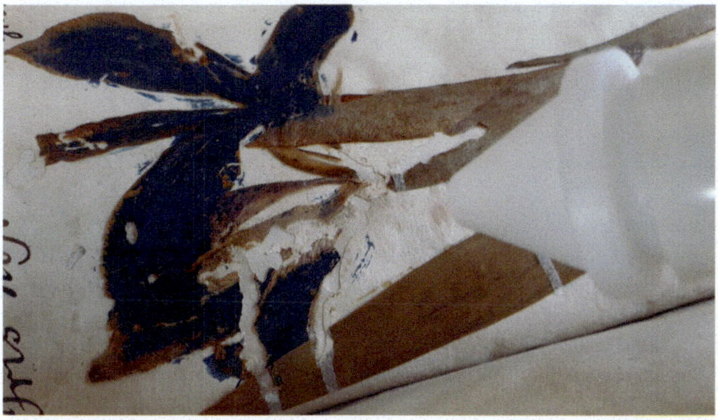

Fig. 5.47 Zeidler herbarium, Main Library of the University of Life Sciences in Lublin, consolidation treatment. (Photo: M. Grenda-Kurmanow)

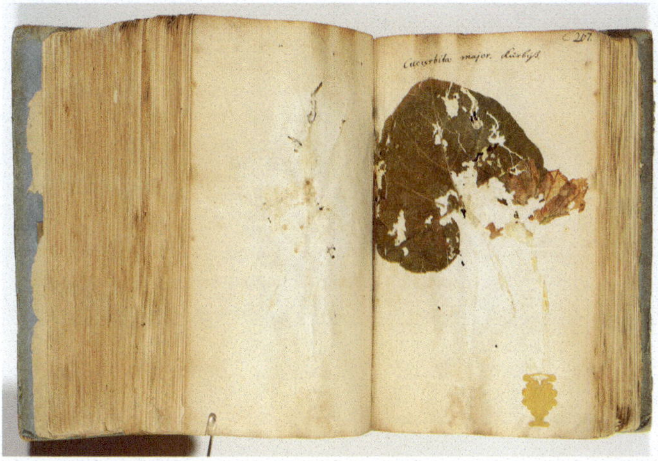

Fig. 5.48 Zeidler herbarium, Main Library of the University of Life Sciences in Lublin, folio 207, before conservation. (Photo: T. Rizov-Ciechański)

as attachments. All attachments were placed in sleeves made of conservation-grade polyester film, which were then placed in acid-free folders. Finally, the text block was reattached to the binding in accordance with the technique found in the object prior to conservation.

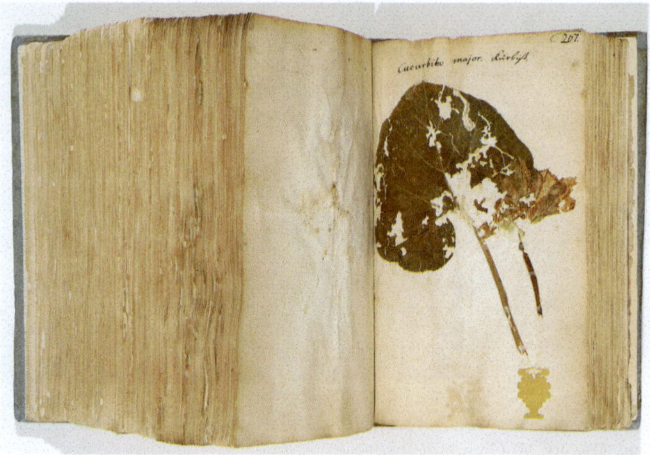

Fig. 5.49 Zeidler herbarium, Main Library of the University of Life Sciences in Lublin, folio 207, after conservation. (Photo: T. Rizov-Ciechański)

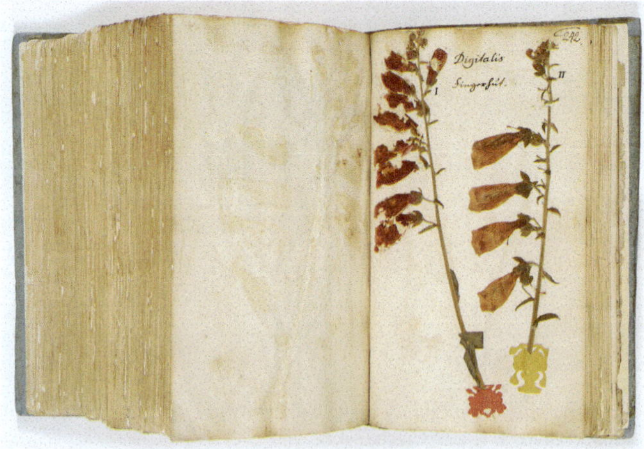

Fig. 5.50 Zeidler herbarium, Main Library of the University of Life Sciences in Lublin, folio 242, after conservation. (Photo: T. Rizov-Ciechański)

5.3 The Helwing/Boretius Herbarium, 1724–45, Herbarium of the Faculty of Biology, University of Warsaw (WA), Ref. WA-KH-13.2.2[26]

5.3.1 *Description*

The herbarium attributed to Helwing or Boretius belongs to the group of the oldest items in the collections of the Herbarium of the Faculty of Biology at the University of Warsaw (WA).[27] Little is known about the history of this object, except that it was most likely created by Andreas Helwing or Matthias Ernest Boretius or was the result of their collaboration and shared naturalist workshop. It is certain that the herbarium was created in Königsberg, where both renowned botanists conducted their scientific work. It is also known that it was part of the collections of the Stadtbibliothek Königsberg. The provenance of the object is confirmed by the watermarks of Johann Adam Riegel's mill in present in paper, as well as the ownership stamp of the library in Königsberg. The stamp is also present in the remaining volumes of herbaria from this collection. These items found their way, in circumstances not fully explained, into the collections of the Herbarium of the Faculty of Biology at the University of Warsaw after 1944. Most of the objects from this collection also bear clear traces of fire. They were therefore most likely removed from the library during the disaster associated with the bombing of Königsberg in 1944. Taking this into account, it can be said that it is truly remarkable that such delicate and complex objects have survived to our times in such good condition.

The herbarium gives the impression of being a working material, a preliminary collection intended to serve as the basis for the creation of a final, fully developed volume.[28] The botanical specimens have not been attached to the substrate, but are instead loosely inserted between the pages of the block (Fig. 5.51). Most specimens (and most likely originally every specimen) have a small label threaded onto them bearing the species name. The labels are made from various types of laid paper, including scraps recovered from earlier manuscripts.[29]

---

[26] Helwing A.J. or Boretius M., untitled, Warsaw, Herbarium of the Faculty of Biology, University of Warsaw (WA), ref. WA-KH-13.2.2, 1724–1745.

[27] Despite different production techniques, the volumes have handwritten reference numbers forming a sequence, probably assigned in the Stadtbibliothek Königsberg, to whose collections they belonged.

[28] The UW Herbarium collection contains a second, analogous volume made in the same way (ref. WA-KH-13.1.4). The remaining Königsberg herbaria from this group are of a completely different character: they are bound in parchment, and in most cases (except for one volume) the specimens are glued to the paper sheets and arranged according to the pre-Linnaean Tournefort system, with a decorative title page for each systematic group. The sheets are numbered, and each specimen is accompanied by a species name. The parchment-bound herbaria are also made on paper from a different mill and contain different watermarks.

[29] Numerous labels reveal fragments of various watermarks in transmitted light, but their fragmentary nature does not allow for precise identification.

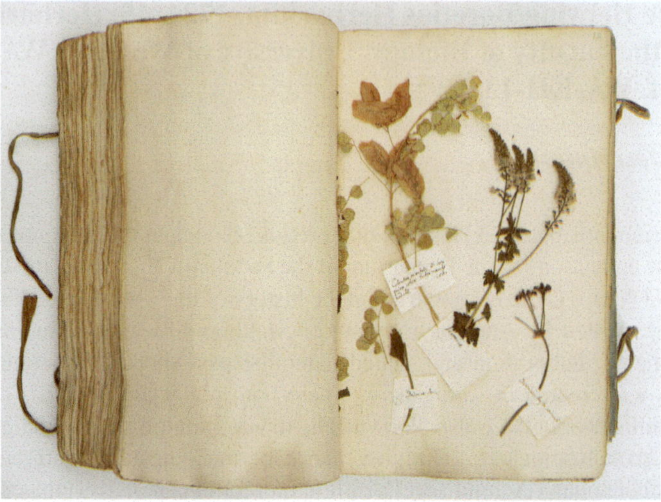

Fig. 5.51 Helwing/Boretius Herbarium, Herbarium of the Faculty of Biology, University of Warsaw (WA), folio 66. Condition before conservation, after pagination. (Photo: T. Rizov-Ciechański)

The tight stitching of a block composed of 115 individual gatherings and its overfilling with numerous specimens (298 items) resulted in significant deformation of both the block itself and the specimens placed between the sheets (Figs. 5.52, 5.53 and 5.54).

The specimens were placed mainly in the centres of the gatherings, which protected them from falling out of the block. However, the arrangement of their distribution was not consistently uniform, indicating that, most likely, specimens had been moved between the block's sheets in the past. This resulted in numerous mechanical damages and losses of plant fragments, and presumably also disrupted the original order of their arrangement. It should be noted that, in the condition in which the object was found, the specimens were not organised in any logical manner; rather, they appeared to have been "thrown" into the gatherings for later use.[30] The fact that the specimens were treated as tools for further work is evidenced by their detailed labelling, and despite the deformation caused by the overfilled block, careful preparation of the specimens as herbarium material was still apparent.

Furthermore, deformation and gaps between the sheets of the block facilitated insect infestation, resulting in numerous losses of specimens and sheets in the form of larval tunnels. Despite the absence of adhesive, which is usually considered the main factor attracting insects, the object bears numerous traces of feeding activity (Figs. 5.55 and 5.56).

[30] In the opinion of Dr. Maja Graniszewska, curator of the UW Herbarium, there is no discernible arrangement of specimens corresponding to any systematic order.

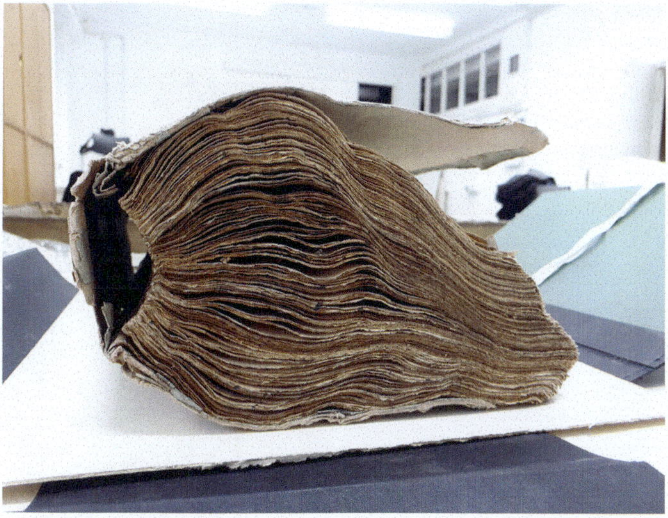

Fig. 5.52 Helwing/Boretius Herbarium, Herbarium of the Faculty of Biology, University of Warsaw (WA), condition before conservation. (Photo: M. Grenda-Kurmanow)

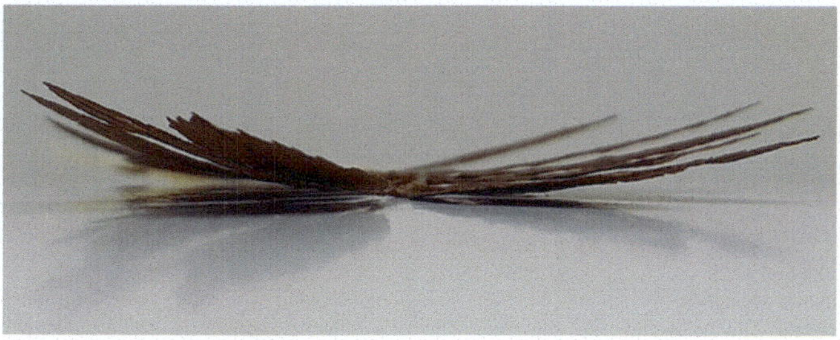

Fig. 5.53 Specimen from the Helwing/Boretius herbarium, Herbarium of the Faculty of Biology, University of Warsaw (WA). Deformation of the specimen. (Photo: M. Grenda-Kurmanow)

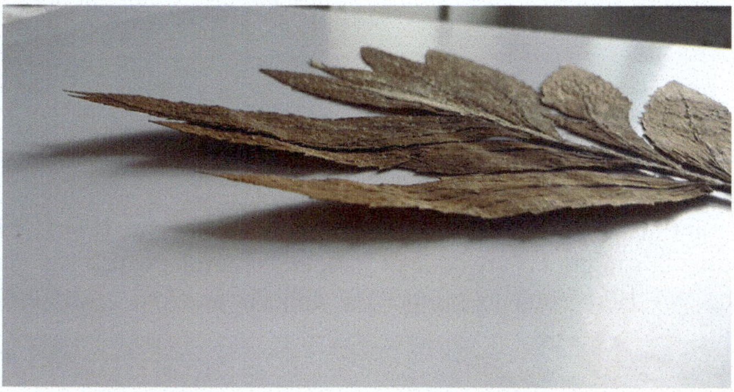

Fig. 5.54 Specimen from the Helwing/Boretius herbarium, Herbarium of the Faculty of Biology, University of Warsaw (WA). Deformation of the specimen. (Photo: M. Grenda-Kurmanow)

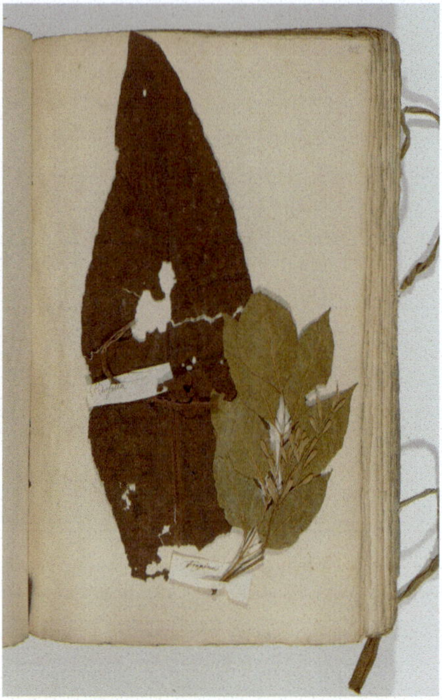

Fig. 5.55 Helwing/Boretius Herbarium, Herbarium of the Faculty of Biology, University of Warsaw (WA), specimen losses caused by insect activity. (Photo: T. Rizov-Ciechański)

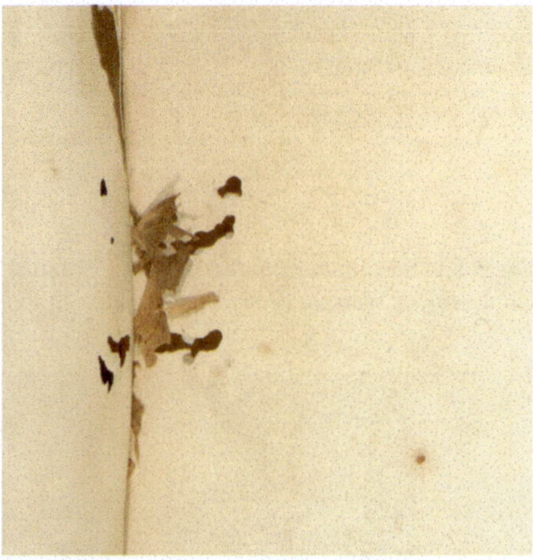

Fig. 5.56 Helwing/Boretius Herbarium, Herbarium of the Faculty of Biology, University of Warsaw (WA), damage caused by insect activity. (Photo: T. Rizov-Ciechański)

Black point discolourations were visible on the block cuts (Fig. 5.57). It was suspected that this might be a residue of mercuric chloride, which was most likely used in the WA Herbarium to protect the collections from insect infestation.[31]

[31] Personal comment of the curator of the Herbarium, Dr. Maja Graniszewska.

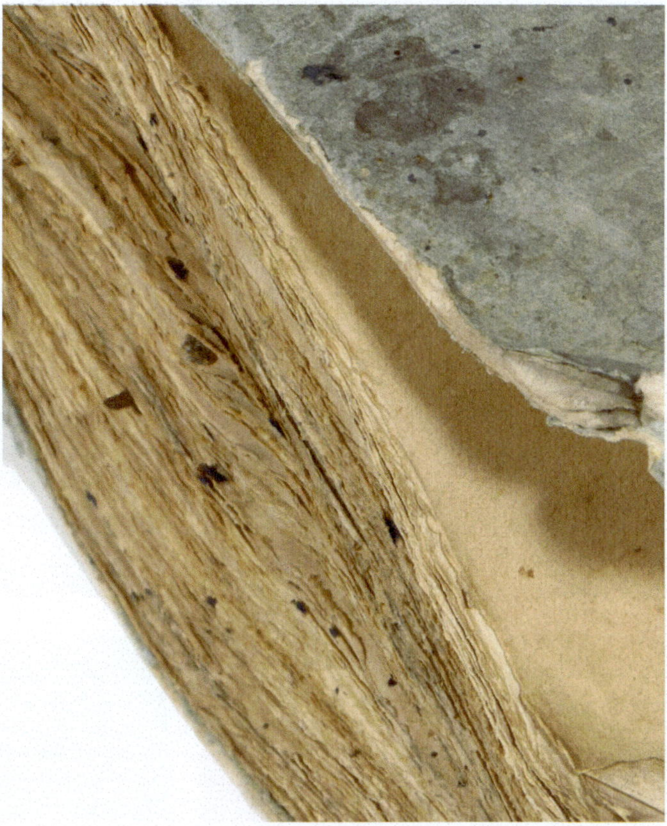

Fig. 5.57 Helwing/Boretius Herbarium, Herbarium of the Faculty of Biology, University of Warsaw (WA), black point discolourations on the block edge. (Photo: T. Rizov-Ciechański)

Numerous iron filings were also present in the paper of the sheets, as well as ink corrosion on many of the labels.

The results of the Ma-XRF[32] analysis (Fig. 5.58, see also Fig. 5.60) demonstrate an example of a dark discolouration, in which a concentration of several metal elements is visible: mercury, zinc, and copper. Bromine, chlorine, and iron are also present, evenly distributed throughout the object. In the case of the examined fragment (the dark discolouration in the first frame and marked with a green circle in the remaining frames), it is difficult to determine unequivocally whether the mercury is a contaminant from a metallic artefact in the paper, or conversely, whether the zinc and copper are contaminants of a mercury-based pesticide. Mercury was also detected in the manuscript layer of this object, and may therefore have been an additive to vitriol in iron gall ink. However, this discolouration is not part of the ink

[32] Ma-XRF analysis, performed by Łukasz Ćwikliński at the Interdisciplinary Centre for Modern Interdisciplinary Technologies (ICNT) in Toruń.

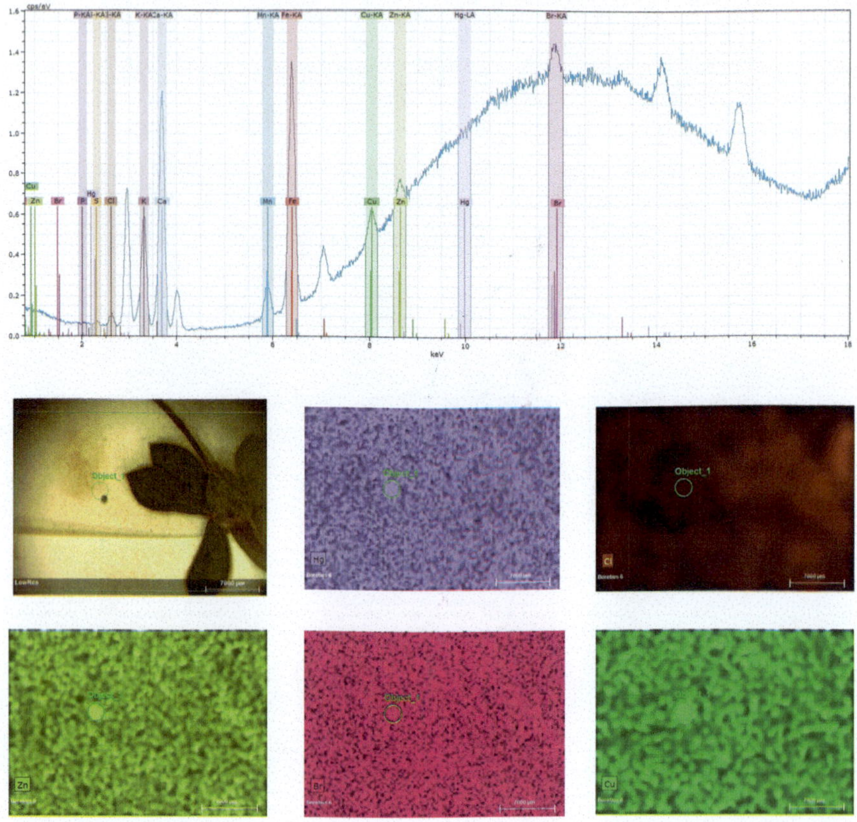

Fig. 5.58 Example of a Ma-XRF spectrum (**a**) and mapping for selected elements for selected elements detected in the Helwing/Boretius herbarium (1724–1745). Fragment in VIS (**b**), mapping of mercury (**c**), chlorine (**d**), zinc (**e**), bromine (**f**), and copper (**g**)

inscription, but rather a structural contamination characteristic of mercuric chloride. It is also known that in the owner's residence, sublimate was used in the collections as a preservation method, so it can be assumed that this result confirms the presence of a biocide. Furthermore, the presence of bromine in all scans suggests the historical use of methyl bromide as a fumigant.

VOC analysis of the Helwing/Boretius herbarium (Fig. 5.59) revealed the presence insecticide available under the name Butocarboxim, belonging to the carbamate group.[33]

As with the other herbaria, the qualitative analysis of the Helwing/Boretius herbarium revealed that among the volatile compounds present within the objects, it is

---

[33] GC/MS-SPME analysis, performed by Prof. Tomasz Sawoszczuk, Kraków University of Economics. The analysis revealed also the presence of arsenic, but its presence was ruled out similar to the case of Zeidler's herbarium.

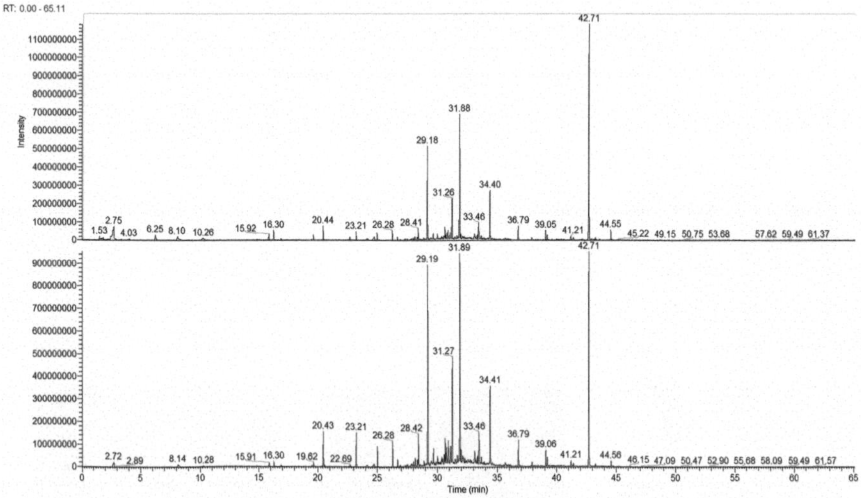

Fig. 5.59 Chromatograms showing VOCs collected inside the Helwing/Boretius herbarium

possible to identify, among others: furfural and acetic acid, which are products of cellulose and hemicellulose degradation; amino acids indicating the degradation of plant material contained within the objects; and essential oils derived from the plants themselves. Analysis for the presence of microbiological volatile organic compounds, which serve as markers of mould activity, excluded the presence of active mould forms.

Analysis of the manuscript layer confirmed the presence of an ink based on iron compounds, most likely iron gall ink,[34] which also contains zinc (Fig. 5.60).

During the preparations for the research and conservation project, a question arose as to why approximately 300 botanical specimens (possibly more in the past) were placed in a very tightly sewn block, and how to address the challenge of preserving the original character of the object while simultaneously ensuring the safety of the botanical specimens.

It has been accepted that the herbarium, as previously mentioned, was preparatory in nature and not a finished work. Interestingly, the binding of the herbarium had a similar construction to that of Zeidler's herbarium. It was therefore concluded that the block was probably intentionally bound in a manner that would allow for easy replacement of the binding.

[34] The presence of iron ions in the +2 oxidation state was also confirmed by testing with bathophenanthroline indicators.

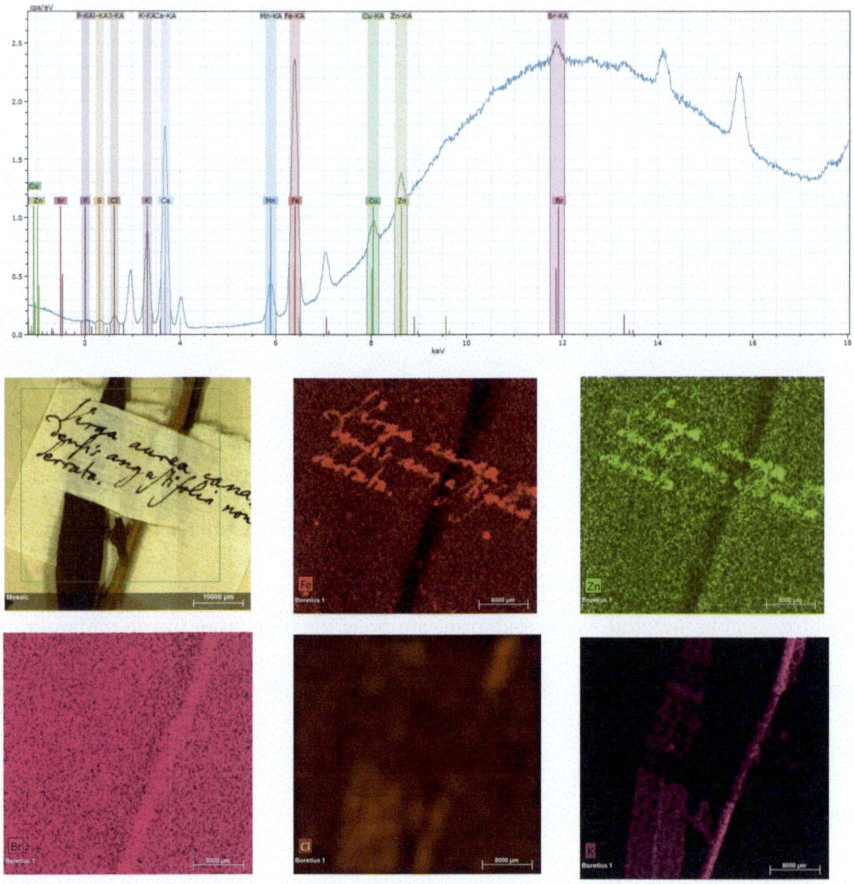

Fig. 5.60 Identification of iron gall ink. Ma-XRF spectrum (**a**) and mapping for selected elements detected in Helwing/Boretius herbarium. Manuscript fragment in VIS (**b**), mapping of iron (**c**), zinc (**d**), bromine (**e**), chlorine (**f**), and potassium (**g**)

5.3.2 Conservation Objectives

As a result of numerous discussions with the Herbarium Curator, it was determined that it would be impossible to preserve the object in its existing form, that is, as botanical specimens loosely inserted between the pages of a tightly bound block, without exposing the plants to further damage and perpetuating their deformation. Moreover, many specimens had become fragmented, and detached leaves, stems, petals, and their fragments had slipped into the gutter, creating a risk of further loss of botanical material. It was therefore clear that the specimens and the block would need to be separated, not only for the duration of the conservation treatments, but also on a permanent basis but in a reversible manner. A decision was thus made to permanently remove the specimens from the block and mount them on individual supports made from acid-free materials. In order to enable the reconstruction of the original arrangement of the specimens, it was decided to introduce pagination and to produce photographic documentation of all pages containing specimens. The conservation of the block itself was planned to be as conservative as possible, in order to preserve the volume as an authentic document of the Prussian naturalists' workshop. Due to extensive damage to the binding, it was decided to separate it from the block to allow for conservation treatments. However, the treatments on the pages of the block were planned without dismantling it.

In the case of the specimens, a decision was made to strive for the maximum possible reassembly of broken specimens by matching preserved fragments. Although current herbarium collection management practice recommends placing broken plant fragments in envelopes (Bridson and Forman 1999, pp. 34–38), in this instance it was considered that the historical nature of the collection and the extent of the damage justified an attempt to reassemble the specimens wherever possible. Furthermore, many specimens consisted solely of fragments, which, if the standard methodology for handling broken botanical specimens were applied, would mean placing all the preserved parts in envelopes. It was determined that such a solution would not be any safer than mounting the fragments on sheets. Fragments that could not be matched were planned to be placed in envelopes attached to the specimen mounts. For the reassembly of specimens, it was necessary to use an adhesive that would not have a destructive effect on the plant genetic material. In addition, as with the previously described herbaria, it was deemed necessary to treat ink corrosion and metal inclusions present in the structure of the sheets, due to their potential catalytic effect on the degradation processes of the herbarium's structural elements.

5.3.3 Conservation Procedures Using a Safe Conservation Methodology and Including Research Findings[35]

The conservation procedures began with the application of pencil pagination and the preparation of photographic documentation, including all sheets containing specimens. Subsequent activities related to the separation of the object's components were carried out in a strictly organised and coordinated manner. Specimens were removed from between the sheets and placed on acid-free cardboard mounts, cut to the size of the block's pages. The mounts were labelled with the numbers of the sheets from which the respective specimens originated. In cases where several specimens were present on a single sheet, an additional sequential number was added in parentheses next to the page number. Small fragments were placed in

[35] Detailed descriptions of all technical analyses results, treatments and specifications of the materials used are included in the conservation report [Grenda-Kurmanow M. (2019c) *Dokumentacja prac konserwatorskich i restauratorskich. Zielnik przypisywany Matthiasowi Boretiusowi lub Andreasowi Helwingowi z I połowy XVIII w., ze zbiorów Zielnika Wydziału Biologii Uniwersytetu Warszawskiego*, conservation report, Warsaw-Kraków].

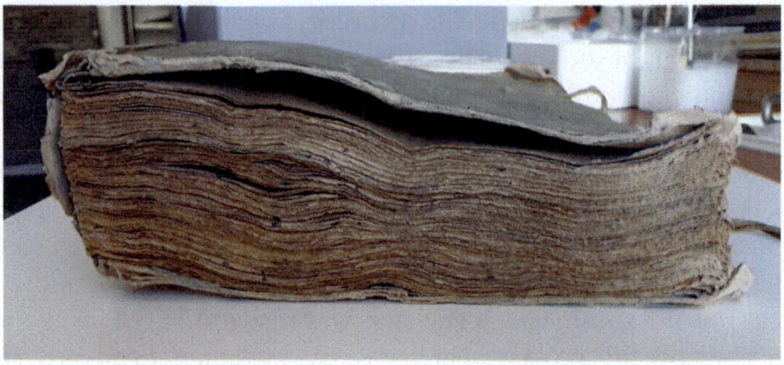

Fig. 5.61 Helwing/Boretius herbarium block, Herbarium of the Faculty of Biology, University of Warsaw (WA), after removal of specimens. (Photo: M. Grenda-Kurmanow)

envelopes made of thin acid-free paper. The mounts were wrapped in thin acid-free paper, and the resulting wrapper was also labelled and stored until conservation procedures could be carried out on the given specimen. The block, together with its binding, changed significantly as a result of the mere removal of the specimens (Fig. 5.61).

The block underwent a series of conservation treatments. Due to damage to the binding, it was separated from the block. A thick layer of dirt and dust, which was removed, had accumulated in the space between the spine of the binding and the spine of the block, as well as on the leaves of the block.

The cover boards were washed, and the blue cover paper, which was also severely degraded, was separated. The boards underwent consolidation and infilling of losses, followed by flattening. Conservation treatments on the block pages were carried out without disassembly, which also included the reinforcement of sewing threads and the spines of gatherings at points of rupture. Only the first and last gatherings were removed, as the sewing in these areas was loose and weakened. The folios were surface cleaned using a soft synthetic bristle brush, latex sponge, and sulphur-free erasers (Fig. 5.62).

Iron inclusions present within the structure of the paper were, in some cases, mechanically removed. Black pinpoint discolourations, most likely resulting from sublimate (mercury chloride), were also mechanically removed. Losses in the paper of the pages and other mechanical damages were repaired using Japanese *mitsumata* paper and purified rice starch paste. A gelatin solution was applied to areas discoloured by the presence of metal particles in the paper. The pH of the text block leaves prior to conservation ranged from 4.6 to 5.4; these were deacidified using the non-aqueous Bookkeeper deacidification agent in spray. After completing conservation treatments on the binding and text block, as well as the conservation of the cover paper, the binding was reassembled with the block in accordance with the original construction scheme (Figs. 5.63 and 5.64).

The accompanying specimen labels were also subjected to conservation. Each label was carefully removed from the specimen and then signed on the reverse in the same manner as the mounts and wrappers. After surface cleaning, the water

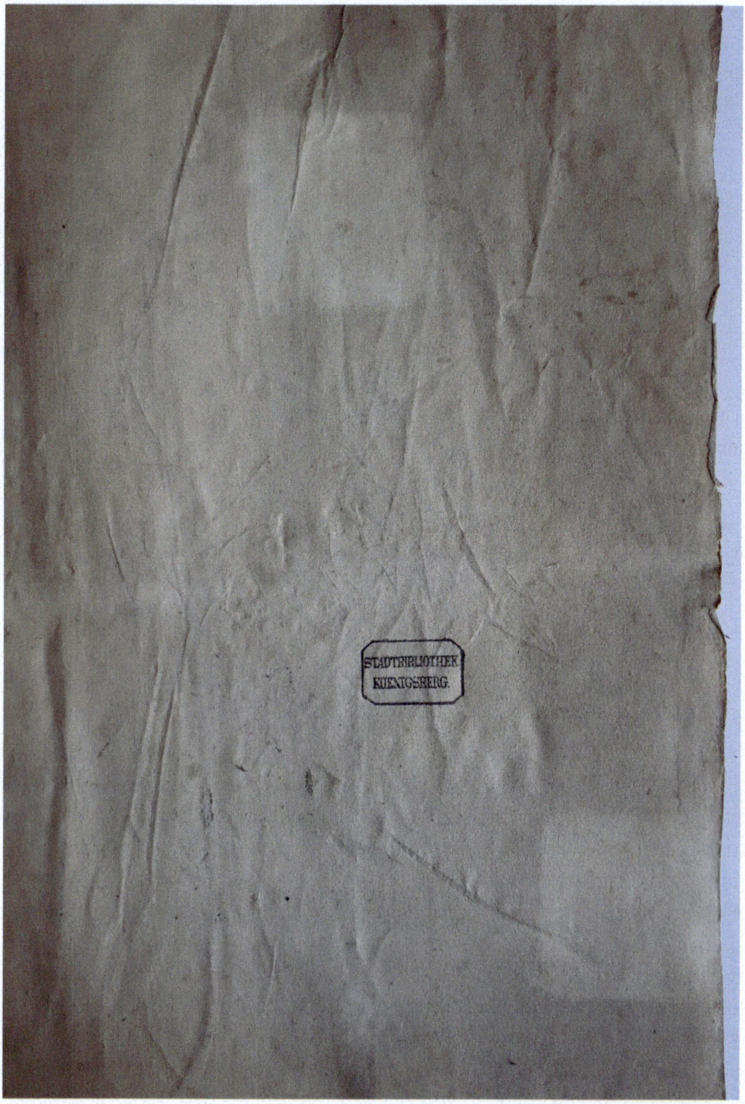

Fig. 5.62 The first page of the Helwing/Boretius herbarium block, Herbarium of the Faculty of Biology, University of Warsaw (WA), during surface cleaning. (Photo: M. Grenda-Kurmanow)

resistance of the manuscript layer was tested. The presence of Fe^{+2} ions was confirmed on selected labels using bathophenantroline strips. The labels were then washed and re-sized with gelatine. Deacidification was not necessary, as the pH of selected labels after aqueous treatment ranged from 6.1 to 7.2. Losses were then filled and mechanical damage repaired using Japanese *kozo* papers. The labels were flattened. Following these procedures, they were re-threaded onto the specimens in

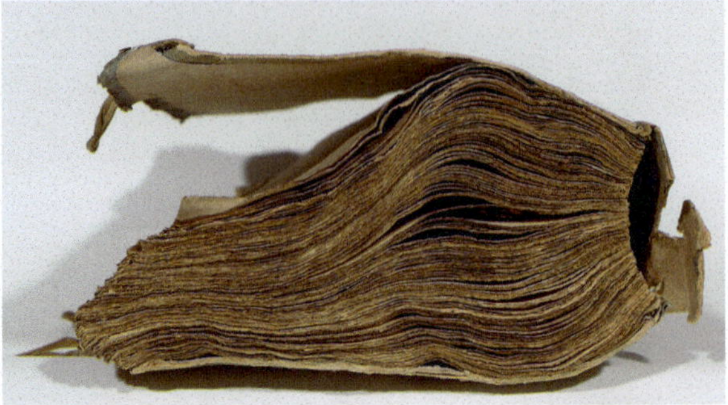

Fig. 5.63 Herbarium block of Helwing/Boretius, Herbarium of the Faculty of Biology, University of Warsaw (WA), before conservation. (Photo: T. Rizov-Ciechański)

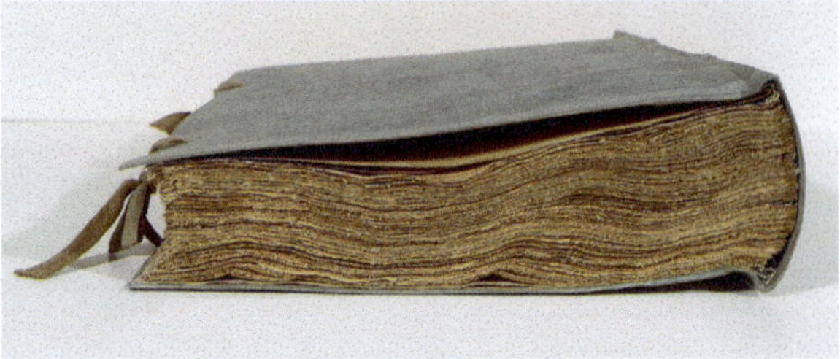

Fig. 5.64 Herbarium block of Helwing/Boretius, Herbarium of the Faculty of Biology, University of Warsaw (WA), after conservation. (Photo: T. Rizov-Ciechański)

accordance with their original arrangement, using photographic documentation taken prior to conservation as a reference.

Subsequently, procedures were carried out on the botanical specimens. No surface cleaning treatments were applied to the specimens. Among the nearly 300 specimens present in the collection, the preserved plants exhibited a wide range of conditions and characteristic structural features that could have been damaged during attempts to clean them with a brush.

Work with each specimen began by placing it on the mount at the intended attachment site. Next, the specimen was secured to the mount without the use of adhesive, following a procedure agreed upon with the owner. If the specimen was complete, the points for incisions to thread the securing strip, cut from acid-free paper, were marked. When determining these points, the principle was to use as few anchor points as possible. The paper strips were threaded through the incisions, leaving free ends on the reverse side of the mount. The free ends of the strip were then flattened by folding them parallel to the surface of the mount (Figs. 5.65 and 5.66). Where it was possible to attach fragments of specimens without the use of adhesive, by securing them next to the main part of the specimen, loose fragments were attached in an analogous manner, by threading the strip (Figs. 5.65, 5.66, and 5.67).

This mounting method is durable while also allowing for very easy disassembly. At the same time, it enabled the flattening of deformed specimens without causing any damage. A different type of mounting was used for a specimen for which strap mounting was not possible. In this case, a pocket was made from conservation-grade polyester, which was closed without the use of adhesives and attached to the backing with a threaded paper strap (Fig. 5.68).

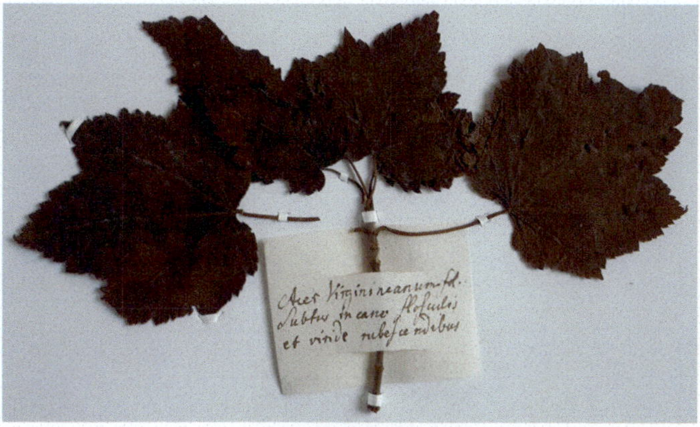

Fig. 5.65 Specimen from the Helwing/Boretius herbarium, Herbarium of the Faculty of Biology, University of Warsaw (WA), adhesive-free mounting, fragments added to the specimen and attached in the same manner. (Photo: M. Grenda-Kurmanow)

Fig. 5.66 Adhesive-free mounting, view from the *verso* of the mount. (Photo: M. Grenda-Kurmanow)

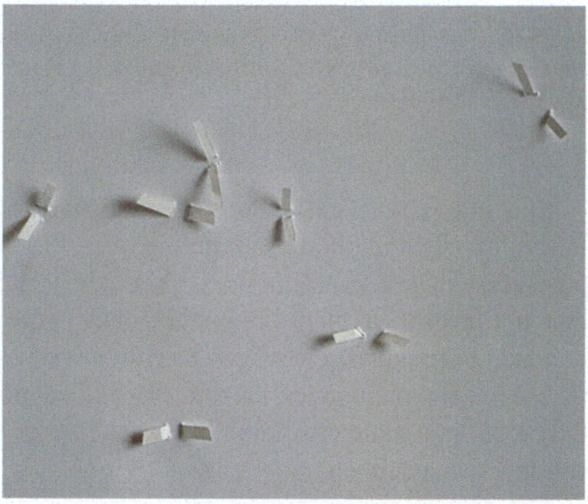

Fig. 5.67 Specimen "reintegrated" by attaching individual fragments in their appropriate positions. (Photo: M. Grenda-Kurmanow)

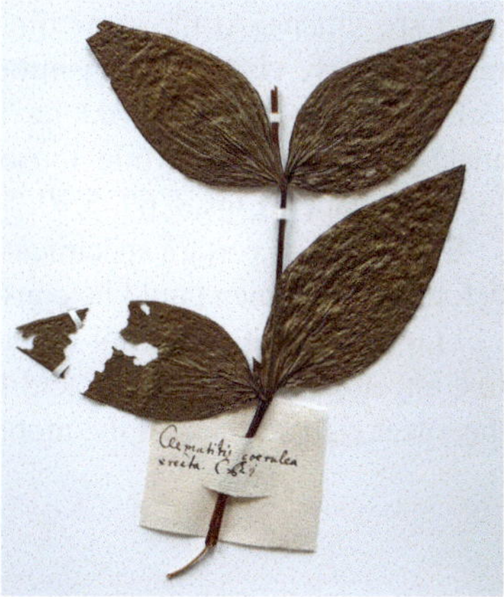

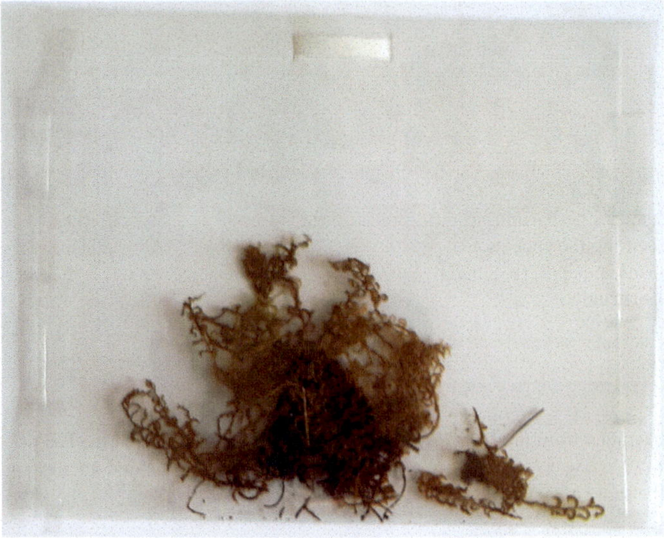

Fig. 5.68 Specimen from the Helwing/Boretius herbarium, Herbarium of the Faculty of Biology, University of Warsaw (WA), mounted in a pocket made of conservation-grade polyester. (Photo: M. Grenda-Kurmanow)

Specimens that had undergone extensive fragmentation, preventing the previously described method of mounting, were first arranged on a support to assess the possibility of reassembling the specimen (Figs. 5.69 and 5.70). If it was possible to match the broken plant fragments, they were then joined using adhesive. The matched fragments were placed face down on nonwoven fabric. Next, along the line where the fragments met, narrow strips of Japanese *kozo* paper were placed across the break, in a manner resembling stitches. Aquazol 200 adhesive was used to consolidate the specimens.

The adhesive proved sufficiently effective that the consolidated specimens could be safely handled for mounting onto the substrate in a manner analogous to the other specimens. At the same time, all damage and fractures within the specimen remain clearly visible in transmitted light (Fig. 5.70b). In many cases, a combined technique was also employed, i.e. fragments that could be mounted separately were attached with strips, while those requiring consolidation were reinforced with Japanese paper (Figs. 5.69, 5.70, 5.71, and 5.72).

In the case of certain specimens, it was necessary to perform multiple such joins before the specimen could be consolidated (Figs. 5.71 and 5.72).

Fragments that could not be matched with certainty were left in labelled acid-free envelopes made of thin acid-free interleaving paper, which were aattached to the lower right corners of the mounts using Aquazol 200 (Figs. 5.70c and 5.72).

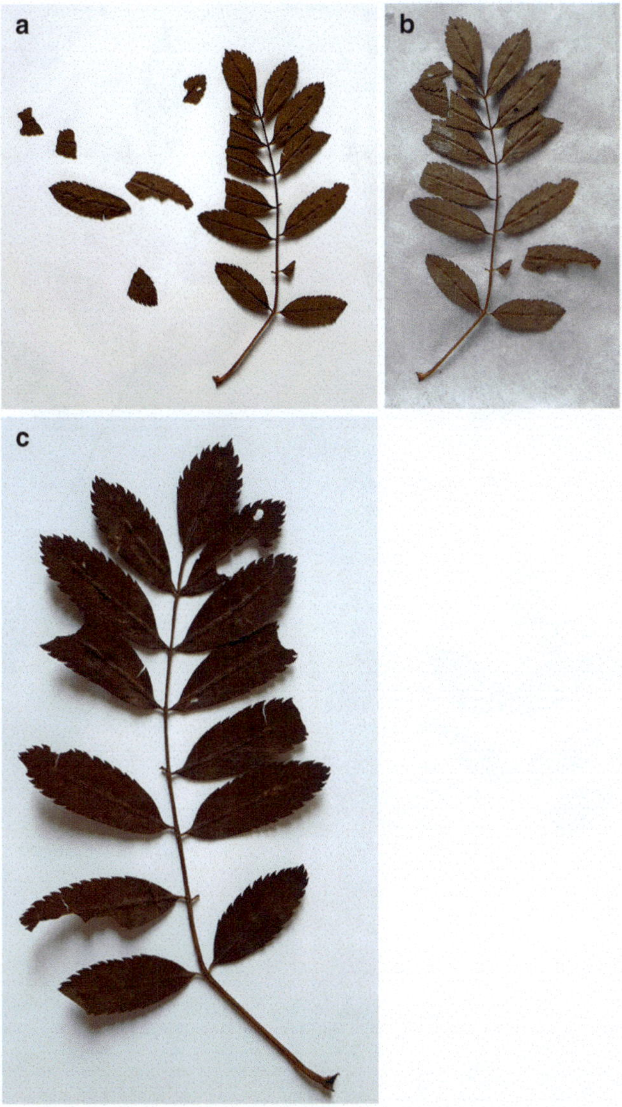

Fig. 5.69 Specimen from the Helwing/Boretius Herbarium, Herbarium of the Faculty of Biology, University of Warsaw (WA); before the application of consolidating reinforcements (**a**), after their application (**b**—*verso*, **c**—*recto* of the specimen). (Photo: M. Grenda-Kurmanow)

After mounting the specimens and envelopes made of thin acid-free paper, simple wrappers were prepared from the same paper in the form of a single folded sheet. Upon completion of all conservation procedures, the volume was placed in a box made of acid-free materials. The specimens on mounts were placed in four identical acid-free boxes.

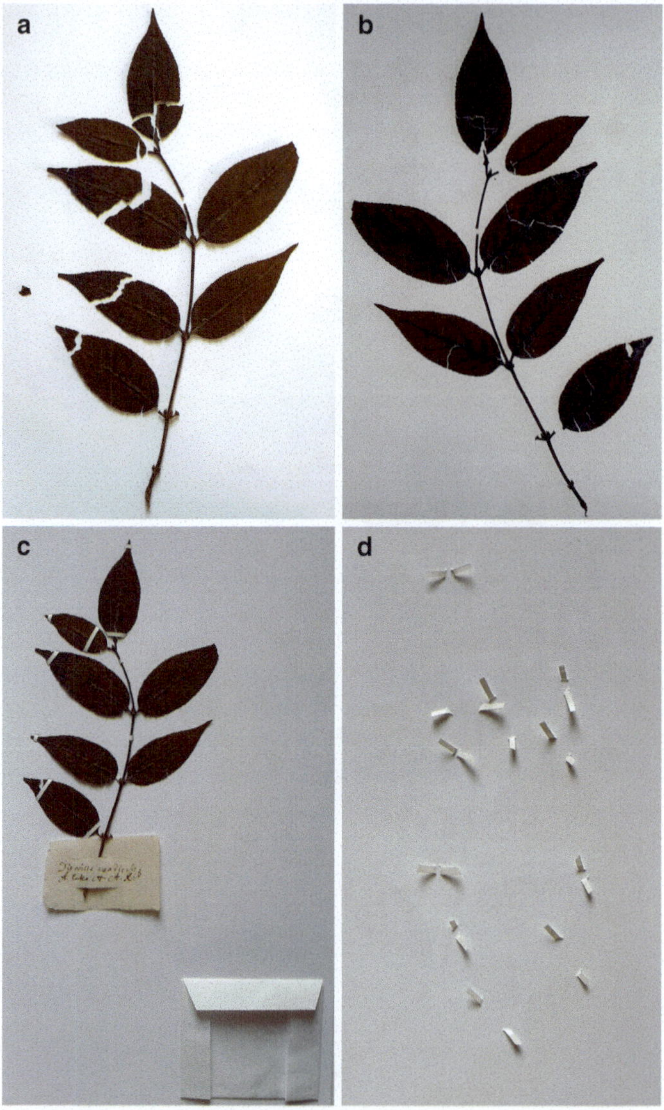

Fig. 5.70 Specimen from the Helwing/Boretius Herbarium, Herbarium of the Faculty of Biology, University of Warsaw (WA); before the application of consolidating reinforcements (**a**); after their application (**b**—view in transmitted light); after the application of consolidating reinforcements and non-adhesive mounting (**c**, **d**); *recto* (**c**); detail of the *verso* of the support (**d**). (Photo: M. Grenda-Kurmanow)

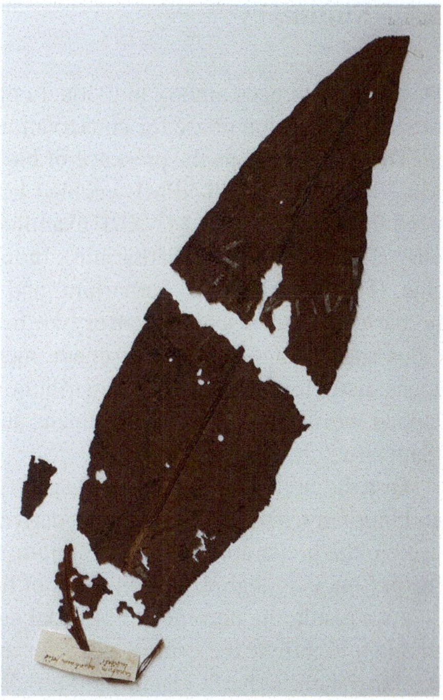

Fig. 5.71 Specimen from the Helwing/Boretius Herbarium, Herbarium of the Faculty of Biology, University of Warsaw (WA), during the process of consolidation mounting. (Photo: M. Grenda-Kurmanow)

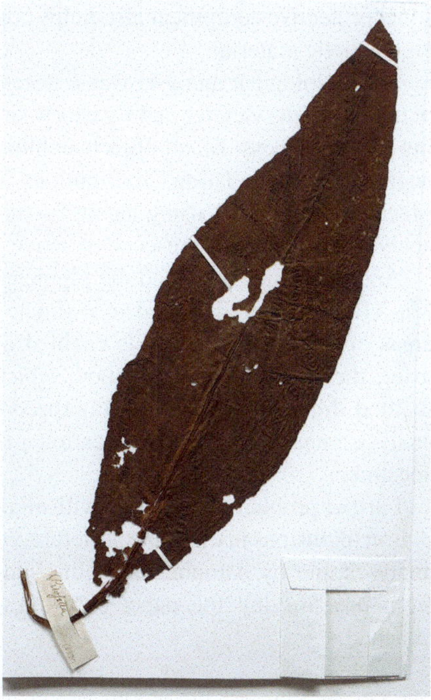

Fig. 5.72 Specimen from the Helwing/Boretius Herbarium, Herbarium of the Faculty of Biology, University of Warsaw (WA), after consolidation with adhesive strips and non-adhesive mounting onto a new substrate. (Photo: M. Grenda-Kurmanow)

5.4 Summary

Despite differences among individual objects, several general issues emerged during the preparation phase for conservation treatment.

The first issue was the presence of biocidal substances in the objects. The use of Ma-XRF and GC/MS-SPME enabled holistic analysis of the objects without the need for sampling. The Ma-XRF examination allowed for the identification of mercury (Helwing/Boretius herbarium), bromine (Helwing/Boretius herbarium), chlorine (Helwing/Boretius herbarium and Czartoryska herbarium), lead (Zeidler herbarium), and arsenic (Czartoryska herbarium), which are components of biocides such as arsenic, lead arsenate, mercuric chloride, and methyl bromide. All scans also clearly showed the distribution of calcium and potassium, which overlapped with the area of the specimens and are macroelements naturally present in plant structures.

Historic herbaria contain a full spectrum of chemical compounds, both organic and inorganic in origin, which may derive from the plants themselves, the materials used in the preparation of the herbarium, its conservation and preservation, or from the presence of degradation products of these materials.

As a result, the presence of biocidal agents was confirmed in all herbaria. These findings highlight the critical need for awareness among conservators and others working with herbaria regarding the risks associated with their use. For each herbarium, the importance of work safety and the necessity of using personal protective equipment when handling the specimens were emphasised. On the other hand, personal protective equipment also helps protect herbaria from contamination with foreign genetic material.

Microbiological analysis was a necessary procedure for all three herbaria, particularly for the Zeidler and Czartoryska collections, due to visible traces of flooding and dampness. As all objects exhibited highly complex structures and varying degrees of degradation, the options for potential disinfection were limited. Mechanical cleaning using alcohol-soaked swabs was considered. However, VOC analysis excluded the presence of active moulds.

Another issue concerned the pigments and dyes present in Zeidler's herbarium. Ma-XRF was initially used to estimate the presence of inorganic compounds in areas of the paint layer. This enabled a more detailed identification of pigments using the microchemical method, which required sampling. When the Ma-XRF method did not yield results, microscopic samples were collected for HPLC/MS analysis, enabling the identification of most of the dyes used to decorate the specimens.

Further problems associated with all objects were ink corrosion and the presence of iron inclusions in the paper structure, confirmed by visible-light, UV and Ma-XRF analyses and by batophenanthroline indicators, as well as the decision to refrain from deacidifying the paper substrates to which the herbarium specimens are attached.

The treatment of the ink corrosion in herbarium collections still needs to be developed. The proposed experimental solution involving nebulization is not perfect, as it humidifies the ink layer; however, it enables the introduction of complexing agents. Another problem is the inability to use wet treatments on objects such as herbaria. Another issue is that gelatin, widely and successfully used to stabilise iron gall ink corrosion, is a natural adhesive, and its use in herbaria may, in many cases, raise concerns about contamination of genetic material. However, the choice of materials used in conservation must provide the long-term stability of all elements.

The acidification of the paper substrate and the presence of transition metal ions, components of inks, result in ongoing ink corrosion and degradation of paper and other herbarium materials, making deacidification a desirable procedure.[36]

Moreover, the acidic environment resulting from substrate degradation may affect the degradation of botanical material by catalysing the destruction of genetic material.[37]

On the other hand, the ability to control the level of alkalisation with Bookkeeper is limited. The optimal pH for herbarium collections has yet to be determined. In the case of over-alkalisation of objects, neutralising this process would be impossible due to the need to avoid water treatments. The treatment would also pose a technical issue: its direct application to herbarium sheets could lead to the accumulation of a white residue on the specimens' surfaces. In most cases, such deposits would be impossible to remove.

Additionally, the presence of large amounts of Prussian blue in certain areas of the Zeidler herbarium precluded the use of deacidifying agents. The use of acid-free interleaves in bound volumes was also not an option due to the risk of overfilling the block structure.

Deacidification was performed only in the Helwing/Boretius herbarium block, as sheets had low pH. The procedure was performed because this block no longer contains botanical specimens. After conservation treatment, each volume was placed in an acid-free box.

Another issue present in all specimens and typical of herbarium objects is deformation of paper and botanical specimens resulting from the combination of dried plants, paper, and adhesive. Deformation of paper in historical objects is generally considered undesirable, and efforts are usually made to eliminate it, typically by humidifying the paper followed by flattening using various methods. In the case of herbaria, however, such procedures are usually entirely inadvisable and could pose a risk to the mounted specimens. Under unfavourable conditions, all layers undergo deformation, degradation, and disintegration, particularly in the Czartoryska Herbarium. With the primary aim of protecting the dried botanical specimens from ongoing deterioration, it is essential to reinforce mechanical damage and carry out infills in a way that preserves the substrate's deformation, thereby providing support to the botanical specimen. The weighting of repairs and reinforcements should

[36] See the section *Acid Hydrolysis* in Chap. 3.

[37] See the section *Degradation of Genetic Material* in Chap. 3.

be carried out using soft padding, such as cotton wool, soft weights, or a suitably soft layer of felt, which allows the object to retain its three-dimensional character during drying and setting of the adhesive. This also implies the need to select a suitable material for infills. It must be sufficiently flexible to allow the deformation, which should be preserved, to be repeated. At the same time, for such procedures, long-fibred paper is preferred as a repair material, as it enables good integration of the infill with the edges of the loss or other area of mechanical damage.

A separate issue concerns direct conservation interventions on botanical specimens. In all the examined collections, numerous broken yet still identifiable fragments of botanical specimens were present, having slid towards the gutter. In some cases, these were very large fragments. The principle applied in modern herbarium collections—that all detached parts of specimens should be placed in a special envelope, which is then attached to the herbarium sheet—often cannot be implemented in the case of historical bound herbaria, where extensive specimen damage is present. Removing a fragment from a given folio significantly impairs its legibility, diminishing its informational value. It is also not possible to non-invasively attach an envelope containing specimen fragments to the folios of a codex. The owners of the collections were unanimous in their desire to be able to use the collections after conservation, and placing specimens as additional attachments in separate envelopes and folders would, in practice, mean their permanent separation from the main object. Regarding the reliability of fragment matching, it was often possible to precisely identify the original location of a given specimen based on the shape of the fragment and the pattern of damage, which could be fitted together like pieces of a puzzle. Original paper deformations, often preserving the outline of stems, were also very helpful in identification, as were discolourations resulting from contact between the plant and the paper substrate, and the layer of adhesive exposed after the specimen had become detached, which often exactly replicated its shape. However, it is important to remember that when matching disconnected fragments, one should avoid acting when hypotheses begin to form. In such instances, reassembling the specimen may resemble the actions of early naturalists, who could reconstruct a specimen's image from several different plants. In cases of identification uncertainty, close collaboration between the conservator and a botanist is essential.

Fragments may be restored to their original location by attaching them with strips of Japanese paper in such a way that adhesive is applied only to the ends of the strip, ensuring that the botanical specimen does not come into direct contact with the adhesive. In particular cases, specimens may also be adhered directly to the substrate. In both cases, adhesives should be used that do not negatively affect the structure of the dried plants. Given the degree of damage to the objects (especially the Czartoryska herbarium) and the low pH of the paper sheets, it can be assumed that the genetic material of the specimens is severely or completely degraded. Naturally, no destructive analyses have been conducted on the historical objects under consideration to confirm this. However, the possibility of conducting such analyses in the future cannot be ruled out. Therefore, it was decided to use various types of synthetic Aquazol adhesive in direct contact with the plants.

A specific issue concerned the planned consolidation, or 'reintegration' of specimens in the Helwing/Boretius herbarium. This collection contained numerous specimens that had become fragmented, but after extracting all fragments from the spines of the gatherings, it became apparent that they could largely be reassembled. Ultimately, the specimens were to be mounted on new supports. In consultation with the owner, a non-adhesive mounting method was selected, involving threading the ends of mounting strips through slits in the backing boards. If the detached fragments of the specimens allowed for such mounting, the "reintegration" of the specimens consisted of arranging them appropriately and individually securing each fragment. However, if the fragments were broken in such a way that separate mounting was impossible, they were joined using Japanese tissue underlays. This, however, required the direct application of adhesive to the botanical specimens. As in previous considerations, Aquazol was chosen for this purpose. Another challenge was consolidating the paint layer in the Zeidler herbarium. As previously described, the paint layer had caused damage to the structure of many botanical specimens, rendering them more brittle and susceptible to further deterioration. It was therefore decided to consolidate the paint layer, guided by the same rationale as for mounting and consolidating the specimens. Aquazol adhesive at low concentration was selected and applied in the form of an ultrasonic mist. The removal of specimens from the Helwing/Boretius block was carried out in a planned and orderly manner, where photographic documentation played a key role. All supports to which the specimens were later mounted were marked with the location from which the specimens originated. In this way, although the object was separated and disassembled, it was thoroughly described and documented to enable its reassembly into its original form, if needed.

Decisions regarding the restoration of botanical specimens to their original locations in the case of the Zeidler and Czartoryska herbaria, as well as the consolidation of specimens from the Helwing/Boretius herbarium, were made in consultation with the owners, who, as previously mentioned, agreed that the removal of especially large and recognisable fragments of specimens would diminish the utility of the historical collections and consign the separated elements to oblivion. It should be emphasised that, for each collection, historical or modern, decisions should be made on an individual basis, guided by the aim of preserving or restoring the authenticity, integrity, and credibility of the object (UNESCO 2015).[38]

[38] See also the section *Ethical and Legal Issues Related to Herbarium Collections* in Chap. 1.

References

Boone T, Kidder L, Russick S (1998) Bookkeeper® for spray use in single item treatments. Book Paper Group Annual 17:29–43

Bridson D, Forman L (1999) The herbarium handbook. Royal Botanic Gardens, Kew

Czartoryska IE (1828) Poczet pamiątek zachowanych w Domu Gotyckim w Puławach. Drukarnia Banku Polskiego, Warsaw, p 99, no 1232

Dauwalder L (2012) Das Herbarium des Felix Platter. Die Erhaltung eines historischen Buch-Herbariums. Dissertation, Fachochshule Bern

Firszt S (2009) Co się stało z cieplickimi zbiorami. Pamiętny rok 1952. Muzeum w Cieplicach vol. 5, Jelenia Góra–Cieplice

Firszt S (2016) Wyniki wstępnej kwerendy w sprawie rozproszonych zbiorów Schaffgotschów. Rocznik Jeleniogórski 18:199–210

Grenda-Kurmanow M (2019a) Dokumentacja prac konserwatorskich i restauratorskich. Herbarium Vivum albo Zielnik naturalnie rosnących zioł, niektorych tu wkleionych, dla lepszego ich rozeznania. Roku 1746 – zielnik Izabeli Czartoryskiej z 1746 roku ze zbiorów Muzeum Narodowego w Krakowie (dawniej w zbiorach Biblioteki Książąt Czartoryskich w Krakowie), dokumentacja konserwatorska, Warszawa–Kraków

Grenda-Kurmanow M (2019b) Dokumentacja prac konserwatorskich i restauratorskich. Zielnik Johanna Friedricha Zeidlera z 1732 roku, ze zbiorów Biblioteki Głównej Uniwersytetu Przyrodniczego w Lublinie, dokumentacja konserwatorska, Warszawa–Lublin

Grenda-Kurmanow M (2019c) Dokumentacja prac konserwatorskich i restauratorskich. Zielnik przypisywany Matthiasowi Boretiusowi lub Andreasowi Helwingowi z I połowy XVIII w., ze zbiorów Zielnika Wydziału Biologii Uniwersytetu Warszawskiego, dokumentacja konserwatorska, Warszawa

Marcotte S, Estel L, Leboucher S, Minchin S (2014) Occurrence of organic biocides in the air and dust at the Natural History Museum of Rouen, France. J Cult Herit 15:68–72

Neevel J (2009) Application issues of the Bathophenanthroline test for iron(II) ions. Restaurator 30(1–2):3–15. https://doi.org/10.1515/rest.002

Neevel JG, Reissland B (2005) Bathophenanthroline Indicator Paper. PapierRestaurierung 6(1):28–36

Ormsby M, Johnson JS, Heald SC, Chang L, Bosworth J (2006) Investigation of solid phase micro-extraction sampling for organic pesticide residues on museum collections. Collect Forum 20(1–2):1–12

Palmer PT (2001) A review of analytical methods for the determination of mercury, arsenic and pesticide residues on museum objects. Collect Forum 16(1–2):25–41

Palmer PT, Martin M, Wentworth G, Caldararo N, Davis L, Kane S, Hostler D (2003) Analysis of pesticide residues on museum objects repatriated to the Hupa tribe of California. Environ Sci Technol 37:1083–1088

Pfister A-L (2008) L'influence des biocides sur la conservations de Naturalia, HEAA Arc, Filière Conservation-restauration, Orientation objets archéologiques et ethnographiques. Dissertation, Hautes écoles spécialisées de Suisse Occidentale

Piekiełko A (1977) Osiemnastowieczny zielnik ze zbiorów Izabeli Czartoryskiej. Studia i materiały z dziejów nauki polskiej B 27:157–174

Purewal V (2001) The identification of four persistent and hazardous residues present on historic plant collections housed within the National Museum and gallery of Wales. Collect Forum 16(1–2):77–86

Purewal V (2012) Novel detection and removal of hazardous biocide residues historically Apllied to herbaria. PhD dissertation,. University of Lincoln

Reissland B, Gaibor P, Ligterink F, Neevel JG (2017) Exploring the late 19th-century landscape of ink manufacturing via a collection of 90 bottles. In: Bridgland J (ed) ICOM-CC 18th triennial conference preprints, Copenhagen, 4–8 September 2017. International Council of Museums, Paris, p Art. 0105

Salmo R, Palmer P, Tribe K (2017) Fast, nondestructive, and cost-effective methods to detect pesticide residues: a case study of several repatriated Karuk Tribe artifacts. Collect Forum 31(1–2):23–33

Sirois J (2001) The analysis of museum objects for the presence of arsenic and mercury: non-destructive analysis and sample analysis. Collect Forum 16(1–2):65–75

Sirois PJ, Sansoucy G (2001) Analysis of museum objects for hazardous pesticide residues: a guide to techniques. Collect Forum 17(1–2):49–66

Sobucki W (2013) Konserwacja papieru. Zagadnienia chemiczne. Ministerstwo Kultury i Dziedzictwa Narodowego, Biblioteka Narodowa, Warszawa

Sobucki W, Macander-Majkowska G, Jeżewska E, Zatorska A (2015) Zastosowanie metody Bookkeeper w konserwacji akwarel, pasteli i innych zabytków na papierze, wykonanych w technikach wrażliwych na wodę: podsumowanie grantu. Notes Konserwatorski 17:139–153

UNESCO (2015) Recommendation concerning the preservation of, and access to, documentary heritage including in digital form https://www.unesco.org/en/legal-affairs/recommendation-concerning-preservation-and-access-documentary-heritage-including-digital-form. Accessed 27 Jan 2026)

Wagner B, Bulska E (2003) Towards a new conservation method for ancient manuscripts by inactivation of iron via complexation and extraction. Anal Bioanal Chem 375:1148–1153. https://doi.org/10.1007/s00216-003-1819-z

Afterword

Herbaria are objects of complex structure and often intricate history. As historical artefacts, they elude classification within established categories of heritage. At the same time, herbaria serve as scientific tools and repositories of biological information. Owing to their complexity and the functions they fulfil, they also pose challenges for their safe use and management. In this book, they are analysed from a multifaceted perspective. The growing popularity of herbaria, reflected in the literature, as well as the development of techniques for analysing genetic material, has led to increased demand for herbaria as sources of genetic information. In the context of conservation and ethics, the preservation of biological information contained within herbaria is of paramount importance. Due to the uniqueness of these objects, this entails significant responsibility for the curators of herbarium collections. The safeguarding of genetic material contained in historical objects imposes distinct standards for working with such items, introducing numerous constraints and further challenges.

A key aspect of preserving historical herbaria is their proper analysis and understanding of the manufacturing techniques and conservation methods used in the past and present. This enables an accurate assessment of the object's condition and the evaluation of the risks associated with its use. One of the most important, fundamental, and useful elements of such analyses is the identification of potentially present biocidal substances. The methodology for detecting the presence of biocides, described in the final section of this book, enables the broadest possible preliminary assessment of biocide contamination in an object without the need for sampling. An important aspect of collection care is also the selection of appropriate materials used for both new specimens and historical herbaria. Specimens incorporated into collections today will become the botanical heritage of future generations; therefore, it is essential to employ conservation methods that will preserve the informational potential of the collections for as long as possible.

This book presents herbaria from historical, ethical, technological, curatorial, and conservation perspectives. It discusses degradation processes, the impact of past collection preservation methods, and conservation issues related to herbaria.

M. Grenda-Kurmanow, *Herbaria*, https://doi.org/10.1007/978-3-032-21904-6

Strategies related to preservation and conservation always require difficult decisions and careful planning for the future of a given object. These decisions should be made with full awareness of all aspects concerning its technology, history, and both its past and intended future functions. At the same time, they should take into account the individual character of the objects, safeguarding their integrity, authenticity, and uniqueness.

I hope this book encourages ongoing research on herbaria, raising awareness among users, especially collection curators, of the importance of these unique archives and the profound impact their daily practices have on genetic heritage.

Index of Cited Herbaria by Location

Basel, Herbaria Basel, Botanisches Institute Universität (BAS), without ref. no., Caspar Bauhin, 1577–1624

Bolonia, Università di Bologna, Erbario Aldrovandi Vol. 001–015, Ulisse Aldrovandi, [*Erbario Aldrovandi*], 1551–1586. http://botanica.sma.unibo.it/. Accessed: 8.01.2026

Bolonia, Università di Bologna, without ref. no., untitled, 1585

Bolonia, Università di Bologna, without ref. no., untitled, 1596

Bern, Burgerbibliothek Bern, ES 70.1–70.9, Felix Platter, [*Das Herbarium des Felix Platter*], 1552

Brescia, Biblioteca Queriniana, Ms.B. V.24, untitled, 15th c

Chantilly, Bibliothèque interuniversitaire de médecine et d'odontologie (BIUM), ms. 2039, Paolo Boccone, [*Herbier*], 1671. http://www.biusante.parisdescartes.fr/boccone/debut.htm, Fol. 15. Accessed: 15.01.2026

Florence, Biblioteca Nazionale di Firenze, Ms. B. V.24, untitled, 15th c

Florence, Museo di Storia Naturale dell'Università di Firenze (FI), without ref. no., Andrea Cesalpino, *Illustratio in Hortum Siccum*, 1555–1563

Florence, Museo di Storia Naturale dell'Università di Firenze (FI), without ref. no., Michele Merini, [*Erbario*], 1540–1545

Gotha, Universitäts- und Forschungsbibliothek Erfurt/Gotha, Codex chartaceus 153–156, Kaspar Ratzenberger, *Herbarius Vivus*, 1598

Heidelberg, B. Giulini, without ref. no., Hieronymus Harder, [*Anfangsherbar*], 1562

Kassel, Naturkundemuseum Kassel (KASSEL), without ref. no., Kaspar Ratzenberger, [*Herbar*], 1556–1592

Kraków, Herbarium of the Institute of Botany, Jagiellonian University (KRA), without ref. no., Jan Antoni Camelin lub Jan Szaster, *Zielnik prawdopodobnie z czasów Syreniusza obejmujący gatunków 269, jako zabytek pamiątkowy*, first half of the 18th c

Kraków, Herbarium of the Institute of Botany, Jagiellonian University (KRA), without ref. no., Andrzej Badurski?, [*Andrzej Badurski Herbarium*], first half of the 18th c

Kraków, Herbarium of the Institute of Botany, Jagiellonian University (KRA), without ref. no., Marian Raciborski, (*Marian Raciborski Herbarium*), 1896–1900

Kraków, National Museum in Kraków, Princes Czartoryski Library, Rkps 2782, *Herbarium Vivum, albo Zielnik naturalnie rosnących zioł niektorych tu wkleionych, dla lepszego ich rozeznania* [*Izabela Czartoryska Herbarium*], 1746

Kraków, National Museum in Kraków, MNK IV-MO-1046/2, Janina Jenko-Sokołowska, [*Album –zielnik w kasecie*], c. 1900

Kraków, Herbarium of the Institute of Botany, Polish Academy of Sciences (KRAM), without ref. no., Józef Jundziłł, [*Józef Jundziłł Herbarium*], 1820s, with specimens dated 18th c. 1876

M. Grenda-Kurmanow, *Herbaria*, https://doi.org/10.1007/978-3-032-21904-6

Kraków, Herbarium of the Institute of Botany, Polish Academy of Sciences (KRAM), separate barcode for each sheet, Józef Mądalski, [*Józef Mądalski Herbarium*], started in 1926, includes specimens from the 19th c. https://rcin.org.pl//dlibra/metadatasearch?action=AdvancedSearchAction&type=-3&val1=recordedBy:%22J.+M%C4%85dalski%22. Accessed: 15.01.2026

Kraków, Herbarium of the Institute of Botany, Polish Academy of Sciences (KRAM), without ref. no., separate barcode for each sheet, Seweryn Udziela, [*Seweryn Udziela Herbarium*], 1890s. https://rcin.org.pl//dlibra/metadatasearch?action=AdvancedSearchAction&type=-3&val1=recordedBy:%22%5C%5BS.+Udziela%5C%5D%22

Leiden, Naturalis Biodiversity Center (L), L. 2077674, Codex Vossianus Germanicus in Folio No. 1 Tom. 1 Pars 2, Francesco Petrollini, *En Tibi Perpetuis Ridentum Floribus Hortum*, 1542–44. https://bioportal.naturalis.nl/result?theme=en_tibi. Accessed: 15.01.2026

Leiden, Naturalis Biodiversity Center (L), (WAG 0271979), [*Clifford Herbarium*], first half of the 18th c

Leiden, Naturalis Biodiversity Center (L), L. 2110004, Petrus Cadé, [*Cadé Herbarium*], 1566. http://www.nationaalherbarium.nl/Cade/. Accessed: 15.01.2026

Leiden, Naturalis Biodiversity Center (L), L. 2077675, Herman Boerhaave, [*Boerhaave Herbarium*], 18th c

Leiden, Naturalis Biodiversity Center (L), L.2077653, Codex Vossianus Germanicus in Folio Vol. 1–IV, Leonhart Rauwolff, *Kreütterbuech*, 1560–1577. https://bioportal.naturalis.nl

Leiden, Naturalis Biodiversity Center (L), L.2077648-L.2077650, Caspar Georg Carl Reinwardt, [*Caspar Georg Carl Reinwardt Herbarium*], 1773–1854

Leiden, Naturalis Biodiversity Center (L), L. 2077627-207730, 2078204-207812, 211011, Philipp Franz von Siebold, [*Siebold Herbarium*], 1823–1830. https://bioportal.naturalis.nl/result?theme=siebold&language=en. Accessed: 8.01.2026

Lindau, Stadtbibliothek, Ma II 182, Hieronymus Harder, *Kreuterbuch*, 1599

Linz, Oberösterreichischen Landesmuseums, without ref. no., Hieronymus Harder, *Kreuterbiechlin*, 1607

London, Linnean Society, LINN 61.19, Carl Linnaeus, *Iris Sibirica*, [part of *Linnaean Herbarium*], before 1741. http://linnean-online.org/817/. Accessed: 21.01.2026

London, Natural History Museum, ref. BM000589107 and BM000589108, Sir Hans Sloane, (*Sloane Herbarium*), 1689

Lublin, Main Library of the University of Life Sciences, Zb. Specj. I Starodruki 14, D. 104.57.646 (vol. I); Zb. Specj. Starodruki XVIII.14; D. 104.57.646 (vol. III), Johann Friedrich Zeidler, *Hortus Perennis/ Immer grünendes/Gewachs-Hautz/das ist:/Aller au(s)s dem hoch Reich graffs Schaff-/gotschitschischen Territorio mais-/tenden Kräutern und Blu-/men//Erster Theil/ zu/ Betrachtung der mannigfaltigen Natur/Belustigung des curieusen Gemüthes/ Preitz(?) des allermeistesten Shönsters/veröffnet/von/Johann Friedrich Zeidler/ Medicinae Practico/ in/ Petersdorf/Anno 1732* (vol. I); *Hortus Perennis/ das ist/ Immer Grunendes GewachsHaus/ Betrachtung der mannigfaltigen Belustigung des curieusen Gemüthes/ Preitz(?) des allermeistesten Shönsters/ veröffnet von Johann Friedrich Zeidler, apotheker/ in Schweidnitz Ao.1751* (vol. III), 1732 (vol. I) and 1751 (vol. III)

Modena, Biblioteca Estense Universitaria, without ref. no., *Erbario Ducale Estense*, 1560?

Monachium, Bayerische Staatsbibliothek, Cod. Icon. 3, Hieronymus Harder, *Kreuterbuch* [*Herbarium Vivum*], 1576–1600. https://opacplus.bsbmuenchen.de/title/BV022466430. Accessed: 8.01.2026

Monachium, Deutsches Museum, without ref. no., Hieronymus Harder, *Kreuterbuch*, 1574–1576

Naples, Biblioteca Nazionale di Napoli, without ref. no., Ferrante Imperato, *Collectio plantarum naturalium*, second half of 16th/the beginning of 17th c

Nürnberg, Nürnberger Stadtbibliothek, Med. 2 194, Georg Forster, 1568

Paris, Muséum national d'histoire naturelle (P), without ref. no., Jehan Girault, 1558 r

Paris, Muséum national d'histoire naturelle (P), without ref. no., Michel Begon, *Herbier Begon*, second half of the 17 c

Paris, Muséum national d'histoire naturelle (P), without ref. no., Albrecht von Haller, [*Herbier Haller*], before 1768
Paris, Muséum national d'histoire naturelle (P), without ref. no., Jean de Thévenot, 1664–1666
Paris, Muséum national d'histoire naturelle (P), without ref. no., Jean-Baptiste Fusée Aublet, [*Herbier Rousseau*], c. 1760
Paris, Muséum national d'histoire naturelle (P), without ref. no., Louise Gailleton, [*Herbier des tranchées*], 1914–1918
Paris, Muséum national d'histoire naturelle (P), MNHN-P-P04892559, Bernard de Retz, 1936
Paris, Muséum national d'histoire naturelle (P), MNHN-P-P04691898 i MNHN-P-P04691899, Jacques Felix, 1939
Poznań, Poznań Society for the Advancement of Arts and Sciences Library, Rkp 880, Eliza Orzeszkowa, [*Eliza Orzeszkowa Herbarium*], 1887–1898
Rome, Biblioteca Angelica, ms. 2344 (Erbario A); ms. 2345–2348 (Erbario B, vol. I–IV), Francesco Petrollini, *Plantarum seu stirpium naturalium*, c. 1532 (Erbario A), 1553 (Erbario B)
Rome, Bibliotheca Apostolica Vaticana, Roma, Pal. Lat. 1276, Hieronymus Harder, 1574
Salzburg, Haus der Natur, without ref. no., Hieronymus Harder, *Kreuterbuch*, 1592
Toruń, Herbarium of the Nicolaus Copernicus University in Toruń (TRN), without ref. no., Wangerin(?) W., *Flora der Provinz Westpreussen*, 1913
Toruń, Herbarium of the Nicolaus Copernicus University in Toruń (TRN), without ref. no., ? Lakowitz., *Flora der Provinz Westpreussen*, 1894
Überlingen, Städtisches Museum Überlingen, without ref. no., Johann Jakob Han, 1578–1594
Überlingen, Städtischen Museum Überlingen, without ref. no., Hieronymus Harder, [*Handherbar*], 1594–1607
Ulm, Stadtarchiv, U 6757, Hieronymus Harder, *Kreuterbuch*, 1594
Vienna, Naturhistorisches Museum, without ref. no., Hieronymus Harder, *Kreuterbuch*, 1599
Warsaw, Central Archives of Modern Records, 63/III/2, Róża Luxemburg, [*Rosa Luxemburg Herbarium*], 1913–1918
Warsaw, National Library, Rps akc. 200/1-2, Georg Andreas Helwing (Jerzy Andrzej Helwing), *Herbarium Vivum Plantarum sponte in Prussia nascentium, Herculeo labore comparatum M. Georgii Andreae Helwingii Pastoris Angerburgensium. et Reg. Societ. Scient. Brand. Membrii* (vol. I); *Florae Napaeisque Sacrum! Civis, amice, advena, qui herbaria amoenitate cupis oblectarier, modestiam et continentiam comites habeas florae custodes, quod rogat, monet, expetit M. Georgius Andreas Helwing, pastor Angeburgensis, operis huius faber* (vol. II), 1695–1705. https://polona.pl/item/herbarium-vivum-plantarum-sponte-in-prussia-nascentium-t-1,Nzk3MTEwOA/3/#info:metadata (vol. I). Accessed: 8.01.2026; https://polona.pl/item/herbarium-vivum-plantarum-sponte-in-prussia-nascentium-t-2,Nzk3MTEwOQ/5/#info:metadata (vol. II). Accessed: 8.01.2026
Warsaw, Herbarium of the Faculty of Biology, University of Warsaw (WA), WA-KH-13.1.1 (vol. I), WA-KH-13.1.2 (vol. II), WA-KH-13.1.4 (vol. IV), WA-KH-13.1.5 (vol. V), Maciej Ernest Borecki (Boretius), *Matth. Ern. Boretii Herbarium vivum, plantarum et florum in Porussia nascentium methodo Tournefortiana, in classes divisum; adscriptis nominibus Plantarum Latinis, Germanicis, Polonicis, cum Indice. Vol. V*, 1712–1738
Warsaw, Herbarium of the Faculty of Biology, University of Warsaw (WA), WA-KH-13.2.1, Jerzy Andrzej Helwing i/lub Maciej Ernest Borecki (Boretius), *Plantar[um] Exotic[um] tom. I*, before 1738
Warsaw, Herbarium of the Faculty of Biology, University of Warsaw (WA), WA-KH-13.2.2, WA-KH-13.2.4, Jerzy Andrzej Helwing i/lub Maciej Ernest Borecki (Boretius), 1724–1745
Warsaw, Herbarium of the Faculty of Biology, University of Warsaw (WA), WA-KH-5.1.–5.10., Michał Fedorowski, [*Ludowe nazwy roślin*], c. 1880a
Warsaw, Herbarium of the Faculty of Biology, University of Warsaw (WA), WA-KH-3, Michał Fedorowski, *Zielnik Litewski*, c. 1880b
Warsaw, Herbarium of the Faculty of Biology, University of Warsaw, W. Winkler, [*Winkler Herbarium*], end of 19th c

Wolfenbüttel, Herzog August Bibliothek, Cod. Guelf. 929 Helmst., Joachim Gagelmann, 1571–1575

Wrocław, Herbarium of the Museum of Natural History (WRSL), without ref. no., Paolo Boccone, [*Paolo Boccone Herbarium*], c. 1689–1695

Wrocław, Herbarium of the Museum of Natural History (WRSL), without ref. no., n.n., *Herbier du Cher*, 19th c

Wrocław, Herbarium of the Museum of Natural History (WRSL), without ref. no., n.n., [*Treviranus Herbarium*], undated

Wrocław, Herbarium of the Museum of Natural History (WRSL), without ref. no., W. Winkler, [*Winkler Herbarium*], 1831

Wrocław, National Ossoliński Institute, Eliza Orzeszkowa, [*Eliza Orzeszkowa Herbarium*] 13967/ II Pal.1890, 1890

Name Index

M. Grenda-Kurmanow, *Herbaria*, https://doi.org/10.1007/978-3-032-21904-6

Subject Index

M. Grenda-Kurmanow, *Herbaria*, https://doi.org/10.1007/978-3-032-21904-6

The manufacturer's authorised representative in the EU is Springer Nature Customer Service Centre GmbH, Europaplatz 3, 69115 Heidelberg, Germany. If you have any concerns regarding our products, please contact ProductSafety@springernature.com

Printed and bound by CPI Group (UK) Ltd, Croydon, CR0 4YY

09/10/2026

02230769-0004